Vladimír Beneš • David Netuka
Editors

Surgical and Interventional Treatment of Cerebral Ischemia

Basic Science to Clinical Practice

Springer

Editors
Vladimír Beneš
Department of Neurosurgery and Neurooncology
First Medical Faculty, Charles University
Prague, Czech Republic

David Netuka
Department of Neurosurgery and Neurooncology
First Medical Faculty, Charles University
Prague, Czech Republic

ISBN 978-3-032-08933-5 ISBN 978-3-032-08934-2 (eBook)
https://doi.org/10.1007/978-3-032-08934-2

This Springer imprint is published by the registered company Springer Nature Switzerland AG
The registered company address is: Gewerbestrasse 11, 6330 Cham, Switzerland

Foreword

Editorial: Surgical and Interventional Management of Ischemic Stroke

Despite significant advances in prevention and treatment, ischemic stroke remains the second leading cause of death, and the third leading cause of death and disability combined worldwide, imposing a substantial socioeconomic burden. Neurosurgeons and neurointerventionists play a pivotal role in both the prevention and management of ischemic stroke, particularly in efforts to restore and optimize cerebral perfusion.

Ischemic stroke may result from either embolic or hemodynamic mechanisms. The location and extent of the ischemic core largely determine the clinical presentation, which can range from devastating neurological impairment to focal deficits or transient ischemic attacks.

Interventions generally serve one of two purposes:

1. **Acute management**, aimed at improving outcomes by reducing intracranial pressure and salvaging at-risk brain tissue
2. **Prevention**, targeting either the initial occurrence or recurrence of stroke

The initial chapters of this volume provide a comprehensive overview of the history, epidemiology, pathophysiology, vascular anatomy, clinical manifestations, and optimal medical strategies for stroke prevention. Subsequent chapters delve into surgical and endovascular interventions, offering a critical and up-to-date analysis of the evidence supporting various indications. Topics covered include, among others, carotid endarterectomy, carotid artery stenting, emergency revascularization, management of restenosis, and considerations for patients undergoing carotid surgery in the context of coronary artery bypass grafting. Each chapter synthesizes the literature and presents practical recommendations or guidelines.

Intracranial occlusive diseases and moyamoya vasculopathies are addressed in dedicated sections, reflecting their unique pathophysiological and therapeutic considerations. The roles of endovascular therapy and flow-augmentation bypass in ischemic stroke management are also explored in depth. Additionally, vertebrobasilar ischemia and pediatric stroke are discussed in separate chapters due to their distinct clinical profiles.

As the field advances toward precision medicine and individualized care, the final chapter outlines future directions in stroke management. It integrates insights from preclinical and clinical research, telemedicine, rehabilitation technologies, artificial intelligence, and public health strategies.

Achieving optimal outcomes for patients with ischemic stroke requires close interdisciplinary collaboration within specialized stroke centers. This book offers current, evidence- or best practice-based recommendations for surgical and interventional strategies across the spectrum of stroke care—from primary prevention to acute treatment and secondary prevention. It will serve as a highly valuable, much-needed, and long-awaited resource for both trainees and specialists, offering a comprehensive overview practical guidance for surgical and interventional management of ischemic stroke, while supporting informed clinical decision-making.

Luca Regli

Professor and Chairman, Department of Neurosurgery
Clinical Science Center University Hospital
and University of Zurich
Zurich, Switzerland

Preface

Cerebral ischemia constitutes the second leading cause of death in developed countries. It ranks among the largest medical markets globally. Nevertheless, neurosurgeons appear to be exhibiting diminished interest in the subject. During the 1980s, significant attention was focused on extracranial-intracranial bypass surgery. A dramatic reduction in involvement was observed after the completion of Barnett's study. Similarly, large-scale carotid surgical trials conducted in the 1990s garnered substantial interest. Subsequently, neurosurgical practice largely shifted toward the subspecialty of vascular surgery. The neurosurgeons focused their interest on aneurysms, arteriovenous malformations, and cavernomas. Endovascular techniques have brought new insights and therapeutic possibilities in the new millennium. These techniques again reduced neurosurgical intervention, except for a limited number of hybrid neurosurgeons.

Recently, the management of cerebral ischemia has primarily been the domain of neurologists, vascular surgeons, and interventional neuroradiologists; neurosurgical involvement is infrequent. Interdisciplinary teams or stroke specialists operate stroke units.

Regardless, the brain is the target of any treatment, and the author firmly believes that neurosurgeons are best suited to address this issue, both intellectually and technically. This book endeavors to rekindle neurosurgical interest in the topic.

The contributing authors are neurosurgeons with expertise in cerebral ischemia. The chapters detail surgical and interventional technique and the processes involved in decision-making. Consequently, some topics are excluded, specifically neurorehabilitation, resocialization, and societal effects of cerebral ischemia. A thorough examination of cerebral ischemia would result in an unwieldy book. The publication applies to all physicians and healthcare professionals treating such patients, as it comprehensively addresses recent surgical and interventional neuroradiology management options.

The book's main goal is to enhance the treatment and preventative measures for stroke patients and those vulnerable to its effects.

Praha, Czech Republic — Vladimír Beneš

Contents

History of Cerebral Ischemia Treatment: "A Generation Which Ignores History Has No Past and No Future"

Vladimír Beneš, Adéla Bubeníková, and David Netuka

1 Introduction

Stroke is a critical medical condition characterized by the abrupt interruption of blood flow to the brain, resulting in acute neurological deficits and potential long-term disability. The evolution of stroke knowledge is paramount for enhancing contemporary therapeutic strategies, improving patient prognoses, and facilitating preventive measures. Stroke represents a significant global health challenge, being one of the leading causes of morbidity and mortality worldwide. According to the World Health Organization, stroke accounts for approximately 11% of all deaths, with an estimated 15 million people suffering a stroke each year; of these, nearly 5 million succumb to the condition, while another 5 million are left permanently disabled [1].

The historical evolution of stroke understanding reflects a dynamic interplay between anatomical insights, pathophysiological discoveries, and therapeutic innovations. From the ancient acknowledgment of apoplexy to the sophisticated interventions available in contemporary clinical practice, the evolution of stroke management underscores the significance of interdisciplinary collaboration in addressing this complex condition [2]. Although strides have been made in stroke care, ongoing challenges persist, particularly in addressing the disparities in access to care and outcomes on a global scale. The continued exploration of cerebrovascular diseases remains essential for enhancing patient outcomes and developing comprehensive strategies for prevention and management. As we build upon the lessons learned from historical milestones, the importance of ongoing research and innovation in stroke medicine cannot be overstated, as it holds the key to mitigating the profound impact of this prevalent condition on individuals and society at large.

This book chapter is essential not only for documenting the historical evolution of stroke understanding but also for providing a comprehensive synthesis of knowledge that informs current clinical practice and future research directions. By elucidating the milestones in the understanding of stroke, this chapter aims to highlight the intricate connections between historical insights and modern treatment methodologies.

2 Definition of Stroke and Early Historical Reports

The early conceptualization of stroke can be traced back to the writings of Hippocrates in the fifth century BC, who employed the term "apoplexy", coming from a Greek word *apoplixia*, to describe a sudden and violent onset of neurological symptoms, reflecting an initial recognition of the acute nature of the condition as described in the Hippocratic Oath (Fig. 1), denoting an individual who experiences a sudden collapse while maintaining cardiac and respiratory functions [3]. An excerpt from the Hippocratic texts provides an account of apoplexy: "The healthy individual is seized by an abrupt sensation of pain, subsequently losing their ability to speak and exhibiting a distinct rattling in the throat. The mouth remains open, and when addressed or stirred, the individual merely groans, exhibiting an inability to comprehend. They may experience profuse urination without awareness. In the absence of fever, death ensues within a week; however, if fever arises, recovery is typically probable". During the Greco-Roman era, apoplexy was a term encompassing conditions such as strokes, epilepsy, and migraines.

V. Beneš (✉) · D. Netuka
Department of Neurosurgery and Neurooncology, First Medical Faculty, Charles University, Prague, Czech Republic
e-mail: beneseva@volny.cz

A. Bubeníková
Department of Neurosurgery, Second Faculty of Medicine, Charles University and Motol University Hospital, Prague, Czech Republic

V. Beneš, D. Netuka (eds.), *Surgical and Interventional Treatment of Cerebral Ischemia*,
https://doi.org/10.1007/978-3-032-08934-2_1

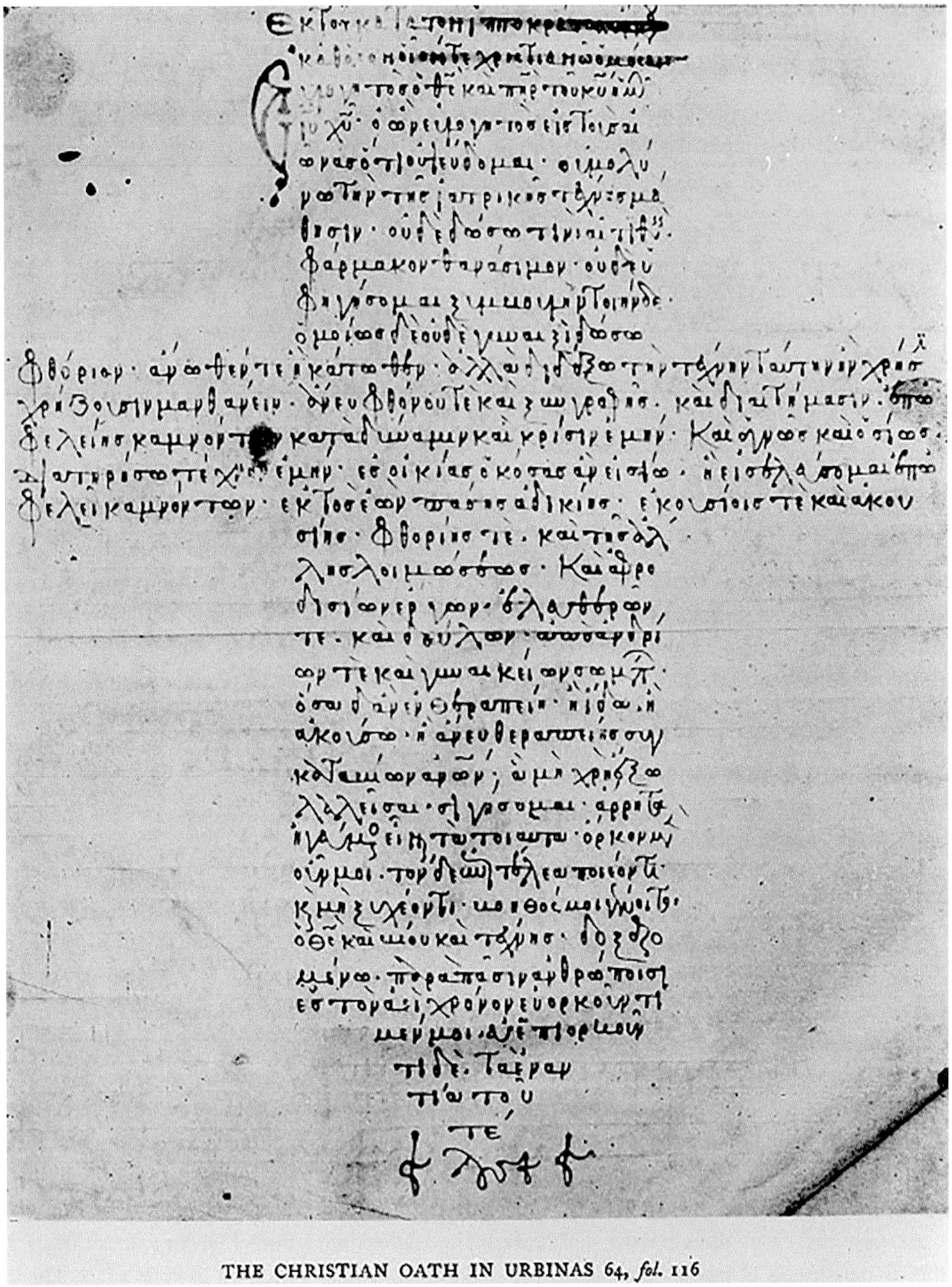

Fig. 1 Hippocratic Oath in Greek from Vatican Manuscript Urbinus 64. folio 116. (Reprinted with CC licence)

2.1 Ancient Times

Hippocrates (circa 460—circa 370 BC) posited that apoplexy resulted from the overheating of cranial blood vessels leading to the influx of phlegm or the accumulation of black bile within the head. This resulted from the hypothesis that there are four humors in a human brain: (1) blood, (2) phlegm, (3) yellow bile, and (4) black bile as articulated in the Hippocratic treatise known as *The Nature of Man* by Polybus, a disciple of Hippocrates [4]. Aretaeus, as one of the most famous antient Greek physicians, was pivotal in documenting the notion that apoplexy affecting one hemisphere of the brain correlates with contralateral paralysis in the body. Claudius Galen (129–216 AD) subsequently asserted that strokes emerged from an imbalance of humors, which obstructed the transmission of the "animal spirit" (Fig. 2). He specifically theorized that blood accumulated in the brain, while phlegm and black bile settled within the cerebral ventricles. He is famous of postulating famous "pneuma" theory which described differences between vital pneuma, which travelled in blood, and psychic pneuma, which went to the brain. Pneuma generally referred to breath, air or spirit, and it was described

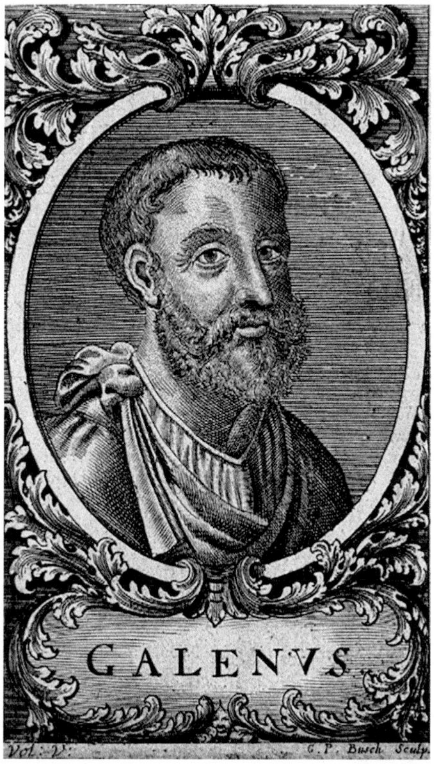

Fig. 2 Portrait of Galen, a Roman and Greek physician, surgeon, and philosopher, considered to be one of the most accomplished of all medical researchers of antiquity, Galen influenced the development of various scientific disciplines, including anatomy, physiology, pathology, pharmacology, and neurology, as well as philosophy and logic. (Reprinted with CC licence [5])

together with basic pulmonary and vascular physiology. Galen's theory also mentions the presence of pneuma along peripheral nerves. Although ancient physicians acknowledged the association between stroke and motor function impairment, the pathophysiological mechanisms underlying cerebrovascular events remained largely undefined.

2.2 Early Modern Period

Muslim scholars made pivotal contributions to the anatomical and physiological understanding of the brain and vascular system, particularly regarding stroke (apoplexy), bridging the knowledge of ancient Greece with the advancements of the Renaissance [4]. Avicenna (Ibn Sina, 980–1037), in his *Canon of Medicine* (1025), provided one of the earliest comprehensive descriptions of cerebrovascular accidents. He identified stroke as a result of impaired cerebral blood flow, referring to it as al-sar'a or apoplexy, and discussed its symptoms and causes, emphasizing the link between vascular disturbances and brain function [6]. Avicenna's work synthesized Greco-Roman medical theories, particularly those of Hippocrates and Galen, and expanded upon them by integrating Islamic medical practices and observations.

Al-Zahrawi (Abulcasis, 936–1013), in his Kitab al-Tasrif, further contributed to neurological and vascular medicine by detailing surgical treatments for cranial injuries and describing hemiplegia, a common result of stroke. Ibn al-Nafis (1213–1288), in his *Commentary on Anatomy* in Avicenna's Canon, advanced knowledge of circulation by accurately describing pulmonary circulation, preceding the discoveries of William Harvey by over three centuries. His work challenged the Galenic understanding of the heart and vascular system, highlighting the role of blood flow in maintaining brain function and health.

The scientific knowledge of these Muslim scholars was transmitted to Europe through translations into Latin during the twelfth century, particularly in centers like Toledo and Salerno. Their works served as essential resources for Renaissance anatomists and physicians, who built upon these foundations to further explore the brain's vascular anatomy and the pathophysiology of stroke. The integration of Greek, Roman, and Islamic medical knowledge facilitated significant advancements in the understanding of stroke as a vascular disorder during the Renaissance.

Following the mediaeval times, from which we have no significant scientific reports not only in neuroscience, but science overall, the Renaissance brought us an enormous number of discoveries across the natural sciences, spanning the 14th to 17th centuries. This era facilitated autopsies, thus advances in anatomy understanding, the translation of ancient texts, and thereby enriching the knowledge pertaining to apoplexy. In 1599, the Oxford English Dictionary referenced "the stroke of the palsy" as synonymous with "the stroke of God's hands". From the seventeenth century onward, the various conditions encapsulated by the term apoplexy began to be investigated individually.

The understanding of stroke could not be possible without a detailed understanding of the vasculature of the brain and its extracranial feeders. Some scholars attribute the first description of the arterial circle, albeit incomplete, to Gabriel Fallopius or Fallopio (1523–1562). In *Observationes Anatomicae* (1561), he delivered a nearly comprehensive account of the arterial polygon with detailed the convergence and subsequent bifurcation of the vertebral arteries, as well as the confluence of the internal branches of the carotid artery [7]. Adriaan van den Spiegel, also known as Adrianus Spigelius (1578–1625) composed an anatomical treatise, though it remained unpublished during his lifetime due to the lack of illustrations. In his will, Spigelius appointed the German physician Daniel Bucretius to oversee the publication of his work. After Spigelius' death, Bucretius began the process of publishing the treatise and managed to acquire 78 out of the 86 original anatomical plates made by Fialetti from Casserius' heirs. To complete the set, he commissioned an additional 20 illustrations from the same artist, which were engraved on copper by Valesio. Consequently, in 1627, the most comprehensive anatomical work of the seventeenth century was published posthumously, titled *De Humani Corporis Fabrica Libri X, Tabulis XCIIX*. This publication, enriched by detailed anatomical descriptions and highly artistic illustrations, became a cornerstone of anatomical knowledge. The title of the book was derived from *De Humani Corporis Fabrica*, written by Spigelius' fellow countryman, Andreas Vesalius (1514–1564, Fig. 3). Bucretius, as the editor, intended this work to serve as a modern update, reflecting the advancements in medical anatomy achieved in the 70 years since Vesalius' treatise [8]. In *Liber X*, there is an illustration that presents the arterial circle at the base of the brain, one of the drawings meticulously produced under Casserius' supervision (Fig. 4). This is recognized as the first published depiction of the arterial circle at the brain's base, printed as *Tabulae X* (Fig. 5), with each anatomical component distinctly labeled with letters for easier identification [8].

Another prominent figure associated with the discovery of the arterial circle at the base of the brain is Johann Vesling (1595–1649). His later editions of *Syntagma Anatomicum* released in 1647 and 1651, included a near-complete depiction of the arterial circle called *Figurae III* (Fig. 6). In 1689, William Cole was the inaugural individual to employ the term "stroke" as a designation for apoplexy. In the seventeenth century, anatomists such as Johann Jakob Wepfer and Thomas Willis advanced the understanding of the cerebral arteries, laying foundational knowledge for subsequent anatomical studies. Meyer and Hieron argue that Johann Jakob Wepfer von Schaffhausen (1620–1695) of Switzerland was, in fact, the true discoverer of the arterial circle, documenting it six years prior to Willis' contributions [10]. In 1658, he

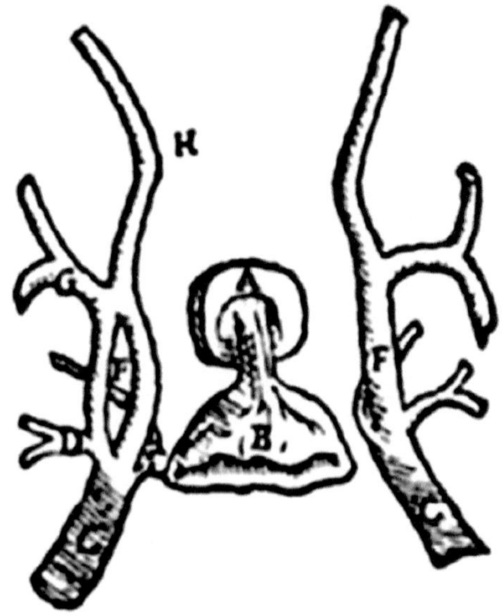

Fig. 4 Graphic representation of the pituitary and arterial vessels in of Vesalius' treatise *De Humani Corporis Fabrica,* in which only few arteries constituting the anterior part of the cerebral artery polygon can be identified. (After Vesalius, 1543)

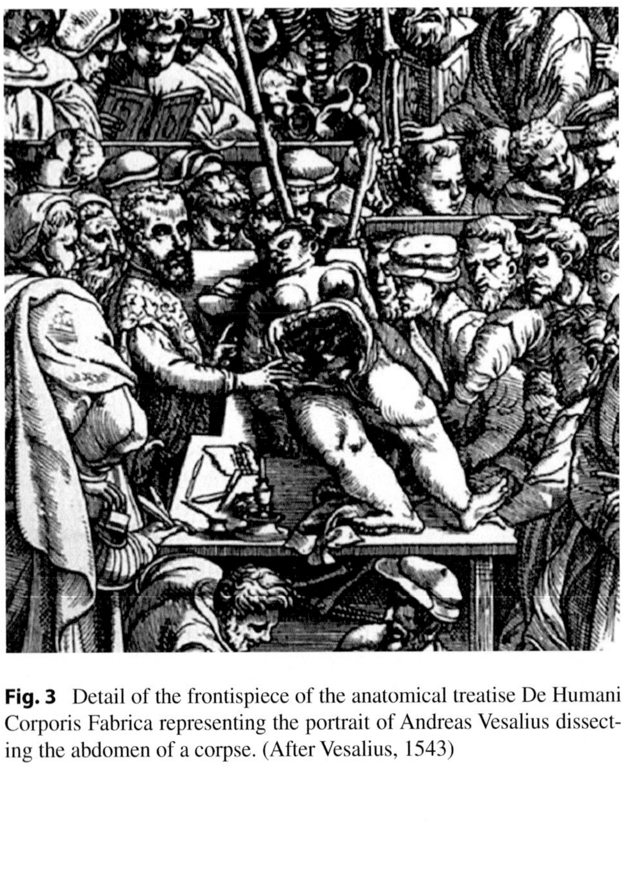

Fig. 3 Detail of the frontispiece of the anatomical treatise De Humani Corporis Fabrica representing the portrait of Andreas Vesalius dissecting the abdomen of a corpse. (After Vesalius, 1543)

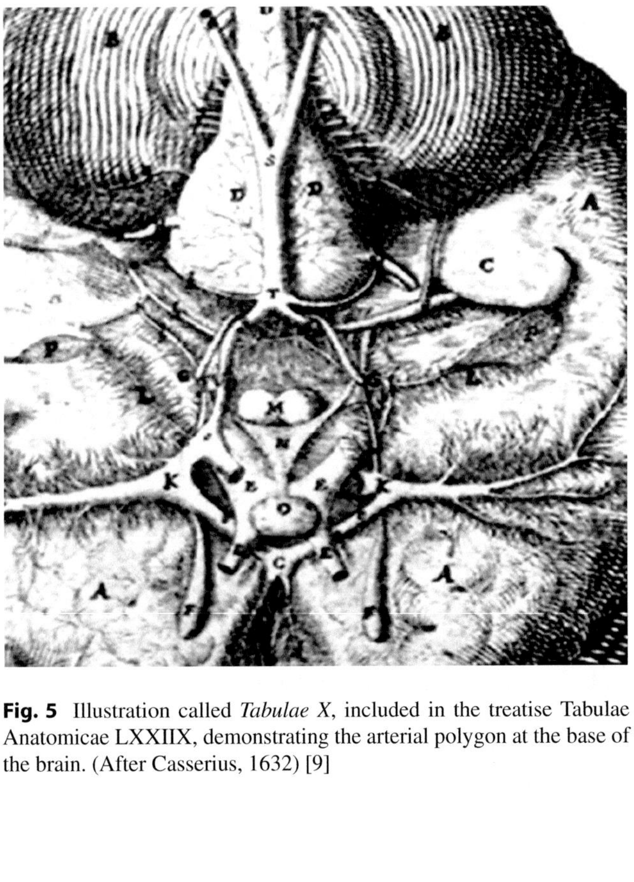

Fig. 5 Illustration called *Tabulae X*, included in the treatise Tabulae Anatomicae LXXIIX, demonstrating the arterial polygon at the base of the brain. (After Casserius, 1632) [9]

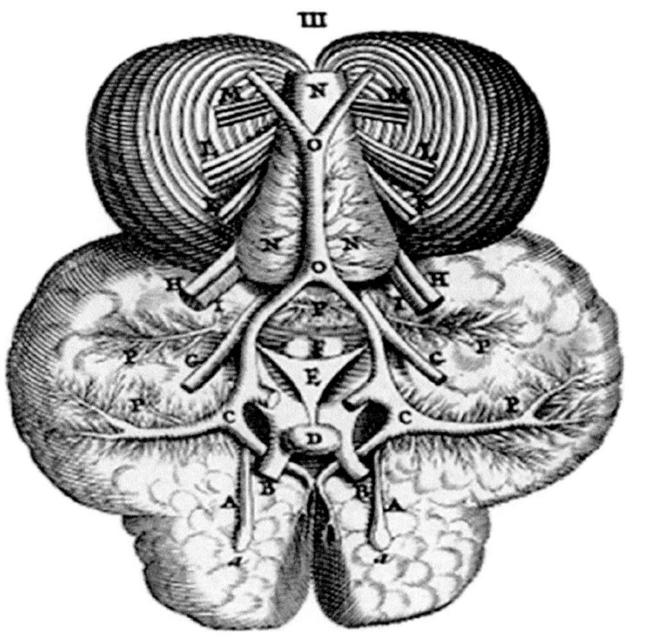

Fig. 6 Illustration called *Figurae III*, included in *Syntagma Anatomicum*, printed in 1647, represents an incomplete arterial polygon. (After Veslingus, 1651) [11]

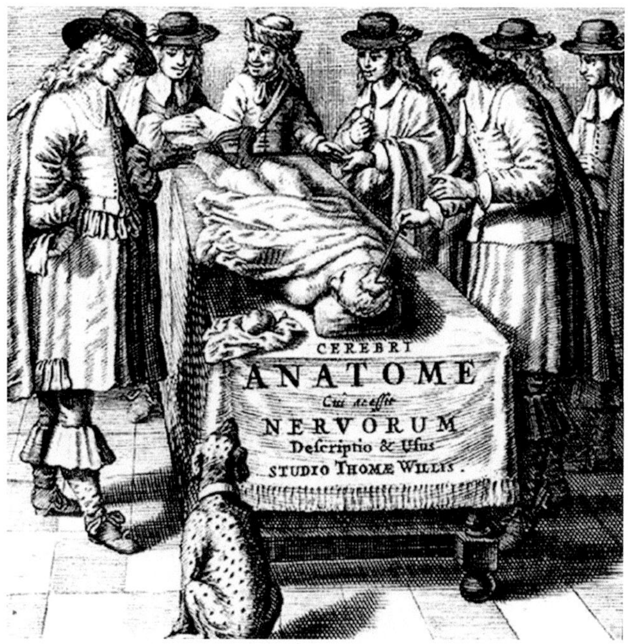

Fig. 7 The cover of the book *De Cerebri Anatome*, edition 1665/1666, published in Amsterdam, shows Thomas Willis' associates, among whom Christopher Wren is noted with the sketchbook and Lower pointing towards the dissection of the head. The drawing shows Thomas Willis, positioned to the left, while the others are looking at him. (After Willis, 1665/1666)

was the first to document carotid thrombosis, both extracranially and intracranially, in a patient with complete occlusion and calcification of the right internal carotid artery. In his *Apoplexia*, also cited as *Historiae apoplecticorum*, he meticulously traced the course of the carotid and vertebral arteries from their origins to the arterial circle at the base of the brain. Additionally, he was among the first to recognize that apoplexy, or stroke, could result from cerebral hemorrhage and he made significant enhancements in anatomical understanding of the brain vasculature since he provided a remarkably precise description of the arterial circle at the brain's base, though his work did not include illustrations. Additionally, *Apoplexia* provided early descriptions of various cerebrovascular events, including completed stroke, progressing stroke, transient ischemic attack (TIA), and reversible ischemic neurological deficit. These observations laid the foundation for future research into cerebrovascular disorders and their clinical manifestations.

In the early seventeenth century, William Harvey (1578–1657) focused his studies on the heart, culminating in his 1628 treatise on blood circulation where he elucidated the principles of blood circulation. Harvey's discovery underscored the necessity of uninterrupted blood flow for maintaining cerebral integrity, thereby establishing a framework for recognizing cerebrovascular accidents as vascular disorders. At the same time, Thomas Willis (1621–1675) shifted focus to brain research. In 1664, Willis published *De Cerebri Anatome*, the most comprehensive and accurate description of the nervous system at the time [12]. This landmark work was the result of collaborative research within The Oxford Experimental Philosophy Club, a group conducting chemical, physical, and anatomical investigations, which later evolved into the Royal Society of London. In *De Cerebri Anatome*, Willis detailed the vascular network at the brain's base, enhanced by Christopher Wren's masterful illustrations (Fig. 7). This work marked a breakthrough in understanding the structure and function of the circular arterial anastomosis. Willis' followers honored him by naming this structure the "circle of Willis", an eponym that has since become one of the most renowned anatomical terms (Fig. 8) [12]. Its discovery signified a major transition from medieval to modern concepts of the brain's vascular anatomy and function. However, it was not until the nineteenth century that the term "stroke" became widely adopted in clinical parlance, accompanied by a burgeoning differentiation between hemorrhagic and ischemic strokes.

In 1856, Rudolf Virchow documented a case of carotid thrombosis that was linked to ipsilateral blindness. Despite this association, he observed that the lumens of both the ophthalmic and central retinal arteries remained patent. Virchow's findings contributed to the understanding of carotid artery pathology, suggesting that visual loss could occur even in the presence of unobstructed blood flow in key ocular arteries, highlighting the complexity of vascular involvement in cerebrovascular events. In fact, Virchow was

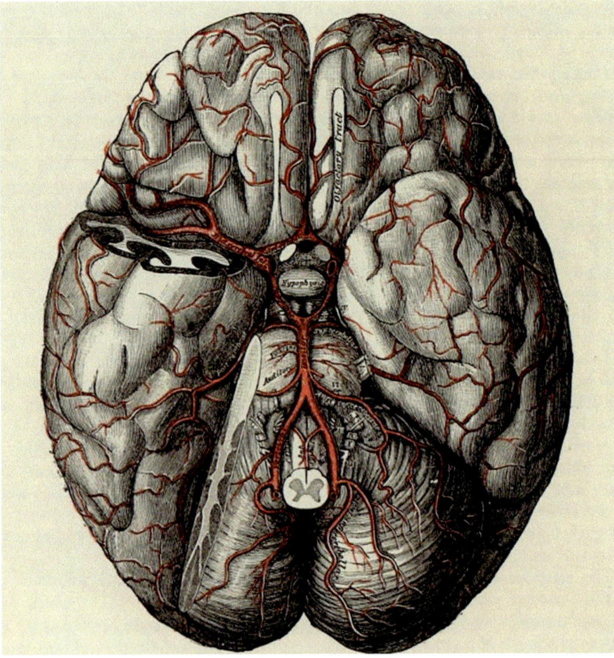

Fig. 8 Brain arterial polygon, also referred to arterial circle or Willis circle in its full beauty. (Reprinted from Gray's Anatomy published in 1929 with CC licence)

the first to introduce the terms "thrombosis" and "embolus," which describe conditions that can reduce blood flow in distal vessels, potentially leading to stroke [13]. His pioneering work laid the foundation for understanding how blood clots (thrombi) and detached clots (emboli) can obstruct circulation. Moreover, Virchow's formulation of the "Virchow's triad," which delineates the contributing factors of venous stasis, vascular injury, and hypercoagulability, laid the groundwork for comprehending the multifactorial nature of stroke pathophysiology. Simultaneously, advancements in diagnostic modalities began to emerge in the nineteenth century, significantly enhancing the clinical approach to stroke. The introduction of the ophthalmoscope by Hermann von Helmholtz in 1851 facilitated the visualization of retinal changes associated with cerebrovascular diseases, allowing for improved understanding of vascular pathology.

By the early twentieth century, clinicians had developed a more nuanced understanding of the distinct mechanisms underlying hemorrhagic and ischemic strokes, leading to the establishment of more targeted therapeutic approaches. Globally renowned clinicians Hans von Chiari (in 1904, Fig. 9) and James Ramsay Hunt (in 1914) conducted autopsies on patients who had endured cerebral infarction and observed that lesions in the cervical carotid artery could be implicated as a potential cause of the stroke, thus implementing the idea that besides intracranial etiology, stroke can result from extracranial cause as well [14]. In 1951, Canadian neurologist Charles Miller Fisher published a series of case reports demonstrating that the etiology of cerebral infarction was often secondary to occlusion of the internal carotid artery.

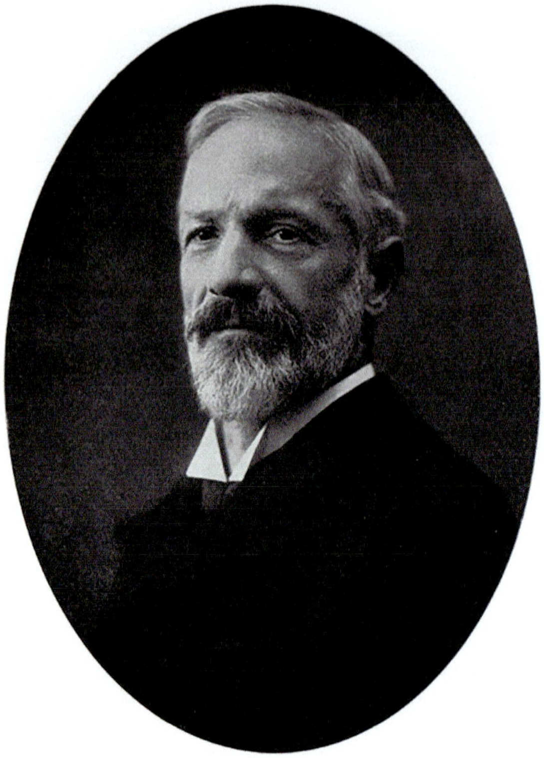

Fig. 9 Portrait of Hans von Chiari (4 September 1851–6 May 1916), a pathologist from Vienna, Austria where he worked as an assistant to Karl Freiherr von Rokitansky and Richard Ladislaus Heschl. In 1878 he received his habilitation in pathological anatomy, and within a few years became an associate professor at the University of Prague. In Prague, he was also superintendent of the pathological-anatomical museum. In 1906 he relocated to the University of Strasbourg as a professor of pathological anatomy. (Reprinted with CC licence)

The advent of cerebral angiography in 1927, pioneered by Portuguese neurologist António Egas Moniz, played an instrumental role in enhancing the understanding of carotid artery disease, thereby facilitating the subsequent development of carotid endarterectomy (CEA) [15]. He primarily used cerebral arteriography for studying brain tumors as a diagnostic technique for detecting occlusive vascular lesions, utilizing sodium iodide as a contrast medium. The first documented case of carotid thrombosis identified through arteriography was reported by Sjöqvist in 1936 [16]. The following year, in 1937, Moniz, along with Lima and de Lacerda, described four patients with occlusion of the cervical portion of the internal carotid artery, confirmed via arteriography. Moniz's pioneering work in cerebral arteriography was groundbreaking and he was twice nominated for the Nobel Prize. He was awarded the prize in 1949 (shared with Rudolf Hess), however, not for his advancements in vascular imaging, but instead for his contributions to prefrontal lobotomy.

The latter half of the twentieth century witnessed a paradigm shift in stroke diagnosis and management with the advent of advanced neuroimaging technologies, including computed tomography (CT) and magnetic resonance imaging (MRI). These imaging modalities revolutionized the diagnostic landscape, enabling prompt differentiation between stroke subtypes and facilitating the timely implementation of targeted interventions. The introduction of thrombolytic therapy, specifically tissue plasminogen activator (tPA) in the 1990s, emerged as a landmark development in the acute management of ischemic stroke, significantly enhancing functional recovery and survival rates [17]. Furthermore, the emergence of endovascular techniques, such as mechanical thrombectomy, has become a cornerstone of treatment for large-vessel occlusions, further improving clinical outcomes.

3 Development of Surgical Technique

The earliest surgical interventions involving the carotid artery were primarily ligation procedures, aimed at controlling trauma or hemorrhage. On December 12, 1785, the famous British surgeon John Hunter ligated an artery that was feeding a popliteal aneurysm [18]. During the procedure he ligated only the proximal side of the artery and left the aneurysm sac untouched. This is frequently viewed as a landmark event in the history of vascular surgery and Hunter lent his name to the eponymous practice of applying ligatures to aneurysmal dilatation of arteries. In 1793, Hebenstreit of Germany, in his translation of Benjamin Bell's *Surgery*, documented a notable case where the carotid artery was damaged during the removal of a scirrhous tumor [19]. To control the ensuing hemorrhage, the surgeon successfully ligated the artery, and the patient survived for many years thereafter. This case is widely regarded as the first recorded instance of carotid artery ligation, marking an important milestone in vascular surgery.

The inaugural reconstruction of the carotid artery was executed in 1951 in Buenos Aires, stemming from the collaborative efforts of Fisher, Murphy, Carrea, and Mollins (Fig. 10) [20]. In the described case report, angiography disclosed significant stenosis of the internal carotid artery above the bifurcation in a patient presenting with symptoms of ischemic stroke. Both arteries were transected 5 mm above the lesion and an anastomosis was performed between the proximal external carotid artery and the distal internal carotid artery. This thus represented the inaugural documentation of an internal-external carotid artery bypass. The patient exhibited recovery from hemiparesis and aphasia, providing the first evidence that reinstating cerebral blood flow post-ischemic stroke could restore motor function. Although this procedure was deemed successful, CEA would soon emerge as the preferred technique for the management of carotid stenosis in subsequent years.

In 1953, Debakey proficiently performed the first CEA on a patient experiencing cerebrovascular insufficiency [21]. It is noteworthy that DeBakey did not utilize angiography to localize the lesion prior to performing his initial endarterectomy; instead, he relied on the prevailing literature suggesting that lesions were commonly situated at the carotid bifurcation. A 53-year-old school bus driver presented with a history of recurring episodes of transient right hemiparesis and dysphasia over a two-year period. Upon examination, he exhibited a mild residual right hemiparesis and weak pulsation in his left carotid artery. Notably, no preoperative arteriogram was performed prior to surgery. During the surgical intervention, a severely stenotic atherosclerotic plaque with an overlay of fresh thrombus was identified, completely occluding the left internal carotid artery. A thromboendarterectomy was performed, which resulted in good retrograde blood flow from both the internal and external carotid arteries. A postoperative arteriogram conducted on the operating table demonstrated patency of the internal carotid artery in both its extracranial and intracranial segments. The patient made a satisfactory recovery and lived for an additional 19 years without experiencing further strokes. He ultimately succumbed to complications related to coronary artery disease on August 17, 1972. Although DeBakey was the first to carry out the procedure, the publication detailing this case did not emerge until 1975. Therefore, Cooley emerged as the first to publish findings on a successful endarterectomy in 1956, marking the initial introduction of a temporary shunt utilized during a CEA procedure [22]. The shunt was constructed from a polyvinyl tube, featuring a 14-gauge needle at its lower end and a 16-gauge needle at the upper end, which was positioned at the internal carotid artery. In addition to the shunt, cerebral protection was enhanced by immersing the patient's head in crushed ice for 30 minutes prior to the procedure. Despite these protective measures, the patient experienced a stroke related to the operation; however, he exhibited a rapid recovery over the following weeks.

The surgical treatment of occlusive lesions in the great vessels arising from the aortic arch developed rapidly alongside advancements in carotid artery surgery. In 1950, Gordon Murray from Toronto successfully restored circulation in a left common carotid artery that was completely occluded at the aortic arch using a probe and specialized instrumentation [23]. In 1954, Davis, Grove, and Julian performed the first innominate artery endarterectomy [24]. Today, bypass procedures, including extrathoracic bypass and endarterectomy, remain the standard surgical treatments for occlusive lesions of the aortic arch vessels.

The external carotid artery-to-internal carotid artery (EC-IC) bypass has a rich and complex history, deeply intertwined with the development of microsurgical techniques for

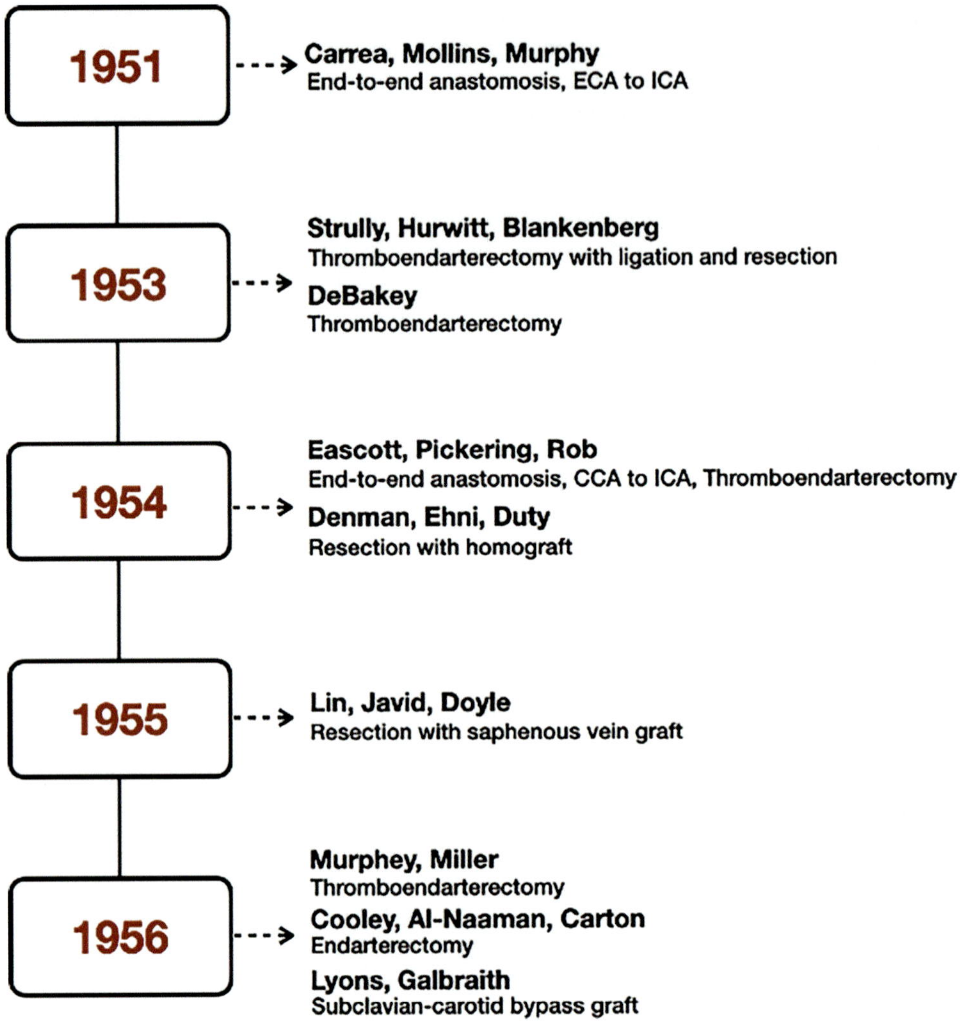

Fig. 10 Summary of the pioneering carotid artery reconstructions for cerebrovascular insufficiency

cerebral revascularization. The earliest conceptualizations of cerebral bypass surgery emerged in the mid-twentieth century, driven by the recognition that ischemic stroke, often caused by atherosclerotic disease of the internal carotid artery, led to significant morbidity and mortality in patients with insufficient collateral cerebral circulation. As direct surgical interventions evolved, the work of early pioneers like Dr. Robert H. Donaghy and Dr. M. Gazi Yasargil laid the foundation for EC-IC bypass surgery [25]. In the early 1960s, Donaghy, a vascular surgeon, and Yasargil [26], a neurosurgeon, introduced microsurgical techniques for direct anastomosis between the superficial temporal artery (STA), a branch of the external carotid artery (ECA), and the middle cerebral artery (MCA) in order to augment cerebral blood flow in patients with symptomatic cerebral ischemia.

One of the first successful EC-IC bypasses was reported by Dr. Yasargil in 1967, in Zurich, Switzerland [27]. The patient, suffering from recurrent TIAs due to a severe stenosis of the ICA, exhibited significant improvement following revascularization through STA-MCA bypass, establishing the procedure as a potential solution for patients with inadequate perfusion from the intracranial vasculature. Throughout the 1970s and early 1980s, the procedure gained traction as a promising intervention for patients with symptomatic cerebrovascular disease that was not amenable to carotid endarterectomy or other revascularization approaches. Surgeons like Dr. Charles G. Drake, a renowned Canadian neurosurgeon, contributed to refining the technical aspects of EC-IC bypass, utilizing it for complex cases of carotid occlusion or intracranial aneurysms where other interventions posed high risk.

In 1969, the Joint Study of Extracranial Arterial Occlusion reported on 2400 CEA procedures performed between 1961 and 1968, revealing a 4.5% surgical mortality rate [28]. However, the exact indications for CEA remained unclear at the time, and the associated risks caused the procedure to take years to become the standard of care. Since then, there has been significant advancement in the treatment of stroke, with the development of various therapeutic alternatives, including endovascular interventions including thrombectomy or the refinement of carotid artery stenting techniques. Additionally, large-scale, randomized clinical trials, such as the North American Symptomatic Carotid Endarterectomy Trial (NASCET) [29] and the European Carotid Surgery Trial (ECST) [30], have rigorously compared these treatments, providing critical evidence that has shaped modern stroke management guidelines.

Regarding the role of EC-IC bypass in the stroke management, the landmark International EC-IC Bypass Study, initiated in 1977 and completed in 1985, fundamentally altered the trajectory of the procedure's adoption [31]. The study was a large, randomized controlled trial that sought to definitively determine the efficacy of EC-IC bypass in preventing recurrent stroke in patients with symptomatic ICA occlusion. The trial enrolled over 1300 patients across multiple centers worldwide, comparing outcomes between patients receiving EC-IC bypass and those managed with medical therapy alone. The results, published in 1985, were surprising to the neurosurgical and stroke communities: the study found no significant reduction in the incidence of stroke in the surgical group compared to the medically treated group, which led to a dramatic decline in the utilization of the procedure. In the 1990s and 2000s, the work of neurosurgeons like Dr. William E. Powers and Dr. Ralph G. Dacey helped to refine patient selection criteria, emphasizing the importance of preoperative hemodynamic assessment [32]. Although EC-IC bypass remains a more limited procedure today, reserved for select cases of symptomatic intracranial stenosis or moyamoya disease, its development represents a critical chapter in the history of stroke surgery. The evolution of this bypass underscores the ongoing refinement of surgical and medical strategies for stroke prevention, reflecting a broader historical trend from invasive procedures toward individualized, image-guided treatment approaches.

4 Conclusion

In conclusion, the historical evolution of stroke understanding underscores the critical interplay between advances in anatomical knowledge, pathophysiological insights, and therapeutic innovations. This chapter has illuminated key milestones that have shaped contemporary practices in stroke management, highlighting the pressing need for ongoing research and education given the high prevalence and substantial morbidity associated with cerebrovascular accidents. As the demand for neurosurgical and endovascular interventions continues to grow, it is imperative to integrate historical insights with modern technological advancements to improve diagnostic accuracy and treatment efficacy. By fostering a comprehensive understanding of stroke's complexities, the medical community can better equip itself to address the challenges posed by this condition, ultimately enhancing patient outcomes and reducing the societal burden of stroke.

References

1. Donkor ES. Stroke in the 21(st) century: a snapshot of the burden, epidemiology, and quality of life. Stroke Res Treat. 2018;2018:3238165.
2. Leak RK, et al. From apoplexy to stroke: historical perspectives and new research frontiers. Prog Neurobiol. 2014;115:1–5.
3. Tsoucalas G, Papaioannou TG, Karamanou M. The Hippocratic doctrine of "the acute brain suffering" as the brain stroke. J Stroke Cerebrovasc Dis. 2019;28(2):412–7.
4. Khuda I, Al-Shamrani F. Stroke medicine in antiquity: the Greek and Muslim contribution. J Family Community Med. 2018;25(3):143–7.
5. Copyright © 2012 Wellcome library, London.
6. Ghaffari F, et al. Avicenna and clinical experiences in canon of medicine. J Med Life. 2022;15(2):168–73.
7. Dumitrescu AM, et al. The discovery of the circle of Willis as a result of using the scientific method in anatomical dissection. Romanian J Morphol Embryol. 2020;61(3):959–65.
8. Bem Junior LS, et al. The anatomy of the brain – learned over the centuries. Surg Neurol Int. 2021;12:319.
9. Casserius, G., Tabulae anatomicae LXXIIX, omnes novae nec ante hac visae. Daniel Bucretius XX quae deerant supplevit & omnium explicationes additit. Impensis & coelo Matthaei Meriani, 1632. Francofurti.
10. Pearce JM. Johann Jakob Wepfer (1620-95) and cerebral haemorrhage. J Neurol Neurosurg Psychiatry. 1997;62(4):387.
11. Veslingus I. Syntagma anatomicum: locis plurimis auctum, emendatum, novisque iconibus diligenter exornatum. Secunda editio ab extrema auctoris manu. Typis Pauli Frambotti Bibliopolae. 1651. Patavii:182–95.
12. Teive HAG, et al. Thomas Willis' legacy on the 400th anniversary of his birth. Arq Neuropsiquiatr. 2022;80(7):759–62.
13. Schiller F. Concepts of stroke before and after Virchow. Med Hist. 1970;14(2):115–31.
14. Tubbs RS, Cohen-Gadol AA. Hans Chiari (1851–1916). J Neurol. 2010;257(7):1218–20.
15. Wilms G, Baert AL. The history of angiography. J Belg Radiol. 1995;78(5):299–302.
16. Johnson HC, Walker AE. The angiographic diagnosis of spontaneous thrombosis of the internal and common carotid arteries. J Neurosurg. 1951;8(6):631–59.
17. Hatcher MA, Starr JA. Role of tissue plasminogen activator in acute ischemic stroke. Ann Pharmacother. 2011;45(3):364–71.
18. Ellis H. John hunter's operation for popliteal aneurysm. J Perioper Pract. 2017;27(6):144–5.
19. Kaufman MH. The excoriation of Benjamin bell: who was 'Jonathan Dawplucker'? J R Coll Physicians Edinb. 2005;35(4):356–64.
20. Estol CJ. Dr C. Miller Fisher and the history of carotid artery disease. Stroke. 1996;27(3):559–66.
21. Hu J, et al. Transcarotid artery revascularization and advances in vascular surgery for carotid artery disease. Surg Technol Int. 2021;39:277–82.
22. Sehgal VS, Ting W. The evolution of carotid surgery. Ann Vasc Surg. 2024;113:287–93.

23. Thompson JE. The evolution of surgery for the treatment and prevention of stroke. Stroke. 1996;27(8):1427–34.
24. Fernandes e Fernandes J, Pedro LM. Extracranial carotid artery disease. In: Liapis CD, et al., editors. Vascular surgery. Berlin, Heidelberg: Springer Berlin Heidelberg; 2007. p. 137–53.
25. Thanapal S, et al. Direct cerebral revascularization: extracranial-intracranial bypass. Asian J Neurosurg. 2018;13(1):9–17.
26. Link TE, et al. Raymond M. P. Donaghy: a pioneer in microneurosurgery: historical vignette. J Neurosurg. 2010;112(6):1176–81.
27. Stienen MN, et al. UniversitätsSpital Zürich: 80 years of neurosurgical patient care in Switzerland. Acta Neurochir. 2018;160(1):3–22.
28. Fields WS, et al. Joint study of extracranial arterial occlusion. V. Progress report of prognosis following surgery or nonsurgical treatment for transient cerebral ischemic attacks and cervical carotid artery lesions. JAMA. 1970;211(12):1993–2003.
29. Ferguson GG, et al. The North American symptomatic carotid endarterectomy trial. Stroke. 1999;30(9):1751–8.
30. Randomised trial of endarterectomy for recently symptomatic carotid stenosis: final results of the MRC European Carotid Surgery Trial (ECST). Lancet. 1998;351(9113):1379–87.
31. The international cooperative study of Extracranial/intracranial arterial anastomosis (EC/IC bypass study): methodology and entry characteristics. The EC/IC Bypass Study group. Stroke. 1985;16(3):397–406.
32. Ashley WW, et al. Flow-assisted surgical cerebral revascularization. Neurosurg Focus FOC. 2008;24(2):E20.

Epidemiology of Stroke

Tatiana Abou-Mrad, Laura Stone McGuire, Richard Bram, Gursant Atwal, Ali Alaraj, and Fady T. Charbel

Abbreviations

AI	Artificial Intelligence
ARIC	Atherosclerosis Risk in Communities
aSAH	Aneurysmal Subarachnoid Hemorrhage
AVM	Arteriovenous Malformation
DALYs	Disability-Adjusted Life Years
HIC	High-Income Countries
ICH	Intracerebral Hemorrhage
IS	Ischemic Stroke
LACI	Lacunar Infarcts
LMCIs	Low- and Middle-Income Countries
MRI	Magnetic Resonance Imaging
OCSP	Oxfordshire Community Stroke Project
PACI	Partial Anterior Circulation Infarcts
PM	Particulate Matter
POCI	Posterior Circulation Infarcts
SES	Socioeconomic Status
TACI	Total Anterior Circulation Infarcts
TOAST	Trial of Org 10,172 in Acute Stroke Treatment
WHO	World Health Organization

T. Abou-Mrad · R. Bram · G. Atwal · A. Alaraj · F. T. Charbel (✉)
Department of Neurosurgery, University of Illinois at Chicago, Chicago, IL, USA
e-mail: fcharbel@uic.edu

L. S. McGuire
Department of Neurosurgery, University of Illinois at Chicago, Chicago, IL, USA

Department of Neurosurgery, University of Wisconsin, Maddison, WI, USA

1 Introduction

Stroke is one of the leading causes of death and long-term disability worldwide, presenting a substantial burden on individuals and healthcare systems. Annually, approximately 15 million strokes occur globally, with over a quarter resulting in fatalities [1]. Stroke ranks as the second most common cause of death, following ischemic heart disease, and accounts for about 10% of all global mortality [2]. Among survivors, at least 30% experience permanent disabilities, contributing significantly to its standing as a leading cause of disability-adjusted life years (DALYs) lost [1].

The repercussions of stroke extend beyond physical impairments to encompass psychological, social, and financial challenges. Lifetime costs per stroke patient range from $59,800 to $230,000, underscoring its economic impact [3]. While stroke predominantly affects individuals aged 65 and older, its outcomes are often severe: approximately one-third of patients die within a year of onset, and more than half of survivors rely on caregivers for daily activities. Strokes also result in secondary conditions, including depression, dementia, and epilepsy. Additionally, as a vascular disease, stroke carries a heightened risk of recurrence or other serious vascular events, with nearly 20% of survivors experiencing such outcomes within a few years of the initial incident [4, 5].

As a complex disease driven by a combination of biological, environmental, and socioeconomic factors, stroke has considerable variation in its incidence and outcomes across populations and regions. Understanding these epidemiological patterns is critical for designing effective prevention strategies and healthcare policies. Recent decades have seen notable advances in stroke prevention and management, fueled by innovations in medical technology, public health initiatives, and research. However, significant challenges persist. The increasing prevalence of risk factors such as obesity and hypertension, healthcare inequalities, and the global effects of urbanization and climate change

V. Beneš, D. Netuka (eds.), *Surgical and Interventional Treatment of Cerebral Ischemia*, https://doi.org/10.1007/978-3-032-08934-2_2

continue to exacerbate the stroke burden. This chapter offers a comprehensive overview of stroke epidemiology, including its global burden, associated risk factors, and prevention strategies. With a specific focus on ischemic strokes (IS), it also explores the socioeconomic and environmental influences on stroke outcomes. By analyzing current trends and future directions, this chapter emphasizes the importance of a multidisciplinary approach in addressing this global health challenge.

2 Definition of Stroke

Stroke refers to an acute brain injury caused by a vascular event, resulting in permanent neuronal damage and functional impairment. It is classified into IS and hemorrhagic stroke. IS occur due to occlusion or significant stenosis of cerebral blood vessels, leading to insufficient blood flow to sustain neuronal function. In contrast, hemorrhagic strokes result from bleeding into or around the brain, often due to aneurysmal rupture, chronic hypertension, arteriovenous malformation (AVM), cerebral amyloid angiopathy, coagulopathies, drug use etc. IS account for 80–90% of all strokes, whereas hemorrhagic strokes comprise 10–20% of all cases but carry higher risks of morbidity and mortality [6].

2.1 Ischemic Stroke

The World Health Organization (WHO) defines stroke as "rapidly developing clinical signs of focal or global cerebral dysfunction lasting 24 hours or more, with no apparent cause other than vascular origin" [7]. IS is primarily caused by thrombosis, embolism, or hypoperfusion. Thrombosis often arises from arterial wall damage caused by atherosclerosis, dissection, or inflammation, leading to thrombus formation at the injury site. This can obstruct blood flow or dislodge, forming emboli that block downstream vessels. Other embolic sources include fat particles from fractures, atherosclerotic plaque rupture, air, amniotic fluid, or fibrous cartilage. Hypoperfusion, on the other hand, occurs when cerebral blood flow diminishes due to triggers such as severe hypotension, sepsis, or cardiac arrest.

Historically, symptoms resolving within 24 hours were classified as a transient ischemic attack (TIA). However, modern imaging techniques like computed tomography (CT) and magnetic resonance imaging (MRI) have revealed ischemic lesions in many TIA cases, which carry similar prognostic risks for death, disability, and recurrence as minor IS [8]. Consequently, the traditional time-based definition of TIA may persist for epidemiological purposes, but clinically, the presence of ischemic lesions should prompt management as an ischemic stroke.

2.2 Hemorrhagic Strokes

Hemorrhagic strokes, including intracerebral hemorrhage (ICH) and aneurysmal subarachnoid hemorrhage (aSAH), account for 8–15% of all stroke cases in Western countries, while Eastern countries, such as Japan and Korea, report higher rates (18–24%). In low- and middle-income countries (LMICs), the incidence of ICH is approximately double that of developed nations (22 versus 10 per 100,000 people) [9, 10]. Spontaneous ICH, the most common form, typically arises from chronic hypertension leading to lipohyalinosis in small cerebral vessels. These hemorrhages often affect regions supplied by perforating arteries, including the pons, cerebellum, basal ganglia, thalamus, and white matter [11]. Non-spontaneous causes should be considered in younger patients or those lacking traditional risk factors such as hypertension or coagulopathy. Common etiologies in these cases include moyamoya disease, AVMs, tumors, and cerebral vein thrombosis. In contrast, aSAH is less common but demonstrates considerable variability in incidence both globally and within the same country.

3 Classification Systems for Ischemic Stroke

IS encompasses several underlying mechanisms, which vary in their clinical presentations, outcomes, and management approaches. This underscores the importance of classification systems in improving IS diagnosis and treatment strategies. This heterogeneity has driven the development of multiple classification systems, each aiming to categorize IS based on the etiology, clinical presentation, and pathophysiological mechanisms.

TOAST Classification

The Trial of Org 10,172 in Acute Stroke Treatment (TOAST) classification system is widely utilized in both clinical practice and research for categorizing IS based on presumed etiology [12]. This system delineates five primary subtypes:

1. **Large Artery Atherosclerosis:** These strokes result from significant atherosclerotic disease in large extracranial or intracranial arteries. Mechanisms include in situ thrombotic occlusion or artery-to-artery embolism. This subtype is more prevalent in certain populations, such as individuals of East Asian descent.
2. **Cardioembolic Stroke:** This subtype arises from emboli originating in the heart, commonly due to atrial fibrillation, valvular heart disease, or infective endocarditis. Cardioembolic strokes are often large, involve cortical regions, and carry a high risk of recurrence if the underlying cardiac condition is untreated.

3. **Small Vessel Occlusion**: Also known as lacunar strokes, these result from occlusion of small perforating arteries, typically due to lipohyalinosis or microatheroma formation. These strokes are often associated with chronic hypertension and diabetes and typically manifest as subcortical syndromes with relatively mild neurological deficits.
4. **Stroke of Other Determined Etiology:** These include a diverse group of etiologies, such as:
   - Recreational drug use (e.g., cocaine, amphetamines).
   - Hematological disorders (e.g., polycythemia, sickle cell disease).
   - Vasculitis (e.g., temporal arteritis).
   - Metabolic conditions (e.g., Fabry disease).
   - Cerebral vasoconstriction syndromes or other uncommon mechanisms.
   - Arterial dissection.
5. **Stroke of Undetermined Etiology:** Despite extensive investigation, the cause of these strokes remains undetermined. Advances in diagnostic techniques, including cardiac monitoring and imaging, are reducing the proportion of cryptogenic strokes by uncovering previously undiagnosed etiologies.

Oxfordshire Community Stroke Project (OCSP) Classification

Another widely used system is the Oxfordshire Community Stroke Project (OCSP) classification, which categorizes IS based on clinical features and the extent of cerebral involvement [13]. This system is particularly valuable in predicting prognosis and guiding early management decisions. The OCSP categories include:

1. **Total Anterior Circulation Infarcts (TACI)**: These strokes involve large areas of the anterior circulation, typically affecting both cortical and subcortical regions. They are associated with severe deficits, including hemiparesis, hemisensory loss, and cortical dysfunction (e.g., aphasia, neglect).
2. **Partial Anterior Circulation Infarcts (PACI)**: These are often considered a less severe form of TACI, as they typically affect a portion of the anterior circulation, leading to more localized deficits.
3. **Lacunar Infarcts (LACI)**: Caused by small vessel disease, these subcortical infarcts produce syndromes such as pure motor or sensory strokes, without cortical signs.
4. **Posterior Circulation Infarcts (POCI)**: These strokes involve the vertebrobasilar system and can result in a wide range of deficits, including cranial nerve abnormalities, ataxia, and visual field defects.

Accurate classification is integral to optimizing stroke management and improving outcomes. Etiology-specific treatments, such as anticoagulation for cardioembolic stroke or revascularization for large vessel atherosclerosis, hinge on proper subtype identification. Additionally, standardized classification systems facilitate clinical research by providing a common framework for patient selection and data interpretation. Classification systems like TOAST and OCSP are essential tools in the diagnosis and management of IS. Continued research and technological advancements are expected to further refine these systems, ultimately enhancing our ability to individualize stroke care and improve patient outcomes. Advances in neuroimaging and molecular diagnostics are paving the way for more refined classification systems. Imaging-based approaches, such as those utilizing diffusion-weighted MRI, allow for precise localization and characterization of infarcts, which may provide additional insights into underlying mechanisms. Furthermore, genetic and biomarker studies are beginning to identify novel subtypes of IS, enhancing our understanding of stroke pathophysiology [14, 15].

4 Global Burden of Stroke

Stroke is a leading global health concern, contributing to approximately 10% of all deaths worldwide, with substantial morbidity reflected in years of life lost (DALYs) [16]. Despite a decline in stroke incidence in high-income countries (HICs), LMICs have seen a sharp increase, driven by disparities in healthcare access, risk factor management, and preventive measures [17]. Between 1970 and 2008, stroke incidence in LMICs more than doubled, surpassing the rates seen in HICs, which saw a 42% decrease over the same period [18]. This decline in HICs can be largely attributed to improvements in healthcare infrastructure, acute stroke care management, and risk factor control. For instance, the Atherosclerosis Risk in Communities (ARIC) study found a 32% decline in stroke incidence among older United States adults, largely due to better cardiovascular risk management [19].

In contrast, stroke-related deaths in LMICs accounted for 85.5% of the global total in 2001, with DALYs lost to stroke nearly seven times higher than in HICs [16]. This stark disparity underscores the growing gap in stroke prevention and outcomes between regions. The global burden of stroke is thus disproportionately concentrated in LMICs, where early case fatality rates have not decreased as significantly as in HICs. This discrepancy is largely due to gaps in healthcare quality and access, compounded by limitations in acute care infrastructure, delayed treatment initiation, and differences in healthcare personnel training [20, 21]. On the other hand, HICs have seen significant advancements in acute stroke care, including the introduction of thrombolytic therapies, endovascular thrombectomy, specialized stroke centers, and improved rehabilitation strategies. These improvements have led to significantly lower early case fatality rates and more favorable outcomes, further highlighting the stark divide in stroke care between regions [16, 18].

Despite significant declines in stroke incidence and mortality rates in HICs, stroke remains a critical health concern, primarily due to the aging populations. As life expectancy increases, the risk of stroke also rises, posing new challenges to healthcare systems. Looking ahead, demographic shifts, such as aging populations, urbanization, and evolving lifestyle factors, are expected to exacerbate the global stroke burden. In the United States, for example, the number of stroke survivors is projected to exceed 10 million by 2030, marking an increase of nearly 3 million from 2018 [22]. This rising prevalence of stroke survivors is poised to place significant pressure on healthcare resources, highlighting the urgent need for comprehensive stroke care management strategies that can address both acute and long-term rehabilitation needs.

5 Risk Factors

Stroke risk factors can be divided into non-modifiable and modifiable categories, each playing a significant role in stroke incidence and outcomes. Non-modifiable risk factors include gender, age, and ethnicity. Age is a particularly strong determinant, with stroke incidence increasing exponentially after the age of 65. While men are generally at higher risk of stroke overall, women tend to experience worse outcomes [23–25]. This disparity is partly attributed to women's longer life expectancy, leading to strokes occurring later in life when comorbidities and frailty are more pronounced. However, studies suggest that poorer functional outcomes in women cannot be fully explained by age or comorbidities [26, 27]. Approximately two-thirds of women with strokes are unpartnered compared to one-third of men, resulting in greater dependency and a higher likelihood of requiring institutional care [28, 29]. Women's dual roles as caregivers and patients, particularly later in life, can also impact their own health and recovery. Further research is warranted to understand the biological and societal factors contributing to these gender-based disparities.

Ethnic disparities in stroke incidence and outcomes are also prominent. Populations of African and South Asian descent, for example, experience higher stroke rates than other ethnic groups, partly due to genetic predispositions and environmental factors [30, 31]. Moreover, studies have shown higher stroke risks among Black, Māori, and Pacific populations compared to white populations [32–34]. While genetic factors are non-modifiable, environmental and socioeconomic factors, both of which are modifiable, play a pivotal role in these disparities and represent critical targets for stroke prevention. Socioeconomic status (SES), in particular, is strongly linked to these disparities, as individuals in lower SES groups are more frequently exposed to stroke risk factors such as hypertension, smoking, and excessive alcohol consumption [35]. Additionally, they often encounter barriers to accessing preventive healthcare and managing these risks effectively, which further contributes to higher stroke incidence and worse outcomes. People from lower SES backgrounds face limited access to healthcare, poorer health literacy, and delays in diagnosis and treatment, all of which elevate stroke mortality rates [17, 36, 37]. Education plays a particularly important role as individuals with higher educational attainment are generally more likely to adopt healthier lifestyles, adhere to medical treatments, and recognize stroke symptoms early, all of which improve stroke outcomes [38]. Environmental factors, such as urbanization and air pollution—especially fine particulate matter (PM2.5)—have also emerged as significant contributors to stroke risk and severity [39].

In addition to addressing these broader determinants, focusing on modifiable risk factors is essential for stroke prevention. Approximately 90% of the population-attributable risk for stroke can be explained by ten key factors: hypertension, physical inactivity, abdominal obesity, unfavorable apolipoprotein B to A1 ratio, smoking, poor diets high in salt, sugar, and trans fats, cardiac conditions, diabetes, psychosocial stress and depression, and excessive alcohol consumption [40]. Among these, elevated blood pressure is the most significant, accounting for nearly 50% of all strokes. Tackling these modifiable risk factors, alongside addressing the environmental and socioeconomic conditions that drive health disparities, is crucial to reducing stroke incidence and improving outcomes across diverse populations.

6 Trends and Future Directions in Stroke Epidemiology

Over recent decades, stroke epidemiology has undergone significant changes, influenced by medical advancements, demographic transitions, and evolving lifestyle patterns. Emerging trends in stroke incidence reveal a troubling rise among younger populations. Hospitalizations for acute ischemic stroke in males aged 20–44 nearly doubled since the 1990s, linked to increasing obesity, diabetes, hypertension, and substance abuse [41–44]. Similarly, the aging population contributes to the overall stroke burden, as age-related conditions like atrial fibrillation and malignancy-associated hypercoagulability heighten stroke risk [45].These demographic and epidemiological shifts call for adaptable prevention strategies that address diverse age groups and their unique risk factors.

Environmental and societal factors are also becoming pivotal in stroke epidemiology. Air pollution, for instance, contributes to over one-eighth of stroke-related deaths globally, with particulate matter exacerbating carotid atherosclerosis and hypertension [46, 47]. The COVID-19 pandemic has further complicated this landscape, with the virus's vascular effects increasing stroke risk, even in asymptomatic younger individuals [48, 49]. These evolving challenges demand innovative approaches to prevention and management.

The future of stroke epidemiology lies in leveraging technology, refining research methodologies, and addressing global disparities. Artificial intelligence (AI) and big data analytics offer transformative potential, enabling predictive modeling, personalized medicine, and real-time monitoring through wearable devices and electronic health records. Standardizing global stroke surveillance and establishing robust data registries can help address inconsistencies, particularly in LMICs, fostering international collaboration for a unified approach to stroke care. Moreover, advancements in genomics and biomarker research promise to enhance early detection and targeted interventions [11, 15]. Meanwhile, the impact of climate change, urbanization, and globalization necessitates proactive public health strategies, from mitigating air pollution to addressing healthcare access in rapidly urbanizing regions.

Equity and inclusion remain paramount for advancing stroke prevention and care. Diverse representation in clinical research and culturally tailored interventions can ensure broader applicability and effectiveness. Additionally, digital health innovations, including telemedicine and mobile health applications, are expanding access to stroke care in underserved areas, while digital platforms facilitate public awareness campaigns [50]. Therefore, sustained advocacy at the global level is critical. With effective application of existing knowledge and cutting-edge advancements, the global community has an opportunity to mitigate the growing burden of stroke and improve outcomes worldwide.

7 Conclusion

Stroke constitutes a major proportion of global health challenges, causing devastating impacts on individuals, healthcare systems, and economies. Its complex etiology, spanning biological, environmental, and socioeconomic factors, highlights the need for a multifaceted approach to prevention, diagnosis, and management disparities persist in stroke incidence and outcomes across populations, driven by inequities in healthcare access, risk factor prevalence, and public health infrastructure. Addressing these challenges requires collaborative global efforts that prioritize primary prevention, early stroke detection, and equitable access to acute and long-term care. Innovations in technology, combined with robust epidemiological research, hold promise for refining our understanding of stroke mechanisms and uncovering novel therapeutics.

References

1. Feigin VL, Brainin M, Norrving B, Martins S, Sacco RL, Hacke W, et al. World Stroke Organization (WSO): global stroke fact sheet 2022. Int J Stroke. 2022;17(1):18–29.
2. Donkor ES. Stroke in the 21(st) century: a snapshot of the burden, epidemiology, and quality of life. Stroke Res Treat. 2018;2018:3238165.
3. Feigin VL, Lawes CMM, Bennett DA, Anderson CS. Stroke epidemiology: a review of population-based studies of incidence, prevalence, and case-fatality in the late 20th century. Lancet Neurol. 2003;2(1):43–53.
4. Aarnio K, Haapaniemi E, Melkas S, Kaste M, Tatlisumak T, Putaala J. Long-term mortality after first-ever and recurrent stroke in young adults. Stroke. 2014;45(9):2670–6.
5. Schneider S, Taba N, Saapar M, Vibo R, Kõrv J. Determinants of long-term health-related quality of life in young ischemic stroke patients. J Stroke Cerebrovasc Dis. 2021;30(2):105499.
6. Boehme AK, Esenwa C, Elkind MSV. Stroke risk factors, genetics, and prevention. Circ Res. 2017;120(3):472–95.
7. Hatano S. Experience from a multicentre stroke register: a preliminary report. Bull World Health Organ. 1976;54(5):541–53.
8. Coutts SB, Hill MD, Campos CR, Choi YB, Subramaniam S, Kosior JC, et al. Recurrent events in transient ischemic attack and minor stroke. Stroke. 2008;39(9):2461–6.
9. Hughes JD, Bond KM, Mekary RA, Dewan MC, Rattani A, Baticulon R, et al. Estimating the global incidence of aneurysmal subarachnoid hemorrhage: a systematic review for central nervous system vascular lesions and meta-analysis of ruptured aneurysms. World Neurosurg. 2018;115:430–47.e7.
10. Wang S, Zou XL, Wu LX, Zhou HF, Xiao L, Yao T, et al. Epidemiology of intracerebral hemorrhage: a systematic review and meta-analysis. Front Neurol. 2022;13:915813.
11. Magid-Bernstein J, Girard R, Polster S, Srinath A, Romanos S, Awad IA, et al. Cerebral hemorrhage: pathophysiology, treatment, and future directions. Circ Res. 2022;130(8):1204–29.
12. Adams HP Jr, Bendixen BH, Kappelle LJ, Biller J, Love BB, Gordon DL, et al. Classification of subtype of acute ischemic stroke. Definitions for use in a multicenter clinical trial. TOAST. Trial of Org 10172 in Acute Stroke Treatment. Stroke. 1993;24(1):35–41.
13. Pittock SJ, Meldrum D, Hardiman O, Thornton J, Brennan P, Moroney JT. The Oxfordshire community stroke project classification: correlation with imaging, associated complications, and prediction of outcome in acute ischemic stroke. J Stroke Cerebrovasc Dis. 2003;12(1):1–7.
14. Traylor M, Farrall M, Holliday EG, Sudlow C, Hopewell JC, Cheng YC, et al. Genetic risk factors for ischaemic stroke and its subtypes (the METASTROKE collaboration): a meta-analysis of genome-wide association studies. Lancet Neurol. 2012;11(11):951–62.
15. Jickling GC, Sharp FR. Biomarker panels in ischemic stroke. Stroke. 2015;46(3):915–20.
16. Global, regional, and national burden of stroke and its risk factors, 1990–2019: a systematic analysis for the Global Burden of Disease Study 2019. Lancet Neurol. 2021;20(10):795–820.

17. Addo J, Ayerbe L, Mohan KM, Crichton S, Sheldenkar A, Chen R, et al. Socioeconomic status and stroke. Stroke. 2012;43(4):1186–91.
18. Feigin VL, Lawes CM, Bennett DA, Barker-Collo SL, Parag V. Worldwide stroke incidence and early case fatality reported in 56 population-based studies: a systematic review. Lancet Neurol. 2009;8(4):355–69.
19. Koton S, Sang Y, Schneider ALC, Rosamond WD, Gottesman RF, Coresh J. Trends in stroke incidence rates in older US adults: an update from the Atherosclerosis Risk in Communities (ARIC) cohort study. JAMA Neurol. 2020;77(1):109–13.
20. Kayola G, Mataa MM, Asukile M, Chishimba L, Chomba M, Mortel D, et al. Stroke rehabilitation in low- and middle-income countries: challenges and opportunities. Am J Phys Med Rehabil. 2023;102(2S Suppl 1):S24–s32.
21. Aguirre AO, Rogers JL, Reardon T, Shlobin NA, Ballatori AM, Brown NJ, et al. Stroke management and outcomes in low-income and lower-middle-income countries: a meta-analysis of 8535 patients. J Neurosurg. 2023;139(4):1042–51.
22. Tsao CW, Aday AW, Almarzooq ZI, Alonso A, Beaton AZ, Bittencourt MS, et al. Heart disease and stroke statistics—2022 update: a report from the American Heart Association. Circulation. 2022;145(8):e153–639.
23. Appelros P, Åsberg S. Chapter 19 – sex differences in stroke. In: Lanzenberger R, Kranz GS, Savic I, editors. Handbook of clinical neurology, vol. 175. Elsevier; 2020. p. 299–312.
24. Wilson ME. Stroke: understanding the differences between males and females. Pflugers Arch. 2013;465(5):595–600.
25. Ali M, van Os HJA, van der Weerd N, Schoones JW, Heymans MW, Kruyt ND, et al. Sex differences in presentation of stroke: a systematic review and meta-analysis. Stroke. 2022;53(2):345–54.
26. Phan HT, Reeves MJ, Gall S, Morgenstern LB, Xu Y, Lisabeth LD. Factors contributing to sex differences in health-related quality of life after ischemic stroke: BASIC (brain attack surveillance in Corpus Christi) project. J Am Heart Assoc. 2022;11(17):e026123.
27. Xu M, Amarilla Vallejo A, Cantalapiedra Calvete C, Rudd A, Wolfe C, O'Connell MDL, et al. Stroke outcomes in women: a population-based cohort study. Stroke. 2022;53(10):3072–81.
28. Reeves MJ, Bushnell CD, Howard G, Gargano JW, Duncan PW, Lynch G, et al. Sex differences in stroke: epidemiology, clinical presentation, medical care, and outcomes. Lancet Neurol. 2008;7(10):915–26.
29. Petrea RE, Beiser AS, Seshadri S, Kelly-Hayes M, Kase CS, Wolf PA. Gender differences in stroke incidence and poststroke disability in the Framingham heart study. Stroke. 2009;40(4):1032–7.
30. Gezmu T, Schneider D, Demissie K, Lin Y, Gizzi MS. Risk factors for acute stroke among south Asians compared to other racial/ethnic groups. PLoS One. 2014;9(9):e108901.
31. Prapiadou S, Demel SL, Hyacinth HI. Genetic and genomic epidemiology of stroke in people of African ancestry. Genes. 2021;12(11):1825.
32. Bonita R, Broad JB, Beaglehole R. Ethnic differences in stroke incidence and case fatality in Auckland, New Zealand. Stroke. 1997;28(4):758–61.
33. Gardener H, Sacco RL, Rundek T, Battistella V, Cheung YK, Elkind MSV. Race and ethnic disparities in stroke incidence in the northern Manhattan study. Stroke. 2020;51(4):1064–9.
34. Ranta A, Jones B, Harwood M. Stroke among Māori in Aotearoa New Zealand and solutions to address persistent inequities. Frontiers in Stroke. 2023;2
35. Chaturvedi A, Zhu A, Gadela NV, Prabhakaran D, Jafar TH. Social determinants of health and disparities in hypertension and cardiovascular diseases. Hypertension. 2024;81(3):387–99.
36. Coughlin SS, Vernon M, Hatzigeorgiou C, George V. Health literacy, social determinants of health, and disease prevention and control. J Environ Health Sci. 2020;6(1)
37. Lindmark A, Eriksson M, Darehed D. Socioeconomic status and stroke severity: understanding indirect effects via risk factors and stroke prevention using innovative statistical methods for mediation analysis. PLoS One. 2022;17(6):e0270533.
38. Che B, Shen S, Zhu Z, Wang A, Xu T, Peng Y, et al. Education level and long-term mortality, recurrent stroke, and cardiovascular events in patients with ischemic stroke. J Am Heart Assoc. 2020;9(16):e016671.
39. Kulick ER, Kaufman JD, Sack C. Ambient air pollution and stroke: an updated review. Stroke. 2023;54(3):882–93.
40. O'Donnell MJ, Xavier D, Liu L, Zhang H, Chin SL, Rao-Melacini P, et al. Risk factors for ischaemic and intracerebral haemorrhagic stroke in 22 countries (the INTERSTROKE study): a case-control study. Lancet. 2010;376(9735):112–23.
41. Ji R, Schwamm LH, Pervez MA, Singhal AB. Ischemic stroke and transient ischemic attack in young adults: risk factors, diagnostic yield, neuroimaging, and thrombolysis. JAMA Neurol. 2013;70(1):51–7.
42. Madsen TE, Khoury JC, Leppert M, Alwell K, Moomaw CJ, Sucharew H, et al. Temporal trends in stroke incidence over time by sex and age in the GCNKSS. Stroke. 2020;51(4):1070–6.
43. Béjot Y, Daubail B, Jacquin A, Durier J, Osseby GV, Rouaud O, et al. Trends in the incidence of ischaemic stroke in young adults between 1985 and 2011: the Dijon Stroke Registry. J Neurol Neurosurg Psychiatry. 2014;85(5):509–13.
44. Yahya T, Jilani MH, Khan SU, Mszar R, Hassan SZ, Blaha MJ, et al. Stroke in young adults: current trends, opportunities for prevention and pathways forward. Am J Prev Cardiol. 2020;3:100085.
45. Kalita J, Bharadwaz MP, Aditi A. Prevalence, contributing factors, and economic implications of strokes among older adults: a study of North-East India. Sci Rep. 2023;13(1):16880.
46. Feigin VL, Roth GA, Naghavi M, Parmar P, Krishnamurthi R, Chugh S, et al. Global burden of stroke and risk factors in 188 countries, during 1990–2013: a systematic analysis for the Global Burden of Disease Study 2013. Lancet Neurol. 2016;15(9):913–24.
47. Global, regional, and national comparative risk assessment of 84 behavioural, environmental and occupational, and metabolic risks or clusters of risks for 195 countries and territories, 1990-2017: a systematic analysis for the Global Burden of Disease Study 2017. Lancet. 2018;392(10159):1923–94.
48. Tu TM, Seet CYH, Koh JS, Tham CH, Chiew HJ, De Leon JA, et al. Acute ischemic stroke during the convalescent phase of asymptomatic COVID-2019 infection in men. JAMA Netw Open. 2021;4(4):e217498-e.
49. Nannoni S, de Groot R, Bell S, Markus HS. Stroke in COVID-19: a systematic review and meta-analysis. Int J Stroke. 2021;16(2):137–49.
50. Verma A, Towfighi A, Brown A, Abhat A, Casillas A. Moving towards equity with digital health innovations for stroke care. Stroke. 2022;53(3):689–97.

Pathophysiology of Cerebral Ischemia

Nikolaos Mouchtouris and Sepideh Amin-Hanjani

1 Cerebral Blood Flow Thresholds in Acute Ischemic Stroke

The brain heavily relies on oxidative metabolism of glucose to meet its energy requirements, utilizing 20% of the body's total oxygen consumption [50]. For that reason, complete arrest of cerebral blood flow (CBF) results in irreversible brain tissue damage within a few minutes [51]. Cerebral metabolic rate of oxygen ($CMRO_2$) represents the brain's utilization of oxygen and energy needs; it is dependent on CBF to transport oxygen from the lungs to the brain, the oxygen-carrying capacity of the blood through hemoglobin, and on the extraction of oxygen from the circulation into brain tissue [18, 26]. The latter is termed oxygen extraction fraction (OEF) and represents the ratio of oxygen consumed by the brain to the oxygen supplied by the circulation [19, 49].

Reduction in CBF below a critical level results in initially reversible and eventually irreversible changes to brain tissue. The hemodynamic stages of decreased CBF are typically grouped into the following three categories: benign oligemia (commonly CBF >17 mL/100 g per minute), penumbra (CBF 10–17 mL/100 g per minute), and infarct core (<10 mL/100 g per minute) [29]. Oligemic tissue refers to brain parenchyma receiving decreased flow without sustaining damage. Penumbra refers to ischemic tissue that is reversibly impaired, but is still viable tissue that may be salvaged. However, if prompt restoration of CBF is not achieved, penumbra may progress to infarct core, which is irreversible, ischemic injury.

In response to reduced CBF, several compensatory mechanisms take place to preserve cerebral metabolism. When tissue is hypoperfused, cerebral autoregulation ensues to compensate for the reduced CBF [16, 36]. The first stage of the response to cerebral hypoperfusion involves maximal vasodilation to maintain adequate CBF. In acute stroke settings, systemic blood pressure has also been noted to transiently increase, and is presumed to be a protective response to improve cerebral perfusion pressure (CPP) [28, 54]. The second stage occurs when adequate CBF is not maintained and oxygen extraction is increased to meet the metabolic need, compensating for the reduced CBF. The third stage starts when the compensatory mechanisms have been exhausted but hypoperfusion persists, resulting in metabolic mismatch. At this stage, patients experience neurological deficits, which will become permanent unless the ischemic penumbra is promptly reperfused. The duration of reduced CBF that can be tolerated by the area at risk varies significantly from patient to patient. The tissue type, presence of collateral circulation, oxygen saturation, blood pressure, glucose levels, temperature, and time to reperfusion are the main factors that affect the time it takes for brain tissue to progress from penumbra to core infarct, which is termed infarct growth rate [47]. More specifically, gray matter (GM) has higher metabolic demand than white matter (WM) and is thereby more susceptible to ischemia when CBF is reduced [6, 9]. As a result, the CBF threshold at which GM becomes penumbra and infarct core is higher than WM [6]. Furthermore, the extent of collateral circulation affects the infarct growth rate, resulting in areas of poor collateral supply to infarct faster. The basal ganglia are an example of tissue that is susceptible to fast progression to infarct core when the lenticulostriate arteries are occluded by a middle cerebral artery occlusion [33]. Lastly, oxygen saturation, blood pressure, glucose, and temperature play a role in both the patient's metabolic demand and the compensatory response to hypoperfusion [47].

2 Cellular/Molecular Pathophysiology

The sudden interruption of cerebral blood flow disrupts the supply of oxygen and glucose to the neurons of the affected tissue. The lack of oxygen and glucose slows down ATP

N. Mouchtouris · S. Amin-Hanjani (✉)
University Hospitals Cleveland Medical Center, Case Western Reserve University School of Medicine, Cleveland, OH, USA
e-mail: sepideh.hanjani@uhhospitals.org

V. Beneš, D. Netuka (eds.), *Surgical and Interventional Treatment of Cerebral Ischemia*,
https://doi.org/10.1007/978-3-032-08934-2_3

synthesis and neurons start to become energy-deficient, which results in oxidative stress-induced damage through the production of reactive oxygen species (ROS) [2]. Normal ATP production occurs through oxidative phosphorylation in mitochondria using glucose as the primary substrate. In ischemic conditions, anaerobic oxidation takes over, using the glucose available in the cytosol to produce ATP. The anaerobic process is significantly less efficient, producing only 2 ATP molecules for each molecule of glucose in contrast to 38 ATP molecules under aerobic conditions [53]. This state of energy deficiency also causes an ionic imbalance in neurons, involving Na^+, Ca^{2+}, and K+, which leads to cell depolarization and glutamate release. The disruption of ionic homeostasis and glutamate release cause ischemic-related excitotoxicity that eventually leads to neuronal apoptosis.

Apoptosis is the process of programmed cell death and is triggered either via the intrinsic or the extrinsic pathway in cerebral ischemia. The intrinsic pathway is initiated when ATP depletion disrupts the ionic homeostasis across cellular membranes. The disrupted Na^+/Ca^{2+} and K^+ channels activate a voltage-dependent Ca^{+2} channel, which releases amino acids in the extracellular space, while accumulating calcium intracellularly and triggering intrinsic apoptosis [14, 30]. The calcium excess also triggers the activation of calpain [12], a protein that promotes the release of proapoptotic factors, such as cytochrome C (Cytc) and apoptosis-inducing factor (AIF), both of which have been implicated in neuronal death.

The extrinsic pathway of apoptosis is also triggered by cerebral ischemia and contributes to neuronal cell death. Ischemia induces a neuroinflammatory response that results in immune cells crossing the disrupted blood-brain barrier (BBB) and accumulating in the ischemic tissue [63]. A number of pro-inflammatory cytokines are released in the injured parenchyma and bind neuronal plasma membranes to activate caspase-mediated apoptosis. These cytokines include interleukin 1β (IL-1β), interleukin-6 (IL-6) tumor necrosis factor α/β (TNF-α/β), and TNF-related apoptosis-inducing ligand (TRAIL), Fas ligand (FasL) [8]. Their targets on the neuronal plasma membranes are called death receptors, some of which are TNF-receptor 1, TRAIL receptor (TRAIL-R), apoptosis antigen-1 (APO1), and Fas receptor. The binding of these ligands onto the membrane receptors initiates a death-inducing signaling cascade that involves the caspase proteins caspase-8 and caspase-3 [22, 42].

The two apoptosis pathways can occur simultaneously and exacerbate the damage of the ischemic injury. In addition, several signaling pathways are involved in modulating the apoptotic processes in ischemia. Most notable are ERK/MAPK and AMPK; ERK/MAP signaling activates metalloproteinase (MMP) expression, which contributes to the ischemia-related BBB disruption and in turn allows for increased extravasation of neuroinflammatory cells into the ischemic tissue. The release of proinflammatory factors aggravates the extrinsic pathway of apoptosis. Further, AMPK signaling has also been associated with apoptosis [23]. Inhibition of AMPK downregulates expression of Cytc and AIF, which in turn blocks apoptosis. Other pathways, such as beta-hydroxybutyrate and SIRT1/NF-κB are neuroprotective and have the potential for minimizing ischemic injury. Beta-hydroxybutyrate suppresses mitochondrial dysfunction and apoptosis [17], while statins have been shown to upregulate SIRT1 and downregulate NF-κB, both of which reduce the apoptotic rate.

3 Blood-Brain Barrier Disruption

The BBB complex protects the central nervous system (CNS) from systemic circulation. It consists of endothelial cells (ECs), tight junctions (TJs) between ECs, pericytes, astrocytic end-feet, and the extracellular matrix (ECM). There are several methods of transport across the BBB complex that are heavily regulated and dependent on the properties of the crossing molecule. Passive diffusion may occur between cells of the BBB complex for small hydrophilic molecules [4], while gases and small lipophilic molecules with size of <400 Da and <8 hydrogen bonds undergo transcellular diffusion [34, 60]. Nutrients such as glucose, fatty acids, amino acids, and nucleotides cross the BBB via carrier-mediated transport, which can be either active or passive diffusion [61]. Lastly, molecules that do not have a specific carrier cross the BBB via receptor-mediated transcytosis [20]. This strict regulation of the BBB complex is enforced through three paracellular multiprotein complexes, the adherens junctions (AJs), TJs, and gap junctions [57].

The initial ischemic insult causes cytotoxic edema, which disrupts the ionic homeostasis. As a result, unregulated sodium influx leads to endothelial cell swelling and initiates the breakdown of the BBB complex [1]. The subsequent cascades that promote the production of ROS, matrix metalloproteinases (MMPs) and inflammatory cytokines are involved in degrading TJs and the ECM of the BBB complex. The influx of ions through the complex causes ionic edema that aggravates the osmotic gradient across the BBB and further exacerbates the extravasation of macromolecules from the circulation into the parenchyma, resulting in vasogenic edema. Vasogenic edema starts to occur within 4–6 hours after the initial ischemic episode [27] and peaks between 48–96 hours, while some studies report increased permeability up to over a week from symptom onset [39]. A few weeks after stroke onset, BBB permeability starts to decrease due to overexpression of TJ proteins and reorganization of the BBB complex. However, the integrity of the

BBB is not always fully restored and permeability may be increased when compared to the general population due to disorganization of the newly generated junctional proteins. As a result, patients with a history of stroke may still be at risk for hemorrhagic transformation even in the later stages of recovery [45].

4 Neuroinflammatory Response

The ischemia-induced BBB disruption is further aggravated by the inflammatory response that occurs after the ischemic insult [5]. Acute stroke causes a compensatory increase in inflammation that consists of neutrophils and monocytes, which in turn damage the TJs of the BBB and increase its permeability during the acute phase [24, 37, 41]. A number of studies have demonstrated that higher levels of systemic inflammation are associated with worse functional outcomes and mortality [10, 43, 48, 62].

There are four main inflammatory mechanisms that are activated after the ischemic insult and contribute to the morbidity of stroke. First, neutrophils and macrophages are recruited to the injured BBB and extravasate into the parenchyma through the degraded TJs [52]. The second mechanism is via the activated neutrophils that secrete pro-inflammatory cytokines and MMPs, MMP-2 and MMP-9 in particular, which exacerbate the BBB permeability by further degrading the TJs and allowing for further immune cell infiltration into the parenchyma [52]. Peripheral immune cell infiltration causes neurotoxicity and further neuronal damage. Third, the production of ROS due to ischemia further worsens the endothelial damage, neutrophil and macrophage activation, and neurotoxicity [40]. Lastly, ROS also activate the microglial NLRP3 (NOD-, LRR- and pyrin domain-containing protein 3) inflammasome, which causes an upregulation of the neuroinflammatory cascades within the parenchyma [25, 56]. This pathway results in microglia-mediated neurotoxicity and neuronal damage within the parenchyma, exponentiating the ischemic injury to the brain.

5 Reperfusion Injury

While restoration of CBF to cerebral territories at risk may decrease the extent of infarct core and ameliorate some of the neurological deficits, revascularization can also induce the overproduction of cytokines and ROS, causing further neurological deterioration, which is termed reperfusion injury. In ischemic injury, ROS are generated by NAPDH oxidase, xanthine oxidase, or the mitochondrial electron transport. When in excess, ROS cause cytotoxicity via lipid peroxidation, protein oxidation, and DNA fragmentation, leading to neuronal cell death [11]. Cerebral reperfusion further stimulates the ROS production and aggravates the cytotoxicity.

NADPH oxidase catalyzes the conversion of oxygen to superoxide by transferring electrons from NADPH. Interestingly, hyperglycemia, hypertension, hypercholesterolemia, and diabetes have been shown to increase the NADPH oxidase activity in endothelial and inflammatory cells, which may explain how these medical comorbidities worsen outcomes in patients [13, 21, 38, 55]. Xanthine oxidase further contributes to ROS overproduction by catalyzing the conversion of hypoxanthine to xanthine, which in turn is converted to uric acid [59]. This process results in overproduction of superoxide radicals, which interfere with membrane integrity, enzyme activity and membrane transport mechanisms [7, 35, 46]. Lastly, the mitochondrial electron transport chain is also involved in superoxide production in cerebral vasculature. Oxidative stress and the subsequent cytotoxicity seen accelerate the superoxide production, while TNF-α, angiotensin II and hyperglycemia are some of the well-known potentiators [3, 15, 44].

Once in excess, ROS cause reperfusion injury by inducing apoptosis through a few mechanisms. Oxidative stress and the ROS overproduction cause the activation of NFκB, which is a key signaling pathway for apoptosis [58]. The PI3K (phosphatidylinositol 3-kinase) and protein kinase B (Akt) signaling pathway is also involved in reperfusion injury. PI3K/Akt is a neuroprotective pathway that inhibits neuroinflammation and neuronal apoptosis, reducing the effect of cerebral infarction. Activation of the PI3K/Akt pathway also inhibits NFκB. However, several studies have shown that the PI3K/Akt pathway is inhibited in ischemic-reperfusion injury animal models [31, 32]. As a result, pro-inflammatory and pro-apoptotic factors are upregulated, and reperfusion injury ensues. The PI3K/Akt pathway is the target of many ongoing trials that aim to enhance its neuroprotective effects and minimize the burden of reperfusion injury.

6 Conclusion

The pathophysiology underlying cerebral ischemia is complex with many neuroprotective and neurotoxic pathways. It is the balance between the competing processes, the initial ischemia followed by reperfusion, the fluctuating BBB permeability and neuro-inflammation in the setting of medical and surgical treatments that determines recovery from stroke. Understanding the pathophysiology of stroke is imperative for developing effective therapies and improving patient outcomes.

References

1. Abdullahi W, Tripathi D, Ronaldson PT. Blood-brain barrier dysfunction in ischemic stroke: targeting tight junctions and transporters for vascular protection. Am J Physiol Cell Physiol. 2018;315(3):C343–56. https://doi.org/10.1152/ajpcell.00095.2018.
2. Andrabi SS, Parvez S, Tabassum H. Ischemic stroke and mitochondria: mechanisms and targets. Protoplasma. 2020;257(2):335–43. https://doi.org/10.1007/s00709-019-01439-2.
3. Ballinger SW. Mitochondrial dysfunction in cardiovascular disease. Free Radic Biol Med. 2005;38(10):1278–95. https://doi.org/10.1016/j.freeradbiomed.2005.02.014.
4. Barar J, Rafi MA, Pourseif MM, et al. Blood-brain barrier transport machineries and targeted therapy of brain diseases. Bioimpacts. 2016;6(4):225–48. https://doi.org/10.15171/bi.2016.30.
5. Bernardo-Castro S, Sousa JA, Bras A, et al. Pathophysiology of blood-brain barrier permeability throughout the different stages of ischemic stroke and its implication on hemorrhagic transformation and recovery. Front Neurol. 2020;11:594672. https://doi.org/10.3389/fneur.2020.594672.
6. Bristow MS, Simon JE, Brown RA, et al. MR perfusion and diffusion in acute ischemic stroke: human gray and white matter have different thresholds for infarction. J Cereb Blood Flow Metab. 2005;25(10):1280–7. https://doi.org/10.1038/sj.jcbfm.9600135.
7. Britnell SR, Chillari KA, Brown JN. The role of xanthine oxidase inhibitors in patients with history of stroke: a systematic review. Curr Vasc Pharmacol. 2018;16(6):583–8. https://doi.org/10.2174/1570161115666170919183657.
8. Cantarella G, Pignataro G, Di Benedetto G, et al. Ischemic tolerance modulates TRAIL expression and its receptors and generates a neuroprotected phenotype. Cell Death Dis. 2014;5(7):e1331. https://doi.org/10.1038/cddis.2014.286.
9. Chen C, Bivard A, Lin L, et al. Thresholds for infarction vary between gray matter and white matter in acute ischemic stroke: a CT perfusion study. J Cereb Blood Flow Metab. 2019;39(3):536–46. https://doi.org/10.1177/0271678X17744453.
10. Cho J, Jeong S, Lee J. Procalcitonin to C-reactive protein ratio is associated with short-term mortality in ischemic stroke patients: preliminary report. Arch Med Sci. 2020;18(2):344–52. https://doi.org/10.5114/aoms.2020.100207.
11. Crack PJ, Taylor JM. Reactive oxygen species and the modulation of stroke. Free Radic Biol Med. 2005;38(11):1433–44. https://doi.org/10.1016/j.freeradbiomed.2005.01.019.
12. Curcio M, Salazar IL, Mele M, et al. Calpains and neuronal damage in the ischemic brain: the swiss knife in synaptic injury. Prog Neurobiol. 2016;143:1–35. https://doi.org/10.1016/j.pneurobio.2016.06.001.
13. Didion SP, Lynch CM, Baumbach GL, et al. Impaired endothelium-dependent responses and enhanced influence of rho-kinase in cerebral arterioles in type II diabetes. Stroke. 2005;36(2):342–7. https://doi.org/10.1161/01.STR.0000152952.42730.92.
14. Dirnagl U, Iadecola C, Moskowitz MA. Pathobiology of ischaemic stroke: an integrated view. Trends Neurosci. 1999;22(9):391–7. https://doi.org/10.1016/s0166-2236(99)01401-0.
15. Doughan AK, Harrison DG, Dikalov SI. Molecular mechanisms of angiotensin II-mediated mitochondrial dysfunction: linking mitochondrial oxidative damage and vascular endothelial dysfunction. Circ Res. 2008;102(4):488–96. https://doi.org/10.1161/CIRCRESAHA.107.162800.
16. Ermine CM, Bivard A, Parsons MW, et al. The ischemic penumbra: from concept to reality. Int J Stroke. 2021;16(5):497–509. https://doi.org/10.1177/1747493020975229.
17. Feng G, Wu Z, Yang L, et al. Beta-Hydroxybutyrate and ischemic stroke: roles and mechanisms. Mol Brain. 2024;17(1):48. https://doi.org/10.1186/s13041-024-01119-0.
18. Fick A. Ueber die Messung des Blutquantum in den Herzventrikeln. Sb Phys Med Ges Wurzburg. 1870:16–7.
19. Gauthier CJ, Hoge RD. Magnetic resonance imaging of resting OEF and CMRO(2) using a generalized calibration model for hypercapnia and hyperoxia. Neuroimage. 2012;60(2):1212–25. https://doi.org/10.1016/j.neuroimage.2011.12.056.
20. Georgieva JV, Hoekstra D, Zuhorn IS. Smuggling drugs into the brain: an overview of ligands targeting Transcytosis for drug delivery across the blood-brain barrier. Pharmaceutics. 2014;6(4):557–83. https://doi.org/10.3390/pharmaceutics6040557.
21. Girouard H, Park L, Anrather J, et al. Angiotensin II attenuates endothelium-dependent responses in the cerebral microcirculation through nox-2-derived radicals. Arterioscler Thromb Vasc Biol. 2006;26(4):826–32. https://doi.org/10.1161/01.ATV.0000205849.22807.6e.
22. Gong Z, Guo J, Liu B, et al. Mechanisms of immune response and cell death in ischemic stroke and their regulation by natural compounds. Front Immunol. 2024;14:1287857. https://doi.org/10.3389/fimmu.2023.1287857.
23. Hu Y, Dong Y, Wu Y, et al. AMPK inhibitor BML-275 induces neuroprotection through decreasing cyt c and AIF expression after transient brain ischemia. Bioorg Med Chem. 2021;52:116522. https://doi.org/10.1016/j.bmc.2021.116522.
24. Jayaraj RL, Azimullah S, Beiram R, et al. Neuroinflammation: friend and foe for ischemic stroke. J Neuroinflammation. 2019;16(1):142. https://doi.org/10.1186/s12974-019-1516-2.
25. Kang R, Gamdzyk M, Lenahan C, et al. The dual role of microglia in blood-brain barrier dysfunction after stroke. Curr Neuropharmacol. 2020;18(12):1237–49. https://doi.org/10.2174/1570159X18666200529150907.
26. Kety SS, Schmidt CF. The nitrous oxide method for the quantitative determination of cerebral blood flow in man: theory, procedure and Normal values. J Clin Invest. 1948;27(4):476–83. https://doi.org/10.1172/JCI101994.
27. Khatri R, McKinney AM, Swenson B, et al. Blood-brain barrier, reperfusion injury, and hemorrhagic transformation in acute ischemic stroke. Neurology. 2012;79(13 Suppl 1):52. https://doi.org/10.1212/WNL.0b013e3182697e70.
28. Kvistad CE, Logallo N, Oygarden H, et al. Elevated admission blood pressure and stroke severity in acute ischemic stroke: the Bergen NORSTROKE study. Cerebrovasc Dis. 2013;36(5–6):351–4. https://doi.org/10.1159/000355685.
29. Latchaw RE, Yonas H-YH, Hunter GJ, et al. Guidelines and recommendations for perfusion imaging in cerebral ischemia: a scientific statement for healthcare professionals by the writing group on perfusion imaging, from the Council on Cardiovascular Radiology of the American Heart Association. Stroke. 2003;34(4):1084–104. https://doi.org/10.1161/01.STR.0000064840.99271.9E.
30. Leng T, Shi Y, Xiong Z, et al. Proton-sensitive cation channels and ion exchangers in ischemic brain injury: new therapeutic targets for stroke? Prog Neurobiol. 2014;115:189–209. https://doi.org/10.1016/j.pneurobio.2013.12.008.
31. Li R, Zheng Y, Zhang J, et al. Gomisin N attenuated cerebral ischemia-reperfusion injury through inhibition of autophagy by activating the PI3K/AKT/mTOR pathway. Phytomedicine. 2023;110:154644. https://doi.org/10.1016/j.phymed.2023.154644.
32. Liu Y, Qu X, Yan M, et al. Tricin attenuates cerebral ischemia/reperfusion injury through inhibiting nerve cell autophagy, apoptosis and inflammation by regulating the PI3K/Akt pathway. Hum Exp Toxicol. 2022;41:9603271221125928. https://doi.org/10.1177/09603271221125928.
33. Loh Y, Towfighi A, Liebeskind DS, et al. Basal ganglionic infarction before mechanical thrombectomy predicts poor outcome. Stroke. 2009;40(10):3315–20. https://doi.org/10.1161/STROKEAHA.109.551705.

34. Lombardo SM, Schneider M, Tureli AE, et al. Key for crossing the BBB with nanoparticles: the rational design. Beilstein J Nanotechnol. 2020;11:866–83. https://doi.org/10.3762/bjnano.11.72.
35. Maciejczyk M, Nesterowicz M, Zalewska A, et al. Salivary xanthine oxidase as a potential biomarker in stroke diagnostics. Front Immunol. 2022;13:897413. https://doi.org/10.3389/fimmu.2022.897413.
36. Markus HS. Cerebral perfusion and stroke. J Neurol Neurosurg Psychiatry. 2004;75(3):353–61. https://doi.org/10.1136/jnnp.2003.025825.
37. Mathias K, Machado RS, Stork S, et al. Blood-brain barrier permeability in the ischemic stroke: an update. Microvasc Res. 2024;151:104621. https://doi.org/10.1016/j.mvr.2023.104621.
38. Matsumoto T, Kobayashi T, Wachi H, et al. Vascular NAD(P)H oxidase mediates endothelial dysfunction in basilar arteries from Otsuka Long-Evans Tokushima Fatty (OLETF) rats. Atherosclerosis. 2007;192(1):15–24. https://doi.org/10.1016/j.atherosclerosis.2006.06.005.
39. Merali Z, Huang K, Mikulis D, et al. Evolution of blood-brain-barrier permeability after acute ischemic stroke. PLoS One. 2017;12(2):e0171558. https://doi.org/10.1371/journal.pone.0171558.
40. Mo Y, Sun Y, Liu K. Autophagy and inflammation in ischemic stroke. Neural Regen Res. 2020;15(8):1388–96. https://doi.org/10.4103/1673-5374.274331.
41. Montaner J, Molina CA, Monasterio J, et al. Matrix metalloproteinase-9 pretreatment level predicts intracranial hemorrhagic complications after thrombolysis in human stroke. Circulation. 2003;107(4):598–603. https://doi.org/10.1161/01.cir.0000046451.38849.90.
42. Muhammad IF, Borne Y, Melander O, et al. FADD (Fas-associated protein with death domain), Caspase-3, and Caspase-8 and incidence of ischemic stroke. Stroke. 2018;49(9):2224–6. https://doi.org/10.1161/STROKEAHA.118.022063.
43. Muir KW, Weir CJ, Alwan W, et al. C-reactive protein and outcome after ischemic stroke. Stroke. 1999;30(5):981–5. https://doi.org/10.1161/01.str.30.5.981.
44. Nishikawa T, Edelstein D, Du XL, et al. Normalizing mitochondrial superoxide production blocks three pathways of hyperglycaemic damage. Nature. 2000;404(6779):787–90. https://doi.org/10.1038/35008121.
45. Ogren J, Irewall A, Bergstrom L, et al. Intracranial hemorrhage after ischemic stroke: incidence, time trends, and predictors in a Swedish Nationwide cohort of 196 765 patients. Circ Cardiovasc Qual Outcomes. 2015;8(4):413–20. https://doi.org/10.1161/CIRCOUTCOMES.114.001606.
46. Orellana-Urzua S, Rojas I, Libano L, et al. Pathophysiology of ischemic stroke: role of oxidative stress. Curr Pharm Des. 2020;26(34):4246–60. https://doi.org/10.2174/1381612826666200708133912.
47. Pensato U, Demchuk AM, Menon BK, et al. Cerebral infarct growth: pathophysiology, pragmatic assessment, and clinical implications. Stroke. 2024; https://doi.org/10.1161/STROKEAHA.124.049013.
48. Pozzilli C, Lenzi GL, Argentino C, et al. Peripheral white blood cell count in cerebral ischemic infarction. Acta Neurol Scand. 1985;71(5):396–400. https://doi.org/10.1111/j.1600-0404.1985.tb03219.x.
49. Rodgers ZB, Detre JA, Wehrli FW. MRI-based methods for quantification of the cerebral metabolic rate of oxygen. J Cereb Blood Flow Metab. 2016;36(7):1165–85. https://doi.org/10.1177/0271678X16643090.
50. Rolfe DF, Brown GC. Cellular energy utilization and molecular origin of standard metabolic rate in mammals. Physiol Rev. 1997;77(3):731–58. https://doi.org/10.1152/physrev.1997.77.3.731.
51. Safar P. Resuscitation from clinical death: pathophysiologic limits and therapeutic potentials. Crit Care Med. 1988;16(10):923–41. https://doi.org/10.1097/00003246-198810000-00003.
52. Sarvari S, Moakedi F, Hone E, et al. Mechanisms in blood-brain barrier opening and metabolism-challenged cerebrovascular ischemia with emphasis on ischemic stroke. Metab Brain Dis. 2020;35(6):851–68. https://doi.org/10.1007/s11011-020-00573-8.
53. Scheinberg P. Survival of the ischemic brain: a progress report. Circulation. 1979;60(7):1600–5. https://doi.org/10.1161/01.cir.60.7.1600.
54. Semplicini A, Maresca A, Boscolo G, et al. Hypertension in acute ischemic stroke: a compensatory mechanism or an additional damaging factor? Arch Intern Med. 2003;163(2):211–6. https://doi.org/10.1001/archinte.163.2.211.
55. Sorescu D, Weiss D, Lassegue B, et al. Superoxide production and expression of nox family proteins in human atherosclerosis. Circulation. 2002;105(12):1429–35. https://doi.org/10.1161/01.cir.0000012917.74432.66.
56. Spronk E, Sykes G, Falcione S, et al. Hemorrhagic transformation in ischemic stroke and the role of inflammation. Front Neurol. 2021;12:661955. https://doi.org/10.3389/fneur.2021.661955.
57. Stamatovic SM, Johnson AM, Keep RF, et al. Junctional proteins of the blood-brain barrier: new insights into function and dysfunction. Tissue Barriers. 2016;4(1):e1154641. https://doi.org/10.1080/21688370.2016.1154641.
58. Stephenson D, Yin T, Smalstig EB, et al. Transcription factor nuclear factor-kappa B is activated in neurons after focal cerebral ischemia. J Cereb Blood Flow Metab. 2000;20(3):592–603. https://doi.org/10.1097/00004647-200003000-00017.
59. Sun M, Jin H, Sun X, et al. Free radical damage in ischemia-reperfusion injury: an obstacle in acute ischemic stroke after revascularization therapy. Oxid Med Cell Longev. 2018;2018:3804979. https://doi.org/10.1155/2018/3804979.
60. Sweeney MD, Zhao Z, Montagne A, et al. Blood-brain barrier: from physiology to disease and back. Physiol Rev. 2019;99(1):21–78. https://doi.org/10.1152/physrev.00050.2017.
61. Tajes M, Ramos-Fernandez E, Weng-Jiang X, et al. The blood-brain barrier: structure, function and therapeutic approaches to cross it. Mol Membr Biol. 2014;31(5):152–67. https://doi.org/10.3109/09687688.2014.937468.
62. Vila N, Filella X, Deulofeu R, et al. Cytokine-induced inflammation and long-term stroke functional outcome. J Neurol Sci. 1999;162(2):185–8. https://doi.org/10.1016/s0022-510x(98)00319-0.
63. Wimmer I, Zrzavy T, Lassmann H. Neuroinflammatory responses in experimental and human stroke lesions. J Neuroimmunol. 2018;323:10–8. https://doi.org/10.1016/j.jneuroim.2018.07.003.

Basic Anatomy of Cerebral Vessels

Igor L. Maldonado, Etienne Dugast, and Christophe Destrieux

1 The Cerebral Arteries

Cerebrovascular anatomy is of great importance to neurologists, neuroradiologists, and neurosurgeons, as the vascular system plays a critical role in maintaining brain function. A thorough understanding enables practitioners to detect abnormalities in cerebral blood supply, recognize possible individual variations, and identify alternative circulatory routes in case of vascular insufficiency. Furthermore, understanding anatomy is crucial for planning open and endovascular neurosurgical procedures, minimizing risks, and preventing complications.

Digital subtraction angiography (DSA), magnetic resonance, and computerized tomography angiography are the primary examination modalities for visualization of cerebral vasculature. Among these, DSA remains the golden standard due to its high level of detail and diagnostic accuracy. Given the complexity of cerebrovascular structures, practitioners must meticulously analyze imaging results to ensure precise interpretation and clinical decision-making.

The brain's arterial supply is maintained by two major systems: the anterior or carotid system and the posterior or vertebrobasilar system (Fig. 1). They are interconnected by the arterial circle of the brain, commonly known as the circle of Willis. This chapter will explore the key components of these systems.

1.1 The Internal Carotid Artery

The cervical portion of the internal carotid artery (ICA) exhibits distinct characteristics that vary with age. In young, healthy individuals, it typically assumes a posterior position relative to the external carotid artery and displays a slight lateral inclination to enter the carotid canal. In lateral imaging, the ICA is easily distinguishable from the external carotid artery thanks to its relative position and the absence of branches. As a rare variant, the ICA may present a thin cervical branch (an ascending pharyngeal artery).

The ICA may elongate and undergo changes in diameter with aging, often resulting in curves, kinks, or loops. In elderly patients, a coronal view is frequently more appropriate to expose the bifurcation. Another key feature of the ICA is the carotid sinus or carotid bulb, the region where the lumen appears enlarged compared to the more distal ICA. This area is a major baroreceptor site and is a common location for atherosclerotic stenosis.

The portion of the cervical ICA located near the parapharyngeal space — a deep region in the neck adjacent to the pharynx — is referred to as the parapharyngeal ICA, with the exact extent of its relationship to this space varying based on individual anatomy and age. This portion is part of the extracranial course of the ICA before it enters the carotid canal (in the petrous part of the temporal bone).

Within the skull, the ICA is divided into multiple segments based on its curves and relative positions. These segments have been classified using various systems, the most widely recognized being those proposed by Fischer, Gibo, and Bouthillier (Figs. 2 and 3) [1–3]. Due to discrepancies among these classification systems, it is essential for practitioners to specify which system they are adopting to ensure accurate communication [4].

The portion of the ICA in the carotid canal is known as the petrous segment. From this segment, tiny branches emerge, including the mandibulovidian, tympanic, or stapedial arteries. These branches are often challenging to

I. L. Maldonado (✉) · E. Dugast · C. Destrieux
Laboratoire d'Anatomie, Faculté de Médecine de Tours, Tours, France

Université de Tours, INSERM, Imaging Brain & Neuropsychiatry iBraiN U1253, Tours, France

CHRU de Tours, Tours, France
e-mail: maldonado@univ-tours.fr; destrieux@univ-tours.fr

V. Beneš, D. Netuka (eds.), *Surgical and Interventional Treatment of Cerebral Ischemia*,
https://doi.org/10.1007/978-3-032-08934-2_4

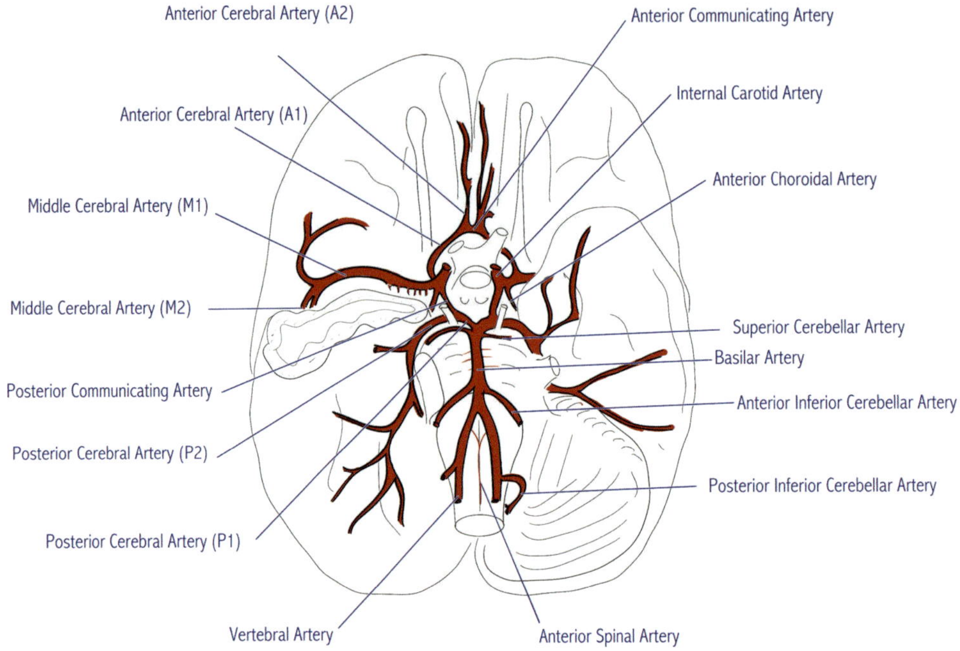

Fig. 1 Basic anatomy of the arteries of the human brain, antero-inferior perspective. Two interconnected systems supply blood to the brain: an anterior carotid system and a posterior vertebro-basilar system

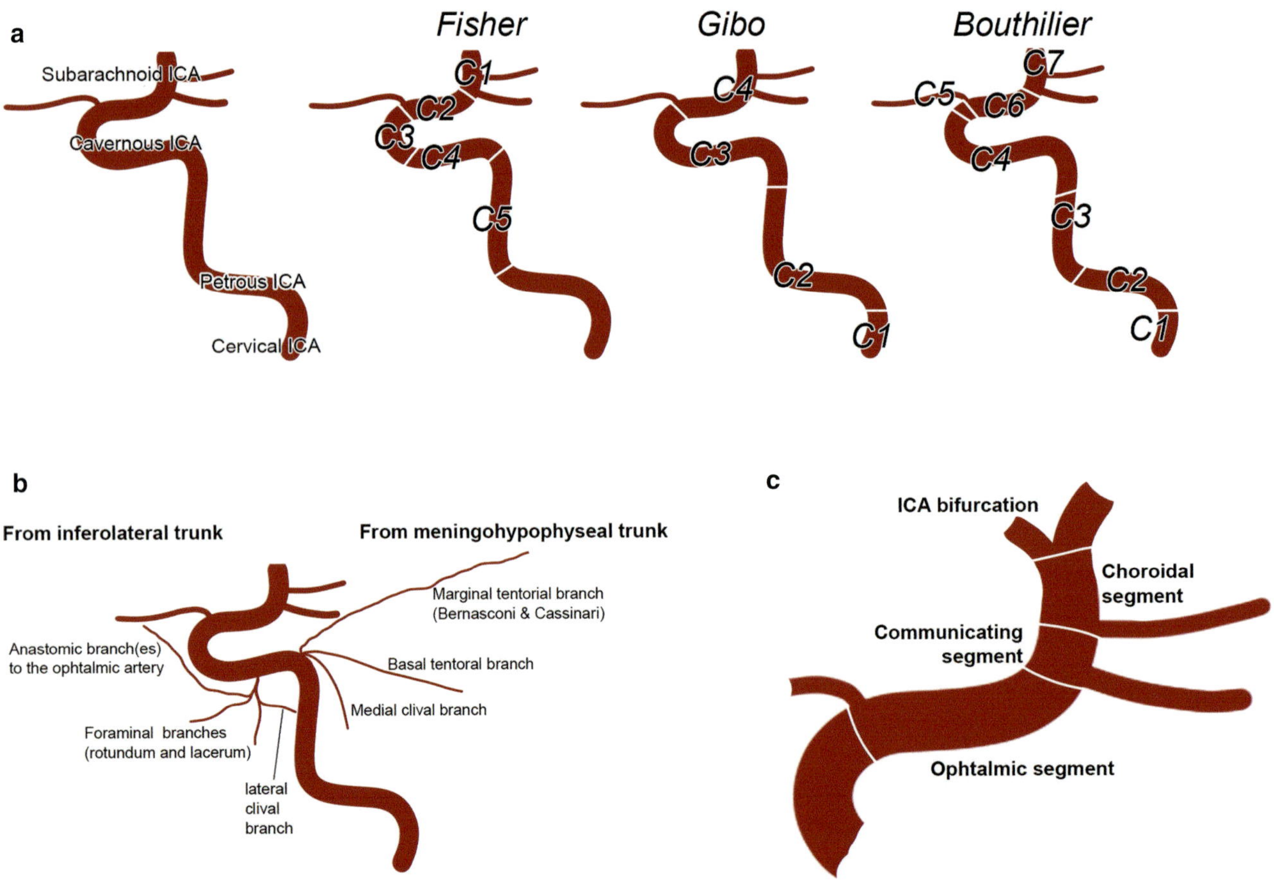

Fig. 2 Internal carotid artery segments, main classification systems. (**a**) Common terminology and correspondence among different numbering systems. (**b**) Intracavernous branches. (**c**) Subarachnoid segments (According to Rhoton et al.). (Reproduced with permission from Maldonado IL. A practical guide to cerebrovascular anatomy. In: Kanaan IN, Beneš V, éditeurs. Neuroanatomy Guidance to Successful Neurosurgical Interventions. Springer Nature Switzerland; 2024. p. 47–57)

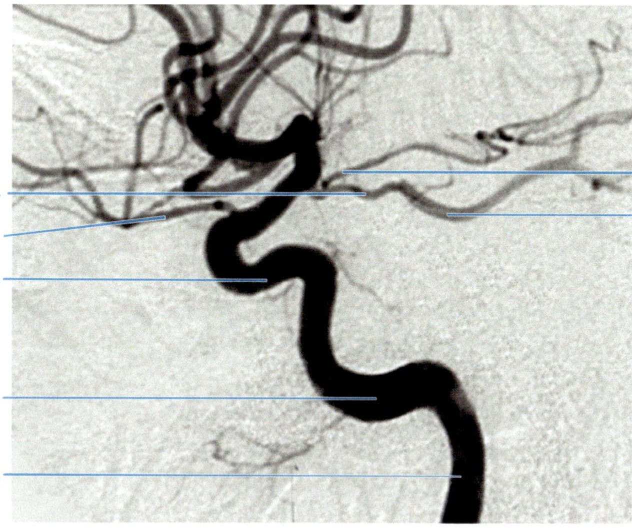

Fig. 3 Internal carotid artery, angiographic aspect. (Reproduced with permission from Maldonado IL. A practical guide to cerebrovascular anatomy. In: Kanaan IN, Beneš V, éditeurs. Neuroanatomy Guidance to Successful Neurosurgical Interventions. Springer Nature Switzerland; 2024. p. 47–57. A lateral view. Please refer to the main text for description)

visualize due to their very small size and variable presence. Some authors have also proposed the term cochlear carotid to denote the initial ascending portion of the ICA in the temporal bone, highlighting the proximity of the artery to the cochlea [5]. The lacerum or pre-cavernous segment follows the petrous segment.

The ICA undergoes two curves within the cavernous sinus, forming the carotid siphon before emerging in the subarachnoid space. The term Gasserian-Clival ICA has been proposed to refer to the initial ascending portion of the ICA within the cavernous sinus (starting at the petrolingual ligament), given its proximity to the lateral border of the clivus (posteriorly) and the Gasserian ganglion (laterally). Similarly, the term sellar carotid has also been proposed by some authors to denote the horizontal portion of this segment, emphasizing the proximity of the ICA to the sella turcica.

The cavernous ICA gives rise to small branches that supply the skull base dura mater, tentorium, cranial nerve foramina, and pituitary gland [6]. These intracavernous branches typically originate from two common trunks: the meningohypophyseal trunk and the inferolateral trunk.

The meningohypophyseal trunk gives rise to branches that supply the dura of the clivus (medial clival branch) and the tentorium. A long branch, the basal tentorial artery, runs along the petrous attachment of the tentorium, while another, the marginal tentorial artery (also known as the artery of Bernasconi and Cassinari), follows the free border of the tentorium. The marginal tentorial artery typically has a wavy appearance along a slight ascendant trajectory. While it may resemble the basal tentorial artery in lateral views, it can be better distinguished in front views, where it outlines the free edge of the tentorium. The inferior hypophyseal artery originates directly from the cavernous ICA or as a branch of the meningohypophyseal trunk [7].

The inferolateral trunk typically gives rise to branches supplying the dura-mater of the clivus, as well as foramina rotundum and lacerum. Its distal branches frequently anastomose with the ophthalmic artery. Less commonly, the marginal tentorial branch arises from the inferolateral trunk instead of the meningohypophiseal trunk. These vessels are typically difficult to visualize but may become prominent under increased flow conditions, such as in skull base tumors, arteriovenous malformations, or fistulas.

The ophthalmic artery is often considered a landmark to denote the superior boundary of the cavernous sinus. This may not be entirely accurate, as the origin of the ophthalmic artery is variable and may be intracavernous [8, 9]. Additionally, the carotid cave, a small extension of the subarachnoid space along the medial aspect of the ICA, should be carefully considered during anatomical assessment.

The central artery of the retina plays a critical role in ocular perfusion. During digital subtraction angiography (DSA), a choroidal blush is often observed in the later phases of contrast passage. Before performing embolization procedures involving the ophthalmic vascular territory, it is essential to confirm the origin of the choroidal blush. This requires selective catheterization of both the internal and external carotid arteries. Such precautions are particularly important due to the frequent presence of anastomoses through the angular branch at the medial canthus of the eye.

The clinoidal segment is a short transitional portion of the ICA that connects the cavernous ICA to its supraclinoidal portions. It is named after its proximity to the anterior clinoidal process, which lies closely against the lateral wall of the artery. This segment is located just before the typical origin of the ophthalmic artery and the superior hypophyseal artery. The term paraclinoid ICA refers to the portions of the ICA located adjacent to the clinoid process, specifically distal to the proximal dural ring and proximal to the posterior communicating artery (PComA). This term includes both the clinoidal and ophthalmic segments of the ICA.

The supraclinoidal segment of the ICA refers to the portion of the ICA located just distal to the clinoidal segment. The supraclinoidal ICA travels through the subarachnoid space and is traditionally divided into four segments: ophthalmic, communicating, choroidal, and carotid termination. The ophthalmic segment extends from the proximal origin of the ophthalmic artery to the proximal border of the ostium of the PComA. The communicating segment spans from the PComA to the proximal border of the ostium of the anterior choroidal artery, while the choroidal segment runs from the anterior choroidal artery to the carotid termination zone. No landmark marks the distal end of the choroidal segment. While the first three segments are more readily identifiable in lateral-view angiograms, providing crucial landmarks for vascular assessment and interventional planning, the carotid bifurcation in anterior and middle cerebral arteries is best depicted in frontal-view.

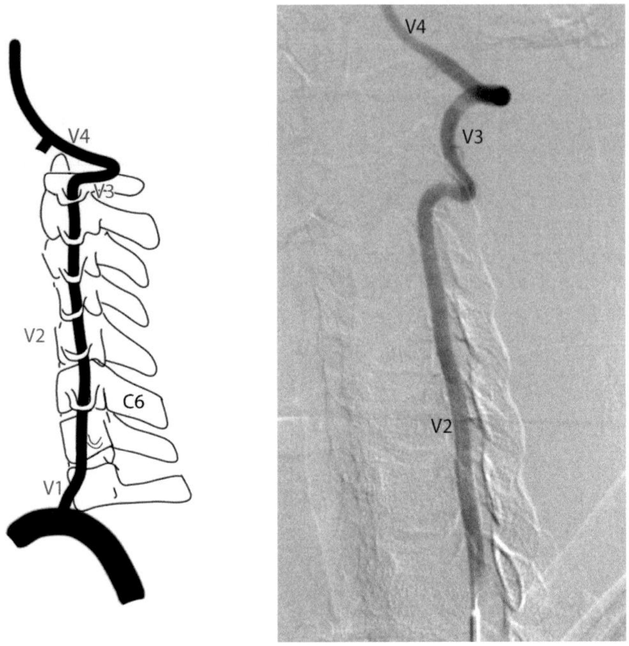

Fig. 4 Vertebral artery segments according to their appearance on digital subtraction angiography. The vertebral artery is divided into four segments: V1 (pre-foraminal segment) extends from its origin at the subclavian artery to the transverse foramen of C6, V2 (foraminal segment) passes through the transverse foramen of C6 to C2, V3 (atlantic or extradural segment) extends from C2 to the dura mater after looping around the atlas, and V4 (intradural or intracranial segment) runs from the dura mater entry to the formation of the basilar artery at the pontomedullary junction

1.2 Vertebral Artery

The vertebral arteries are branches of the subclavian artery and play an essential role in irrigating the central nervous system. They ascend through the transverse foramina of the cervical vertebrae, generally from C6 to C1, before piercing the atlantooccipital membrane and entering the cranial cavity through the foramen magnum. The anterior and posterior spinal arteries, and the posterior inferior cerebellar arteries (PICA) emerge before the vertebral arteries converge to form the basilar artery.

The vertebral artery is divided into four segments (Fig. 4): V1 (pre-foraminal) extends from its origin at the subclavian artery to the transverse foramen of C6, V2 (foraminal) passes through the transverse foramina of C6 to C2, V3 (atlantic or extradural) extends from C2 to the dura mater after looping around the atlas, and V4 (intradural or intracranial) runs from the dura mater entry to the formation of the basilar artery at the pontomedullary junction.

The cervical branches of the vertebral arteries play an essential role in the arterial supply of structures in the cervical region, including muscles and bones. These muscular branches are a source of (often insufficient) collateral circulation in cases of chronic obstructive disease. A posterior meningeal artery may rarely arise from the vertebral artery's intracranial segment, near its dural penetration at the foramen magnum, and ascend with a wavy course supplying the dura mater of the posterior cranial fossa. This variant is, however, less common than an origin from the ascending pharyngeal artery.

Within the cranial cavity, the vertebral arteries run along the anterior surface of the medulla, give origin to the posterior inferior cerebellar artery (PICA), and converge at the lower edge of the bridge to form the basilar artery. A phenomenon of vertebral dominance is sometimes observed, characterized by asymmetry in diameter and blood flow between the vertebral arteries. The larger vertebral artery will provide most of the arterial supply to the posterior circulation and be responsible for significant contrast medium washing phenomena during DSA when the contralateral vertebral artery is injected.

A dominant left vertebral artery is more frequent than a right dominant one. In extreme situations, the non-dominant artery (usually the right one) is continuous with the PICA, and only a tiny connection with the contralateral vertebral artery persists. These variants have significant clinical implications, especially in arterial stenosis or dissection cases, where a compromised dominant artery can lead to more severe ischemic deficits in the vertebrobasilar territory.

Proximal variants are persistent carotid-vertebrobasilar anastomoses as a remnant from embryonic development. During carotid opacification in DSA, a persistent trigeminal artery produces opacification of both the ICA and the superior third of the basilar ramification tree, including the entire posterior cerebral artery. Other rare remnants are the otic, hypoglossal, and proatlantal arteries [10].

1.3 External Carotid Artery

Despite its primary function being the irrigation of extracranial structures, the external carotid artery plays a crucial role in the development of routes for collateral circulation. When a significant stenosis concerns the ICA, the external carotid artery may provide some compensatory supply through anastomoses with intracranial territory and attenuate neurological deficits in chronic cerebrovascular disease. A typical site is the angular artery, a terminal branch of the facial artery that connects with the dorsal branch of the ophthalmic artery near the medial canthus, allowing blood flow to be inverted in the ophthalmic artery and redirected to brain structures.

The facial, ascending pharyngeal, and maxillary arteries stand out among the branches of the external carotid artery that participate in intra-extracranial anastomoses. A detailed description of these connections is out of the scope of this chapter.

1.4 Anterior Choroidal Artery

The anterior choroidal artery (AChA) is a branch of the internal carotid artery and plays a crucial role in irrigating deep structures of the brain. It originates distal to the junction of the internal carotid artery with the posterior communicating artery and follows a posterolateral and slight ascending course towards the inferior horn of the lateral ventricle. During its course, it gives off branches to important brain formations, including the optic tract, the globus pallidus, the internal capsule, and the spinothalamic tract.

This artery has strategic vascularization, supplying critical functional areas, such as the posterior limb of the internal capsule, where corticospinal motor fibers pass. Obstructions in the anterior choroidal artery can cause severe neurological syndromes, including contralateral hemiparesis, sensory deficits, and visual disturbances despite a relatively small volume of ischemic tissue. Its detailed recognition is essential in neurosurgical interventions and neurovascular procedures, especially in approaching deep tumors and skull base surgery.

The anterior choroidal artery exhibits significant variability in its course and distribution. In some circumstances, it can anastomose with branches of the middle cerebral artery or one of the posterior choroidal arteries.

1.5 Anterior Cerebral Artery

The anterior cerebral artery (ACA) is one of the major arteries supplying the medial aspect of the cerebral hemisphere, particularly the frontal and parietal lobes (Fig. 5). It plays a crucial role in perfusing structures involved in sensorymotor functions and also cognitive and limbic processes. The anterior cerebral artery is subdivided into five segments in the direction of the blood flow (Fig. 6): A1 or pre-communicating, A2 or post-communicating (infracallosal), A3 or precallosal (around the genu of the corpus callosum), A4 callosomarginal (supracallosal), and A5 or the terminal segment. The bifurcation in the pericallosal and callosomarginal branches is usually in the A3 segment. The terminal distal branch of the anterior cerebral artery—the posterior pericallosal artery –often anastomoses with a distal branch of the posterior cerebral artery.

Few perforators originate near the communicating artery and may be destined for the fornix, septal area, anterior cingulate gyrus, and corpus callosum. The anterior cerebral artery contributes with medial lenticulostriate branches, one of which is particularly long and recurrent and penetrates the anterior perforated substance irrigating basal nuclei, especially the head of caudate: the long striate artery (also known as recurrent artery of Heubner). This artery is a branch of the A2 segment in most cases.

In the medial aspect of the cerebral hemisphere, the pericallosal artery courses along or close to the sulcus of the corpus callosum, while the callosomarginal artery reaches the cingulate sulcus. One of its branches crosses the precuneus, while a more anterior one penetrates the marginal branch of the cingulate sulcus. The paracentral lobule is located above the cingulate sulcus, anterior to the marginal branch, and posterior to the paracentral branch of the cingulate sulcus. The superior extremity of the central sulcus is located in the superior and posterior portion of the paracentral lobule and contains the central branch of the middle cerebral artery. Notably, the paracentral lobule contains the contralateral lower limb's somatotopic motor and sensory maps.

1.6 Anterior Communicating Artery

The anterior communicating artery (AComA) is a crucial component of the cerebral arterial circle (Circle of Willis), connecting the left and right anterior cerebral arteries (ACA). This small yet functionally significant artery enables collateral circulation between the two hemispheres, ensuring adequate blood supply in cases of vascular compromise, such as internal carotid artery occlusion. Perforators that arise directly from the AComA are usually very small. Part of the arterial supply of the optic chiasma is derived, however, from delicate AComA branches directed posteriorly and inferiorly. The anterior communicating artery is a common site for intracranial aneurysms, which account for a significant proportion of subarachnoid hemorrhages.

Variants of the anterior communicating complex are frequent, with varying diameters of the anterior communicating artery and asymmetric pre-communicating (A1)

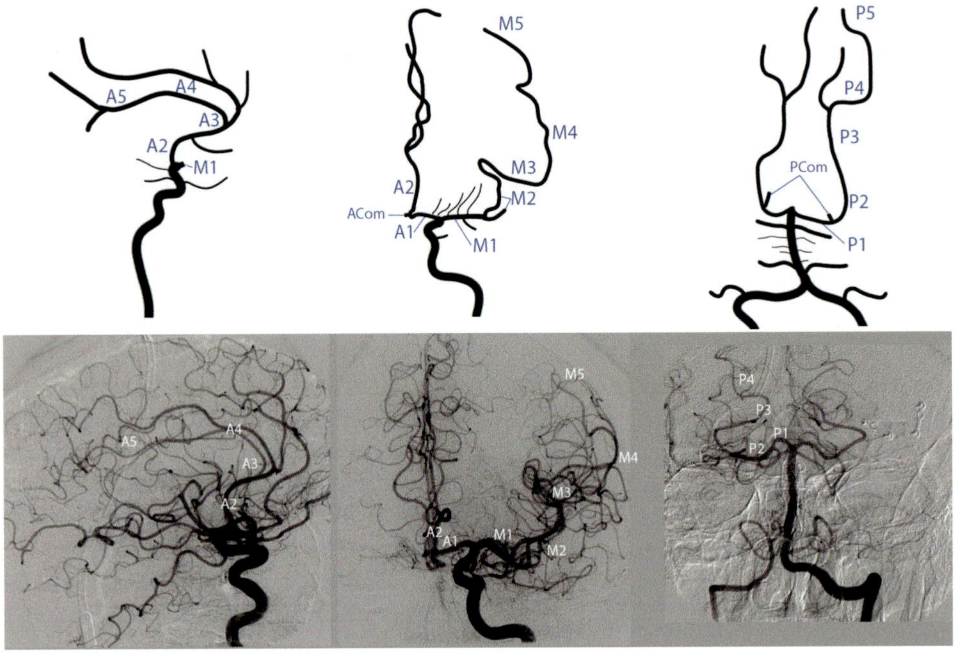

Fig. 5 Segments of the anterior, middle, and posterior cerebral arteries, according to their appearance on digital subtraction angiography. The anterior cerebral artery is subdivided into five segments: A1 (pre-communicating), A2 (post-communicating/infracallosal), A3 (precallosal, around the genu of the corpus callosum), A4 (supracallosal), and A5 (terminal) segments. The middle cerebral artery consists of M1 (horizontal/sphenoidal), M2 (insular), M3 (opercular), M4 (cortical), and M5 (terminal) segments. The posterior cerebral artery is divided into P1 (pre-communicating), P2 (post-communicating), further classified into P2A (peduncular/crural) and P2P (ambient), P3 (quadrigeminal), and P4 (cortical/terminal/calcarine). These classifications are crucial for understanding cerebrovascular anatomy, aiding in neuroimaging interpretation, surgical planning, and stroke management

Fig. 6 Main vascular territories of the human cerebral hemisphere in axial and coronal views. According to the classical anatomical works of Testut and Latarjet (1899) [15]

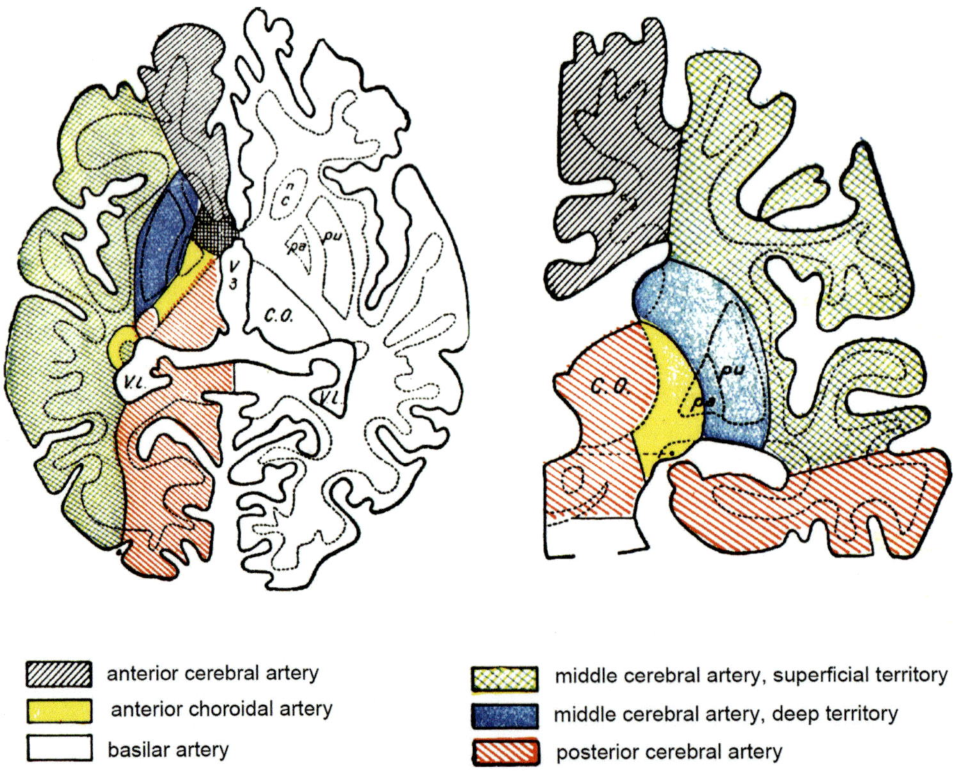

segments, leading to a dominance phenomenon where the flow from one of the ICAs fills both A2 segments [11]. Surgical or endovascular disconnection of the anterior communicating artery is reserved for cases where both A1 segments are functional without significant hypoplasia or asymmetry. Azygos A2 and duplications of certain elements are not uncommon. The so-called Wilder's thermal artery appears as a third post-communicating segment from the anterior communicating artery. Interestingly, it is often directed to the paracentral lobule.

1.7 Middle Cerebral Artery

The middle cerebral artery (MCA) irrigates the lateral aspects of the frontal, temporal, and parietal lobes, including the primary motor and sensory cortices for the face and upper limbs, as well as key language areas (Broca's and Wernicke's in the dominant hemisphere). The middle cerebral artery is subdivided into segments, as follows: M1 (horizontal or sphenoidal portion), M2 (insular), M3 (opercular), M4 (cortical), and M5 (terminal) branches. The curves of the middle cerebral artery serve as useful anatomical landmarks, with the transition from M1 to M2 indicating the location of the limen insulae.

On the superior aspect of the M1, lateral lenticulostriate arteries emerge and penetrate the anterior perforated space behind the olfactory stria. In open surgery, the olfactory tract is a valuable landmark that can be followed until the carotid bifurcation. Classically, the right lenticulostriate arteries assume an S-shape and the left have an inverted S-shape. The lenticulostriate arteries are bounded by neighboring structures such as the optic pathways medially and part of the uncus laterally.

In angiograms, the M2 branches frame the cortex of the insula laterally. Vascular deflections in the circular sulcus of the insula identify the boundaries of the insula and are visible in both front and lateral views. In lateral view, these deflections draw the so-called "Sylvian triangle.". The sides of the triangle correspond roughly to the insula's superior, anterior, and inferior limiting sulcus. The so-called posterior Sylvian point corresponds to the posterior-most deflection, covered by the supramarginal gyrus. The posteromedial extremity of the most posterior of the transverse temporal gyri points to that region.

The M3 and M4 branches contour the frontoparietal and temporal opercular parts. Then the cortical branches receive the names of the regions they irrigate: orbitofrontal, prefrontal, precentral, central, anterior and posterior parietal, angular (generally form the inferior division), temporo-occipital, posterior middle, anterior temporal, and temporopolar. Typically, distal cortical branches provide pial anastomoses between the territories of the anterior and middle cerebral arteries.

Importantly, the angular branch of the middle cerebral artery follows the general direction of the lateral sulcus, crosses the supramarginal gyrus, and reaches the angular gyrus. It is usually a relatively large branch that deals with higher functions, such as language circuits and visuospatial integration mechanisms, respectively, in most individuals' left and right hemispheres. The three or four middle cerebral artery branches above and anterior to it are also destined to eloquent cortex, including primary motor and sensory cortices.

Given the disposition of the cortical and projection fiber somatotopy, middle cerebral artery infarctions are classically associated with disproportionate hemiparesis with brachial predominance and different degrees of language disturbance. Lesion to the inferior parietal lobule has been associated with visuospatial integration difficulties and hemineglect, especially in the non-dominant hemisphere. One or two branches are destined to the Wenicke's area in the posterosuperior portion of the temporal lobe. More anterior temporal infarctions may spare the Wernicke's area, but due to the presence of optical radiations, they may be associated with visual field defects of the superior contralateral quadrant.

1.8 Basilar Artery

The basilar artery is a fundamental vessel of the posterior circulation, formed by the union of the left and right vertebral arteries at the level of the pontomedullary junction. It courses along the ventral aspect of the pons, giving rise to several critical branches that supply the brainstem, cerebellum, and posterior cerebral structures. Among its major branches are the anterior inferior cerebellar arteries (AICA), the superior cerebellar arteries (SCA), and the posterior cerebral arteries (PCA), which collectively ensure perfusion to vital neural structures, including the thalamus, midbrain, and occipital lobes.

The basilar artery is crucial for maintaining brainstem function. Its branches provide perfusion to essential nuclei controlling respiration, cardiovascular regulation, and consciousness. Basilar artery occlusion is a life-threatening condition that can lead to catastrophic neurological deficits. Early recognition and intervention through thrombolysis or mechanical thrombectomy are critical for improving outcomes in such cases. In elderly individuals, the artery may exhibit a dolichoectatic course characterized by elongation and widening, which increases the risk of compressive symptoms, ischemia, or aneurysm formation.

The basilar artery gives rise to several perforating branches supplying the brainstem and adjacent structures.

Paramedian, short circumferential, and long circumferential perforators penetrate the pontine parenchyma, providing critical blood flow to the corticospinal tracts, cranial nerve nuclei, and reticular formation. The paramedian perforators originate from the midline and supply the medial pons, while the short and long circumferential arteries perfuse the lateral pons and part of the superior cerebellum. Advanced imaging techniques, including high-resolution magnetic resonance imaging, have improved the visualization of these perforators, aiding in diagnosing and managing cerebrovascular diseases affecting the brainstem.

1.9 Posterior Cerebral Artery

The posterior cerebral artery (PCA) is a critical vessel supplying blood to the occipital lobe, the inferior part of the temporal lobe, and various deep structures of the brain. Its anatomy is an important consideration in neurovascular procedures and imaging. Four segments of the PCA are usually described: P1 (pre-communicating), P2 (post-communicating), P3 (quadrigeminal), and P4 (cortical/terminal, calcarine). The P2 segment can be subdivided into an anterior portion, namely P2A (peduncular or crural), and a posterior portion, P2P (ambient).

The pre-communicating P1 segment relates to the interpeduncular fossa. Its perforators penetrate the posterior perforated space between the two cerebral peduncles, many of which are thalamoperforators. Sometimes, a thalamic artery originates exclusively or predominantly on one side, the so-called Percheron's artery [12]. The P1 segment is related inferiorly to the third nerve, which emerges above the superior cerebellar artery.

Among the cortical branches of the PCA are the perisplenial, parietooccipital, calcarine arteries, and two or more temporal branches. The periesplenial artery non-rarely continues as a posterior pericallosal artery and provides a site of anastomosis with the ACA territory. In this situation, the operator may have the position of the splenius visualizable in a lateral angiographic view.

One horizontal branch enters the calcarine fissure (the calcarine artery) and a postero-superior one enters the parietal occipital sulcus (the parieto-occipital artery). The lingula, forming the inferior lip of the calcarine fissure, and the boundaries of the cuneus and precuneus are also recognizable thanks to this ramification pattern in a lateral view angiogram. A medial (more proximal) and a lateral (more distal) posterior choroidal artery arise from the P2 segment of the PCA in most cases. Less frequently, the medial posterior choroidal artery (MPChA) can sometimes originate from the P1 segment.

Anatomical variations are frequent. Some cases show a dominant flow from the ICA, while others show a dominant flow from the vertebrobasilar system. In this case, better opacification of the PComA and poor opacification of the P2 segment will be seen on DSA when the contrast medium is injected in the ICA, demonstrating the presence of a functional P1 segment.

More evident asymmetry comes from PComA unilateral hypoplasia, P1 hypoplasia, or fetal variant. In the fetal variant, the PCA originates from the posterior aspect of the intracranial ICA, and the P1 is very hypoplasic (or absent). The PComA may also be associated with an infundibular formation (enlarged origin, non-rarely seen at the origin of the anterior choroidal artery).

1.10 Posterior Communicating Artery

The posterior communicating artery (PComA) is an important link between the internal carotid artery and the posterior cerebral artery, contributing to the cerebral circle of the brain (Fig. 7) and serving as a key pathway for collateral

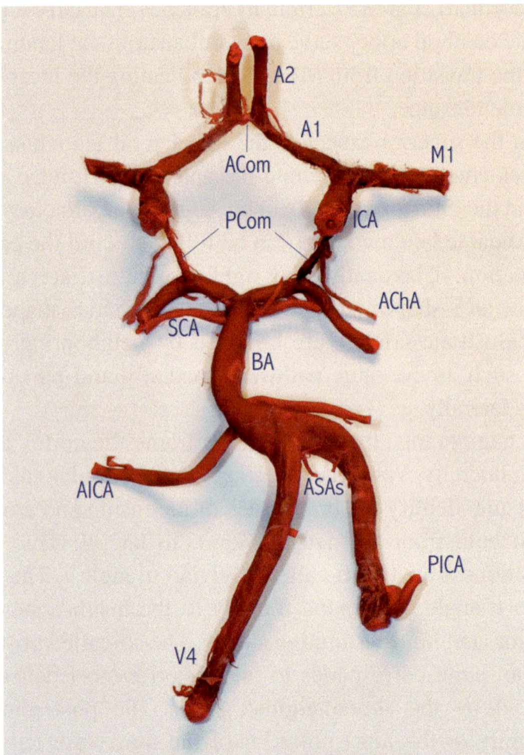

Fig. 7 Arterial circle of the brain (Willis' polygon and afferents). Acrylic injection of a real specimen. AChA, anterior choroidal artery; ACom, anterior communicating artery; AICA, anterior inferior posterior cerebellar artery; ASAs, anterior spinal artery (origins); A1, pre-communicating anterior cerebral artery; A2 post-communicating anterior cerebral artery; BA, basilar artery; M1 horizontal (sphenoidal) middle cerebral artery; M2 insular middle cerebral artery; P1, pre-communicating posterior cerebral artery, P2 post-communicating posterior cerebral artery; PCom, posterior communicating artery, PICA, posterior inferior cerebellar artery; SCA, superior cerebellar artery

circulation. The posterior communicating artery displays a distinct change in direction and diameter as it approaches the posterior cerebral artery on angiograms. The posterior communicating artery gives rise to several small but clinically significant perforators. These arteries penetrate the posterior perforated substance and supply deep structures, including part of the hypothalamus, anterior thalamus, subthalamic region, and portions of the internal capsule. The tuberothalamic (aka premamillary) artery is often the most prominent, supplying the anterior part of the thalamus and the mammillary bodies.

The vascular supply from the PComA perforators meets the territory of the anterior choroidal artery and thalamoperforators from the P1 segment, creating potential local anastomotic networks. Variations in the number and distribution of these perforators can influence stroke patterns, particularly in cases of PComA hypoplasia or occlusion. Their small caliber and deep penetration make them vulnerable to ischemia during aneurysm clipping or other neurosurgical interventions near the PComA. The posterior communicating artery is a frequent site for aneurysm formation, particularly at its junction with the internal carotid artery. Given its involvement in normal and pathological cerebral circulation, the PComA is of great interest in vascular neurology, neurovascular surgery, and endovascular treatment planning.

2 Overview of Cerebral Veins

The cerebral venous anatomy plays a crucial role in maintaining adequate cerebral perfusion, ensuring efficient removal of metabolic wastes and regulating intracranial pressure. Unlike the arterial circulation, the cerebral venous system is highly variable and lacks valves, making it particularly susceptible to pathologies such as cerebral venous thrombosis, venous infarction and disturbances in cerebrospinal fluid dynamics. In the context of ischaemic stroke, understanding venous drainage is essential for optimising perfusion strategies, interpreting imaging findings and identifying secondary complications such as venous stasis or haemorrhagic transformation.

The cerebral venous system (Fig. 8) comprises a superficial and a deep system [13, 14]. They all ultimately drain into dural sinuses and the internal jugular vein, and present with considerable inter-individual morphological variability.

The superficial cerebral veins are found mainly on the outer surface of the brain's hemispheres and are responsible for draining blood from the cortex. They are generally grouped into three categories based on their position relative to the lateral sulcus: superior, middle (superficial sylvian), and inferior superficial veins. Most superior veins are located above the lateral sulcus and include the prefrontal, frontal, parietal, and occipital veins. They drain into the superior sagittal sinus (mostly) or to the transverse sinus. The superficial middle cerebral vein runs along the lateral sulcus. It may have a plexiform appearance. It usually drains forward into the sphenoparietal sinus, which connects to the cavernous sinus, or posteriorly directly into the transverse sinus. The veins of the inferior group are relatively thin and vary in number. A group of uncal veins, found on the inner side of the temporal lobe, drain into the basal vein, while veins on the ventral aspect of the temporal lobe drain into the cavernous sinus, the basal vein, or the transverse sinus. Two important superficial anastomotic veins interconnect venous territories: the superior anastomotic vein (vein of Trolard) running upward from the middle cerebral vein to the superior sagittal sinus, and the inferior anastomotic vein (vein of Labbé) running downward from the middle cerebral vein to the transverse sinus. These anastomotic veins play a key role in balancing venous drainage across different parts of the brain.

The basal veins (of Rosenthal) drain into the deep system (vein of Galen). Each basal vein originates below the anterior perforated substance, where three primary tributaries converge: the anterior cerebral vein (draining blood from the medial frontal lobe, anterior cingulum, and anterior part of the corpus callosum), the olfactory vein (on the inferior surface of the frontal lobe), and the deep middle cerebral vein

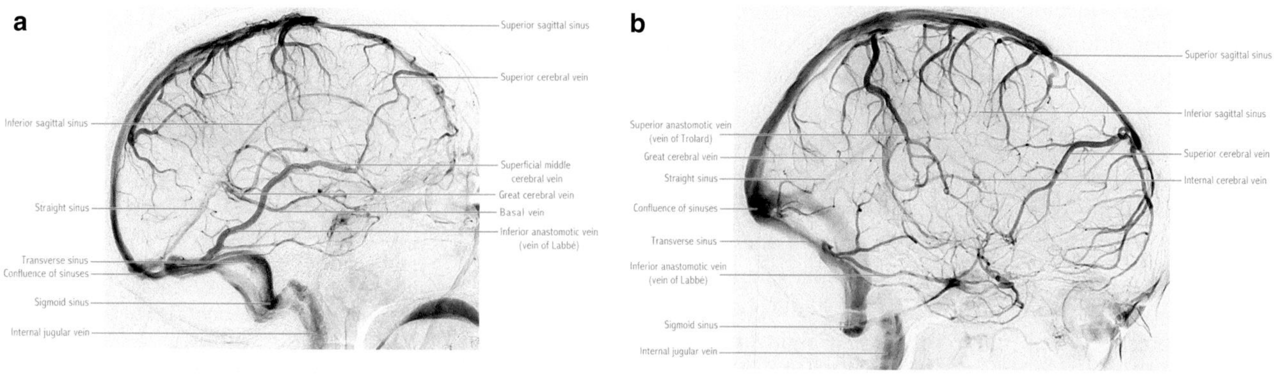

Fig. 8 Cerebral venous anatomy on lateral view digital subtraction angiography (DSA). Key venous structures are labeled. See text for details

(emerging from the insular region near the limen insulae). From their origin, each basal vein courses posteriorly, gradually increasing in size along its pre-peduncular, latero-peduncular, and terminal portions. Ultimately, the basal vein drains into the great cerebral vein and receives several tributaries along its pathway. These tributaries are variable but typically include inferior thalamostriate veins, uncal, inferior ventricular, inferior choroidal, peduncular, and medial and lateral mesencephalic veins.

The two internal cerebral veins each originate at the level of the interventricular foramen, by the junction of three smaller veins. The thalamostriate vein (aka superior thalamosstriate vein or terminal vein), is the most significant one, originating from venules draining the thalamus, striatum (caudate and lenticular nuclei), and deep white matter, running from back to front in the thalamo-caudate sulcus along the inferior wall of the lateral ventricle. The superior choroidal vein, which arises from venules of the choroid plexus and third ventricle, drains part of the fornix and corpus callosum. The anterior septal vein, near the corpus callosum, forms from venules draining the head of the caudate nucleus, the genu of the corpus callosum, and the septum pellucidum. The internal cerebral veins travel horizontally, with a slight inferior concavity, passing through the transverse fissure, curving around the splenium of the corpus callosum in an upward course before converging at the midline to form the great cerebral vein. Important tributaries drain into each internal cerebral vein: the posterior septal vein, the lateral ventricular vein, the (multiple) lateral direct veins, and veins from the caudate nucleus and thalamus. The great cerebral vein, or great vein of Galen, originates at the junction of the two internal cerebral veins, between the splenium of the corpus callosum above and the pineal gland below. It drains into the straight sinus after a short course, concave superiorly, following the convexity of the splenium. The great cerebral vein often receives tributaries including the posterior veins of the corpus callosum (which also drain part of the posterior cingulate gyrus and precuneus), veins of the midbrain and upper cerebellum.

The venous sinuses of the dura mater are endothelial-lined channels located within the dura, serving as the brain's final drainage pathway. They include unpaired median sinuses, paired lateralized sinuses, and accessory sinuses. The superior sagittal sinus, the longest and widest, runs along the attached margin of the falx cerebri from the foramen cecum anteriorly to the confluence of sinuses posteriorly, receiving cortical veins and the superior anastomotic vein. The inferior sagittal sinus, smaller and running along the free edge of the falx cerebri, drains venules from the corpus callosum and medial cerebral hemispheres and joins the great cerebral vein to form the straight sinus. The straight sinus courses posteriorly and inferiorly, draining into the confluence of sinuses, where it meets the superior sagittal and occipital sinuses. From the confluence arise the transverse sinuses, which run laterally along the tentorium, receiving the superficial middle cerebral, temporal, superior petrosal, and cerebellar veins, before continuing as sigmoid sinuses near the parieto-occipital suture. The sigmoid sinuses, S-shaped, curve medially and inferiorly toward the jugular foramen, where they become the internal jugular veins.

The cavernous sinuses, located lateral to the sella turcica, are reticulated venous spaces receiving blood from the sphenoparietal sinuses, orbit and face. The sphenoparietal sinuses course along the posterior border of the lesser wing of the sphenoid to drain into the cavernous sinuses. The superior petrosal sinuses run along the petrous ridge of the temporal bone, draining into the transverse sinuses, while the inferior petrosal sinuses, narrower and located along the petroclival fissure, empty into the sigmoid sinuses. The superior petrosal sinus receives drainage from Dandy's vein, commonly synonymous with the superior petrosal vein, which collects blood from the lateral brainstem, cerebellopontine angle, and anterior surfaces of the cerebellum, forming a critical component of the posterior fossa venous outflow. The occipital sinus, along the falx cerebelli, drains into the confluence. The basilar plexus, a venous network on the posterior surface of the clivus, connects with both the inferior petrosal sinuses and the internal vertebral venous plexus.

The cerebral venous system is a complex and highly variable network with critical implications for stroke physiopathology and management. While arterial occlusion remains the primary focus in ischaemic stroke, venous dysfunction may exacerbate ischaemic injury, influence collateral flow, and contribute to stroke-related complications. Detection of venous abnormalities on imaging and understanding their impact on cerebral haemodynamic are also essential to improve patient outcomes.

References

1. Bouthillier A, Van Loveren HR, Keller JT. Segments of the internal carotid artery: a new classification. Neurosurgery. 1996;38:425–33.
2. Gibo H, Lenkey C, Rhoton A Jr. Microsurgical anatomy of the supraclinoid portion of the internal carotid artery. J Neurosurg. 1981;55:560–74.
3. Fischer E. Die Lageabweichungen der vorderen Hirnarterie im Gefäßbild. Zentralblatt Für Neurochir. 1938;3:300–13.
4. Maldonado IL. A practical guide to cerebrovascular anatomy. In: Kanaan IN, Beneš V, editors. Neuroanat Guid success Neurosurg Interv [Internet]. Cham: Springer Nature Switzerland; 2024. p. 47–57. [Cited 2025 Mar 5]. Available from: https://link.springer.com/10.1007/978-3-031-59838-8_5.
5. Abdulrauf S, Ashour A, Marvin E, Coppens J, Kang B, Hsieh TY, et al. Proposed clinical internal carotid artery classification system. J Craniovertebr Junction Spine. 2016;7:161.
6. Morris P. Practical neuroangiography. 2nd ed. Philadelphia: Lippincott Williams & Wilkins; 2007.

7. Cironi KA, Decater T, Iwanaga J, Dumont AS, Tubbs RS. Arterial supply to the pituitary gland: a comprehensive review. World Neurosurg. 2020;142:206–11.
8. Matsumura Y, Nagashima M. Anatomical variations in the origin of the human ophthalmic artery with special reference to the cavernous sinus and surrounding meninges. Cells Tissues Organs. 1999;164:112–21.
9. Michalinos A, Zogana S, Kotsiomitis E, Mazarakis A, Troupis T. Anatomy of the ophthalmic artery: a review concerning its modern surgical and clinical applications. Anat Res Int. 2015;2015:1–8.
10. Namba K. Carotid-vertebrobasilar anastomoses with reference to their segmental property. Neurologia medico-chirurgica. 2017;57:267–77.
11. Lasjaunias P, Berenstein A, Ter Brugge KG. Clinical vascular anatomy and variations. Springer; 2001.
12. Percheron G. The anatomy of the arterial supply of the human thalamus and its variations. J Neurol Surg Cent Eur Neurosurg. 1973;128:93–125.
13. Rhoton AL. The cerebral veins. Neurosurgery. 2002;51:S1–159–205.
14. Kılıç T, Akakın A. Anatomy of cerebral veins and sinuses. In: Caso V, Agnelli G, Paciaroni M, editors. Front Neurol Neurosci [Internet]. Basel: KARGER; 2007. p. 4–15. [Cited 2025 Apr 10]. Available from: https://karger.com/books/book/2601/chapter/5747086.
15. Testut L. Traité d'anatomie humaine. Tome deuxième – angéiologie, système nerveux central. Paris: Octave Doin; 1899.

Clinical Symptomatology of Ischemic Stroke

Roman Herzig and Libor Šimůnek

1 Introduction

Acute ischemic stroke (AIS) is usually caused by a sudden occlusion of a cerebral artery, or cervical artery supplying the brain, leading to hypoperfusion and reduced oxygen supply to the brain with subsequent neuronal damage. Occlusions of cerebral veins and sinuses belong among the less frequent AIS causes. Clinical manifestation depends mainly on the AIS localization and the volume of the affected brain tissue, which are associated with the involved vascular territory. Occlusion of the internal carotid arteries (ICA), middle cerebral arteries (MCA), and anterior cerebral arteries (ACA) or their branches results in anterior circulation stroke (ACS), accounting for approximately 70–80% of all AIS. Posterior circulation stroke (PCS) refers to any infarction localized in the regions supplied by the vertebrobasilar arterial system, with a reported prevalence ranging from 20 to 30%. Although the most common symptoms of ACS and PCS are well described, reliably distinguishing between them can be challenging, as PCS causes a broader spectrum of less specific symptoms than ACS [19].

2 General Symptoms of Ischemic Stroke

Ischemic stroke presents with a variety of symptoms that depend on the affected vascular territory and the extent of brain tissue damage [3, 6, 11, 12, 20, 22]. Common symptoms include sudden onset of:

- **Hemiparesis or hemiplegia**: Weakness or paralysis on one side of the body. The Oxford Muscle Grading Scale is widely used for assessing muscle strength in clinical settings (Table 1) [9].
- **Facial droop**: Drooping of one side of the face. The central lesion of the facial nerve affects the lower part of the face.
- **Speech disturbances**
  - **Aphasia**: Difficulties with speech production or comprehension (usually associated with the lesions of the dominant hemisphere).
  - **Dysarthria**: Problems with articulation (slurred speech).
- **Neglect syndrome** (associated with the lesions of the non-dominant hemisphere)
- **Other disorders of higher nervous activity**
- **Memory problems**
- **Forced gaze deviation toward the lesion site**
- **Visual disturbances**: Loss of vision in one eye, visual field deficits in both eyes, diplopia.
- **Balance and coordination difficulties:** Ataxia, vertigo, or unsteadiness.
- **Sensory deficits**: Numbness or altered sensation.
- **Headache** with sudden onset
- **Nausea and vomiting**
- **Altered consciousness**: Qualitative or quantitative impairment, ranging from confusion to coma.

R. Herzig (✉) · L. Šimůnek
Department of Neurology, Faculty of Medicine in Hradec Králové, Charles University, Hradec Králové, Czech Republic

Department of Neurology, Comprehensive Stroke Center, University Hospital Hradec Králové, Hradec Králové, Czech Republic
e-mail: libor.simunek@fnhk.cz

V. Beneš, D. Netuka (eds.), *Surgical and Interventional Treatment of Cerebral Ischemia*,
https://doi.org/10.1007/978-3-032-08934-2_5

Table 1 Oxford Muscle Grading Scale

Grade	Muscle movement
0/5	No detectable muscle contraction.
1/5	Visible or palpable muscle contraction, but no movement occurs.
2/5	Movement through the full range with gravity eliminated (considered poor strength).
3/5	Movement through the full range against gravity only (considered fair strength).
4/5	Movement through the full range against gravity with some resistance (considered good strength).
5/5	Movement through the full range against gravity with full resistance (considered normal strength).

3 Stroke Symptoms by Affected Artery

3.1 Anterior Circulation Syndromes

3.1.1 Anterior Cerebral Artery (ACA) Syndrome

Occlusion of the ACA leads to characteristic deficits due to ischemia in the medial frontal and parietal lobes, including [6, 20]:

- **Contralateral leg weakness and sensory loss** (greater than arm or facial involvement).
- **Prefrontal syndrome:** Behavioral and personality changes, including apathy, lack of initiative (abulia), confusion, and impaired judgment.
- **Urinary incontinence**: Related to disruption of cortical micturition centers.

3.1.2 Middle Cerebral Artery (MCA) Syndrome

MCA occlusion is the most common ischemic stroke and presents with [6, 20, 22]:

- **Contralateral hemiparesis:** More pronounced weakness in the arm than in the leg.
- **Contralateral weakness of the lower part of the face** (central lesion)
- **Contralateral sensory loss**—hemianesthesia or hemihypoesthesia
- **Aphasia** (dominant hemisphere involvement):
  - **Broca's aphasia**: Non-fluent, effortful speech with preserved comprehension.
  - **Wernicke's aphasia**: Fluent but meaningless speech with impaired comprehension.
  - **Global aphasia**: Severe deficits in both expression and comprehension.
  - **Conduction aphasia**: Fluent speech with preserved comprehension but difficulty in repeating phrases.
  - **Transcortical aphasia**: Preserved repetition with deficits in expression (motor) or comprehension (sensory).
- **Neglect syndrome** (non-dominant hemisphere involvement): Inattention to the contralateral side of the body or environment.

Table 2 Summary of symptoms based on occlusion of particular segments of the middle cerebral artery

MCA segment	Symptoms
M1 segment	Contralateral hemiparesis, contralateral sensory loss, aphasia, and homonymous hemianopsia
M2 segment (inferior trunk)	Contralateral weakness/sensory loss, neglect syndromes, and cognitive deficits
M2 segment (superior trunk)	Contralateral weakness/sensory loss with a focus on the arm and face
Lenticulostriate branches	Pure hemiparesis or pure hemianesthaesia

- **Contralateral homonymous hemianopsia**: Loss of the same half of the visual field in both eyes.

1. The occlusion of different MCA segments can lead to a variety of neurological deficits, reflecting the specific areas supplied by each segment (Table 2) [18].

3.1.3 Internal Carotid Artery (ICA) Syndrome

A combination of the deficits seen in ACA and MCA syndromes.

3.2 Posterior Circulation Syndromes

Involvement of the posterior circulation affects the brainstem, cerebellum, and occipital lobes.

3.2.1 Posterior Cerebral Artery (PCA) Syndrome

PCA occlusion results in deficits related to the occipital lobe and medial temporal structures [20, 22]:

- **Contralateral homonymous hemianopsia**: Loss of the same half of the visual field in both eyes with macular sparing.
- **Visual agnosia**: Difficulty recognizing objects despite normal visual acuity.
- **Anton's syndrome**: Cortical blindness with denial of visual deficits.
- **Memory impairments**: Due to medial temporal lobe involvement.
- **Thalamic symptoms**: Hypersomnolence, cognitive deficits, and ataxia may occur if deep structures are involved.

3.2.2 Anterior Inferior Cerebellar Artery (AICA) Syndrome—Lateral Pontine Syndrome

AICA supplies blood to parts of the cerebellum and brainstem, and its occlusion can result in a variety of neurological symptoms [7, 13]:

- **Ipsilateral facial paralysis affecting the entire half of the face** (nuclear lesion)
- **Ipsilateral facial sensory loss**

- **Contralateral pain and temperature sensory loss**
- **Ipsilateral hearing loss and/or tinnitus**
- **Vertigo**
- **Nausea and vomiting**
- **Ipsilateral limb ataxia**
- **Ipsilateral Horner's syndrome**—ptosis, miosis, anhidrosis
- **Nystagmus**
- **Dysarthria**

3.2.3 Posterior Inferior Cerebellar Artery (PICA) Syndrome—Lateral Medullary Syndrome, Wallenberg Syndrome

PCA supplies blood to the posterior part of the cerebellum and parts of the medulla oblongata [8].

- **Ipsilateral facial pain and temperature sensory loss**
- **Contralateral body pain and temperature sensory loss**
- **Dysphagia**
- **Dysarthria**
- **Ipsilateral Horner's syndrome**—ptosis, miosis, anhidrosis
- **Vertigo**
- **Nausea and vomiting**—frequently associated with vertigo
- **Nystagmus**—severe rotatory
- **Ipsilateral ataxia of the extremities**

3.2.4 Superior Cerebellar Artery (SCA) Syndrome

The SCA supplies the superior part of the cerebellum as well as the dentate nucleus, and midbrain, and its occlusion can result in [16]:

- **Ipsilateral limb ataxia**
- **Contralateral body pain and temperature sensory loss**
- **Vertigo**
- **Nausea and vomiting**
- **Nystagmus**
- **Dysarthria**
- **Headache**

3.2.5 Basilar Artery (BA) Syndromes

The occlusion of specific segments of the BA can lead to a range of neurological symptoms, depending on the location and extent of the occlusion [2, 5, 10]:

Proximal and Mid Basilar Artery Occlusion

- **Locked-in syndrome:** This devastating condition arises from bilateral pontine ischemia, characterized by:
  - **Quadriplegia:** Complete paralysis of all four limbs.
  - **Preserved consciousness:** Patients are fully aware.
  - **Inability to speak**
  - **Preserved vertical eye movements**, while horizontal movements are often lost.
- **Decreased consciousness:** Altered levels of consciousness can occur due to brainstem involvement.
- **Alternating hemiplegia (crossed hemiplegia)** is a form of hemiplegia with ipsilateral cranial nerve lesions and contralateral hemiplegia or hemiparesis of extremities.
- **Cranial nerves lesions:** Dysfunction of cranial nerves (ipsilateral to the side of the lesion due to the impairment of their nuclei) can lead to various deficits, including:
  - **Dysphagia**
  - **Dysarthria**
  - **Oculomotor dysfunction**
- **Motor dysfunction:** While motor function is often severely impaired (plegia), some patients may exhibit preserved motor function in certain muscle groups.

Distal Basilar Artery Occlusion (Top of the Basilar Syndrome)

- **Visual disturbances:**
  - **Diplopia**
  - **Visual field deficits**—due to ischemia affecting the occipital lobes and visual pathways
- **Behavioral changes:** Patients may experience altered mental status, including confusion or hallucinations.
- **Somnolence:** Patients may present with excessive sleepiness or dream-like states.
- **Oculomotor dysfunction:** Similar to proximal occlusions—patients may exhibit eye movement abnormalities.

General Symptoms Across All Basilar Artery Occlusions

Regardless of the specific segment affected, common symptoms associated with BA occlusion include:

- **Severe dizziness or vertigo:** Often described as a spinning sensation.
- **Ataxia**—due to cerebellar involvement
- **Weakness or numbness:** Particularly on one side of the body or bilateral weakness, depending on the extent of ischemia.
- **Severe headache:** Sudden-onset headaches are common in acute occlusions.
- **Nausea and vomiting**

3.2.6 Subclavian Steal Syndrome

Subclavian steal syndrome manifests by a combination of neurological and upper extremity symptoms primarily due to altered blood flow dynamics with reversed blood flow in the vertebral artery due to subclavian artery stenosis or occlusion. The severity and nature of symptoms can vary widely among patients, often exacerbated by physical exertion or specific head movements, and include [21]:

- **Ipsilateral arm claudication:** Patients often experience pain, fatigue, or discomfort in the affected arm during exertion. Numbness or tingling may occur in the arm due to inadequate blood supply.
- **Vertebrobasilar insufficiency symptoms**:
  - **Vertigo**—often exacerbated by head movements
  - **Nausea and vomiting**
  - **Drop attacks—**sudden episodes of weakness leading to falls without warning, particularly when exerting the arms.
  - **Visual disturbances**—blurred vision, diplopia, or transient vision loss in one or both eyes
  - **Headache:** Patients may report headaches, which can be associated with changes in blood flow dynamics.
  - **Focal neurological deficits:** may occur due to reduced perfusion in areas supplied by the posterior circulation.

4 Lacunar Infarcts

These are small, deep infarcts typically resulting from the occlusion of small penetrating arteries. Common locations include the basal ganglia, thalamus, internal capsule, and brainstem. Symptoms from small vessel occlusions can sometimes be subtle and may not present as dramatic deficits compared to larger vessel strokes; thus, they can be easily overlooked. Lacunar infarcts often present with [6, 15, 20]:

- **Pure hemiparesis**—often due to infarcts in the posterior limb of the internal capsule
- **Pure hemianesthesia**—typically resulting from thalamic infarcts
- **Ataxic hemiparesis**—a combination of weakness and limb ataxia, often due to lesions in the pons or corona radiata
- **Dysarthria–clumsy hand syndrome**—usually associated with infarcts in the AICA territory or related areas
- **Cognitive and behavioral changes:** Infarcts in certain regions, particularly in the thalamus or basal ganglia, can lead to cognitive deficits, confusion, or changes in behavior.
- **Visual disturbances:** Depending on the specific vascular territory involved, visual field deficits may occur in the case of the involvement of areas supplied by small branches of the PCA.

5 Symptoms of Cerebral Sinus Occlusion

The occlusion of cerebral sinuses, particularly in the context of cerebral venous sinus thrombosis (CVST), can lead to a range of symptoms due to impaired venous drainage and increased intracranial pressure [4, 17, 23].

5.1 General Symptoms of Cerebral Sinus Occlusion

- **Headache:** Present in approximately 90% of cases, headaches can be severe and may develop gradually or suddenly. They are often described as the worst headache ever experienced or may resemble a thunderclap headache.
- **Nausea and vomiting:** These symptoms are common and can accompany headaches due to increased intracranial pressure.
- **Seizures:** Seizures occur in about 40% of patients, often presenting as focal seizures that may generalize.
- **Altered mental status:** Patients may experience confusion, decreased consciousness, or even coma in severe cases.
- **Focal neurological deficits:** Focal symptoms may arise depending on the affected brain regions.
- **Visual symptoms:** Blurred vision or diplopia can occur, especially if there is increased pressure affecting cranial nerves.
- **Papilledema:** Swelling of the optic disc due to increased intracranial pressure may be observed during an eye examination.

5.2 Symptoms Related to the Occlusion of Specific Cerebral Sinuses

5.2.1 Superior Sagittal Sinus Thrombosis

Symptoms may include:

- **Headache—often severe**
- **Seizures**
- **Focal neurological deficits**
  - **Monoparesis or paraparesis of lower limbs**
  - **Aphasia**
- **Caput medusae sign**—visible enlargement of veins on the surface of the head (especially in children)

5.2.2 Cavernous Sinus Thrombosis

This condition can present with:

- **Headache**—severe, particularly around the eyes
- **Eye pain and swelling (proptosis)**
- **Diplopia**—due to cranial nerve palsies.
- **Altered consciousness**—in the case of a significant intracranial pressure increase

5.2.3 Transverse Sinus Thrombosis

Symptoms may include:

- **Headache**
- **Tinnitus**
- **Symptoms related to increased intracranial pressure**
- **Focal deficits**—may occur if there is associated venous infarction in the cerebellum or brainstem

5.2.4 Sigmoid Sinus Thrombosis

Symptoms may include:

- **Unilateral ear pain**
- **Hearing loss**
- **Headache**
- **Visual disturbances**
- **Signs of increased intracranial pressure**

5.2.5 Vein of Galen Thrombosis

This rare condition can lead to **severe neurological deficits** due to impaired drainage from deep structures of the brain, potentially causing **significant developmental delays** or **cognitive impairment in pediatric cases**.

6 Clinical Assessment of Stroke Severity

The National Institutes of Health Stroke Scale (NIHSS) is standardly used to assess the severity of neurological deficits in ischemic strokes [14]. However, NIHSS underestimates clinical severity in PCS, and patients presenting with low NIHSS may be considered ineligible for reperfusion therapies. Thus, a modified version of the NIHSS, the Posterior NIHSS (POST-NIHSS) was developed to improve NIHSS prognostic accuracy for PCS patients with mild-moderate symptoms [1].

7 Conclusion

Prompt recognition of stroke symptoms is critical for effective treatment. The specific symptoms can guide healthcare providers in identifying which artery is affected, allowing for targeted interventions to restore blood flow and minimize brain damage. Immediate medical attention is essential when stroke symptoms are observed.

References

1. Alemseged F, Rocco A, Arba F, on behalf of the Basilar Artery Treatment and Management (BATMAN) Collaboration Investigators, et al. Posterior National Institutes of Health Stroke Scale improves prognostic accuracy in posterior circulation stroke. Stroke. 2022;53(4):1247–55. https://doi.org/10.1161/STROKEAHA.120.034019.
2. Available from URL: https://www.emdocs.net/em3am-basilar-artery-occlusion/
3. Available from URL: https://emedicine.medscape.com/article/1916852-overview
4. Available from URL: https://en.wikipedia.org/wiki/Cerebral_venous_sinus_thrombosis
5. Available from URL: https://www.healthline.com/health/stroke/basilar-artery-stroke#symptoms
6. Available from URL: https://www.msdmanuals.com/professional/neurologic-disorders/stroke/ischemic-stroke
7. Available from URL: https://www.neuropt.org/docs/default-source/vsig-english-pt-fact-sheets/aica-stroke3ca035a5390366a68a96ff00001fc240.pdf?sfvrsn=f0a35343_0
8. Available from URL: https://www.ninds.nih.gov/health-information/disorders/wallenbergs-syndrome
9. Available from URL: https://www.physio-pedia.com/Oxford_Scale
10. Available from URL: https://radiopaedia.org/articles/acute-basilar-artery-occlusion
11. Available from URL: https://www.ssmhealth.com/services/neurosciences/stroke/ischemic-stroke
12. Available from URL: https://www.yalemedicine.org/conditions/ischemic-stroke
13. Available from URL: https://en.wikipedia.org/wiki/Anterior_inferior_cerebellar_artery
14. Brott T, Adams HP Jr, Olinger CP, et al. Measurements of acute cerebral infarction: a clinical examination scale. Stroke. 1989;20(7):864–70. https://doi.org/10.1161/01.STR.20.7.864.
15. Chen Z, Mo J, Xu J, et al. Risk profile of ischemic stroke caused by small-artery occlusion vs. deep intracerebral hemorrhage. Front Neurol. 2019;10:1213. https://doi.org/10.3389/fneur.2019.01213.
16. Erdemoglu AK, Duman T. Superior cerebellar artery territory stroke. Acta Neurol Scand. 1998;98(4):283–7. https://doi.org/10.1111/j.1600-0404.1998.tb07310.x.
17. Gokey R, Das JM. Venous sinus thrombosis. Treasure Island (FL): StatPearls Publishing; 2024.
18. Gruber P, Valbuena P, Sassenburg R, et al. Anatomical distribution and clinical significance of middle cerebral artery M2 segment vessel occlusions and its cortical branches in acute ischaemic stroke patients. BMJ Neurol Open. 2023;5(2):e000450. https://doi.org/10.1136/bmjno-2023-000450.
19. Halúsková S, Herzig R, Krajíčková D, et al. Acute management should be optimized in patients with less specific stroke symptoms. J Clin Med. 2021;10(5):1143. https://doi.org/10.3390/jcm10051143.
20. Hui C, Tadi P, Suheb MZK, et al. Ischemic stroke. Treasure Island (FL): StatPearls Publishing; 2024.
21. Kikkeri NS, Nagalli S. Subclavian steal syndrome. Treasure Island (FL): StatPearls Publishing; 2024.
22. Musuka TD, Wilton SB, Traboulsi M, et al. Diagnosis and management of acute ischemic stroke: speed is critical. CMAJ. 2015;187(12):887–93. https://doi.org/10.1503/cmaj.140355.
23. Tadi P, Behgam B, Baruffi S. Cerebral venous thrombosis. Treasure Island (FL): StatPearls Publishing; 2024.

Best Medical Treatment

Roman Herzig and David Školoudík

1 Introduction

The occlusion of cerebral arteries due to atherosclerosis, cardioembolism, or small vessel disease primarily causes an ischemic stroke (IS) or transient ischemic attack (TIA). In rare cases, IS may also occur due to the occlusion of cerebral sinuses and veins. Patients with a history of IS or TIA are at an increased risk of recurrent stroke and cardiovascular events, including myocardial infarction. The rate of recurrent stroke following IS has been reported to range between 9% and 15% after 1 year and between 27% and 40% at 10 years, dependent on stroke etiology. Following TIA, 6% of patients suffer from stroke, and 12% from stroke or TIA within 1 year. Medical treatment for IS or TIA (in addition to specific acute recanalization therapy, i.e., intravenous thrombolysis) focuses mainly on secondary prevention to achieve long-term compensation for vascular risk factors and reduce the risk of recurrent stroke. For this purpose, primarily antiplatelet, anticoagulant, and hypolipidemic therapies and management of blood pressure (BP) and diabetes mellitus (DM) are used. Lifestyle modifications must also accompany the best medical treatment [2, 5, 13].

2 Antiplatelet Therapy

Antiplatelet agents are essential in the management of noncardioembolic strokes or TIA. Recommendations on the indication of antiplatelets to reduce the risk of recurrent stroke and other cardiovascular events while minimizing the risk of bleeding are based on the analysis of studies comparing aspirin with placebo, cilostazol with placebo, ticlopidine with placebo, aspirin plus dipyridamole with placebo, and aspirin plus dipyridamole with aspirin monotherapy [5, 11]:

- In patients with previous IS or TIA, long-term use of antiplatelet monotherapy (aspirin 50 to 325 mg daily or clopidogrel 75 mg daily) is recommended.
- The addition of a low-dose direct oral anticoagulant (DOAC) to an antiplatelet can be considered to optimize the treatment of coronary artery disease or peripheral arterial disease in people with a history of IS or TIA more than 1 month previously.
- The use of antiplatelet therapy, and not a DOAC, is suggested in patients with an embolic stroke of an undetermined source.

The indications for short-term dual antiplatelet therapy in patients with IS or TIA are presented in Table 1 [4, 11].

The ABCD^2 score is defined in Table 2 [8].

The number needed to treat (NNT) for antiplatelet therapy to prevent one recurrent stroke in patients with noncardioembolic IS, compared to placebo, varies depending on the specific antiplatelet agent and treatment regimen used. For example, the NNT for aspirin compared to placebo in preventing one recurrent stroke within 2–4 weeks in patients with IS is 140 [9]. In other studies, the efficacy of antiplatelet drugs was generally compared with each other, not against a placebo.

R. Herzig (✉)
Department of Neurology, Faculty of Medicine in Hradec Králové, Charles University, Hradec Králové, Czech Republic

Department of Neurology, Comprehensive Stroke Center, University Hospital Hradec Králové, Hradec Králové, Czech Republic

D. Školoudík
Centre for Health Research, Department of Clinical Neurosciences, Faculty of Medicine, University of Ostrava, Ostrava, Czech Republic

V. Beneš, D. Netuka (eds.), *Surgical and Interventional Treatment of Cerebral Ischemia*,
https://doi.org/10.1007/978-3-032-08934-2_6

Table 1 Indications for short-term dual antiplatelet therapy in patients with ischemic stroke or transient ischemic attack

Antiplatelets and doses	Length of time of medication administration	Indications
Aspirin (100 mg/d) + Clopidogrel (loading dose 300 mg, then 75 mg/d)	21 days (early initiation ideally within 12–24 hours and at least within 7 days of symptom onset; followed by antiplatelet monotherapy)	Non-cardioembolic minor IS (NIHSS score ≤ 3) in the past 24 hours
		Non-cardioembolic high-risk TIA (ABCD^2 score ≥ 4) in the past 24 hours
Aspirin (100 mg/d) + Ticagrelor (loading dose 180 mg, then 2x90 mg/d)	30 days (followed by antiplatelet monotherapy)	Non-cardioembolic mild to moderate IS (NIHSS ≤ 5) in the past 24 hours
		Non-cardioembolic high-risk TIA (ABCD^2 score ≥ 6 or with intracranial atherosclerosis or ICA stenosis ≥ 50%) in the past 24 hours

ICA internal carotid artery, *IS* ischemic stroke, *NIHSS* National Institutes of Health Stroke Scale, *TIA* transient ischemic attack

Table 2 ABCD^2 score

	Risk factor		Score
A	Age ≥ 60 years		1
B	Blood pressure elevation on first assessment after TIA (systolic ≥ 140 mmHg or diastolic ≥ 90 mmHg)		1
C	Clinical symptoms	Unilateral weakness	2
		Speech impairment without weakness	1
D	Duration of symptoms	≥ 60 minutes	2
		10–59 minutes	1
D	Diabetes mellitus		1

TIA transient ischemic attack

3 Anticoagulation Therapy

For cardioembolic strokes, anticoagulation therapy is critical but is generally delayed until the subacute phase to minimize hemorrhagic transformation risks. Early anticoagulation may be considered after imaging confirms the absence of significant hemorrhagic transformation of large infarcts. Guidelines [11] recommend initiating oral anticoagulation between 2–14 days post-stroke in patients with atrial fibrillation (AF) to balance hemorrhagic and embolic risks. However, in patients with stroke at high risk of hemorrhagic conversion in the setting of AF, it is reasonable to delay the initiation of oral anticoagulation beyond 14 days to reduce the risk of intracranial hemorrhage. In contrast, in patients with TIA and nonvalvular AF, it is reasonable to initiate anticoagulation immediately after the index event to reduce the risk of recurrent stroke. The following anticoagulants may be used [11]:

- DOACs:
  - Preferred to warfarin in patients with nonvalvular AF or atrial flutter and IS or TIA for long-term anticoagulation due to lower rates of intracranial hemorrhage and non-inferior efficacy to reduce the risk of recurrent stroke regardless of whether the AF pattern is paroxysmal, persistent, or permanent.
- Warfarin is indicated in patients with IS or TIA and:
  - valvular AF (moderate to severe mitral stenosis or any mechanical heart valve) to reduce the risk of recurrent stroke or TIA. Target INR is adjusted based on individual risk profiles.
  - left ventricle thrombus for at least 3 months to reduce the risk of recurrent stroke
  - left atrial or left atrial appendage thrombus in the setting of ischemic, nonischemic, or restrictive cardiomyopathy and left ventricle dysfunction for at least 3 months to reduce the risk of recurrent stroke or TIA.
- In patients with AF and stroke or TIA who have end-stage renal disease or are on dialysis, it may be reasonable to use warfarin or apixaban (dose adjusted if indicated) for anticoagulation to reduce the chance of recurrent stroke.

For the anticoagulants used as the initial treatment of acute cardioembolic stroke, the NNT is approximately 51 to prevent one recurrent IS within 7 to 14 days compared to placebo [14]. In patients with nonvalvular AF and previous stroke or TIA, the NNT is 17 to prevent one recurrent IS over one year compared to aspirin [16].

4 Hypolipidemics

Clinical trials and meta-analyses demonstrated risk reduction in recurrent vascular events in patients suffering from IS or TIA treated with hypolipidemics, reflected in the following recommendations [5]:

- Patients who have had an IS or TIA should be prescribed statins to lower their cholesterol.
- Lipid-lowering treatments should aim to keep the low-density cholesterol level <1.4 mmol/l to reduce the risk of major cardiovascular events [3].
- In patients who do not achieve the recommended LDL-C targets despite taking a maximally tolerated statin dose

for at least 6 weeks, adding ezetimibe to the therapy should be considered.

- In patients who do not achieve the recommended LDL-C targets on a maximally tolerated dose of statin and ezetimibe, a combination with a proprotein convertase subtilisin/kexin type 9 (PCSK9) inhibitor is recommended [3].

As shown in the SPARCL study, the NNT of patients treated with atorvastatin 80 mg daily versus placebo in the secondary prevention of stroke or TIA for five years to prevent one stroke is 46 [1].

5 Management of Blood Pressure

Arterial hypertension is a key risk factor for stroke. BP level has a log-linear relationship with the risk of stroke. A 20-mmHg systolic or 10-mmHg diastolic increase in BP is associated with an approximate doubling of the risk of stroke. Elevated BP after IS or TIA is also a risk factor for recurrence [10, 12]. Thus, compensation of arterial hypertension is crucial to reduce the recurrence of both IS and TIA [5]:

- Patients who have had an IS or TIA should be prescribed medication to lower their BP if this is raised.
- Treatment should aim to achieve a BP level <130/80 mmHg except in some patients at an increased risk of problems, such as the very elderly, people with kidney problems, and those with severe stenoses of the large cerebral vessels.
- Treatment initiation with a combination of two BP-lowering drugs, usually containing either a thiazide-like diuretic (such as indapamide) or a calcium channel blocker (such as amlodipine or felodipine), combined with an inhibitor of the renin-angiotensin system (ACE inhibitor or angiotensin 2 receptor blocker), is likely to be beneficial for most patients, with consideration of monotherapy where there are potential risks of arterial hypotension, such as in frail, elderly people and people with borderline arterial hypertension.
- Monitoring BP at home is likely to achieve better long-term BP control.

6 Management of Diabetes Mellitus

Patients with DM are at a two-fold increased risk of stroke, and the relative risk of stroke is reported to increase by approximately 15% with each 1% increase in glycated hemoglobin (HbA1c) level [7, 15]. Intensive control of blood glucose levels in patients with DM reduces the risk of microvascular complications such as retinopathy, nephropathy, and neuropathy. The following recommendations regarding DM management are valid in patients with IS or TIA and DM [5]:

- Treatment should aim to achieve an HbA1c level of <53 mmol/mol (7%) to reduce the risk of microvascular and macrovascular complications. However, this target may need to be individualized based on the duration of DM, age, and comorbidities.
- Pioglitazone is suggested to be used in patients with insulin resistance or type 2 DM to reduce the risk of recurrent stroke, but this should be balanced against an increased risk of broken bones, heart failure, and bladder cancer.

7 Specific Clinical Scenarios

7.1 Cerebral Edema

Osmotic therapy with mannitol and hypertonic saline is recommended to reduce intracranial pressure in patients with significant edema threatening brainstem compression.

7.2 Arterial Dissection

In patients with IS or TIA who are <3 months after an extracranial carotid or vertebral arterial dissection, treatment with antithrombotic therapy (either aspirin or warfarin) for at least 3 months is indicated to prevent recurrent stroke or TIA [11].

7.3 Cerebral Venous Thrombosis [6]

- In adult patients with acute cerebral venous thrombosis (CVT), including pregnant and puerperal patients and patients with intracerebral hemorrhage at baseline, treatment with low-molecular-weight heparin (LMWH) in therapeutic dosage is recommended during the acute phase, followed by oral anticoagulation with warfarin for 3–12 months after CVT to prevent recurrent CVT and other venous thromboembolic events.
- In patients with acute CVT and Behçet's disease and other inflammatory diseases (e.g., systemic lupus erythematosus), steroids may be used to improve outcomes.
- Women of fertile age and prior CVT should be informed about the risks of combined hormonal contraception and advised against its use.
- Prophylaxis with subcutaneous LMWH during pregnancy/puerperium is suggested for pregnant women with a previous history of CVT and without contraindication for prophylaxis or indication for anticoagulation in therapeutic dosage.

8 Conclusion

The management of IS and TIA involves a multifaceted approach focused on preventing recurrence through medical therapies and lifestyle modifications. Antiplatelets, anticoagulants, and hypolipidemic agents, as well as the management of BP and diabetes mellitus, are crucial for the secondary prevention of IS and TIA. Individualized care based on the etiology of stroke, patient comorbidities, and overall health status, timing of intervention, and evidence-based approaches should be emphasized. While significant advances have been made in acute and secondary prevention strategies, future research should explore optimizing treatment combinations and addressing disparities in global stroke care.

References

1. Amarenco P, Bogousslavsky J, Callahan A 3rd, Stroke Prevention by Aggressive Reduction in Cholesterol Levels (SPARCL) Investigators, et al. High-dose atorvastatin after stroke or transient ischemic attack. N Engl J Med. 2006;355(6):549–59. https://doi.org/10.1056/NEJMoa061894.
2. Amarenco P, Lavallée PC, Labreuche J, TIAregistry.org Investigators, et al. One-year risk of stroke after transient ischemic attack or minor stroke. N Engl J Med. 2016;374(16):1533–42. https://doi.org/10.1056/NEJMoa1412981.
3. Authors/Task Force Members; ESC Committee for Practice Guidelines (CPG); ESC National Cardiac Societies. 2019 ESC/EAS guidelines for the management of dyslipidaemias: lipid modification to reduce cardiovascular risk. Atherosclerosis. 2019;290:140–205. https://doi.org/10.1016/j.atherosclerosis.2019.08.014.
4. Dawson J, Merwick A, Webb A, for the European Stroke Organisation, et al. European Stroke Organisation expedited recommendation for the use of short-term dual antiplatelet therapy early after minor stroke and high-risk TIA. Eur Stroke J. 2021;6(2):CLXXXVII–CXCI. https://doi.org/10.1177/23969873211000877.
5. Dawson J, Béjot Y, Christensen LM, et al. European Stroke Organisation (ESO) guideline on pharmacological interventions for long-term secondary prevention after ischaemic stroke or transient ischaemic attack. Eur Stroke J 2022; 7(3): I-XLI. DOI: https://doi.org/10.1177/23969873221100032.
6. Ferro JM, Bousser M-G, Canhão P, for the European Stroke Organization, et al. European stroke organization guideline for the diagnosis and treatment of cerebral venous thrombosis—endorsed by the European Academy of Neurology. Eur Stroke J. 2017;2(3):195–221. https://doi.org/10.1177/2396987317719364.
7. Folsom AR, Rasmussen ML, Chambless LE, et al. Prospective associations of fasting insulin, body fat distribution, and diabetes with risk of ischemic stroke. The Atherosclerosis Risk in Communities (ARIC) Study Investigators. Diabetes Care. 1999;22(7):1077–83. https://doi.org/10.2337/diacare.22.7.1077.
8. Johnston SC, Rothwell PM, Nguyen-Huynh MN, et al. Validation and refinement of scores to predict very early stroke risk after transient ischaemic attack. Lancet. 2007;369(9558):283–92. https://doi.org/10.1016/S0140-6736(07)60150-0.
9. Kamarova M, Baig S, Patel H, et al. Antiplatelet use in ischemic stroke. Ann Pharmacother. 2022;56(10):1159–73. https://doi.org/10.1177/10600280211073009.
10. Kaplan RC, Tirschwell DL, Longstreth WT Jr, et al. Blood pressure level and outcomes in adults aged 65 and older with prior ischemic stroke. J Am Geriatr Soc. 2006;54(9):1309–16. https://doi.org/10.1111/j.1532-5415.2006.00838.x.
11. Kleindorfer DO, Towfighi A, Chaturvedi S, et al. 2021 guideline for the prevention of stroke in patients with stroke and transient ischemic attack: a guideline from the American Heart Association/American Stroke Association. Stroke. 2021;52(7):e364–467. https://doi.org/10.1161/STR.0000000000000375.
12. Lewington S, Clarke R, Qizilbash N, Prospective Studies Collaboration, et al. Age-specific relevance of usual blood pressure to vascular mortality: a meta-analysis of individual data for one million adults in 61 prospective studies. Lancet. 2002;360(9349):1903–13. https://doi.org/10.1016/s0140-6736(02)11911-8.
13. Li L, Yiin GS, Geraghty OC, et al. Oxford Vascular Study. Incidence, outcome, risk factors, and long-term prognosis of cryptogenic transient ischaemic attack and ischaemic stroke: a population-based study. Lancet Neurol. 2015;14(9):903–13. https://doi.org/10.1016/S1474-4422(15)00132-5.
14. Paciaroni M, Agnelli G, Micheli S, et al. Efficacy and safety of anticoagulant treatment in acute cardioembolic stroke: a meta-analysis of randomized controlled trials. Stroke. 2007;38(2):423–30. https://doi.org/10.1161/01.STR.0000254600.92975.1f.
15. Selvin E, Bolen S, Yeh H-C, et al. Cardiovascular outcomes in trials of oral diabetes medications: a systematic review. Arch Intern Med. 2008;168(19):2070–80. https://doi.org/10.1001/archinte.168.19.2070.
16. van Walraven C, Hart RG, Singer DE, et al. Oral anticoagulants vs aspirin in nonvalvular atrial fibrillation: an individual patient meta-analysis. JAMA. 2002;288(19):2441–8. https://doi.org/10.1001/jama.288.19.2441.

Radiologic Diagnosis of Cerebral Ischemia: Diagnostics

Tatiana Abou-Mrad, Laura Stone McGuire, Richard Bram, Gursant Atwal, Ali Alaraj, and Fady T. Charbel

Abbreviations

2D	Two-dimensional
3D	Three-dimensional
ASPECTS	Alberta Stroke Program Early CT Score
CBF	Cerebral blood flow
CBV	Cerebral blood volume
CE	Contrast-enhanced
Cow	Circle of Willis
CT	Computed tomography
CTA	Computed tomography angiography
CTP	Computed tomography perfusion
DSA	Digital subtraction angiography
DWI	Diffusion-weighted imaging
Dyna CT	Dynamic computed tomography
ECD	Ethyl cysteinate dimer
FPCT	Flat panel computed tomography
FRE	Flow-related enhancement
HMPAO	Hexamethylpropyleneamine oxime
ISR	In-stent restenosis
MMD	Moyamoya disease
MOSTA	Multiple overlapping thin-slab angiography
MRA	Magnetic resonance angiography
MRI	Magnetic resonance imaging
MTT	Mean transit time
NOVA	Noninvasive optimal vessel analysis
PC	Phase-contrast
PET	Positron emission tomography
QMRA	Quantitative magnetic resonance angiography
RF	Radiofrequency
SAH	Subarachnoid hemorrhage
SONIA	Stroke outcomes and neuroimaging of intracranial atherosclerosis
SPECT	Single-photon emission computed tomography
TCD	Transcranial doppler
TOF	Time-of-flight
VENC	Velocity encoding
VWI	Vessel wall imaging

T. Abou-Mrad · R. Bram · G. Atwal · A. Alaraj · F. T. Charbel (✉)
Department of Neurosurgery, University of Illinois at Chicago, Chicago, IL, USA
e-mail: fcharbel@uic.edu

L. S. McGuire
Department of Neurosurgery, University of Illinois at Chicago, Chicago, IL, USA

Department of Neurosurgery, University of Wisconsin, Maddison, WI, USA

1 Introduction

Neurovascular imaging has advanced significantly since cerebral angiography was first performed in 1927 [1]. Over decades, technological refinements have revolutionized the diagnosis and management of cerebrovascular diseases. Computed tomography (CT) and magnetic resonance imaging (MRI) have emerged as reliable, non-invasive alternatives to traditional methods, with modern techniques integrating functional and hemodynamic data [2–5]. This progress has enhanced diagnostic accuracy, improved treatment planning, and expanded therapeutic windows for cerebral ischemia.

Currently, noninvasive neurovascular imaging techniques can be broadly categorized into those based on CT or MRI. These include computed tomography angiography (CTA), CT perfusion (CTP), single-photon emission computed tomography (SPECT), magnetic resonance angiography (MRA), magnetic resonance perfusion imaging and vessel wall imaging (VWI). Each of these modalities offers unique strengths and limitations, depending on the clinical scenario and the specific diagnostic needs. Despite these advancements, digital subtraction angiography (DSA) remains the gold standard in certain scenarios, particularly for complex or peripheral lesions. This chapter provides an

V. Beneš, D. Netuka (eds.), *Surgical and Interventional Treatment of Cerebral Ischemia*,
https://doi.org/10.1007/978-3-032-08934-2_7

overview of the available neuroimaging techniques used in the diagnosis of cerebral ischemia.

2 Computed Tomography Techniques

Since their inception in the 1970s, CT technologies have undergone significant advancements in imaging technology and computational methods, enhancing our ability to visualize cerebrovascular anatomy and assess neurophysiological states [6]. These developments have improved the imaging of cerebrovascular anatomy and hemodynamic properties in both normal and pathological states, enhancing diagnostic accuracy and therapeutic decision-making in various cerebrovascular conditions, especially cerebral ischemia.

2.1 Computed Tomography Angiography

The standard CTA protocol begins with a non-contrast-enhanced (CE) head CT to establish baseline imaging. This is followed by the administration of a nonionic intravenous contrast agent at a rate of 3–4 mL/s. A built-in scanning delay, either empirically set at 25 s or triggered by contrast detection in the aortic arch, ensures optimal timing for capturing thin slices (2.5 mm thickness) with high spatial resolution. The imaging field typically extends from the aortic arch to the circle of Willis (CoW), providing detailed visualization of major cerebrovascular structures. This enables the identification of stenosis, thrombus, or dissection (Fig. 1). CTA also visualizes the primary intracranial vessels, such as the M1 segment of the middle cerebral artery, aiding in confirming the affected vascular territory and guiding targeted chemical or mechanical thrombolysis. Postprocessing at dedicated workstations generates reformatted images, including three-dimensional (3D) reconstructions and maximum intensity projections.

The speed and efficiency of CTA make it an indispensable tool in acute stroke management protocols. Its ability to swiftly acquire and reconstruct detailed vascular images significantly impacts clinical decision-making, particularly in cases of acute ischemia. CTA is critical in evaluating patients eligible for intra-arterial thrombolysis, a therapeutic intervention that can halt neurological deterioration and improve long-term outcomes. Beyond acute settings, CTA has gained prominence as a noninvasive diagnostic tool for detecting carotid and intracranial stenosis in patients with chronic ischemic conditions. Studies demonstrate that CTA achieves detection rates for intracranial stenosis nearly equivalent to those of DSA [7, 8].

One of CTA's key advantages is its ability to visualize bony anatomy in relation to vascular structures, making it invaluable for planning interventions. However, its limitations include difficulty differentiating between severe stenosis (>90%) and total occlusion [9], often necessitating confirmation via DSA. Furthermore, CTA excels in detecting vascular abnormalities but has reduced sensitivity for small foci or microangiopathic disease and cannot provide dynamic hemodynamic data, such as flow rates or collateral circulation [10, 11]. These limitations are particularly relevant in complex anatomical regions or peripheral lesions, where DSA remains indispensable due to its dynamic and high-resolution capabilities. Emerging hybrid systems combining CTA with advanced techniques like perfusion imaging are

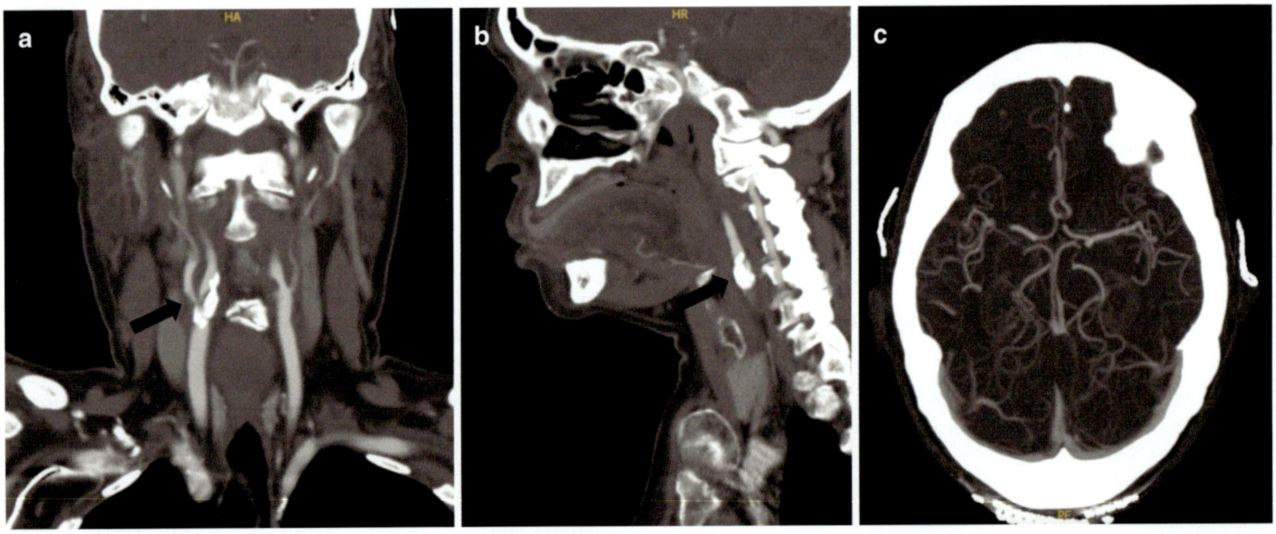

Fig. 1 A 68-year-old female was evaluated for right eye vision loss. Contrast-enhanced CT angiography (CTA) of the carotid arteries (**a**: anteroposterior, **b**: right lateral) demonstrated heavy atherosclerotic calcification and plaque at the right carotid bifurcation, with 70–79% narrowing at the origin of the right internal carotid artery (black arrows). (**c**) Maximum intensity projection image of CTA illustrates the intact internal cerebral vasculature, including the Circle of Willis, in high detail

improving the evaluation of ischemic regions, particularly in resource-rich settings. Such innovations expand CTA's role in cerebrovascular diagnostics and therapeutic planning, complementing traditional imaging modalities while addressing some of its inherent limitations.

2.2 CT Perfusion

Since its introduction, CT perfusion (CTP) has evolved to provide critical functional and physiological insights that complement anatomical imaging, revolutionizing the management of cerebrovascular diseases. Recent advancements in imaging technology, including sophisticated software algorithms and hardware improvements in helical CT scanners, have enabled the seamless integration of CTP into standard stroke protocols at many institutions. These developments have optimized the acquisition and processing of high-quality perfusion data, reducing scanning times, and enhancing spatial resolution. Consequently, CTP has become an indispensable tool in the rapid evaluation and triage of stroke patients, aiding in timely therapeutic decision-making and expanding eligibility for reperfusion therapies [12].

Dynamic CE CT, the most widely used CTP technique, employs bolus tracking to capture the dynamic passage of iodinated contrast through cerebral vasculature. The procedure begins with unenhanced imaging on a helical scanner, typically followed by perfusion imaging of two to four selected brain sections. These regions are often chosen based on initial findings from non-contrast CT, with the basal ganglia being a preferred site due to its inclusion of vascular territories supplied by the anterior, middle, and posterior cerebral arteries. During the scan, a bolus of iodinated contrast is injected intravenously, and transient increases in attenuation are recorded as the contrast perfuses through the cerebral parenchyma. Time-attenuation curves are then generated by tracking changes in contrast density. Using mathematical deconvolution techniques, key perfusion parameters including cerebral blood volume (CBV), cerebral blood flow (CBF), mean transit time (MTT), and time-to-peak enhancement are derived [13]. These metrics are integral in differentiating between salvageable ischemic tissue (penumbra) and irreversibly infarcted tissue (core infarct), which guide treatment strategies and predict outcomes [14, 15].

An alternative approach to perfusion imaging is perfused blood volume mapping, which subtracts unenhanced CT images from CTA images to create blood volume maps of the entire brain. This technique offers the advantage of whole-brain coverage, facilitating global assessment of cerebral perfusion. However, its inability to quantify critical parameters like CBF and MTT limits its utility in identifying the ischemic penumbra. As a result, perfused blood volume mapping is less commonly employed in routine clinical practice [16].

Flat panel CT (FPCT) is increasingly used in the angiography suite, serving both diagnostic and interventional purposes. FPCT excels in generating high-resolution CBV maps, offering superior vascular and soft tissue visualization compared to conventional CTA techniques. It requires lower doses of contrast and provides slightly improved spatial resolution, which is especially beneficial for post-endovascular treatment follow-ups [17]. However, FPCT is less effective in detecting small blood volumes or early ischemic changes, and has difficulty measuring CBF due to the extended acquisition time required [18]. Nonetheless, innovations such as Dynamic CT (DynaCT, Siemens Medical Solutions) have expanded FPCT's utility. Unlike regular FPCT, Dynamic CT provides time-resolved imaging, enabling real-time assessment of blood flow dynamics. This high-resolution technique is particularly valuable for evaluating stent placement and assessing intracranial atherosclerotic disease [19–21].

In CTP, the infarct core is characterized by prolonged MTT and Time-to-maximum (Tmax; time to reach maximum contrast enhancement), markedly reduced CBF (<30%), and moderately decreased CBV (<40%). In contrast, the ischemic penumbra, which typically surrounds the infarct core, also demonstrates prolonged MTT and Tmax but is distinguished by only moderately reduced CBF and near-normal or even increased CBV due to autoregulatory vasodilation (Fig. 2) [16, 22, 23]. Notably, relying solely on CBF to visually assess the infarct core can lead to overestimation, as the penumbra may also exhibit reduced CBF. Therefore, MTT and CBV are considered safer parameters for visual assessment. Color-coded perfusion maps derived from deconvolution algorithms allow rapid identification of the penumbra. These maps are critical for determining whether thrombolysis or clot retrieval is warranted, balancing the risks and benefits of intervention. Refinements are ongoing to improve differentiation between benign oligemia (where CBF reductions recover without intervention) and true ischemic penumbra, with MTT showing promise as a distinguishing factor [24].

The combination of CTP with CTA provides robust data, enabling clinicians to rapidly identify obstructed vessel sites and assess tissue viability. Retrospective studies have highlighted CTP's superior accuracy in detecting infarct extension compared to non-CE CT and standard CTA imaging [25, 26]. Additionally, the correlation between MTT and thrombolytic therapy outcomes underscores the importance of perfusion imaging in guiding acute stroke management [27]. Nonetheless, while CTP has demonstrated significant benefits, delays in initiating reperfusion therapy due to advanced imaging requirements remain a concern. However, studies indicate that these delays do not adversely impact

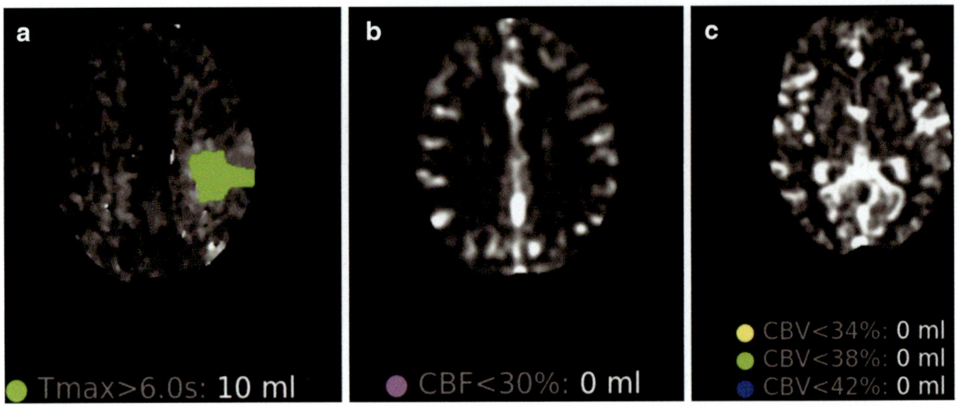

Fig. 2 A 75-year-old female sustained a right middle cerebral artery (MCA) stroke. CT perfusion maps (**a**: Tmax; **b**: CBF; **c**: CBV) demonstrate a large area of abnormally increased Tmax in the left lateral parietal area within the left MCA distribution (total volume of 10 mL), with preserved CBF and CBV. This is indicative of ischemic penumbra

clinical outcomes, hemorrhage rates, or final infarct volumes, supporting the continued integration of timely CTP imaging into acute stroke protocols [28, 29].

2.3 Single-Photon Emission Computed Tomography

SPECT is a functional imaging modality that employs a gamma-emitting radioisotope, such as technetium 99m, bound to a delivery agent like hexamethylpropyleneamine oxime (HMPAO) or ethyl cysteinate dimer (ECD) that enable its transport across the blood-brain barrier following intravenous injection. Once the isotope enters the brain tissue, it becomes metabolized and trapped within cells, with its uptake directly proportional to CBF at the time of administration [30, 31]. This feature allows imaging to be conducted for several hours post-injection.

Although SPECT provides valuable perfusion data, it does not directly quantify CBF unless combined with invasive techniques like an indwelling arterial line. As a result, a semiquantitative approach is often employed. This involves comparing the relative uptake of the radioisotope in the region of interest—typically the suspected ischemic area—to an unaffected control region. However, interpreting these comparisons can be challenging. For instance, patients with acute stroke often exhibit underlying chronic ischemia, which may hinder the differentiation between acute and chronic perfusion deficits. Additionally, dynamic fluctuations in CBF within unaffected regions may further complicate interpretation [32].

SPECT has demonstrated clinical utility in identifying both acute and chronic ischemic lesions and in detecting areas at risk of infarction (Fig. 3). The modality is particularly valuable in assessing the ischemic penumbra, especially in settings where advanced imaging options like CT and MR perfusion are unavailable [33]. Despite its reliance on semiquantitative data, SPECT exhibits good sensitivity and specificity for detecting ischemia [34]. In addition to its role in stroke detection, SPECT has been instrumental in identifying delayed neurological deficits caused by vasospasm after subarachnoid hemorrhage (SAH) [35, 36]. It is also employed to assess patient tolerance to hypoperfusion within specific vascular territories, aiding decisions regarding revascularization procedures [37, 38]. SPECT's practical advantages include its accessibility and cost-effectiveness compared to other functional imaging modalities like positron emission tomography (PET) or advanced MRI techniques. Most stroke centers are equipped with SPECT capabilities, and the preparation of injection kits is straightforward, allowing for rapid generation of perfusion maps in acute and chronic ischemia.

However, SPECT has limitations. Its non-anatomical representation of cerebral perfusion necessitates integration with CT or MRI for a comprehensive evaluation of vascular territories [32]. Recent technological advancements, such as hybrid imaging systems (e.g., SPECT/CT or SPECT/MRI), have further enhanced its diagnostic capabilities. These systems combine functional perfusion data with detailed anatomical imaging, facilitating precise localization of ischemic regions and improving diagnostic accuracy [39]. Additionally, semiquantitative data cannot be standardized across patients or institutions, limiting SPECT's generalizability and hindering the establishment of universal guidelines for radioisotope uptake. Furthermore, its spatial resolution is lower than that of modalities like PET or CTP, which may affect the precision of findings [40]. Ongoing advancements in radiopharmaceuticals and quantitative SPECT techniques hold promise for improving diagnostic accuracy and standardization [41]. For example, arterial input function modeling is emerging as a tool to enable more precise CBF quantification, enhancing the clinical applicability of SPECT. These developments highlight the evolving role of SPECT in the diagnosis and management of cerebral ischemia, particularly in resource-limited settings where its affordability and practicality make it indispensable.

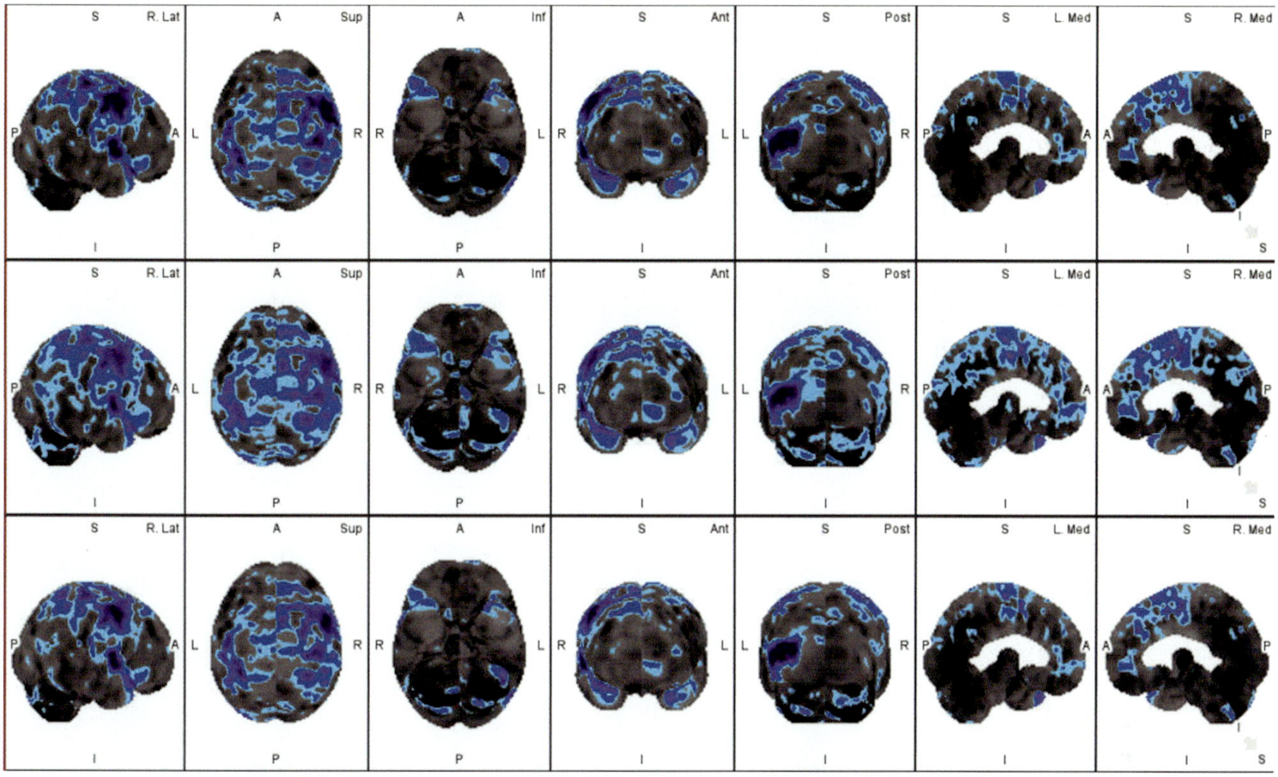

Fig. 3 A 49-year-old female with history of multiple prior strokes and known right carotid occlusion underwent SPECT imaging for evaluation of perfusion defect. Images were acquired 30 min after the injection of 27.4 mCI of radiolabeled cerebral perfusion agent (HMPAO), revealing decreased perfusion to the left temporal, parietal, and occipital lobes with preserved perfusion of the left frontal lobe, along with global decreased perfusion in the right cerebral hemisphere with preserved perfusion of the right occipital lobe. (L = left, R = right, Lat = lateral, Sup = superior, I = inferior, Post = posterior, Ant = anterior, Med = medial)

3 Magnetic Resonance Imaging-Based Techniques

MRI has revolutionized neurovascular imaging, offering unparalleled versatility for diagnosing and monitoring cerebrovascular conditions. Advances in high-field strength MRI, MRA technology, and postprocessing algorithms, have significantly enhanced image quality while reducing acquisition and processing time [42–44]. These improvements have enabled a detailed and noninvasive assessment of vascular anatomy and flow dynamics, making MRI an essential tool for evaluating cerebrovascular diseases.

3.1 Magnetic Resonance Angiography

MRA utilizes radiofrequency (RF) excitation pulses and magnetic gradients to visualize variations in proton spine. MRI depends on the application of repeated RF excitation pulses to a selected slice. Stationary tissues subjected to these pulses experience saturation, leading to reduced signal intensity. However, moving tissues, such as blood, are less affected by saturation, causing them to appear brighter in the resulting images. MRA employs three main approaches: time-of-flight (TOF), phase-contrast (PC), and CE MRA. TOF and PC techniques achieve direct visualization of blood vessels by exploiting the dynamic properties of flowing blood relative to surrounding static tissues. In contrast, CE MRA relies on intravenous contrast agents and does not depend on flow dynamics [45].

Time-of-Flight Imaging

TOF imaging operates on the principle of flow-related enhancement (FRE), where the movement of blood through a given section results in heightened signal intensity compared to surrounding stationary tissue. This technique relies on gradient-recalled echoes, producing hyperintense vessels that create "white blood" images [46]. There are two main modalities of TOF imaging: two-dimensional (2D) and 3D. The 2D TOF technique captures a single slice at a time, making it well-suited for regions with slow or complex flow. In contrast, 3D TOF acquires data from a volume or slab of tissue in a single pass, enabling higher spatial resolution and thinner slices (Fig. 4a). However, 3D TOF is susceptible to the "entry slice effect," where flow-related enhancement is most prominent in the initial slice but diminishes deeper into

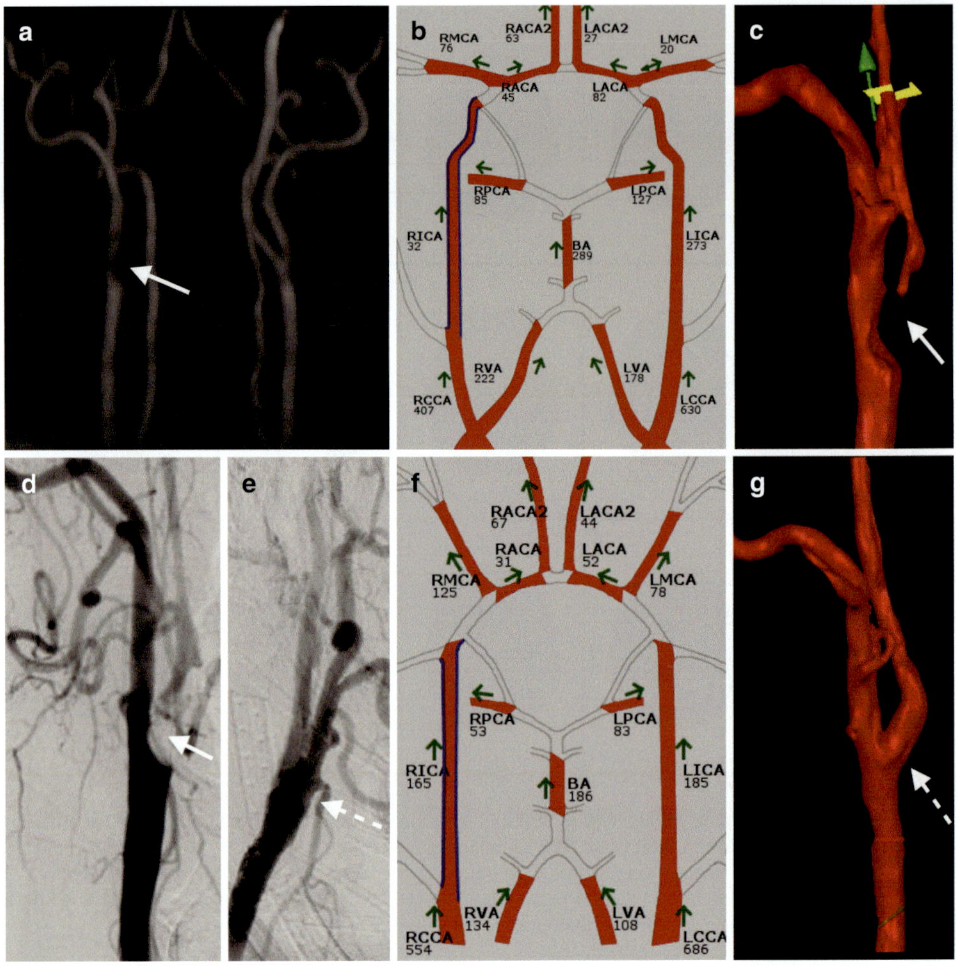

Fig. 4 A 65-year-old male presented with a right middle cerebral artery (MCA) ischemic stroke. (**a**) Time-of-flight magnetic resonance angiography (TOF MRA) revealed severe (90%) stenosis of the right internal carotid artery (ICA) at its origin. (**b**) Noninvasive Optimal Vessel Analysis (NOVA) quantitative MRA (QMRA) demonstrated markedly reduced flow in the right ICA (32 mL/min) compared to the left (273 mL/min). (**c**) A 3D anatomic reconstruction clearly depicted the right ICA stenosis. (**d**) Digital subtraction angiography (DSA) showing the pre-procedure severe ICA stenosis and (**e**) post-cerebral endarterectomy restoration of flow. (**f**, **g**) NOVA QMRA confirmed reconstitution of flow in the right ICA following the procedure

the slab as blood becomes progressively saturated. To address this limitation, specialized techniques such as multiple overlapping thin-slab angiography (MOTSA) have been developed to preserve signal intensity across slices [47, 48]. TOF imaging is most effective in areas with high blood flow velocities and when vessels are perpendicular to the imaging plane. However, it faces challenges in cases of slow or in-plane flow, often resulting in signal loss. In such cases, contrast agents can help increase signal intensity.

Phase-Contrast Imaging

PC imaging leverages both the magnitude and phase of MRI signals to quantify motion, including blood flow velocity and direction. This method involves acquiring two separate images: one with a bipolar gradient applied in a specific direction and another with the gradient reversed. Subtracting these images isolates phase differences caused by motion, allowing flowing blood to be distinguished from static tissue, making it appear hyperintense.

The ability of PC imaging to provide quantitative flow data is one of its most significant advantages. Flow velocity is encoded using velocity encoding (VENC), which corresponds to the velocity producing a 180-degree phase shift. By carefully selecting a VENC value slightly higher than the expected flow velocity, signal-to-noise ratio is maximized, and artifacts are minimized. This optimization enhances the accuracy and reliability of flow measurements. Quantitative phase-contrast MRA (QMRA) has become indispensable in neurovascular imaging due to its non-invasive measurement of volumetric blood flow. A landmark advancement in this field came in 2000 when Zhao et al. introduced a 3D localization technique that formed basis for the Noninvasive Optimal Vessel Analysis (NOVA) protocol developed by VasSol [49]. This protocol has become widely accepted for assessing intracranial blood flow. The QMRA process starts with the acquisition of axial 2D or 3D TOF MRA images, which are then transferred to a workstation with NOVA software. Using a marching cube algorithm, the software creates a 3D surface-rendering of the cerebral vasculature, including the CoW. A line-fitting algorithm determines the scan line for a double-oblique scan using gates 2D PC MRA, ensuring accurate flow measurement. The generated flow report provides detailed metrics, such as mean volumetric flow rates for each vessel of interest. While both 1.5-T and 3-T MRI units can perform PC MRA, the latter offers superior image quality and sensitivity, allowing better differentiation of small arteries and veins. In the context of cerebral ischemia, QMRA is valuable for assessing areas with compromised blood flow, such as stenosis or collateral circulation (Fig. 4). Additionally, it has proven particularly useful in detecting in-stent restenosis (ISR), as it is not affected by stent-related artifacts: a flow reduction of over 25% detected by QMRA can indicate early ISR, while reductions of 50% or greater are associated with symptomatic ISR [50, 51].

Despite its advantages, PC imaging faces challenges. Complex flow patterns at vascular branch points or sharp curvatures, and distal stenoses, can lead to signal loss. Additionally, the pulsatile nature of blood flow, especially in the intracranial circulation, may introduce artifacts. Cardiac cycle-triggered acquisition, which synchronizes image capture with specific phases of the cardiac cycle, helps reduce these motion artifacts and improves image quality.

Contrast-Enhanced Imaging

Unlike TOF and PC imaging, CE MRA relies on the intravenous administration of paramagnetic agents to shorten the T1 relaxation time of blood, thereby enhancing signal intensity. This approach is analogous to conventional x-ray angiography, where the blood vessels are visualized based on the filling of the lumen with contrast material, rather than relying on flow dynamics. CE MRA is particularly useful in scenarios involving slow flow, tortuous or branching vessels, or when detailed visualization of luminal surfaces and atherosclerotic plaque morphology is needed [52, 53]. By timing the contrast bolus with image acquisition, CE MRA achieves high spatial and temporal resolution, circumventing flow-related artifacts and offering a level of detail comparable to invasive angiographic techniques [54].

3.2 Magnetic Resonance Perfusion and Diffusion Imaging

MR perfusion imaging provides valuable insights into CBF through indirect measurements, helping assess neurovascular integrity. This technique is particularly essential for understanding brain perfusion dynamics in both acute and chronic ischemic conditions [55]. The procedure involves the intravenous injection of a gadolinium-based contrast agent into the antecubital vein at a rate of approximately 5 mL/s. The contrast bolus passes through the capillary bed of the brain, while a rapid gradient echo, echo planar imaging sequence captures multiple brain volumes during its first passage. The entire acquisition is completed in less than a minute, enabling real-time evaluation of perfusion dynamics. Temporal changes in signal intensity induced by the contrast agent are analyzed to generate perfusion parameter maps, including CBV, CBF, and MTT [55, 56].

MR perfusion imaging is particularly valuable for assessing functional brain tissue viability, making it indispensable in ischemic stroke management. It provides critical information about blood flow dynamics, allowing clinicians to identify areas of reduced perfusion. When combined with diffusion-weighted imaging (DWI), this approach achieves even greater diagnostic precision. DWI is an advanced MRI technique that measures water diffusion within brain tissue, making it highly sensitive to early cellular injury [57]. It identifies regions with cytotoxic edema, where restricted water diffusion corresponds to ischemic brain tissue. The integration of MR perfusion and DWI allows for a comprehensive evaluation of the ischemic cascade, facilitating the precise differentiation between the core infarct and the ischemic penumbra therapies [58, 59]. However, it is important to recognize that the DWI/MR perfusion combination can be time-consuming, especially for intubated or agitated patients where logistic challenges and motion artifacts may delay treatment. In such cases, CTP may offer a practical alternative. This underscores the importance of integrating clinical judgment with imaging modality selection in the time-sensitive context of cerebral ischemia.

3.3 Vessel Wall Imaging

VWI has emerged as a valuable non-invasive MRI technique for investigating plaque composition and the structural changes in arterial walls in intracranial vascular diseases. Unlike traditional imaging techniques that focus primarily on the lumen, VWI enables direct visualization of the vessel wall and atherosclerotic plaques, providing critical insights into their composition and stability [60]. This is particularly useful in detecting early-stage atherosclerosis, where traditional MRA or CTA may overlook subtle changes in intracranial arteries. By addressing this gap, VWI reduces reliance on invasive procedures like DSA while providing a detailed assessment of vessel pathology [61].

High-resolution imaging at 3T field strength has further enhanced VWI's diagnostic capabilities, especially for conditions such as moyamoya disease (MMD) [62, 63]. Its ability to provide detailed anatomical visualization alongside assessment of plaque burden, stenosis severity, collateral vessel development, and vascular remodeling makes it a powerful tool for evaluating cerebrovascular health. The non-invasive nature of VWI also facilitates monitoring of chronic cerebrovascular conditions, stroke risk stratification, and assessment of treatment efficacy [60, 61]. As precision imaging evolves (especially with the integration of ultra-high-field (7T) imaging), VWI is poised to revolutionize

62. Han C, Li M-L, Xu Y-y, Ye T, Xie C-F, Gao S, et al. Adult moyamoya-atherosclerosis syndrome: clinical and vessel wall imaging features. J Neurol Sci. 2016;369:181–4.
63. Kesav P, Krishnavadana B, Kesavadas C, Sreedharan SE, Rajendran A, Sukumaran S, et al. Utility of intracranial high-resolution vessel wall magnetic resonance imaging in differentiating intracranial vasculopathic diseases causing ischemic stroke. Neuroradiology. 2019;61:389–96.
64. Rutland JW, Delman BN, Gill CM, Zhu C, Shrivastava RK, Balchandani P. Emerging use of ultra-high-field 7T MRI in the study of intracranial vascularity: state of the field and future directions. AJNR Am J Neuroradiol. 2020;41(1):2–9.
65. Shaban S, Huasen B, Haridas A, Killingsworth M, Worthington J, Jabbour P, et al. Digital subtraction angiography in cerebrovascular disease: current practice and perspectives on diagnosis, acute treatment and prognosis. Acta Neurol Belg. 2022;122(3):763–80.
66. Cloft HJ, Joseph GJ, Dion JE. Risk of cerebral angiography in patients with subarachnoid hemorrhage, cerebral aneurysm, and arteriovenous malformation. Stroke. 1999;30(2):317–20.
67. Hankey GJ, Warlow CP, Molyneux AJ. Complications of cerebral angiography for patients with mild carotid territory ischaemia being considered for carotid endarterectomy. J Neurol Neurosurg Psychiatry. 1990;53(7):542–8.

Thoracic Outlet Syndrome, Subclavian Artery Transposition

Libor Janoušek, Jozef Kováč, Petra Dubská, Jaroslav Chlupáč, and Karol Sutoris

Abbreviations

ATOS	Arterial Thoracic Outlet Syndrome
DASH	Disabilities of the Arm, Shoulder, and Hand score
NSAIDs	Nonsteroidal Anti-Inflammatory Drugs
NTOS	Neurogenic Thoracic Outlet Syndrome
PTA	Percutaneous Transluminal Angioplasty
ROM	Range of Motion
TENS	Transcutaneous Electrical Nerve Stimulation
TOS	Thoracic Outlet Syndrome
VATS	Video-Assisted Thoracoscopic Surgery
VTOS	Venous Thoracic Outlet Syndrome

L. Janoušek (✉)
Transplantation Surgery Department, Institute for Clinical and Experimental Medicine, Prague, Czech Republic

First Faculty of Medicine, Charles University, Prague, Czech Republic
e-mail: lija@ikem.cz

J. Kováč
Radiodiagnostic and Interventional Radiology Department, Institute for Clinical and Experimental Medicine, Prague, Czech Republic
e-mail: joko@ikem.cz

P. Dubská · K. Sutoris
Transplantation Surgery Department, Institute for Clinical and Experimental Medicine, Prague, Czech Republic
e-mail: dubp@ikem.cz; sutk@ikem.cz

J. Chlupáč
Transplantation Surgery Department, Institute for Clinical and Experimental Medicine, Prague, Czech Republic

Department of Anatomy, Second Faculty of Medicine, Charles University, Prague, Czech Republic
e-mail: jacu@ikem.cz

1 Thoracic Outlet Syndrome

1.1 Introduction

Thoracic outlet syndrome (TOS) is a relatively rare syndrome (1–3 per 100,000) [1].

TOS was first characterized by Rob and Standeven in 1958. TOS is a nonspecific diagnosis representing many symptoms caused by the compression of the neurovascular structures that pass through the thoracic outlet. TOS is divided into four different types: a venous variant (VTOS), arterial (ATOS), traumatic, and true neurogenic (NTOS). The most common type is neurogenic thoracic outlet syndrome, accounting for over 90% of all. Patients from the 1958 study suffered from a wide range of symptoms, caused by venous, arterial, or nerve compression. These symptoms included pain, numbness, and paresthesia of the neck, upper back, and upper extremities. The thoracic outlet comprises three main structures: first rib, scalene muscles, and the clavicle with their fibrous tissues.

Both nonsurgical and surgical treatments are available to patients with TOS.

1.2 Epidemiology and Pathophysiology

Neurogenic TOS is the most common form of this syndrome, and it is diagnosed in patients between 30 and 40 years of age. Symptoms arise as a result of neck trauma, including falls, automobile accidents (resulting in hyperextension of the neck or a limb), and repetitive stress injuries caused by fibrous tissues [2].

Venous TOS is the second most common type, most frequently seen in people who do manual labor involving overhead work as well as in competitive athletes, swimmers, and bodybuilders. Risk factors include repetitive hyperabduction and extension of the arm resulting in compression of the tho-

V. Beneš, D. Netuka (eds.), *Surgical and Interventional Treatment of Cerebral Ischemia*,
https://doi.org/10.1007/978-3-032-08934-2_8

racic outlet. TOS will often become symptomatic when the patient reaches a hypercoagulable state. Patients typically present with VTOS at a young age. Axillo-subclavian thrombosis can be described in patients as old as 65 years. The prevalence is higher among men, typically affecting their dominant arm [3].

Arterial TOS is the result of congenital abnormalities (cervical rib, first rib, fibromatous tissues, and muscular bands). ATOS in the cervical rib affects up to 1% of the population, and 75% of such cases occur in women, 5% of patients who undergo surgery for TOS will have anomalous anatomy. ATOS remains the most common cause of acute arterial thrombosis of the upper extremities in patients younger than 40 years of age.

TOS manifests due to the compression of vascular and nervous structures in the thoracic outlet. Anatomic abnormalities are perpetrators of increased pressure and tissue changes in the region. Cervical ribs, which typically arise from the seventh cervical vertebrae, are one of the most common causes of thoracic outlet syndrome. Eighty five percent of neurogenic TOS is caused by abnormal ribs. Moreover, neck trauma often precedes NTOS.

Soft tissue components and anatomical abnormalities are also major contributors to TOS.

1.3 Prevention, Screening, and Diagnosis

TOS and tissue abnormalities cause repetitive stress injuries in the vascular wall and surrounding nerve bundle. Symptoms with a positive elevated arm test or Adson maneuver can facilitate diagnosis, especially with disappearance of the pulse wave.

While arterial and venous TOS are easily diagnosed with noninvasive imaging, diagnosing neurological TOS remains more difficult and controversial. Photoplethysmography and Doppler ultrasound are helpful in monitoring the radial artery when it is subjected to provocative maneuvers. For both arterial and venous TOS, duplex ultrasound examinations, especially when combined with provocative maneuvers, can consistently demonstrate anatomic compression of vascular structures. Computed tomography and magnetic resonance imaging can identify aneurysmal degeneration of the subclavian artery and anatomy while simultaneously providing visualization of the contralateral thoracic outlet. These diagnostic procedures can also verify subclavian vascular thrombosis. Magnetic resonance can identify an abnormal attachment of muscles and other soft tissue structure abnormalities, which cause brachial plexus compression. Electrophysiology and nerve conduction testing can detect chronic neurologic changes in small hand muscles and diminished amplitude of the ulnar nerve. Not all patients with symptoms of TOS experience changes in nerve structure. Traditional electrophysiological assessment provides little diagnostic value.

1.4 Relevant Anatomy of the Thoracic Outlet

TOS presents a complex anatomical challenge for surgeons, and treating it requires detailed knowledge of the neurovascular structures and their potential compression points. This chapter examines the critical anatomical structures targeted during surgical intervention for TOS. The superior opening of the bony thorax is commonly referred to as the thoracic outlet. The proper anatomical term "superior thoracic aperture" and "thoracic outlet" will be used in the text interchangeably to describe the regional anatomy.

1.4.1 Anatomical Boundaries of the Thoracic Outlet

The thoracic outlet region is located within the lower neck, just above and behind the clavicle. This region can be described as a confined and dynamic space through which critical neurovascular structures (subclavian vessels and brachial plexus) must pass from the central origins in the central thorax through the axilla to their peripheral termini in the upper extremity. A thorough understanding of its boundaries is essential for successful surgical decompression.

More accurately, the thoracic outlet is bounded by the clavicle anteriorly, the first thoracic rib posteriorly, the insertion of the pectoralis minor muscle to the coracoid process of the scapula laterally, and the sternum medially [4, 5]. It consists of three clinically significant topographic areas that comprise potential compression sites and surgical targets:

1. **Interscalene triangle** (i.e., scalene triangle, scalene fissure)—above the clavicle;
2. **Costoclavicular space** (cervicoaxillary canal)—between the clavicle and first rib; and
3. **Subcoracoid space** (i.e., pectoralis minor, subpectoral, retropectoral) space—below the clavicle.

Anatomical variations and anomalies are common in this thoracic outlet region, and they may predispose individuals to compression of the neurovascular bundle, leading to the development of TOS itself. Many of these variations can be attributed to the embryologic origins of the structures forming the thoracic outlet. Therefore, a thorough understanding of both the anatomy and embryology of this region is essential for identifying clinical manifestation of TOS.

Arterial (ATOS) and neurogenic (NTOS) forms are typically caused by a narrowing of the interscalene or costoclavicular spaces, often involving the anterior and middle scalene muscles or the first rib. In venous TOS (VTOS), compression occurs within the anterior costoclavicular space, involving structures such as the anterior scalene muscle, first rib, costocoracoid ligament, and subclavius tendon. Additionally, compression in the subcoracoid space, beneath the pectoralis minor muscle, can result in so-called pectoralis minor syndrome.

1.4.2 Interscalene Triangle: Primary Compression Site

The interscalene triangle is considered one of the principal sites for nerve and blood vessel compression, which leads to TOS. Therefore, this site is a critical anatomical focal point for TOS surgery [5–7]. This space is formed by the following:

- Anterior scalene muscle anteriorly: originating from the cervical spine vertebrae and running vertically to the top of the anterior first rib;
- Middle scalene muscle posteriorly: originating from the cervical vertebrae and attaching to the top of the mid-portion of the first rib; and
- First rib inferiorly: forms the base of the triangle.

Directly behind the scalene fat pad (a thick fatty layer in the lower neck) lies the anterior scalene muscle. The narrow vertical space between the anterior and middle scalene muscles, with the first rib at the base, creates the scalene triangle through which the brachial plexus and subclavian artery pass [4]. The subclavian vein, however, runs anterior to this compartment, which is an important distinction for surgical planning [7].

1.4.3 Costoclavicular Space: Secondary Compression Site

The costoclavicular space is one of three main anatomical regions involved in TOS, where neurovascular structures can become compressed. Its boundaries are the following:

- Clavicle anteriorly;
- First rib posteriorly;
- Costoclavicular ligament (rhomboid ligament, Halsted's ligament) medially: attached below to the upper and medial part of the cartilage of the first rib. It ascends at an angle posteriorly and laterally, and is fixed above to the costal tuberosity on the inferior aspect of the clavicle; and
- Subclavius muscle laterally: a small triangular muscle, placed between the clavicle and the first rib (part of anterior wall of the axilla) [4].

This space is particularly important because it comprises the brachial plexus, subclavian artery, and subclavian vein. Compression in this region, often due to poor posture, trauma, or repetitive overhead activities, can contribute to neurological and vascular symptoms in TOS [5, 6].

1.4.4 Subcoracoid Space: Tertiary Compression Site

The subcoracoid space is another topographic region where TOS can occur, particularly pectoralis minor syndrome. The boundaries of the subcoracoid space comprise the following:

- Pectoralis minor muscle anteriorly: arising from the upper margins and ventral surfaces of the third, fourth, and fifth ribs near their costal cartilages, and from the aponeuroses covering the intercostalis spaces. Its tendon is attached to the medial border and cranial surface of the coracoid process of the scapula;
- Ribs and anterior scapula posteriorly;
- Coracoid process of the scapula superiorly; and
- Upper ribs inferiorly [4].

This space is clinically significant because compression of the brachial plexus, subclavian artery, or axillary vein beneath the pectoralis minor muscle can lead to neurovascular symptoms similar to those of TOS. In addition to the above-mentioned causes, hypertrophy of the pectoralis minor muscle can also play a role in compression [5, 6].

1.4.5 Neurovascular Structures at Risk

Understanding the precise arrangement of neurovascular structures is crucial for safe and effective surgical treatment of TOS.

The brachial plexus passes through the interscalene triangle, positioned posteriorly and laterally to the subclavian artery. It then continues through the costoclavicular space and subcoracoid space. The anatomy of the brachial plexus can vary significantly, with prefixed and postfixed plexuses potentially associated with cervical or first rib anomalies. During embryological development, the brachial plexus, in effect, separates what was once a common scalene muscle into the anterior and middle components, which would explain why anatomical variations are common in this region [4].

The subclavian artery passes posteriorly to the anterior scalene muscle and through the scalene triangle alongside the brachial plexus. Meanwhile, the subclavian vein passes anteriorly to the anterior scalene muscle and does not traverse the interscalene triangle [6]. All of these structures then pass underneath the clavicle through the costoclavicular space.

After passing through the costoclavicular space, the vessels continue through the subcoracoid space, where the subclavian artery and vein become the axillary artery and vein, respectively [5].

1.4.6 Common Anatomical Variations, Anomalies, and Contributing Factors

Surgical decompression for TOS often targets anatomical anomalies that predispose the region to neurovascular compression. Various congenital or acquired anatomical abnormalities can further compromise the thoracic outlet; this would come in the form of the presence of a cervical rib, congenital soft tissue abnormalities, long C7 transverse process, fibrous bands or muscular anomalies (e.g., a broad scalene attachment or hypertrophied scalenes), clavicular hypomobility, scoliosis or elevated scapula, and functionally acquired anatomical changes [7–9]. From a developmental and functional perspective, it is best to distinguish between muscular, osseous, and connective tissue anomalies (fibrous bands).

In the 1970s, a pioneering surgeon named David Roos developed a classification system for anomalous structures within the thoracic outlet, which eventually expanded to include up to 14 variants [10]. However, significant overlap between individual classifications and other anatomical descriptions led to its decline. The system was ultimately deemed overly complex and of uncertain relevance to clinical or surgical treatment.

In the 8th gestational week, the scalene muscles develop from a common scalene muscle, which is later separated into distinct components by the brachial plexus. This developmental pattern explains the high frequency of muscular variations in this region [4, 10]:

- Interdigitating muscle fibers that connect the anterior and middle scalene muscles in 75% of dissections of TOS patients, creating a sling that traps the brachial plexus and subclavian artery (Type 4 band of Roos);
- Scalenus minimus: a supernumerary muscle passing between the subclavian artery and brachial plexus, potentially irritating the lower trunk; and
- Scalenus pleuralis: this may present as a residual ligament rather than a true muscle [1].

An abnormally anterior insertion of the anterior scalene muscle may compress the subclavian vein against the subclavius tendon, a situation particularly relevant in venous TOS [4]. A rare accessory muscle slip (Langer's arch) can compress the distal axillary structures.

Cervical ribs, which are supernumerary ribs arising from the C7 vertebra, occur in approximately 0.5–1% of the population. Their presence tightens the scalene triangle and elevates the thoracic outlet, forcing the subclavian artery and brachial plexus to ascend over the supernumerary rib [4, 9].

The following fibrous bands can contribute to TOS and require surgical attention:

- Outlet bands: ligamentous bands extending from the neck of the first rib to its inner surface;
- Roos' bands: classification system of various fibromuscular connections, with Types 1, 3, 5 and 11 being the most common [4, 9–11].

1.5 Conservative Management of TOS

Conservative management remains the first-line treatment for the majority of TOS, with a focus on relieving symptoms through non-surgical interventions. This chapter explores various conservative approaches, including physical therapy, lifestyle modifications, and medical interventions, aimed at effectively managing TOS and improving patient quality of life.

1.5.1 Physical Therapy

Physical therapy is a cornerstone of conservative treatment for TOS. A well-designed rehabilitation program targets postural correction, muscle imbalances, and nerve mobilization. Key components include the following:

- **Postural training**: patients are educated on proper posture to minimize compression of the thoracic outlet. Techniques such as scapular retraction exercises and ergonomic modifications are emphasized;
- **Stretching exercises**: gentle stretching of the scalene muscles, pectoralis minor, and surrounding soft tissues helps alleviate tension and improve mobility;
- **Strengthening exercises**: strengthening the trapezius, rhomboids, and serratus anterior enhances scapular stability and reduces strain on the brachial plexus;
- **Nerve gliding techniques**: mobilization exercises aid in reducing nerve entrapment and improving neural conductivity [12–16].

1.5.2 Lifestyle Modifications

Lifestyle changes play a critical role in symptom management. Patients are advised to take part in the following:

- **Ergonomic adjustments**: modifying workspaces, adjusting chair height, and using ergonomic keyboards can prevent exacerbation of symptoms;
- **Activity modification**: avoiding repetitive overhead movements and heavy lifting reduces strain on the thoracic outlet; and
- **Weight management**: maintaining a healthy body weight decreases mechanical compression and inflammation.

1.5.3 Medical Interventions & Adjunct Therapies

Conservative management may also involve pharmacological and adjunct therapies, and include the following:

- **Pain management**: nonsteroidal anti-inflammatory drugs (NSAIDs) and muscle relaxants can help alleviate discomfort;
- **Physical modalities**: heat therapy, ultrasound, and transcutaneous electrical nerve stimulation (TENS) can provide symptom relief; and
- **Manual therapy**: soft tissue manipulation and myofascial release techniques may be incorporated to improve circulation and reduce muscle tightness.

Studies have assessed the effectiveness of various conservative treatments, including multidisciplinary care, orthosis application, and exercise programs [17–20]. The outcomes of such treatment have ranged from subjective satisfaction to objective improvements in range of motion (ROM) and grip strength. Key outcome criteria included the following:

- Symptom relief, compliance with exercise, and recurrence of symptoms;
- Reduction in work disability, pain relief, and functional improvement; and
- Sensory and motor disturbances, ability to perform daily activities, and return to work rates.

A suitable combination of exercise, orthosis application, and a multidisciplinary approach yields positive results. Although orthotic use may provide benefits, its long-term comfort and impact on quality of life remain a concern. Patient education is essential in fostering adherence to rehabilitation programs and encouraging active participation in recovery. A multidisciplinary strategy that involves various healthcare professionals can optimize treatment effectiveness and improve patient outcomes [21]. In regards to conservative TOS management, future research should focus on refining treatment protocols, ensuring homogeneous sample selection, and investigating long-term treatment efficacy. Additionally, research should aim to identify the most effective therapeutic methods in order to minimize treatment duration while maximizing long-term relief and functional recovery.

1.6 Endovascular Treatment of TOS

Endovascular reconstruction of the subclavian artery can be used to prevent downstream sequelae of arterial or venous thoracic outlet syndrome (A/VTOS), which include functional impairment and even amputation due to distal arterial embolization. Catheter-directed therapy may be performed either as an adjunct to open surgery or after it, to identify and treat subclavian arterial or venous pathology (as shown in Figs. 1, 2, 3, 4, and 5). Clinical data demonstrate that initial endovascular treatment, proposed as first-line therapy for highly symptomatic patients or those with failed conservative management, improves symptoms in approximately 75% of cases, thereby avoiding the need for acute surgery. In cases where local thrombolytic therapy leads to suboptimal recanalization, the procedure is followed by percutaneous balloon angioplasty (PTA).

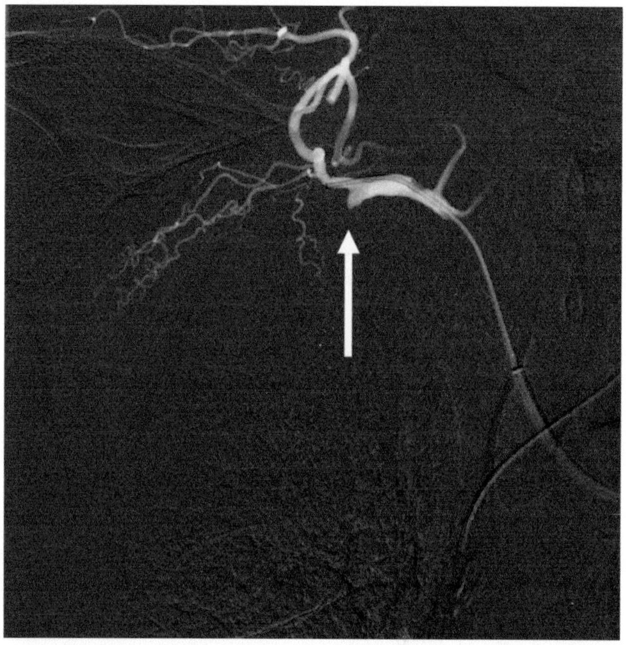

Fig. 1 Arterial TOS—right subclavian artery thrombosis (digital subtraction angiography finding)

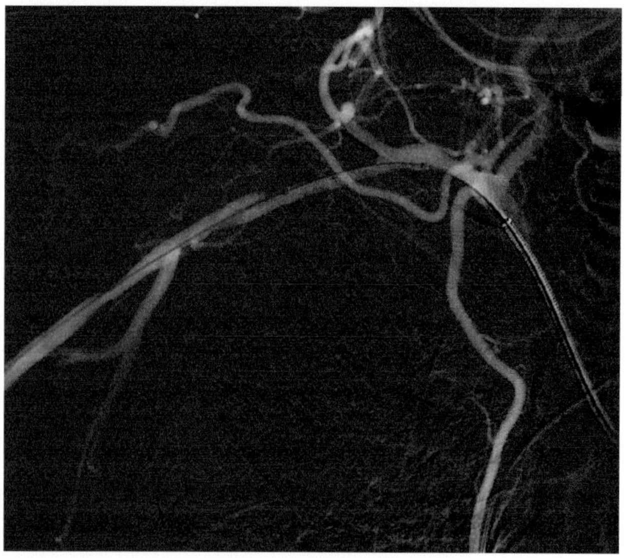

Fig. 2 Right subclavian artery percutaneous angioplasty

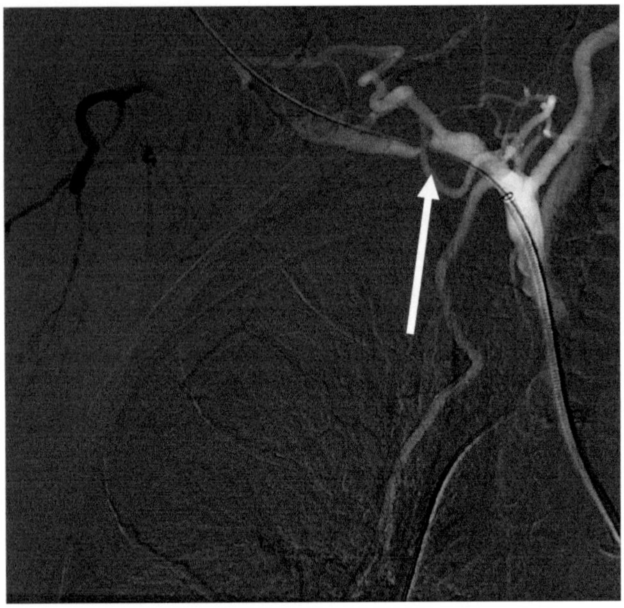

Fig. 3 Right upper limb elevated (digital subtraction angiography finding): recurrent ATOS (patient underwent acute first rib resection)

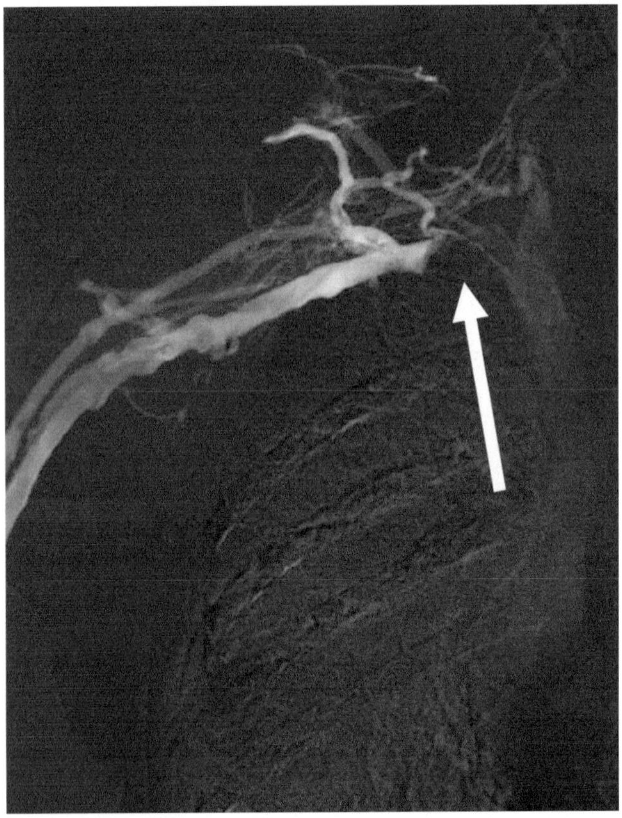

Fig. 4 Venous TOS—right subclavian vein thrombosis (digital subtraction angiography finding)

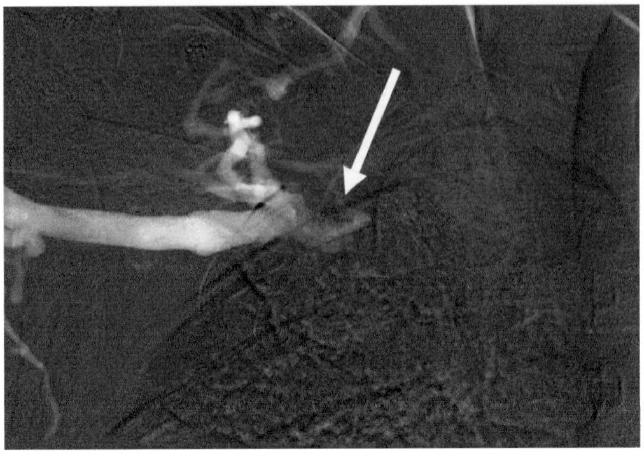

Fig. 5 Right upper limb elevated (digital subtraction angiography finding): recurrent VTOS (patient underwent first rib resection)—1-month follow-up

1.7 Surgical Treatment of TOS

Surgery for TOS consists of decompression of the anterior shoulder region, usually with resection of the first rib. TOS surgery outcome is dependent on appropriate patient selection. The current consensus suggests that surgery should take place only after conservative treatment fail or in cases of vascular complications [12–14].

Several surgical techniques have been described for the treatment of TOS. The transaxillary and supraclavicular approaches are most commonly employed for resection of the first rib and scalene muscles. In recent years, the development of advanced technologies—such as endoscopic or robotic-assisted first rib resection as well as arthroscopic pectoralis minor release—has helped overcome some of the limitations associated with traditional methods [22]. However, despite ongoing debate, there is currently no definitive evidence supporting the superiority of one surgical approach over another. This report examines the various surgical approaches for TOS management, comparing their long-term outcomes, complications, and overall efficacy.

1.7.1 Transaxillary Approach

The transaxillary approach is one of the most commonly utilized techniques for TOS decompression. This approach involves accessing the first rib between the pectoralis major and latissimus dorsi muscles in the axilla, with the patient positioned laterally [6]. The assistant holds the patient's arm using a wrist lock position for stability and to minimize fatigue. Another way to achieve this proper position is with the aid of the Machleder retractor TRIMANO FORTIS Support Arm [23].

The incision is made between the pectoralis major and latissimus dorsi muscles, just below the axillary hair line [22], allowing for quick and straightforward access to the first rib and anterior scalene muscle without the need for muscle dissection. Using electrocautery, the anterior and middle scalene muscles are carefully dissected from their attachments on the first rib. The rib is then elevated from the underlying pleura and resected using a rongeur, oscillating micro-saw, or rib cutter to minimize the risk of pleural injury. Optimal visualization is achieved with the assistance of lighted retractors and a surgical headlight [24]. Additionally, this technique results in a cosmetically favorable incision.

This approach offers several advantages. A study comparing various approaches found that transaxillary first rib resections resulted in shorter post-operative hospital stays and fewer complications when compared to more invasive approaches like the transthoracic method [25]. However, this procedure has its limitations in terms of exposure and visualization.

One critical factor affecting long-term outcomes of the transaxillary approach is the completeness of the first rib resection [26, 27]. The presence of a long posterior first rib stump was the strongest predictor of poor long-term results, with reoperation being necessary in selected cases where the stump required removal [26, 27].

1.7.2 Supraclavicular Approach

The supraclavicular approach provides direct access to the brachial plexus and allows for thorough decompression.

A scalenotomy via the supraclavicular approach (with or without first rib resection) is performed through a transverse incision 1–2 cm superior to the clavicle, followed by dissection of the platysma. The lateral head of the sternocleidomastoid muscle and the scalene fat pad are carefully dissected to preserve the supraclavicular nerve. Once exposed, the scalene muscles and brachial plexus are explored. Anterior and middle scalenectomies are performed using electrocautery, often followed by first rib resection. The supraclavicular approach offers superb access when performing neurolysis, as well as for resection of the scalene muscles, fibrous bands, first rib, and any cervical rib, if present [22].

Compared to the transaxillary approach, the supraclavicular approach offers superior visualization and direct access to the thoracic outlet structures within a shallow operative field, enhancing both the safety and feasibility of performing a scalenectomy. Therefore, some evidence suggests the supraclavicular approach may be superior to the transaxillary method. A comparative study found that "the supraclavicular approach seems to be the more effective technique of the two because it offers the surgeon better access to the brachial plexus and a direct view" [27, 28]. These studies also reported that the supraclavicular approach resulted in more favorable surgical outcomes and lower reoperation rates when compared to transaxillary procedures [27, 28].

The supraclavicular approach is particularly advantageous when large abnormal bony structures, neurologic symptoms, and/or severe limb ischemia are present [29].

1.7.3 Infraclavicular Approach

This approach is primarily utilized in the management of VTOS, which is typically diagnosed through venography, computed tomography, or ultrasonography to detect stenosis or thrombosis of the axillary-subclavian vein, as seen in conditions such as Paget-Schroetter syndrome (effort thrombosis). This technique requires a scalenectomy of the middle and anterior scalene muscles to expose the first rib [6, 22].

The transverse incision is made 1–2 cm below the clavicle. The pectoralis major muscle is either preserved or released from the clavicle to access the subclavian muscle, which is then excised. This exposes the subclavian vein and the first rib for further exploration. The infraclavicular approach enables resection of the subclavian muscle, the anterior portion of the first rib, the costoclavicular ligament, and the anterior scalene muscle—all potential sources of subclavian vein compression. This technique offers excellent exposure of the subclavian vein within a shallow operative field, facilitating subclavian venolysis and reconstruction when necessary. Additionally, by extending the infraclavicular incision, a pectoralis minor tenotomy can be performed to address pectoralis minor syndrome.

While the infraclavicular approach offers convenient access to the anterior aspect of the costoclavicular space, it provides limited exposure to the posterior portion of the first rib and the middle scalene muscle. As a result, performing neurolysis through this approach is challenging, making it less suitable for the treatment of NTOS. Therefore, exclusive application of the infraclavicular approach is typically reserved for managing VTOS or pectoralis minor syndrome. From a cosmetic standpoint, the infraclavicular incision is generally more favorable than the supraclavicular incision though it is not as aesthetically discreet as the incision employed in the transaxillary approach [22].

1.7.4 Other Surgical Approaches

Although not applied very often, there are several other approaches for TOS decompression [22]:

- Posterior approach: via a longitudinal periscapular incision between the spinous processes and the medial border of the scapula; rarely implemented as an initial operation (limited to reoperations);
- Combined approaches: these include transaxillary with supraclavicular or supraclavicular with infraclavicular (paraclavicular);

- Endoscopic-assisted transaxillary approach (arthroscopic): technically demanding;
- Transthoracic approach: less commonly implemented than transaxillary procedures due to higher complication rates and longer operative time [25];
- Video-assisted thoracoscopic surgery (VATS) & robotic-assisted first rib resection: with/without robotic assistance, involves opening the pleural cavity, placement of a pleural drain is required—considered a disadvantage of this approach; and limiting its use to thoracic surgeons with advanced training and expertise in the procedure [22, 30, 31].

1.7.5 Overall Success Rates

Surgical treatment for TOS provides generally favorable long-term functional outcomes across the various approaches. A multicenter retrospective cohort study with follow-ups ranging from 1 to 11 years found that complete relief of symptoms was reported postoperatively in 54% of patients, with symptoms improving in 90% [32].

A meta-analysis summarizing outcomes from multiple studies showed that improvement to Derkash's classification category excellent/good was achieved in 90% of the arterial and venous TOS groups [32]. The same analysis demonstrated a 28.3 point improvement in the Disabilities of the Arm, Shoulder, and Hand (DASH) score after surgical treatment for neurogenic TOS.

Studies with longer follow-up periods continue to show positive results. One study with follow-ups ranging from 11 to 21 years found that 80–90% of patients reported sustained recovery with minor or no residual symptoms and normal working ability [33]. Although 51.9% of these patients had some level of residual symptoms, most were willing to undergo surgery again if given the choice [33].

When directly comparing the transaxillary and supraclavicular approaches, there are no significant differences in average operative time (151.3 ± 54.1 min versus 126.1 ± 36.1 min) or length of hospital stay (2.3 ± 1.9 days versus 2.4 ± 1.4 days) between the groups [34].

In terms of symptom resolution, the same study reported that 49% of patients experienced complete resolution of symptoms, 46% had partial improvement, and 5% had no improvement; there were no differences in symptom resolution between either approach [34].

However, some evidence suggests differences in specific outcomes. A separate study found that persistent pain and symptoms were significantly more common in patients who underwent the transaxillary approach. There were also more permanent and transient brachial plexus injuries in the cases than in those of the supraclavicular approach; however, the difference was not statistically significant [27].

1.7.6 Complications Across Surgical Approaches

The risk of serious complications from TOS surgery is generally low. A multicenter retrospective cohort study reported no 30-day mortality, with reoperation due to bleeding in only 1.8% of patients, and 9% of patients developing pneumothorax [32].

As for immediate complications, the prevalence of opening the pleural cavity and/or pneumothorax, hemothorax, and vessel injuries appears to be identical for both the transaxillary and supraclavicular approaches [27]. Minor complications are reported in about 6% of patients regardless of approach, with major complications occurring at an identical rate (6%) [34].

Brachial plexus injury after first rib resection does occur, but reports vary widely across studies. In a multi-institution database study, brachial plexus injuries were reported in only 0.6% of patients with neurogenic TOS following transaxillary first rib resection [6]. However, another study reported a brachial plexus injury prevalence of 9% and 4% after transaxillary and supraclavicular first rib resection, respectively [6].

1.7.7 Factors Affecting Long-Term Surgical Outcomes

Among the factors influencing long-term results, the following are worth mentioning:

- TOS type: vascular forms have better outcomes than neurogenic types;
- Timing: early surgery (≤3 months) leads to more favorable results;
- Technique: complete resection of the first rib is critical; residual rib stumps are linked to recurrence; and
- Patient factors: poorly defined neurological symptoms, depression, or misdiagnoses may impede surgical success.

The type of TOS appears to affect surgical outcomes significantly. Functional outcomes as measured by DASH scores are typically better in vascular forms of TOS (arterial and venous) when compared to neurogenic TOS [6, 32]. A meta-analysis found clinical success rates of ≥90% for patients with vascular forms of TOS and 60–80% for those with neurogenic TOS [32].

Evidence suggests that early treatment (≤3 months) could result in better functional outcomes than could be achieved with delayed treatment (>6 months). This benefit may be due to the prevention of further nerve degeneration and muscle wasting caused by prolonged compression at the thoracic outlet [32].

Completeness of first rib resection is crucial for long-term success. A study with a mean follow-up of 99 months found that the presence of a long posterior first rib stump, identified and evaluated through a chest X-ray, was the strongest determinant of long-term results [26]. When patients with recurring symptoms underwent reoperation to remove the remaining rib stump, the results were excellent in all cases [26].

Certain patient factors appear to influence outcomes. Patients suffering from poorly systematized neurological symptoms in the arm tend to have less favorable results and should be either denied surgery or made aware that postoperative results might be disappointing [29]. Additionally, impediments to successful outcomes include major depression or comorbid conditions that can skew an initial diagnosis [6].

1.7.8 Persistent Functional Impairment

Despite generally positive outcomes, it is important to note that some degree of functional impairment often persists even after successful TOS surgery. A study using the QuickDASH questionnaire found that TOS patients continue to experience a higher degree of functional impairment when compared to the general population despite surgical treatment. While most patients reported improvement in their symptoms, only 39% had a mean QuickDASH score of 10 or lower (comparable to that of the general population) [32].

At 6 months post-surgery, one study found that 53% of patients with arterial TOS continued to express at least mild complaints related to the hand, arm, and shoulder [35].

1.7.9 Conclusion

The evidence suggests that surgical decompression for TOS is beneficial to most patients, with clinical improvement reported in up to 90% of cases and complete symptom resolution in approximately 50–60% of patients. Long-term outcomes remain favorable, with 80–90% of patients reporting sustained recovery even 10–20 years after surgery.

While no single surgical approach has definitively proven superior to all others, each treatment offers distinct advantages. The supraclavicular approach provides superior visualization and access to the brachial plexus, potentially resulting in better outcomes for NTOS. The transaxillary approach may offer reduced hospital stays and is preferred by many surgeons for first rib resections due to its lower complication rates when compared to more invasive approaches.

Emerging robotic-assisted and minimally invasive techniques show promise in reducing complications (particularly brachial plexus injuries) while maintaining favorable outcomes. However, these approaches require specialized training and equipment.

A specific surgical approach should be selected based on the type of TOS, patient anatomy, the need for additional procedures, and required level of surgical expertise. Regardless of the approach, a complete first rib resection appears to be a key factor in ensuring long-term success and preventing symptom recurrences.

2 Subclavian Artery Transposition

2.1 Introduction

Subclavian artery transposition is typically indicated for symptomatic isolated proximal occlusive lesions of the subclavian arteries. Moreover, reconstruction of the subclavian artery is increasingly employed to maintain perfusion to the vertebral circulation and the left upper extremity, while simultaneously extending the proximal neck landing zone in preparation for thoracic aortal endograft deployment.

This technique not only ensures preservation of upper limb, vertebral, and internal mammary artery flow, but proximal ligation of the subclavian artery also serves to reduce the risk of type II endoleaks (retrograde filling via a culprit branch vessel).

2.2 Surgical Procedure

Cervical reconstruction is typically performed via a transverse cervical incision placed superior to the clavicle. Meticulous dissection is essential to avoid injury to the external jugular vein. The common carotid artery is mobilized medially, in conjunction with the vagus nerve, as reflected in Fig. 6. On the left side, the thoracic duct and associated lymphatic vessels are identified, ligated, and divided to prevent chyle leak. The subclavian artery and its proximal branches are dissected posterior to the clavicle. Adequate control of the vertebral and internal mammary arteries is imperative. Particular care must be taken to preserve surrounding sympathetic nerve fibers and avoid iatrogenic injury.

Once proximal control is achieved, the subclavian artery is transected and an end-to-side anastomosis is created with the common carotid artery. In situations where direct arterial transposition is not technically feasible due to anatomical or pathological constraints, a prosthetic bypass conduit may be utilized as an alternative revascularization strategy (the resulting angiographic finding is shown in Fig. 7). Novel bioengineered vascular grafts [36] and innovative patency surveillance strategies [37] are currently under investigation.

In selected cases, the operating surgeon may choose not to revascularize the left subclavian artery, opting instead to deploy either the covered or bare-wire segment of the stent-

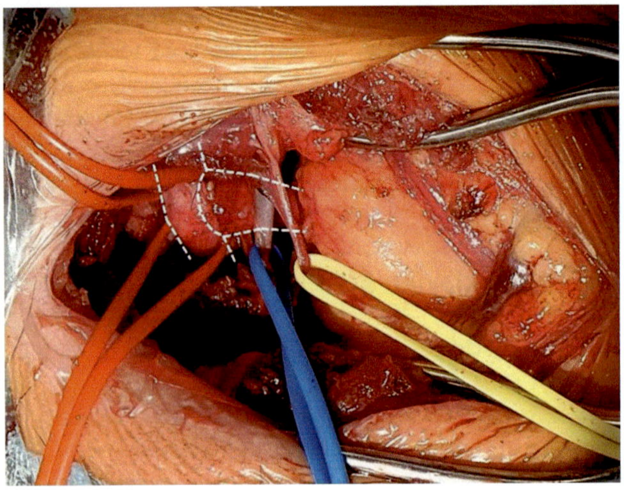

Fig. 6 Subclavian artery transposition to the common carotid artery on the left side performed using a supraclavicular approach and an end-to-side anastomosis. This prophylactic procedure was conducted prior to the deployment of a thoracic aorta endograft covering the left subclavian artery. Red rubber loops indicate the common carotid artery, the blue rubber loop indicates the internal jugular vein, and the yellow rubber loop indicates the phrenic nerve. (Courtesy of Dr. Jaroslav Chlupáč, MD, PhD, IKEM, Prague, Czech Republic)

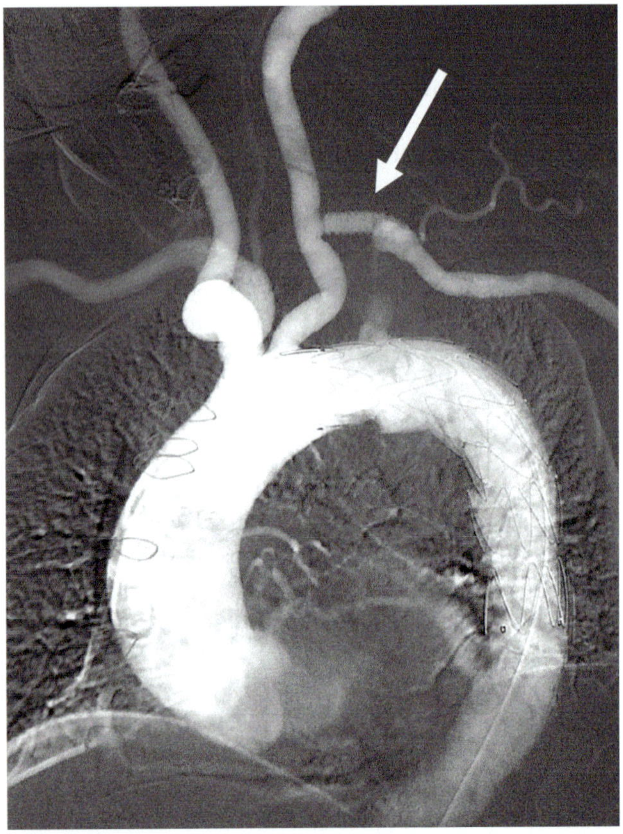

Fig. 7 Carotico-subclavian by pass (on the left side), preserving mammary artery and preventing upper limb ischemia, done prior to endograft deployment in the thoracic aorta (digital subtraction angiography finding)

graft across its origin, depending on the clinical context and device design itself.

Acknowledgements Supported by the project National Institute for Research of Metabolic and Cardiovascular Diseases (Programme EXCELES, ID Project No. LX22NPO5104)—Funded by the European Union—Next Generation EU and by the Ministry of Health of the Czech Republic (Grant No. NW24J-02-00061, Grant No. NW24-09-00184). All rights reserved.

Supported by the grant reg. No. FW10010514 funded by the Technology Agency of the Czech Republic

Supported by the project reg. No. G 9053-Funded by the Institutional Support for Long-term Conceptual Development of the IKEM, research organization

We wish to thank Brian Kavalir for his copy-editing services.

Declarations

Competing Interests The author(s) has no competing interests to declare that are relevant to the content of this manuscript.

Ethics Approval The author(s) declares that this manuscript does not include primary research with human participants.

References

1. Illig KA, Rodriguez-Zoppi E. How common is thoracic outlet syndrome? Thorac Surg Clin. 2021;31(1):11–7.
2. Chang DC, Lidor AO, Matsen SL, Freischlag JA. Reported in-hospital complications following rib resections for neurogenic thoracic outlet syndrome. Ann Vasc Surg. 2007;21(5):564–70.
3. Freischlag J, Orion K. Understanding thoracic outlet syndrome. Scientifica (Cairo). 2014;2014:248163.
4. Connolly MR, Auchincloss HG. Anatomy and embryology of the thoracic outlet. Thorac Surg Clin. 2021;31(1):1–10.
5. Camporese G, Bernardi E, Venturin A, Pellizzaro A, Schiavon A, Caneva F, Strullato A, Toninato D, Forcato B, Zuin A, Squizzato F, Piazza M, Stramare R, Tonello C, Di Micco P, Masiero S, Rea F, Grego F, Simioni P. Diagnostic and therapeutic management of the thoracic outlet syndrome. Review of the literature and report of an Italian experience. Front Cardiovasc Med. 2022;9:802183.
6. Jones MR, Prabhakar A, Viswanath O, Urits I, Green JB, Kendrick JB, Brunk AJ, Eng MR, Orhurhu V, Cornett EM, Kaye AD. Thoracic outlet syndrome: a comprehensive review of pathophysiology, diagnosis, and treatment. Pain Ther. 2019;8(1):5–18.
7. Hooper TL, Denton J, McGalliard MK, Brismée JM, Sizer PS Jr. Thoracic outlet syndrome: a controversial clinical condition. Part 1: anatomy, and clinical examination/diagnosis. J Man Manip Ther. 2010;18(2):74–83.
8. Li N, Dierks G, Vervaeke HE, Jumonville A, Kaye AD, Myrcik D, Paladini A, Varrassi G, Viswanath O, Urits I. Thoracic outlet syndrome: a narrative review. J Clin Med. 2021;10(5):962.
9. Laulan J, Fouquet B, Rodaix C, Jauffret P, Roquelaure Y, Descatha A. Thoracic outlet syndrome: definition, aetiological factors, diagnosis, management and occupational impact. J Occup Rehabil. 2011;21(3):366–73.
10. Roos DB. Congenital anomalies associated with thoracic outlet syndrome. Anatomy, symptoms, diagnosis, and treatment. Am J Surg. 1976;132(6):771–8.
11. Juvonen T, Satta J, Laitala P, Luukkonen K, Nissinen J. Anomalies at the thoracic outlet are frequent in the general population. Am J Surg. 1995;170(1):33–7.

12. Illig KA, Donahue D, Duncan A, Freischlag J, Gelabert H, Johansen K, Jordan S, Sanders R, Thompson R. Reporting standards of the Society for Vascular Surgery for thoracic outlet syndrome. J Vasc Surg. 2016;64(3):e23–35.
13. Crosby CA, Wehbé MA. Conservative treatment for thoracic outlet syndrome. Hand Clin. 2004;20(1):43–9.
14. Watson LA, Pizzari T, Balster S. Thoracic outlet syndrome part 2: conservative management of thoracic outlet. Man Ther. 2010;15(4):305–14.
15. Collins E, Orpin M. Physical therapy management of neurogenic thoracic outlet syndrome. Thorac Surg Clin. 2021;31(1):61–9.
16. Balderman J, Abuirqeba AA, Eichaker L, Pate C, Earley JA, Bottros MM, Jayarajan SN, Thompson RW. Physical therapy management, surgical treatment, and patient-reported outcomes measures in a prospective observational cohort of patients with neurogenic thoracic outlet syndrome. J Vasc Surg. 2019;70(3):832–41.
17. Lindgren KA. Conservative treatment of thoracic outlet syndrome: a 2-year follow-up. Arch Phys Med Rehabil. 1997;78(4):373–8.
18. Nakatsuchi Y, Saitoh S, Hosaka M, Matsuda S. Conservative treatment of thoracic outlet syndrome using an orthosis. J Hand Surg Br. 1995;20(1):34–9.
19. Luu D, Seto R, Deoraj K. Exercise rehabilitation for neurogenic thoracic outlet syndrome: a scoping review. J Can Chiropr Assoc. 2022;66(1):43–60.
20. Ohman JW, Thompson RW. Thoracic outlet syndrome in the overhead athlete: diagnosis and treatment recommendations. Curr Rev Musculoskelet Med. 2020;13(4):457–71.
21. Balakatounis KC, Angoules AG, Panagiotopoulou KA. Conservative treatment of thoracic outlet syndrome (TOS): creating an evidence-based strategy through critical research appraisal. Curr Orthop. 2007;21(6):471–6.
22. Suzuki T, Kimura H, Matsumura N, Iwamoto T. Surgical approaches for thoracic outlet syndrome: a review of the literature. J Hand Surg Glob Online. 2022;5(4):577–84.
23. Alkhani M, Arsicot M, Oliny A, Millon A, Della Schiava N, Bordet M. Thoracic outlet syndrome: single-center experience on the transaxillary approach with the aid of the TRIMANO Arthrex arm. J Vasc Surg Cases Innov Tech. 2023;10(2):101400.
24. Tracci MC. Thoracic outlet syndrome: transaxillary approach. Oper Tech Thorac Cardiovasc Surg. 2011;16(4):267–77.
25. Toso C, Robert J, Berney T, Pugin F, Spiliopoulos A. Thoracic outlet syndrome: influence of personal history and surgical technique on long-term results. Eur J Cardiothorac Surg. 1999;16(1):44–7.
26. Mingoli A, Feldhaus RJ, Farina C, Cavallari N, Sapienza P, di Marzo L, Cavallaro A. Long-term outcome after transaxillary approach for thoracic outlet syndrome. Surgery. 1995;118(5):840–4.
27. Hosseinian MA, Loron AG, Soleimanifard Y. Evaluation of complications after surgical treatment of thoracic outlet syndrome. Korean J Thorac Cardiovasc Surg. 2017;50(1):36–40.
28. Donahue DM. Supraclavicular first rib resection. Oper Tech Thorac Cardiovasc Surg. 2011;16(4):252–66.
29. Degeorges R, Reynaud C, Becquemin JP. Thoracic outlet syndrome surgery: long-term functional results. Ann Vasc Surg. 2004;18(5):558–65.
30. Minervini F, Kestenholz P, Scarci M, Mayer N. Robotic-assisted thoracoscopic surgery first rib resection-surgical technique. J Thorac Dis. 2024;16(10):7086–95.
31. Zehnder A, Lutz J, Dorn P, Minervini F, Kestenholz P, Gelpke H, Schmid RA, Kocher GJ. Robotic-assisted thoracoscopic resection of the first rib for vascular thoracic outlet syndrome: the new gold standard of treatment? J Clin Med. 2021;10(17):3952.
32. Peek J, Vos CG, Ünlü Ç, Schreve MA, van de Mortel RHW, de Vries JPM. Long-term functional outcome of surgical treatment for thoracic outlet syndrome. Diagnostics (Basel). 2018;8(1):7.
33. Nuutinen H, Kärkkäinen JM, Mäkinen K, Aittola V, Saari P, Pesonen J. Long-term outcome over a decade after first rib resection for neurogenic thoracic outlet syndrome. Interact Cardiovasc Thorac Surg. 2021;33(5):734–40.
34. Aboul Hosn M, Goffredo P, Man J, Nicholson R, Kresowik T, Sharafuddin M, Sharp WJ, Pascarella L. Supraclavicular versus transaxillary first rib resection for thoracic outlet syndrome. J Laparoendosc Adv Surg Tech A. 2020;30(7):737–41.
35. Köse S, Özdemir S. Evaluation of functions after surgical treatment in patients with arterial thoracic outlet syndrome using QuickDASH. Turk Gogus Kalp Damar Cerrahisi Derg. 2021;29(1):70–6.
36. Bačáková L, Chlupáč J, Filová E, Musílková J, Tomšů J, Wu YC, Svobodová L, Pražák Š, Brož A. Vascular damage and repair – are small-diameter vascular grafts still the "Holy Grail" of tissue engineering? Physiol Res. 2024;73(Suppl 1):S335–63.
37. Maly S, Janousek L, Bortel R, Sebek J, Hospodka J, Skapa J, Fronek J. NIRS-based monitoring of kidney graft perfusion. PLoS One. 2020;15(12):e0243154.

Carotid Endarterectomy Randomized Trials: Overview

David Pakizer and David Školoudík

1 Introduction

We systematically searched the PubMed database with the search equation "carotid AND endarterectomy AND (randomized OR randomised)" to include all published RCTs in our chapter. No search limitations were implied except for the study sample size of >30 patients and narrowing the article type only to "clinical trial" and "randomized controlled trial". The search was made from the beginning of the database (1976) to October 1, 2024 and 616 articles were identified. After exclusion based on title/abstract, the final 327 RCTs were included in this chapter. Additionally, systematic reviews and meta-analyses on RCTs of CEA were included, a citation search of key studies was conducted and an additional 25 studies were added. In CEA vs BMT and CEA vs CAS subchapters are listed all retrieved RCTs. In the rest of subchapters, only the major studies are listed and meta-analyses of RCTs are presented. Finally, substudies of large RCTs are not presented to reduce the length of this chapter.

2 Carotid Endarterectomy Versus Best Medical Treatment

2.1 Symptomatic Carotid Artery Trials

Several RCTs have investigated the efficacy of CEA in symptomatic patients with internal carotid artery (ICA) stenosis. From the first successful CEA performed by Michael DeBakey in 1953 [1], it took almost 20 years to complete the first RCT (initiated in 1959) supporting CEA for patients with symptomatic carotid artery disease, shaping clinical practice and improving outcomes for patients at risk of stroke [2]. Together with a trial halted prematurely in 1984 after 41 patients were enrolled because of a surgical morbidity and mortality rate of 35% [3], they laid the foundation for major studies published in the 1990s. The key trials are listed below, their settings are in Table 1 and their results are in Table 2.

2.1.1 The Joint Study of Extracranial Arterial Occlusion, 1970 [2, 4]

- **Sites**: USA and Uruguay, 24 centers
- **Participants**: 316 patients (enrolled 1962–1968 and selected from 1237 patients) with transient cerebral ischemic attacks (TIA), no neurological deficit, and varied degrees of stenosis, randomly allocated to surgical or nonsurgical treatment (169 vs 147 patients).
- **Results**: 42-month follow-up; surgical group: 38% TIA, 4% stroke, 46.6% no symptoms; nonsurgical group: 54.5% TIA, 12.4% stroke, 28.2% no symptoms.
- **Mortality rates**: The survival rates of 68% and 61%, respectively, were not significantly different in 1225 patients randomized to surgery/no surgery [4]. Operative mortality and morbidity of 11.4% was reported in 316 patients (CEA vs BMT) [2].
- **Conclusion**: The first RCT supporting CEA for symptomatic patients, particularly those with high-grade stenosis. Still, many patients had symptoms in the vertebrobasilar artery territory.

2.1.2 Veteran Affairs Symptomatic Trial (Cooperative Studies Program 309), 1991 [5]

- Study details and detailed results in Tables 1 and 2, respectively. Prematurely terminated due to the results of the NASCET and ECST.
- **Key findings**: CEA significantly lowered the incidence of ipsilateral strokes, particularly in patients with >70% stenosis. Duplex ultrasonography showed poor accuracy compared with angiography over intermediate ranges of stenosis, with frequent underestimation of the stenotic lesion.

D. Pakizer · D. Školoudík (✉)
Faculty of Medicine, University of Ostrava, Ostrava, Czech Republic

V. Beneš, D. Netuka (eds.), *Surgical and Interventional Treatment of Cerebral Ischemia*,
https://doi.org/10.1007/978-3-032-08934-2_9

Table 1 Details on the setting of symptomatic CEA vs BMT trials

	NASCET, 1991 [6, 7]	ECST, 1998 [9]	VACSP 309, 1991 [5]
Sites	USA, Canada; 50 centers	12 European countries; 97 centers	USA; 16 centers
Participants	Hemispheric or retinal TIA or nondisabling stroke within 120 days before entry	Hemispheric or retinal TIA or nondisabling stroke within 6 months before entry	Hemispheric or retinal TIA or nondisabling stroke within 120 days before entry (only male veterans)
Stenosis	0–99%	0–99%	50–99%
Stenosis measurement	Residual lumen/normal lumen distal to stenosis	Residual lumen/estimate of normal lumen at level of stenosis	Residual lumen/normal lumen distal to stenosis
Center qualification	<6% 30 days stroke and death (50 consecutive CEAs over prior 2 years)	–	>25 CEAs/year over prior 3 years with <6% 30 days morbidity/mortality
Medical treatment in control group	Antiplatelet (usually aspirin 1300 mg/day), antihypertensive, antilipid, antidiabetic therapy	Aspirin, antihypertensive treatment, advice to stop smoking	Enteric-coated aspirin (325 mg orally once daily)
First outcomes	Stroke, death	Disabling stroke, fatal stroke, perioperative death	Stroke, death, crescendo TIA
Follow-up	8 years	6.1 years (mean)	11.9 months (mean)

Table 2 Results of major symptomatic CEA vs BMT trials

	NASCET 70–99%, 1991 [7]		NASCET <70%, 1998 [6]		ECST, 1998 [9]		VACSP 309, 1991 [5]	
Groups	CEA (n = 328)	BMT (n = 331)	CEA (n = 1108)	BMT (n = 1118)	CEA (n = 1807)	BMT (n = 1211)	CEA (n = 91)	BMT (n = 101)
Age; years	65 (media)	66 (media)	66 (media)	66 (media)	62.5 (mean)	62.3 (mean)	66 (mean)	63.8 (mean)
Male sex; %	68	69	71	69	72	72	100	100
TIA; %	67	69	40	37	50	49	37	39
Stroke; %	33	31	42	45			24	23
Amaurosis fugax; %			12	13	25	26	38	38
Retinal infarct; %			6	5	6	6		
Perioperative period (0–30 days)								
Minor event; %	3.7	2.4	4	1			2.2	5.9
Major event; %	1.5	0.6	1.6	1.4	2.2	0.1	1.1	0
Fatal event; %	0.3	0.3	1.2		1.2	0		
Death; %	0.3	0					3.3	0
Follow-up	**2 years**		**5 years (50–69%)**		**3 years (80–100%)**		**11.9 months**	
Any ipsilateral stroke; %	9	26	15.7	22.2			1.1	12.9
Any stroke; %	12.6	27.6	23.9	32.3			1.1	12.9
Any stroke and death; %	15.8	32.3	33.2	43.3			1.1	12.9
Major/fatal ipsilateral stroke; %	2.5	13.1			6.8	20.6	1.1	3
Any major/ fatal stroke; %	3.7	13.1			8.5	22.4	1.1	3
Any major stroke and death; %	8	18.1	18.3	25.2	14.9	26.5	1.1	3
Death; %	4.6	6.3			8.8	10.5	0	0

- **Limitations**: Generalizability of findings (only male veterans), small sample size (192 patients in the CEA vs BMT study) follow-up duration (mean 11.9 months).

2.1.3 North American Symptomatic Carotid Endarterectomy Trial (NASCET), 1991 [6, 7]

- Study details and detailed results in Tables 1 and 2, respectively.
- **Key findings**: CEA highly benefited patients with 70–99% stenosis. The benefits were less clear for patients with 50–69% stenosis, suggesting a more conservative approach. No benefit was found for patients with <50% stenosis.
- **Long-term outcomes**: In patients with 70–99% stenosis, CEA was long-term efficacious, moderately beneficial for BMT patients with delayed CEA, and with high risk of occlusion for BMT patients [8].

2.1.4 European Carotid Surgery Trial (ECST), 1998 [9]

- Study details and detailed results in Tables 1 and 2, respectively.
- **Key findings**: The trial reported a 30% reduction in the risk of stroke or death at 5 years for patients undergoing CEA compared to those receiving BMT alone (the highest benefit for patients with >80% stenosis).
- **Long-term outcomes**: The benefits of CEA persist over time, with a notable decrease in stroke rates even years after the procedure.

2.1.5 Other

A pilot study of early CEA for acute stroke: 7 sites in Manchester (UK), published in 1997 [10]. From 593 patients with TIA/recent stroke (<7 days) and 70–99% stenosis, only 16 patients were randomized (9 for BMT vs 7 for CEA). In the CEA group, only 3 patients had no postoperative complications (1 patient died). No statistical analyses were conducted.

Carotid stump syndrome and ICA occlusion [11]: 40 patients were enrolled and randomized in the BMT and CEA groups. For 4 months of follow-up, only one vascular event occurred in BMT patients and one patient died from CEA patients. CEA of carotid stump syndrome was a safe procedure (on a small sample size) but its benefit over BMT is unclear.

2.1.6 Conclusion

A meta-analysis from NASCET and ECST trials showed that the benefit from CEA depends not only on stenosis degree but also on several other clinical characteristics such as delay to surgery after the presenting event. Ideally, the procedure should be done within 2 weeks of the patient's last symptoms [12]. The data from RCTs showed a clear high benefit for CEA over BMT in the management of patients with symptomatic stenosis >70% despite the lack of a recent RCT considering the development of BMT.

2.2 Asymptomatic Carotid Artery Trials

After successfully proven trials in favor of CEA in symptomatic patients, the role of CEA in preventing stroke in asymptomatic carotid stenosis was unclear or nonbeneficial. The first published RCTs from 1984 are listed (and in Tables 3 and 4) and the major and latest trials published from the 1990s are presented in more detail below (and in Tables 5 and 6).

2.2.1 The Walter Reed Army Medical Centre Study (WRAMC), 1984 [13]

- **Key findings**: The first RCT for asymptomatic carotid stenosis compared BMT with CEA on 29 patients with a follow-up for 3 years and no history of cerebrovascular symptoms or deaths was found. Therefore, concluded that there is no need for intervention unless symptoms develop.
- **Limitation**: CEA or lack of aspirin could cause a difference in outcome etween the BMT and CEA groups.

2.2.2 L'Association Universitaire de Recherche en Chirurgie Trial (L'AURC), 1989 [14, 15]

- **Key findings**: 230 patients were included and the comparison between CEA and aspirin groups showed a reduction in neurologic accidents in the surgical group, significant after a follow-up of about 45 months.
- **Limitation**: The French multicenter study conducted in 1883–1989 was never fully published as the data in Tables 3 and 4 were derived directly from the principal investigator and were inconsistent with little published trial material.

2.2.3 Carotid Artery Stenosis with Asymptomatic Narrowing: Operation Versus Aspirin (CASANOVA), 1991 [16]

- **Sites**: Germany, 10 centers; recruited/randomized: 410 patients.

Table 3 Characteristics of the first smaller RCTs for asymptomatic stenosis

Study (year)	Nr of patients CEA	Nr of patients BMT	Male; %	Age; mean	Stenosis degree; %	Follow-up; mean (years)	Aspirin as the BMT; mg/day CEA	Aspirin as the BMT; mg/day BMT
WRAMC, 1984 [13]	15	14	72	64	Mean 72	3	None	1300
L'AURC, 1989[a] [14, 15]	128	109	73	64	≥70	5	1000	1000
CASANOVA, 1991[b] [16]	206	204	73	55	≥50–≤90	3	975 + dipyridamole	975 + dipyridamole
MACE, 1992 [18]	36	35	58	–	≥50	2	None	80
VA CSP 167, 1993 [19]	211	233	100	65	≥50	4	1300	1300

[a]Trial completed but never fully published (data available from the principal investigator);
[b]Protocol stipulation resulted in nearly half of the patients in the non-surgical group undergoing CEA

- Patients were randomized to CEA (group A) and BMT (group B). However, none of them was purely surgical or nonsurgical as group A involved CEA in 87% and group B in 43% of patients (complicated randomization). Moreover, >26% of patients received a contralateral CEA before entry into the study.
- **Key findings**: No significant differences between the two groups were found, leading the authors to conclude that there is no difference between CEA + BMT and BMT. However, this conclusion is not substantiated by this trial. Due to a small number of randomized patients, the odds ratio for outcome events was 0.94 not excluding the possibility of reduction risk as high as 43% by CEA.
- **Limitations**: Study design, randomization process, small randomized sample size (low statistical power), protocol violation in 17% of randomized patients with no adequate explanation, high mortality of >27% [17].

Table 4 Results of the first smaller RCTs for asymptomatic stenosis

	Ipsilateral stroke plus perioperative stroke or death; %		All ipsilateral stroke (including perioperative); %		All stroke and death; %	
Study, year	CEA	BMT	CEA	BMT	CEA	BMT
WRAMC, 1984 [13]	0	0	0	0	0	0
L'AURC, 1989[a] [14, 15]	3.9	13.8	3.1	13.8	6.3	14.7
CASANOVA, 1991[b] [16]					27.2	27.5
MACE, 1992 [18]	8.3	0	5.6	0	8.3	0
VA CSP 167, 1993 [19]	8	20.6	8	20.6	41.2	44.2

[a]Trial completed but never fully published (data available from the principal investigator)
[b]Protocol stipulation resulted in nearly half of the patients in the nonsurgical group undergoing CEA

2.2.4 Mayo Asymptomatic Carotid Endarterectomy Study (MACE), 1992 [18]

- **Key findings**: Compared CEA (no aspirin) and low-dose aspirin (80 mg), terminated prematurely because of high numbers of myocardial infarctions (MI; >22%) in the CEA group, from which aspirin was withheld.
- **Limitation**: CEA or lack of aspirin could cause a difference in outcome between the BMT and CEA groups; premature termination (only 71 patients randomized out of planned 1890).

2.2.5 Veteran Affairs Asymptomatic Trial (Cooperative Studies Protocol 167), 1993 [19]

- **Sites**: USA, 11 centers; CEA + aspirin vs BMT (aspirin); 444 males included.
- **Key findings**: CEA reduced the overall incidence of ipsilateral neurologic events in a selected group of male patients with asymptomatic carotid stenosis. No significant influence of CEA on the combined incidence of S + D was found but a modest effect could not be excluded due to sample size.

Table 5 Details on the setting of major asymptomatic CEA vs BMT trials

	ACAS, 1995 [20]	ACST, 2004 [21]	SPACE-2, 2022 [23]
Sites	USA, Canada; 39 centers	30 countries (international, mainly European); 126 centers	Austria, Germany, Switzerland; 36 centers
Participants	Enrollment 1987–1993; 1662 patients (66% male; mean age 67 years)	Enrollment 1993–2003; 3120 patients (66% male; mean age 68 years)	Enrollment 2009–2014; 513 patients (75% male; mean age 69 years)
Stenosis	≥60%	≥60%	50–99% (NASCET), ≥70% (ECST)
Imaging modality	Ultrasound	Ultrasound	Ultrasound
Surgical group	CEA, aspirin 325 mg daily	CEA as soon as possible, standard medical treatment including antiplatelet drugs	CEA/CAS + BMT (aspirin 100 mg, clopidogrel 75 mg, and statins only in CAS)
Medical group	Aspirin 325 mg daily	No CEA unless symptoms occurred, standard medical treatment including antiplatelet drugs	Medication recommended by current treatment guidelines and modification of lifestyle factors
Primary outcomes	Ipsilateral stroke or any perioperative stroke or death	Perioperative stroke or death; non-perioperative stroke	Any stroke or death from any cause within 30 days
Follow-up	Median 2.7 years	Mean 3.4 years	5 years
Notes	Generalizability: 683 non-randomized but likely eligible patients underwent CEA by ACAS surgeons during the trial period	Generalizability: unknown number of eligible patients not randomized. In CEA group only half had CEA within 1 month and 88% by 1 year. In BMT group 6% had CEA after 1 year, and 18% by 5 years, because of symptoms in about half.	Low sample size due to premature termination of enrolment (study power reduced to 23.15% for CEA/BMT vs BMT, leaving the study ineffectual to detect a significant difference between treatments), small number of endpoint events

Table 6 Results of major asymptomatic carotid CEA vs BMT trials

Groups	ACAS, 1995 [20] CEA (n = 825)	ACAS, 1995 [20] BMT (n = 834)	ACST, 2004 [21] CEA (n = 1560)	ACST, 2004 [21] BMT[a] (n = 1560)	SPACE-2, 2022 [23] CEA (n = 203)	SPACE-2, 2022 [23] BMT (n = 113)
Death; %	0.4	0.1	1	0.1	0	0
Disabling stroke; %	1.9	0.2	0.6	0.2	0.5	0
Non-disabling stroke; %			1	0.4	2.0	0
Death or any stroke; %	2.3	0.4	2.6	0.7	2.5	0
Follow-up	**Median 2.7 years**		**Median 3.4 years**		**5 years[b]**	
Any ipsilateral stroke; %			0.8	4	2	2.7
Any stroke; %			2.7	7.7	5.3	6.5
Death; %					6.4	7.1
Non-disabling stroke; %	3.3	4.7	1.8	5.2	3.9	3.5
Death or disabling stroke; %	12.1	13.9	1.9[c]	5.8[c]	7.4	8.9
Death or any stroke; %	15.4	18.6			11.3	12.4
5-year risk (%) of stroke or procedural morbidity	5.1	11	6.4	11.7	–	–

[a]Immediate CEA (CEA group) vs Deferral CEA (BMT group)
[b]Follow-up results based on Kaplan-Meier estimates of cumulative incidence of outcome events within 5 years
[c]Only disabling or fatal stroke (the worst stroke after randomization)

2.2.6 Asymptomatic Carotid Atherosclerosis Study (ACAS), 1995 [20]

- **Key findings**: The aggregate 5-year risk for ipsilateral stroke and any perioperative stroke or death was 5.1% for CEA patients and 11.0% for BMT patients (aggregate risk reduction of 53%). The benefit of CEA was more pronounced in patients with ≥70% stenosis and a smaller absolute benefit was shown for patients with 60–69% stenosis.
- **Long-term outcomes**: The long-term follow-up suggested that the benefits of CEA in reducing the risk of stroke persisted over the study duration.

2.2.7 The Asymptomatic Carotid Surgery Trial (ACST), 2004 [21]

- **Key findings**: In <75-year-old asymptomatic patients with >70% stenosis on ultrasound, immediate CEA halved the net 5-year stroke risk from 12% to 6% (including the 3% perioperative hazard).
- **Long-term outcomes (ACST-1, 2010)** [22]: Combining perioperative events and strokes, net risks were 6.9% vs 10.9% at 5 years (gain 4.1%, 2.0–6.2) and 13.4% vs 17.9% at 10 years (gain 4.6%, 1.2–7.9) both in favor of CEA group. Successful CEA for asymptomatic patients <75 years of age reduces 10-year stroke risks (50% reduction in disabling/fatal strokes).

2.2.8 Stent-Protected Angioplasty in Asymptomatic Carotid Artery Stenosis Versus Endarterectomy (SPACE-2), 2022 [23]

- **Design**: Initially designed as three-arm trial including one group for BMT alone (randomization 2·9:2·9:1; 2008), the study design was amended (due to slow recruitment; 2013) to become two substudies: CEA + BMT vs. BMT alone (SPACE-2a) and CAS + BMT vs. BMT alone (SPACE-2b), both in 1:1 randomization [24].
- **Key findings**: CEA + BMT or CAS + BMT were not superior to BMT alone regarding any S + D risk within 30 days or ipsilateral stroke over 5-year follow-up (should be interpreted with caution given its limitations, particularly the small sample size and the small number of endpoint events).
- **Long-term outcomes**: During the 5-year follow-up period, 3 ipsilateral strokes occurred in the CAS + BMT and BMT alone group, with 0 in the CEA + BMT group.
- **Notes**: Despite the conclusion, study results also support CEA. A significant association was found between BMT alone and ipsilateral TIA 30 days after randomization. Moreover, BMT-alone patients were more likely to have progressive stenosis and restenosis, compared to the CEA group. Finally, the SPACE-2a and SPACE-2b subsets (CEA vs CAS) were unlikely to be directly comparable, as the intervention was decided before randomization (between the chosen intervention or BMT alone).

2.2.9 Asymptomatic Carotid Artery Stenosis Study (AMTEC), 2015 [25]

- **Setting**: Russia, 3 centers; 55 patients with stenosis 70–79% (on ultrasound and computed tomography [CT]/magnetic resonance imaging [MRI]) enrolled 2009–2013.
- **Intervention**: CEA + modern BMT (antiplatelet therapy, atorvastatin, antihypertensive therapy; additionally, lifestyle modification training) vs modern BMT alone.
- **Endpoints**: Primary—nonfatal ipsilateral S + D from any cause; secondary—nonfatal stroke, carotid revascularization, death.

- **Results**: Prematurely stopped after a median follow-up of 3.3 years (max 5.0 years). The 3.3-year cumulative primary event rates were 6.5% and 37.5% in favor of CEA and the secondary endpoint was 12.9% and 50.0% in favor of CEA.
- **Key findings**: The first study that evaluated modern BMT. CEA as an initial management strategy could reduce the risk of death and major cerebrovascular events when added to modern BMT.

2.2.10 Meta-analyses of RCTs on Symptomatic or Asymptomatic CEA Versus BMT

- **CEA for asymptomatic carotid stenosis** (5223 patients, 3 RCTs; 2005): CEA reduced ipsilateral stroke risk and any stroke by 30% over 3 years, despite 3% perioperative S + D rate. The absolute risk reduction is only 1% annually for the first follow-up years [26].
- **Optimal management** of **asymptomatic** carotid artery stenosis (14,310 patients, 7 RCTs; 2023): Modern BMT (post-2000) showed reductions in major stroke, combined stroke, and mortality to CEA. The overall risk reductions are low and data were unavailable to assess subgroups that may benefit from intervention. However, BMT can potentially reduce the requirement for CEA in asymptomatic carotid stenosis [27].
- **Asymptomatic** stenosis **CEA vs BMT** for **women with ≥60% stenosis** (2182 female patients, 4 RCTs; 2021): CEA conferred no benefit over BMT for long-term rates of S + D (OR 0.91; 95%CI: 0.61–1.37) and modestly (3%) increased perioperative S + D risk [28].

2.2.11 Ongoing CEA Versus CAS RCTs

- **The 2nd European Carotid Surgery Trial (ECST-2)** [29]
  - **Characteristics**: CEA/CAS + BMT vs BMT alone (modern optimized medical treatment) for symptomatic and asymptomatic carotid stenosis.
  - **Sites**: Europe and Canada, 30 centers.
  - **Setting**: Non-inferiority RCT with blinded outcome adjudication of the primary outcome and 1:1 allocation to the two treatment arms balanced by minimization.
  - **Participants**: ≥50% stenosis and a low-to-intermediate estimated 5-year stroke risk, defined as Carotid Artery Risk score <20%.
  - **Outcomes**: Primary—stroke in any territory at any time, or periprocedural death attributed to carotid revascularization; secondary—any other perioperative and postoperative complications, cognition, and quality-adjusted life year (QUALY) with cost analysis.
  - **Notes**: Initially designed for 2000 patients, recruitment was suspended after 429 were enrolled, allowing for a planned interim analysis and devising a path forward for the study. It had become clear that reaching the planned enrollment was no longer practical, and there were difficulties with funding.
  - **Progress**: Initiated in 2012, recruitment suspended in 2019, interim 2-year results presented in 2023 and published in mid-2025 [30].
- **Carotid Revascularization, Endarterectomy Versus Stent Trial-2 (CREST-2)** [31]
  - **Characteristics**: (1) CEA + BMT vs. BMT alone (SPACE-2A) and (2) CAS + BMT vs. BMT alone (SPACE-2B) for asymptomatic carotid stenosis.
  - **Sites**: USA, Canada, Spain, Israel; 142 centers.
  - **Setting**: A set of 2 separate 2-arm RCTs where one trial compares intensive BMT with and without CAS and the other compares intensive medical management with and without CEA. The CREST-2 Registry was established to ensure patient safety and give stenting the best possible chance of demonstrating net benefits in stroke prevention.
  - **Participants**: 2486 of 2480 enrolled participants (≥70% stenosis, >35 years old). Enrollment in the CAS: completed in August 2024; enrollment in the CEA: completed in September 2023; the registry has enrolled 9830 patients providing the most contemporary results for transfemoral CAS
  - **Outcomes**: Primary—composite of stroke and death within 44 days after randomization and stroke ipsilateral to the target vessel after that, up to 4 years; Secondary—change in cognition and differences in major and minor stroke.
  - **Progress**: Initiated in 2014, enrollment completed in August 2024, results expected in 2026.
- **Endarterectomy Combined With Optimal Medical Therapy (OMT) vs OMT Alone in Patients With Asymptomatic Severe Atherosclerotic Carotid Artery Stenosis at Higher-than-average Risk of Ipsilateral Stroke (ACTRIS)** [32]
  - **Characteristics**: CEA + BMT vs BMT alone (modern optimized medical treatment) for asymptomatic carotid stenosis.
  - **Sites**: France; 23 centers.
  - **Participants**: >70% stenosis (NASCET), age >50 years old, ≥1 marker of ipsilateral stroke risk based on imaging vulnerability criteria (e.g. echolucent plaque or microembolization on ultrasound, silent brain infarction or intraplaque hemorrhage on MRI, etc.)
  - **Outcomes**: Primary—any ipsilateral stroke within 6 years after randomization or procedural (within 30 days after revascularization) stroke or death; secondary—any other perioperative and postoperative complications and QUALY.
  - **Notes**: Timely enrollment was not possible and ACTRIS will likely be underpowered because stroke

rates in such patients have not first been measured with current BMT alone.
- **Progress**: Initiated in 2016, recruitment started and was suspended in 2019, 43 enrolled patients with study status "completed" on clinicaltrial.gov to October 2024. No information about the results anticipated date release.

2.2.12 Conclusion

CEA proved beneficial over BMT in the management of asymptomatic carotid stenosis for stroke risk reduction, particularly in patients with ≥70% stenosis. However, with improvements in BMT in the past 20 years, the stroke risk declined markedly. The stroke risk in asymptomatic patients with >50% stenosis declined from 3% in the ACAS trial to only 0.34% annually in the OxVasc study published in 2010 [33]. Some individuals with asymptomatic carotid stenosis and high-risk carotid plaque characteristics detected by non-invasive imaging modalities should be considered for CEA but rethinking the management of asymptomatic carotid stenosis patients based on modern BMT is necessary [34, 35].

3 Carotid Endarterectomy Versus Carotid Angioplasty with Stenting

In the 1980s, carotid endovascular treatment (angioplasty and stenting; CAS) was developing, and The first RCT in that field was finished prematurely in 1998 due to the high occurrence of postoperative stroke (in 5 of 7 CAS patients; 0 in CEA patients) and many ethical dilemmas encountered in the performance of this study [36]. The first substantial trial results comparing CAS with CEA in symptomatic patients (and 3% of asymptomatic) were reported in 2001 and many others followed due to the fast development of endovascular techniques and instruments [37]. The following paragraphs list all major RCTs comparing CEA with CAS in patients with both symptomatic and asymptomatic (and in Tables 7a, and 7b [details], 8a, and 8b [detailed results]), only symptomatic (and in Tables 9a, and 9b [details], 10a, and 10b [detailed results]), and only asymptomatic (and in Tables 11 [details] and 12 [detailed results]) carotid stenosis.

3.1 Symptomatic and Asymptomatic Patients

3.1.1 Carotid and Vertebral Artery Transluminal Angioplasty Study (CAVATAS), 2001 [37]

- **Key findings**: Major outcome events within 30 days did not differ significantly between CAS and CEA. At 1 year after treatment, 70–99% ipsilateral carotid stenosis was more usual after CAS (14% vs 4%, $p < 0.001$). No substantial difference in ipsilateral stroke in 3 years follow-up (adjusted HR 1.04, 95%CI 0.63–1.70, $p = 0.9$).

Table 7a Details on CEA vs CAS trials setting of symptomatic and asymptomatic patients

	CAVATAS, 2001 [37]		SAPPHIRE, 2004 [38]		TESCAS-C, 2006 [40]	
	CEA (n = 253)	CAS (n = 251)	CEA (n = 167)	CAS (n = 167)	CEA (n = 84)	CAS (n = 82)
Sites	Europe, Australia, Canada; 22 centers		USA; 29 centers		China; Multicenter	
Co-intervention	Aspirin		Aspirin (81 or 325 mg/day), clopidogrel (75 mg/day only for CAS)		Aspirin and clopidogrel or ticlopidine	
Stenosis for inclusion; %	NA		>50 (symptomatic), >80 (asymptomatic)		>50 (symptomatic), >70 (asymptomatic)	
Imaging of stenosis before treatment	Ultrasound (first) + MRA/CTA		Ultrasound		Ultrasound	
Stent implementation; %	–	26	–	100	–	NA
Ballon angioplasty alone; %	–	74	–	0	–	NA
Cerebral protective devices; %	–	0	–	95.6	–	100
Amaurosis fugax; %	25	24	NA	NA	NA	NA
TIA; %	39	37	34	31.1	NA	NA
Retinal infarct; %	1	2	NA	NA	NA	NA
Stroke; %	26	25	23.8	27.1	NA	NA
No symptoms; %	3	4	72.3	70.1	NA	NA
Male sex; %	70	69	67.1	66.9	NA	NA
Mean age; years	67	67	72.6	72.5	63	63
Mean stenosis; %	85.1	86.4	NA	NA	NA	NA

Table 7b Details on CEA vs CAS trials setting of symptomatic and asymptomatic patients

	Beijing, 2009 [41]		CREST, 2010 [42]		Beijing, 2013 [44]	
	CEA (n = 20)	CAS (n = 20)	CEA (n = 1240)	CAS (n = 1262)	CEA (n = 35)	CAS (n = 28)
Sites	China; 1 center		USA, Canada; 117 centers		China; 2 centers	
Co-intervention	Aspirin (75 mg/day) or clopidogrel (75 mg/day)		Aspirin (325 mg/bid), clopidogrel (75 mg/bid or 450 mg if CAS within 48 h) [both daily after treatment] or ticlopidine (250 mg/bid)		Aspirin (300 mg/day), clopidogrel (75 mg/day)	
Stenosis for inclusion; %	≥50 (symptomatic), ≥70 (asymptomatic)		Symptomatic: ≥50 (angiography), ≥70 (ultrasound, CTA/MRA if 50–69% on ultrasound); asymptomatic: ≥60 (angiography), ≥70 (ultrasound), ≥80 (CTA/MRA if 50–69% on ultrasound)		≥50 (symptomatic), ≥70 (asymptomatic)	
Imaging of stenosis before treatment	Ultrasound, CTA or DSA		Ultrasound, angiography, MRA, CTA		CTA or MRA	
Stent implementation; %	–	NA	–	100	–	100
Ballon angioplasty alone; %	–	NA	–	0	–	0
Cerebral protective devices; %	–	91.3	–	96.1	–	100
Amaurosis fugax; %	NA	NA	NA	NA	NA	NA
TIA; %	NA	NA	NA	NA	NA	NA
Retinal infarct; %	NA	NA	NA	NA	NA	NA
Stroke; %	40	30	NA	NA	NA	NA
No symptoms; %	25	30	47.3	47.1	NA	NA
Male sex; %	85	75	66.4	63.9	65.7	67.9
Mean age; years	64	66.8	69.2	68.9	70	68.3
Mean stenosis; %	NA	NA	NA	NA	73.4	73.6

Table 8a Outcomes of CEA vs CAS trials of symptomatic and asymptomatic patients

	CAVATAS, 2001 [37]		SAPPHIRE, 2004 [38]		TESCAS-C, 2006 [40]	
	CEA (n = 253)	CAS (n = 251)	CEA (n = 151)	CAS (n = 159)	CEA (n = 84)	CAS (n = 82)
Outcome events within 30 days						
Death; %	2	3	2	1.6	NA	NA
Disabling stroke; %	4	4	2	0.6	Odds ratio = 0.68 (95% CI 0.11–4.15) favors CAS	
Non-disabling stroke; %	4	4	1.3	3.1		
Death or disabling stroke; %	5.9	6.4	4	1.3	NA	NA
Death or any stroke; %	9.9	10	5.3	3.8	11.9[a]	9.8[a]
Mean duration; years	**1.98**	**1.95**	**1**	**1**	**0.5**	**0.5**
Death; %	0.8	0.4	12.6	6.9	NA	NA
Disabling stroke; %	0.8	0	4	0.6	NA	NA
Non-disabling stroke; %	2.4	2	4	5.7	NA	NA
Death or disabling stroke; %	1.6	0.4	16.6	7.5	NA	NA
Death or any stroke; %	4	2.4	20.5	13.2	19.1[a]	22[a]

[a]Together with myocardial infarction
Neurological complications (detailed data NA)

- **Notes**: The rate of S + D within 30 days of treatment was higher in both groups (10%) than reported in ECST and NASCET (6.3%) and very likely represents the clinical practice unlike those from both major clinical trials.

3.1.2 Stenting and Angioplasty with Protection in Patients at High Risk for Endarterectomy (SAPPHIRE), 2004 [38]

- The first RCT on CAS with an emboli-protected device.
- **Key findings**: CEA is not inferior to CEA. At 1 year, revascularization was repeated in fewer patients after CAS than CEA.
- **Long-term outcomes** [39]: At 3 years, no significant difference was shown in long-term outcomes (S + D incidence CAS/CEA: 24.6% vs 26.9%).
- **Notes**: Enrolled only patients at high surgical risk (generalizability); 310 patients treated of 334 randomized; early termination (slow enrollment); substantial loss to follow-up.

Table 8b Outcomes of CEA vs CAS trials of symptomatic and asymptomatic patients

	Beijing, 2009 [41]		CREST, 2010 [42]		Beijing, 2013 [44]	
	CEA (n = 23)	CAS (n = 23)	CEA (n = 1240)	CAS (n = 1262)	CEA (n = 35)	CAS (n = 28)
Outcome events within 30 days						
Death; %	Risk ratio = 3 (95% CI 0.129–69.515) favors CEA		0.3	0.7	2.9	0
Disabling stroke; %	4.3[a]	8.7[a]	0.6	0.9	2.9	7.1
Non-disabling stroke; %	1.7	3.2	1.7	3.2		
Death or disabling stroke; %	NA	NA	0.9	1.6	NA	NA
Death or any stroke; %	NA	NA	2.6	4.8	5.7	7.1
Mean duration; years	**1.5**	**1.5**	**Median 2.5 (4-years study period + periprocedural)**		**1**	**1.1**
Death; %	NA	NA	12.6	11.3	0	0
Disabling stroke; %	0	0	1.3	2.3	2.9	3.6
Non-disabling stroke; %	0	0	7.3	8.5		
Death or disabling stroke; %	NA	NA	13.9	13.6	NA	NA
Death or any stroke; %	NA	NA	20.5	21.5	2.9	3.6

[a]Neurological complications (detailed data NA)

Table 9a Details on the setting of CEA vs CAS trials of symptomatic patients

	Leicester, 1998 [36]		WALLSTENT, 2001 [45]		Kentucky 1, 2001 [46]		EVA-3S, 2006 [48, 49]		SPACE, 2006 [50]	
	CEA (n = 10)	CAS (n = 7)	CEA (n = 112)	CAS (n = 107)	CEA (n = 51)	CAS (n = 53)	CEA (n = 259)	CAS (n = 261)	CEA (n = 584)	CAS (n = 599)
Sites	UK; 1 center		USA; NA centers		USA; 1 center		France; 30 centers		Germany, Austria, Switzerland; 35 centers	
Co-intervention	Aspirin		Aspirin (325 mg/bid), ticlopidine (250 mg/bid)		Aspirin (325 mg), clopidogrel (75 mg)		Aspirin (100–300 mg/day) and clopidogrel (75 mg/day) or ticlopidine (500 mg/day)		Aspirin (100 mg/day), clopidogrel (75 mg/day)	
Stenosis for inclusion; %	70–99		60–90		>70		≥60		≥50 (NASCET) or ≥70 (ECST)	
Imaging of stenosis before treatment	Ultrasound		Ultrasound		Ultrasound		Angiography or both ultrasound and MRA		Ultrasound	
Stent implementation; %	–	100	–	NA	–	100	–	100	–	100
Ballon angioplasty alone; %	–	0	–	NA	–	0	–	0	–	0
Cerebral protective devices; %	–	0	–	0	–	0	–	91.9	–	NA
Amaurosis fugax; %	30	14.3	NA	NA	19.6	22.6	14.3	12.6	15.2	15.9
Retinal infarct; %	0	0	NA	NA	0	0	1.9	2.3		
TIA; %	30	28.6	68	65	64.7	60.4	30.1	36.4	31	29.5
Stroke; %	40	57.1	NA	NA	15.7	17	53.7	48.7	43	44.4
Male sex; %	40	71.4	62	66	NA	NA	78	72.4	71.6	72
Mean age; years	66.7	68	70	66.5	69.6	66.4	70.3	69.1	68.2	67.6
Mean stenosis; %	81.5	82.9	75	76	88.2	82.4	NA	NA	NA	NA

Table 9b Details on the setting of CEA vs CAS trials of symptomatic patients

	BACASS, 2008 [52]		Regensburg, 2008 [53]		ICSS, 2010 [55]		CREST, 2011 [57]	
	CEA (n = 10)	CAS (n = 10)	CEA (n = 44)	CAS (n = 43)	CEA (n = 857)	CAS (n = 853)	CEA (n = 653)	CAS (n = 668)
Sites	Switzerland; 1 center		Germany; 1 center		Europe, Australia, New Zealand, Canada; 50 centers		USA, Canada; 117 centers	
Co-intervention	Aspirin, clopidogrel		Aspirin (100 mg/day), clopidogrel (75 mg/day)		Combination of aspirin and clopidogrel was recommended		Aspirin (325 mg/bid), clopidogrel (75 mg/bid or 450 mg if CAS within 48 h) [both daily after treatment] or ticlopidine (250 mg/bid)	
Stenosis for inclusion; %	70–99		>70		>50		≥50 (angiography), ≥70 (ultrasound, CTA/MRA if 50–69% on ultrasound)	
Imaging of stenosis before treatment	Ultrasound, MRA		Ultrasound		Noninvasive imaging including ultrasound		Ultrasound, angiography, MRA, CTA	
Stent implementation; %	–	100	–	100	–	100	–	100
Ballon angioplasty alone; %	–	0	–	0	–	0	–	0
Cerebral protective devices; %	–	100	–	0	–	72	–	NA
Amaurosis fugax; %	50	0	29.5	18.6	17	17	NA	NA
Retinal infarct; %	NA	NA	NA	NA	3	3	NA	NA
TIA; %	10	10	40.9	53.5	35	32	NA	NA
Stroke; %	40	90	36.4	27.9	44	46	NA	NA
Male sex; %	90	80	NA	NA	71	70	65.4	64.1
Mean age; years	71	69	68.4	67.9	70	70	68.8	68.8
Mean stenosis; %	82	84.5	85.1	84.7	NA	NA	NA	NA

3.1.3 Trial of Endarterectomy versus Stenting to Carotid Atherovascular Stenosis-China (TESCAS-C), 2006 [40]

- **Key findings**: CAS was not inferior to CEA.
- **Notes**: Only abstract and information from meta-analyses were available, not the full text in Chinese.

3.1.4 Beijing Trial, 2009 [41]

- **Key findings**: No significant difference between CEA and CAS in early and midterm outcomes but hospitalization costs in China were much higher in CAS.
- **Notes**: 40 patients but 46 treatments (6 bilateral stenoses); only limited detailed results from the Chinese article are available.

3.1.5 Carotid Revascularization Endarterectomy vs. Stenting Trial (CREST), 2010 [42]

- **Key findings**: No difference between CEA and CAS in risk of stroke, MI, or death but higher stroke risk with CAS and higher MI risk with CEA during the periprocedural period.
- **Long-term outcomes**: The low absolute risk of recurrent stroke suggests that both CAS and CEA are clinically durable and may also reflect advances in BMT.
- **At 10 years** [43]: No significant difference between CEA/CAS for the risk of periprocedural stroke, myocardial infarction, or death and subsequent ipsilateral stroke.

3.1.6 Beijing Trial, 2013 [44]

- **Key findings**: The efficacies and safety of CAS and CEA are similar in treating high-risk carotid stenosis patients with <4% S + D rates for both procedures.
- **Notes**: Short-term follow-up, underpowered sample size.

3.2 Only Symptomatic Patients

3.2.1 Leicester Trial, 1998 [36]

- Significantly higher rate of microemboli in CAS (284 vs 12 in CEA; $p = 0.015$).
- Terminated due to harm (71% stroke in the CAS group).

3.2.2 WALLSTENT trial, 2001 [45]

- Results were never fully published (only an abstract); CAS was not equivalent to CEA; stopped early (planned enrollment: 700 patients)—harm from CAS.

Table 10a Outcomes of CEA vs CAS trials of symptomatic patients

	Naylor, 1998 [36]		WALLSTENT, 2001 [45]		Kentucky 1, 2001 [46]		EVA-3S, 2006 [48, 49]		SPACE, 2006 [50, 51]	
	CEA (n = 10)	CAS (n = 7)	CEA (n = 112)	CAS (n = 107)	CEA (n = 51)	CAS (n = 53)	CEA (n = 259)	CAS (n = 261)	CEA (n = 584)	CAS (n = 599)
Outcome events within 30 days										
Death; %	0	0	NA	NA	2	0	1.2	2	0.86	0.17
Disabling stroke; %	0	42.9	NA	NA	0	0	0.4	2.7	2.91	4.01
Non-disabling stroke; %	0	28.6	NA	NA	0	0	2.3	7.7	2.2	2.5
Death or disabling stroke; %	0	42.9	NA	NA	2	0	1.5	3.4	3.77	4.67
Death or any stroke; %	0	71.4	4.5	12.1	2	0	3.9	9.6	6.51	7.68
Follow-up										
Mean duration; years (nr of patients if changed)	**NA**	**NA**	**0.9**	**1**	**2**	**2**	**3.6 (n = 262)**	**3.5 (n = 265)**	**2 (n = 573)**	**2 (n = 563)**
Death; %			NA	NA	2	0	13	13.6	4.9	6.2
Disabling stroke; %			0.9	3.7	0	0	3.8	3.8	2	2.3
Non-disabling stroke; %			NA	NA	0	0				
Death or disabling stroke; %			NA	NA	2	0	NA	NA	NA	NA
Death or any stroke; %			3.6	12.1	2	0	16.8	17.4	7.8[a]	9.4[a]

[a]Only ipsilateral ischemic strokes

Table 10b Outcomes of CEA vs CAS trials of symptomatic patients

	BACASS, 2008 [52]		Regensburg, 2008 [53]		ICSS, 2010 [55, 56]		CREST, 2011 [57]	
	CEA (n = 10)	CAS (n = 10)	CEA (n = 44)	CAS (n = 43)	CEA (n = 821)	CAS (n = 828)	CEA (n = 653)	CAS (n = 668)
Death; %	0	0	0[a]	0[a]	0.5	1.3	0	0.5
Disabling stroke; %	0	0	0[a]	2.3[a]	1.7	4.3	0.9	1.2
Non-disabling stroke; %	10	0			1.3	1.7	2.3	4.3
Death or disabling stroke; %	0	0	NA	NA	2.2	3.1	0.9	1.7
Death or any stroke; %	10	0	0[a]	2.3[a]	3.4	7.4	3.2	6
Mean duration; years (nr of patients if changed)	**3.6**	**4**	**5.3**	**5.5**	**Median 4.2 (CEA/n = 811 vs CAS/n = 752)**		**NA**	**NA**
Death; %	10	10	29.5	23.3	14.6[b]	16.6[b]		
Disabling stroke; %	0	0	0	9.3	4.8	7.4		
Non-disabling stroke; %	0	0						
Death or disabling stroke; %	10	10	NA	NA	3.3[c]	3.2[c]		
Death or any stroke; %	10	10	29.5	32.6	19.1[b]	22.5[b]		

[a]1-year results (30 days results NA)
[b]On intention-to-treat population (CEA/n = 857 vs CAS/n = 853)
[c]Fatal or disabling stroke

3.2.3 Kentucky Trial 1, 2001 [46]

- **Key findings**: CAS is equivalent to CEA in reducing stenosis without increased risk for death/stroke. Because of shortened hospitalization (3.8 days vs 5.6 days in CEA) and convalescence (return to full activity within 1 week: 80% vs 67% in CEA), CAS challenges CEA if cost reduction can be achieved.
- **Long-term outcomes** [47]: CAS and CEA are equally effective in the long-term prevention of ipsilateral ischemic stroke. The combined risk for ipsilateral stroke and MI incidence was higher in CEA vs CAS (HR 5.702; vs 3.996) at 10-year follow-up.
- **Notes** [47]: Together with asymptomatic patients from Kentucky Trial 2: Of 91% (n = 173) initially enrolled

Table 11 Details on the setting of CEA vs CAS trials of asymptomatic patients

	Kentucky 2, 2004 [58]		CREST, 2011 [57]		ACT I, 2016 [59]		Haifa, 2017 [60]		ACST-2, 2021 [61]	
	CEA (n = 42)	CAS (n = 43)	CEA (n = 587)	CAS (n = 594)	CEA (n = 364)	CAS (n = 1089)	CEA (n = 68)	CAS (n = 68)	CEA (n = 1814)	CAS (n = 1811)
Sites	USA, monocentric		USA, Canada; 117 centers		USA, 67 centers		Israel, monocentric		33 (mostly European countries + Brazil, USA, Canada, Kazakhstan, Israel, China, Japan, Argentina, Egypt); 130 centers	
Co-intervention	Aspirin (325 mg) and clopidogrel (75 mg)		Aspirin (325 mg/bid), clopidogrel (75 mg/bid or 450 mg if CAS within 48 h) [both daily after treatment] or ticlopidine (250 mg/bid)		Aspirin (325 mg/daily), clopidogrel (only for CAS, NA mg daily)		Patients already on any appropriate medical treatment (e.g. statin, aspirin, diabetes management, and blood pressure-lowering medication), clopidogrel (75 mg/daily)		Management of patients were left to the discretion of the clinician and usually included antithrombotic, antihypertensive, and lipid-lowering therapy	
Stenosis for inclusion; %	>80		≥60 (angiography), ≥70 (ultrasound), ≥80 (CTA/MRA if 50–69% on ultrasound)		70–99 (if no >60% contralateral carotid stenosis)		>70		≥60	
Imaging of stenosis before treatment	Angiography		Ultrasound, angiography, MRA, CTA		Ultrasound or angiography		Ultrasound and CTA or MRA		Ultrasound and CTA or MRA	
Stent implementation; %	–	100	–	100	–	100	–	100	–	100
Ballon angioplasty alone; %	–	0		0	–	0	–	0	–	0
Cerebral protective devices; %	–	0	–	NA	–	85	–	100	–	85
Male sex; %	NA	NA	67.5	63.8	70	70	71	66	70	70
Mean age; years	69.9	66.6	69.6	69	NA	NA	68	69	NA	NA
Mean stenosis; %	85.6	86.3	NA	NA	NA	NA	NA	NA	NA	NA

patients monitored for 10 years, 87 (50.2%) died; the majority (54%) from nonvascular conditions (lack of information about the risk profile of patients). Death related to all strokes was uncommon (6/173; 3.5%), slightly more prevalent in CAS (5/90; 5.7%) than in CEA (1/83; 1.1%).

3.2.4 Endarterectomy versus Angioplasty in Patients with Symptomatic Severe Carotid Stenosis (EVA-3S), 2006 [48]

- **Key findings**: The rates of death/stroke at 1 and 6 months were lower with CEA than with CAS (incidence at 6 months: 6.1% vs 11.7%).
- **Long-term outcomes** [49]: CAS is as effective as CEA for middle-term prevention but CAS needs to be improved before being used as an alternative.
- **Notes**: Early termination (futility and harm); slightly unbalanced randomization; 504 patients treated from 527 randomized.

3.2.5 Stent-Supported Percutaneous Angioplasty of the Carotid Artery versus Endarterectomy (SPACE), 2006 [50]

- **Key findings**: SPACE failed to prove the non-inferiority of CAS compared with CEA for the periprocedural complication rate (6.34% in CEA vs 6.84 in CAS).
- **Long-term outcomes** [51]: After 2 years of follow-up, no difference was found between CEA and CAS for recurrent ipsilateral ischemic strokes but recurrence stenosis was significantly higher after CAS.
- **Notes**: Stopped prematurely (funding issues).

Table 12 Outcomes of CEA vs CAS trials of asymptomatic patients

	Kentucky 2, 2004 [58]		CREST, 2011 [57]		ACT I, 2016 [59]		Haifa, 2017 [60]		ACST-2, 2021 [61]	
	CEA (n = 42)	CAS (n = 43)	CEA (n = 587)	CAS (n = 594)	CEA (n = 364)	CAS (n = 1089)	CEA (n = 68)	CAS (n = 68)	CEA (n = 1814)	CAS (n = 1811)
Death; %	0	0	0	0	0.3	0.1	0	0		
Disabling stroke; %	0	0	0.3	0.5	0.3	0.5	1.5	2.9	0.4	0.3
Non-disabling stroke; %	0	0	1	2	1.1	2.4			1.6	2.7
Death or disabling stroke; %	0	0	1	2	0.6	0.6	NA	NA	1	0.9
Death or any stroke; %	0	0	1.4	2.5	1.7	2.9	1.5	2.9	2.7	3.7
Mean duration; years	**2**	**2**	**NA**	**NA**	**4**	**4**	**2.2; (n = 67)**	**2.2; (n = 65)**	**4.9**	**4.9**
Death; %	0	0			NA	NA	6	6.2	17.3	18.2
Disabling stroke; %	0	0			NA	NA	0	0	1.4	1.6
Non-disabling stroke; %	0	0			NA	NA			1.9	2.7
Death or disabling stroke; %	0	0			NA	NA	NA	NA	18.7	19.8
Death or any stroke; %	0	0			NA	NA	6	6.2		

3.2.6 Basel Carotid Artery Stenting Study (BACASS), 2008 [52]

- **Key findings**: CAS and CEA seem to be comparably safe (no disabling strokes, death, MI). Data useful for meta-analysis are provided (with long-term results).
- **Notes**: Recruitment was stopped when the center started randomizing participants in the ICSS trial; only 20 patients.

3.2.7 Regensburg Trial, 2008 [53, 54]

- **Key findings**: The first long-term follow-up study initiated in 1999 found that CEA was superior to CAS for stroke (0% vs 9.5%, resp.), >70% restenosis (0% vs 18.8%, resp.), and re-intervention rates (0% vs 15.6%, resp.) over 5.5 years.
- **Notes**: No embolic protection device in CAS; early recruitment (1999–2002: quick CAS evolving); randomization stopped early (SPACE trial initialization).

3.2.8 International Carotid Stenting Study (ICSS), 2010 [55]

- **Key findings**: Risks of any stroke (65 vs 35 events; HR 1.92, 1.27–2.89) and any death (19 vs 7; HR 2.76, 1.16–6.56) were higher in CAS vs CEA at 120 days. CEA should remain the treatment of choice for patients suitable for surgery.
- **Long-term outcomes** [56]: At a median follow-up of 4.2 years, the incidence of the primary endpoint (any fatal/disabling stroke) was virtually identical in the two groups. Nevertheless, an excess of any stroke was observed in CAS, with a 5-year cumulative risk of 15.2% vs 9.4% in CEA, although functional disability and QUALY did not differ between groups.

3.2.9 Carotid Revascularization Endarterectomy vs. Stenting Trial—by symptom status (CREST), 2011 [57]

- Only the CREST results on symptomatic patients; for the main study results see a subchapter headline "Symptomatic and Asymptomatic Patients"
- **Key findings**: No significant differences between CAS/CEA in asymptomatic patients.

3.3 Only Asymptomatic Patients

3.3.1 Kentucky Trial 2, 2004 [58]

- **Key finding**: CAS and CEA may be equally effective and safe (n = 85).
- **Long-term outcomes** [47]: CAS and CEA are equally effective in the long-term prevention of ipsilateral ischemic stroke. The combined risk for ipsilateral stroke and

MI incidence was higher in CEA (HR 2.27) at 10-year follow-up.

- **Notes** [47]: Together with symptomatic patients from Kentucky Trial 1: Of 91% (n = 173) initially enrolled patients monitored for 10 years, 87 (50.2%) died; the majority (54%) from nonvascular conditions (lack of information about the risk profile of patients). Death related to all strokes was uncommon (6/173; 3.5%), slightly more prevalent in CAS (5/90; 5.7%) than in CEA (1/83; 1.1%).

3.3.2 Carotid Revascularization Endarterectomy vs. Stenting Trial—by symptomatic status (CREST), 2011 [57]

- Only the CREST results on symptomatic patients; for the main study results see a subchapter headline "Symptomatic and Asymptomatic".
- **Key findings**: No significant differences between CAS/CEA by asymptomatic status.

3.3.3 Asymptomatic Carotid Trial I (ACT I), 2016 [59]

- **Characteristics**: Randomization 3:1 (CAS vs CEA), patients aged ≤79 years, not at high risk for surgical complications.
- **Key findings**: CAS was non-inferior to CEA at 1 year regarding the primary composite end point of death, stroke, and MI within 30 days or ipsilateral stroke within 365 days after the procedure. The rates of stroke and survival after the procedure did not differ significantly between both groups over 5 years.
- **Long-term outcomes**: The cumulative 5-year rate of stroke-free survival was 93.1% in the CAS group and 94.7% in the CEA group (p = 0.44).
- **Notes**: Prolonged enrollment period (2005–2013), early termination.

3.3.4 Haifa Trial, 2017 [60]

- **Key findings**: No difference in short- and long-term results between the two groups. Thirty-day morbidity included one stroke in each group with no MI.
- **Long-term outcomes**: Long-term results up to 5 years included 4 deaths in each group; none from stroke. One TIA was noted after CAS, and 3 cases of restenosis were found in CEA and one in CAS.

3.3.5 Second Asymptomatic Carotid Surgery Trial (ACST-2), 2021 [61]

- **Key findings**: There was no significant difference in the risk of adverse, procedure-related events for CAS and CEA. For both treatments, 1% of patients had a disabling stroke or died within 30 days and 2% had a non-disabling stroke.
- **Long-term outcomes**: Similar number of strokes in CAS and CEA over the 5-year follow-up. Fatal or disabling stroke occurred in 2.5% CEA/CAS patients. 92% of all-cause mortality (330/CAS vs 313/CEA deaths) was not from stroke.
- **Notes**: The highest level of evidence to date—for asymptomatic patients who are good candidates for CAS and CEA, both procedures are comparable concerning disabling and fatal events.

3.4 Cognition

3.4.1 Comparison of domain-specific cognitive function after carotid endarterectomy and stenting, 2015 [62]

- **Sites**: Monocentric (USA)
- **Settings**: >80% stenosis, asymptomatic patients; tests to assess the cognitive domains of attention, memory, mood, visual-spatial skills, motor ability, processing speed, and executive functioning ≤10 days preoperatively and postoperatively at 6 weeks and 6 months.
- **Key findings**: Baseline cognitive performance was similar between CAS (n = 29) and CEA (n = 31). Carotid revascularization improves memory and attention within the 6 months after CEA/CAS. CAS showed improvements in cognitive processing speed, executive functioning, and motor function compared to CEA.

3.4.2 Randomized clinical trial comparing neurological outcomes after carotid endarterectomy or stenting, 2015 [63]

- **Sites**: Monocentric (Czech Republic)
- **Settings**: >70% stenosis, asymptomatic/symptomatic patients; neurological examination, cognitive function tests, and brain MRI were undertaken before and 24 h after intervention.
- **Results**: Of 150 patients (73 in CAS vs 77 in CEA), new MRI infarctions were found significantly more frequently after CAS (49% vs 25%) as well as lesion volume. Stroke/TIA occurred once in CEA and twice in CAS.
- **Key findings**: A higher risk of silent infarction on brain MRI after CAS than CEA, but without measurable change in cognitive function.

3.5 Sonolysis

3.5.1 Sonolysis in Prevention of Brain Infarction During Carotid Endarterectomy and Stenting (SONOBUSTER), 2016 [64]

- **Sites**: Multicentric (Czech Republic); **Inclusion**: symptomatic/asymptomatic ICA stenosis ≥70%, patient aged 40–80 years, no MRI/CTA contraindications.
- **Aim**: Whether intraoperative sonolysis alters the risk of new brain ischemic lesions during CEA or CAS (randomization 1:1).

- **Key findings**: Of the 487 screened patients, new brain ischemic lesions on post-procedure MRI were significantly less frequent in sonolysis group (n = 121) vs control group (31.4% vs. 47.1%; p = 0.018). Sonolysis and CEA were identified as independent predictors of reduced brain ischemic risk. Stroke or TIA occurred in one sonolysis patient and three control patients. No differences were found in post-intervention cognitive test scores.
- **Outcome**: This study provides Class II evidence that sonolysis during CEA/CAS reduces the risk of new brain ischemic lesions.

3.5.2 SONOlysis in prevention of Brain InfaRctions During Internal carotid Endarterectomy (SONOBIRDIE), 2024 [65, 66]

- **Sites**: Europe, 16 centers (recruitment 2015–2022)
- **Methods**: Patients with stenosis ≥70% aged 40–85 years with a clinical indication for CEA, were randomized either to sonolysis or to a sham procedure. Neurological exams and MRI were performed both before and after CEA to detect any stroke, mini-stroke or death within 30 days.
- **Results**: Of 1004 patients (mean age of 68 years, 31% of women), 507 were randomized to the sonolysis group. Sonolysis during CEA was associated with a significant reduction in risks of stroke, mini-stroke, or death at 30 days (2.2% vs. 7.6%). The same was seen for both symptomatic strokes (1.8% vs. 7.5%) and new ischemic lesions on MRI (8.6% vs. 17.4%).
- **Key findings**: Sonolysis using diagnostic 2-MHz probe is safe and significantly reduces the risk of stroke/TIA and silent brain infarctions detected using brain MRI. In clinical practice, this could mean not only an increase in the safety of CEA but also an expansion of indications for this procedure.
- **Notes**: Stopped due to "clear evidence" of effectiveness in 2020.

3.6 Others

- **Effect of treatment** of ICA stenosis **on blood pressure** [67]: In the first 24 h after the procedure, hypotension occurred (75%/CEA vs 76%/CAS; hypertension: 11%/CEA vs 13%/CAS) with significant fall in blood pressure at 1 h after the procedure in both groups (24/16 mm Hg fall in CEA/CAS) but only sustained in CAS.
- Therapeutic effect on **hemodynamics** in patients with high-risk carotid stenosis (CEA/n = 65 vs CAS/n = 65): After an operation, carotid intima-media thickness, plaque areas, and carotid artery resistance indexes in both groups decreased significantly, and the carotid artery peak blood flow velocities increased significantly. CAS can effectively promote patency of carotid blood flow, and exertion of its effect is related to lowering lipid and inflammatory factor expression. The postoperative 3-month followed-up mortality rate was significantly lower in CAS (1.5% vs 9.2 in CEA) [68].
- **Neuropsychological consequences** of CEA (n = 24)/CAS (n = 21): CAS is not associated with greater cognitive deterioration than CEA (6 and 30 days after the treatment for both groups: no difference in S100β protein values and cognitive changes) [69].
- Comparison of CEA and repeated CAS for **in-stent restenosis** (CERCAS trial) [70]: 31 patients with in-stent stenosis >80% were randomized to re-CAS or CEA and followed for 1 year. While mild restenosis was more common in the CAS group, severe restenosis, clinical complications, and recurrent vascular events were similar in both groups. Longer-term data are needed.

3.7 Meta-analyses of RCTs on Symptomatic or Asymptomatic CEA Versus CAS

3.7.1 Symptomatic and Asymptomatic Carotid Stenosis

- CEA vs CAS and **short-term and long-term outcomes** (7477 patients, 13 RCTs; 2011): Significantly less frequent stroke events after CEA in the long-term context (OR 1.37 for stroke; OR 1.25 for S + D both in CAS). CEA seems superior to CAS, but in some subgroups, e.g. <68-year-old patients, CAS/CEA results seem equivalent [71].
- **Long-term efficacy and safety** of CAS vs CEA (7000 patients with follow-up at least 4 years, 8 RCTs; 2017): CEA was found to be superior to CAS for short- and long-term outcomes, although CEA was associated with a higher risk of periprocedural MI [72].
- **Overview of primary and secondary analyses** of 20 RCTs (3467 asymptomatic and 5797 symptomatic patients, 20 RCTs/126 publications; 2019): CAS confers higher rates of 30-day S + D than CEA. After 30 days, ipsilateral stroke is virtually identical for CEA and CAS. New white matter lesions were significantly more common after CAS (52% vs. 17%) and were associated with higher rates of late stroke/TIA (23% vs. 9%) with no evidence of late cognitive impairment. Restenoses were more common after CAS (10%) without increased late ipsilateral stroke risk. Restenoses (70–99%) after CEA were associated with a small but significant increase in late ipsilateral stroke (OR 3.87) [73].
- **CEA vs CAS for treatment** of symptomatic/asymptomatic stenosis (9753 patients, 22 RCTs; 2020): CAS for symptomatic stenosis is associated with higher risk of peri-

procedural S + D than CEA, mostly attributed to increased minor, non-disabling strokes in patients >70 years. Beyond the periprocedural period, CAS/CEA are both effective in preventing recurrent stroke but combining procedural safety and long-term efficacy in preventing recurrent stroke still favors CEA. A small increase in periprocedural S + D risk with CAS than CEA was found in asymptomatic patients but CIs of treatment effects were wide (further data from asymptomatic stenosis RCTs are needed). >50% restenosis was more common in CAS [74].

- **Asymptomatic restenosis** after carotid interventions and its relationship with **recurrent ipsilateral stroke** (6965 patients, 11 RCTs; 2017): The weighted incidence of restenosis >70% was 5.8% after "any" CEA, 4.1% after patched CEA, and 10% after CAS. CAS patients with untreated asymptomatic >70% restenosis had an extremely low rate of late ipsilateral stroke (0.8% over 50 months), and CEA patients had significantly higher risk of late ipsilateral stroke (vs. patients with no restenosis; only 5% at 37 months). 97% of all late ipsilateral strokes after CAS and 85% after CEA occurred in patients without evidence of high restenosis/occlusion [75].

3.7.2 Only Symptomatic Carotid Stenosis

- **Body mass index (BMI)** and outcome after revascularization (1969 patients, 4 RCTs; 2017): BMI was not associated with periprocedural S + D risk but BMI 25–30 is associated with lower postprocedural risk than BMI 20–25. Observations were similar for CAS/CEA [76].
- **Early CEA/CAS** (4138 patients, 4 RCTs individual patient-level data; 2017): In the association between timing of treatment (0–7 days and >7 days after the qualifying neurological event) and the 30-day risk of S + D after CAS/CEA, CAS was associated with a substantially higher periprocedural risk during the first 7 days after the onset of symptoms (8.3% vs 1.3% in CEA; adjusted RR 6.7, 95% CI 2.1–21.9). Early CEA is safer than CAS for preventing future strokes [77].
- **Long-term outcomes** of CAS vs CEA (4754 patients followed up to 12.4 years, 4 RCTs individual patient-level data; 2019): After the periprocedural period, the annual rates of ipsilateral stroke per person-year were similar for both treatments: 0.60% (95% CI 0.46–0.79) for CEA, 0.64% (0.49–0.83) for CAS. However, combined peri-/post-procedural risks favored CEA, with treatment differences at 1, 3, 5, 7, and 9 years all ranging in 2.8–4.1% [78].

3.7.3 Only Asymptomatic Carotid Stenosis

- **CEA vs CAS or BMT in asymptomatic** patients with significant carotid stenosis (8771 patients, 10 RCTs; 2019): CEA is associated with a lower early all-stroke risk compared to CAS. Other early/late outcomes did not show any difference between both methods. CEA showed a benefit over BMT against long-term ipsilateral stroke, although early outcomes are worse in CEA. No study ever compared CAS to BMT alone [79].
- Evaluating the **overlapping meta-analyses** of RCTs (5 meta-analyses, 2023): The clinical findings favor CEA over CAS in terms of minor and overall stroke incidence and stroke-related mortality rates. However, CAS was superior to CEA in the events of cranial nerve injury during the intervention. No significant difference between CEA and CAS in ipsilateral stroke and MI events was found.

3.8 Conclusion

RCTs of CEA vs 1st generation CAS indicated that CEA is safer in the peri-procedural period, with the difference driven mainly by 30-day minor strokes. However, recent trials showed that improved intra-procedural cerebral protection in CAS and 2nd generation stents (plaque-sequestrating, anti-embolic) may significantly reduce intra-procedural plaque-related embolism and eliminate post-procedural cerebral embolism. Today, improvements in stent delivery systems, stent design including micromesh stents, and retrograde flow design continue and promise better CAS outcomes. Additionally, transcarotid artery revascularization (TCAR), a hybrid procedure that involves stenting of CCA/ICA via remote surgical access to the CCA used particularly in the USA from 2015, may represent an alternative treatment to CEA and CAS in the future but no RCT is available (the proposed CREST-3 multicenter 30-day endpoint trial comparing TCAR to CEA/CAS was abandoned by industry sponsors) [80].

Contemporary guidelines, which recommend that interventions may be appropriate if performed with a risk <3%, are based on RCTs completed in the 2000s and should now be considered outdated. Therefore, CEA/CAS is recommended to be reserved for patients with symptomatic severe stenosis or asymptomatic patients at higher stroke risk with BMT than with intervention [81]. With improvements in medical therapy in the past 20 years, stroke risk in patients, particularly with asymptomatic carotid stenosis, has declined markedly. The impact of modern BMT should be reflected by RCT results soon.

In patients with high-grade asymptomatic carotid stenosis, contemporary level A evidence was not available before SPACE-2 to guide treatment decisions for those patients. Unfortunately, SPACE-2 failed, and level A evidence should be available in 2026 (CREST-2 results) to provide more precision in the choice of treatment. For high-grade symptomatic stenosis, also no contemporary level A evidence is available to guide those patient treatments [82]. TCAR can be a promising prospective alternative to CEA and CAS (included in the ECST-2 trial) but well-designed RCTs with large sample sizes and no problems with long-term funding are warranted. Whatever the choice of invasive treatment, careful attention to medical management of risk factors is of utmost importance for physicians and patients.

4 Carotid Endarterectomy and Anesthesia

4.1 The Largest RCTs

4.1.1 General Anesthesia Versus Local Anesthesia for Carotid Surgery (GALA), 2008 [83]

- **Key results**: No definite difference was observed between GA and LA (n = 3526). Both groups did not significantly differ in life quality, hospital stay length, or the primary outcome in the prespecified age subgroups, contralateral carotid occlusion, and baseline surgical risk. In consultation with the patient, the anesthetist and surgeon should decide which technique to use individually.

4.1.2 Optimization of Cerebral Oxygenation Based on Regional Cerebral Oxygen Saturation Monitoring, 2024 [84]

- **Interventions**: (A) Cerebral oxygenation optimization based on rSO_2 monitoring using near-infrared spectroscopy (n = 437) vs (B) standard care (n = 442).
- **Key results**: Optimization of cerebral oxygenation based on rSO_2 did not reduce the occurrence of cerebral ischemic lesions postoperatively compared with controlled hypertensive therapy.

An overview of RCTs comparing GA with LA is presented in Tables 13a, 13b, and 13c.

A meta-analysis of RCTs that compared LA vs GA for CEA in 4839 patients (16 RCTs; 2021) found that LA makes little to no difference in stroke risk and may not reduce death risk (both within 30 days of surgery when compared to GA). Details are provided in Table 14 [85].

The efficacy and safety of LA versus that of GA for patients undergoing CEA is still a debatable topic as only one large sample size RCT in this topic is available with several study limitations [83]. The execution of a well-designed, large-scale, randomized, multicenter study is recommended when comparing the effects of LA with GA for CEA patients [86]. To conclude, no overall significant difference was found between LA and GA in published RCTs.

Table 13a Overview of RCTs directly comparing local with general anesthesia and presenting their perioperative outcomes

	Forssell, 1989 [96]		Sbarigia, 1999 [97]		Binder, 1999 [98]		McCarthy, 2004 [99, 100]	
	LA (n = 56)	GA (n = 55)	LA (n = 55)	GA (n = 52)	LA (n = 27)	GA (n = 19)	LA (n = 88)	GA (n = 88)
Characteristics	Sweden (1985–1987); cross-overs: 8 LA performed under exclusions during trial, no losses to follow-up		Italy (1995–1998); cross-overs: 2 exclusions during trial, 18 losses to follow-up		Austria (1999); block randomization, cross-over (yes but unclear number of excluded during trial), no losses to follow-up		UK (2004); cross-over not reported, no losses to follow-up	
Intervention	Cervical block and skin infiltration with bupivacaine and mepivacaine or adrenaline	Thiopental, isoflurane and bupivacaine or adrenaline skin infiltration	Superficial and deep cervical block with bupivacaine	Alfentanil + propofol or sodium thiopental + fentanyl + isoflurane or vecuronium + nitrous oxide	Superficial and deep block with bupivacaine	Thiopental, vecuronium, fentanyl	Superficial cervical block: bupivicaine, lignocaine, adrenaline	Midazolam, fentantyl or alfentinl, propofol; end-tidal isofluorane
Mean age, years	65	67	69	70	73	68	72	71
Male; %	71	64	87	89	NA	NA	68	61
Hypertension; %	70	64	80	71	NA	NA	NA	NA
Coronary artery disease; %	46	55	49	54	NA	NA	NA	NA
Previous MI/ heart failure, %	NA	NA	13	17	NA	NA	NA	NA
Asymptomatic patient; %	14	13	20	21	0	0	14	7
Indication for stroke/retinal; %	39	47	14	14	NA	NA	35	37
Indication for TIA/amaurosis fugax; %	43	38	66	65	NA	NA	51	56
Follow-up; days	3	3	30	30	2	2	3	3
Events within 30 days of operation								
Any stroke; %	7.1	3.6	0	3.8	0	0	3.4	3.4
Death; %	0	1.8	0	5.5	0	0	0	0
Stroke or death; %	7.1	5.5	0	7.7	0	0	3.4	3.4
MI; %	3.6	1.8	1.8	3.8	0	0	2.3	2.3
Local hemorrhage; %	1.8	10.9	0	5.8	3.7	5.3	NA	NA
Arteries shunted; %	8.9	45.5	9.1	11.5	100	100	NA	NA

MI myocardial infarction, *TIA* transient ischemic attack

Table 13b Overview of RCTs directly comparing local with general anesthesia and presenting their perioperative outcomes

	Kasprzak, 2006 [101]		Mrozek, 2007 [102]		GALA, 2008 [83]		Mazul-Sunko, 2010 [103]	
	LA (n = 91)	GA (n = 95)	LA (n = 40)	GA (n = 40)	LA (n = 1773)	GA (n = 1753)	LA (n = 29)	GA (n = 28)
Characteristics	Germany (2006); cross-over: 6 participants changed from LA to GA, no losses to follow-up		Czech Republic (2007); no cross-over, no losses to follow-up		24 countries, 95 centers (1999–2007); cross-over: 5.3% GA participants and 4.2% LA participants received the opposite treatment allocation to that allocated at randomization, 0.09% losses to follow-up (3/3523)		Croatia (2010); no information on cross-over and losses to follow-up	
Intervention	Superficial and deep cervical plexus block by 0.5% bupivacaine + 1% prilocaine	Fentanyl, etomidate, vecuronium, isoflurane	Superficial and deep cervical block by 0.5% bupivacaine under neurostimulator	Intravenous etomide, thiopental, atracurium, midazolam, fentanyl and atracurium	Deep and superficial cervical plexus block + local infiltration (e.g. with bupivacaine)	Intravenous access, arterial line under local anesthetic; muscle relaxant, opiate analgesia	Superficial cervical plexus block by levobupivacaine (1.5 mg/kg) and supplemental infiltration with 1% lidocaine	Etomidate, fentanyl, vecuronium with isoflurane; reversal with neostigmine and atropine
Mean age, years	69	69	67	67	69	70	66	66
Male; %	67	61	55	87.5	71	70	90	86
Hypertension; %	NA	NA	NA	NA	78	76	88	89
Coronary artery disease; %	NA	NA	NA	NA	35	37	NA	NA
Previous MI/heart failure, %	NA	NA	NA	NA	5	5	3	0
Asymptomatic patient; %	NA	NA	NA	NA	38	39	NA	NA
Indication for stroke/retinal; %	NA	NA	NA	NA	22	22	38	29
Indication for TIA/amaurosis fugax; %	NA	NA	NA	NA	31	30	3	0
Follow-up; days	NA	NA	NA	NA	30, 365	30, 365	NA	NA
Events within 30 days of operation								
Any stroke; %	2.2	1.1	0	0	3.7	4	0	0
Death; %	0	1.1	0	0	1.1	1.5	0	0
Stroke or death; %	2.2	2.1	0	0	4.2	4.6	0	0
MI; %	0	0	0	0	0.5	0.2	0	0
Local hemorrhage; %	2.2	4.2	0	0	8.5[a]	8.3[a]	NA	NA
Arteries shunted; %	20.9	10.5	15	87.5	14.3	42.9	3.4	82.1

MI myocardial infarction, *TIA* transient ischemic attack
[a]Wound hematoma, cerebral hemorrhage 0.4% (LA) vs 0.6% (GA)

Table 13c Overview of RCTs directly comparing local with general anesthesia and presenting their perioperative outcomes

	Moritz, 2010 [104]		Hussein, 2017 [105]		Orlický, 2019 [106]	
	LA (n = 48)	GA (n = 48)	LA (n = 15)	GA (n = 15)	LA (n = 105)	GA (n = 105)
Characteristics	Germany (2010); cross-over: 2 participants from LA to GA but these 2 participants were excluded from study; exclusion during trial: 6 (2 withdrawal of consent, 4 incomplete data); losses to follow-up not reported		Egypt (2013–2015); cross-over and losses to follow-up not reported; exclusion during trial: 2 allergic reaction, 1 severe vagal response, 1 ventricular tachycardia, 2 severe hypotension		Czech Republic (2015–2016); no cross-over, no losses to follow-up	
Intervention	Superficial and deep cervical block by 1% prilocaine	Fentanyl, propofol, rocuronium and anesthesia maintain by inspired sevoflurane, bolus fentanyl	Superficial and deep cervical plexus block using 0.5% bupivacaine + 2% lidocaine	Propofol and fentanyl	Cervical plexus block with local infiltration	Received either gaseous volatile anesthetic agents with muscle relaxant or total intravenous anesthesia
Mean age, years	NA	NA	65	65	68	63
Male; %	71	69	67	67	64	67
Hypertension; %	60	60	NA	NA	85	86
Coronary artery disease; %	40	38	NA	NA	38	31
Previous MI/ heart failure, %	25	23	NA	NA	13	8
Asymptomatic patient; %	50	42	NA	NA	40	40
Indication for stroke/retinal; %	10	19	NA	NA	NA	NA
Indication for TIA/amaurosis fugax; %	23	33	NA	NA	NA	NA
Follow-up; days	NA	NA	NA	NA	30	30
Any stroke; %	0	0	NA	NA	1.9[a]	2.9[a]
Death; %	0	2	0	0	0	0
Stroke or death; %	0	2	NA	NA	1.9[a]	2.9[a]
MI; %	0	4	NA	NA	0	0
Local hemorrhage; %	NA	NA	NA	NA	8.6	1.9
Arteries shunted; %	16.7	10.4	NA	NA	12.4	6.7

MI myocardial infarction, *TIA* transient ischemic attack
[a]Together with TIA

Table 14 Major findings from the robust meta-analysis comparing LA to GA [85]

Outcomes within 30 days from surgery	Relative effect; odds ratio (95% confidence interval)	Number of patients (number of randomized trials)	Quality of the evidence based on GRADE approach
Any stroke	0.91 (0.66–1.26)	4663 (13)	+ + + – (moderate)
Death	0.61 (0.35–1.06)	4421 (12)	+ + – – (low)
Ipsilateral stroke	1.03 (0.71–1.48)	3733 (2)	+ + – – (low)
Stroke or death	0.85 (0.62–1.16)	4391 (11)	+ + + – (moderate)
Myocardial infarction	1.53 (0.67–3.47)	4567 (12)	+ + – – (low)
Local hemorrhage	0.99 (0.79–1.25)	4186 (6)	+ + + – (moderate)
Arteries shunted	0.25 (0.22–0.29)	4133 (8)	+ + – – (low)

GRADE grading of recommendations assessment, development and evaluation

5 Carotid Endarterectomy and Closure Techniques

5.1 The Largest RCTs

5.1.1 CEA with Primary Closure and Patch Angioplasty with Saphenous Vein, Jugular Vein, and PTFE, 1996 [87]

- **Intervention**: (A) primary closure (n = 135) vs (B) PTFE patch (n = 134) vs (C) vein patch (saphenous vein and jugular vein) (n = 130).
- **Key findings**: Both vein and PTFE patches were superior to primary closure. Patching was also significantly superior in lowering the incidence of early postoperative stenosis. When patching is deemed necessary, a saphenous vein or PTFE may be appropriate.
- **Long-term outcomes (30 months)** [88]: Patching significantly lowered the incidence of late recurrent stenoses, especially in women.

5.1.2 EVERsion Carotid Endarterectomy Versus Standard Trial (EVEREST), 1998 [89]

- **Setting**: Italy, 7 centers; enrolled 1994–1997.
- **Intervention**: (A) Eversion (n = 678) vs (B) standard CEA (n = 675).
- **Key findings**: The incidence of major technical defects during CEA is low, yet the perioperative neurological prognosis of patients with major defects warranting revision is poor. Completion angiography or angioscopy and possible correction of defects did not protect per se from an unfavorable early outcome after CEA.
- **Long-term outcomes** [90]: No significant differences were found in late outcomes between the eversion and standard techniques at the mean 33-month follow-up.

5.2 Ongoing RCTs

- **Stroke Prevention and Educational Awareness Diffusion group and the Surgical Treatment of Acute Cerebral Ischemia Italian (SPREAD-STACI) Trial** [91]
  – **Characteristics**: Urgent CEA (<48 h) vs delayed CEA (48 h to 15 days) after symptom onset; a total of 456 patients (228/group) is needed.
  – **Outcomes**: Primary—reduction in all types of stroke, acute MI or death; secondary—reduction of ipsilateral ischemic stroke, identification of predictive risk factors, confirmation of no different rate for hemorrhagic/ischemic complications between groups.
  – **Sites**: Italy; **Status**: initiated 2012, no updates.

A network meta-analysis published in 2021 compared data from 23 RCTs (4440 patients) when investigating seven different retrieved closure techniques in CEA (primary carotid closure, n = 753; eversion CEA, n = 431; vein patch closure, n = 973; PTFE patch, n = 948; Dacron patch, n = 828; bovine pericardium patch, n = 249; and polyurethane patch, n = 258). Eversion CEA and patching with bovine pericardium or PTFE is associated with a lower incidence in both short-term and late undesired outcomes following CEA and seems to represent the best choice compared with other carotid closure techniques [92].

Using combined RCT and observational studies data, eversion CEA was superior to conventional CEA regarding peri-operative outcomes (stroke, death, death/stroke) and late restenosis but was similar to patched CEA in both early and late outcomes (16,246 eversion CEAs vs 33,251 conventional CEAs from 5 RCTs and 20 observational studies; 2017) [93].

Finally, routine carotid patching or eversion CEA was superior to primary closure (level 1 evidence). No significant differences were found between the preferential use of several patch materials. The rates of significant post-CEA stenosis for CEA with patching were similar to that with eversion CEA, and both were superior to primary closure based on RCTs review from 2021 [94].

6 Carotid Endarterectomy and Heart

- **Coronary Artery Bypass graft surgery in patients with Asymptomatic Carotid Stenosis (CABACS) Trial, 2022** [95]
  - **Sites**: Germany and the Czech Republic, 17 centers; enrollment 2010–2014.
  - **Key findings**: Only 129 asymptomatic patients with carotid stenosis ≥80% (by ECST) were enrolled. At 30 days, the rate of any stroke or death in the intention-to-treat population was 18.5% in patients receiving synchronous CEA + CABG vs 9.7% in patients receiving isolated CABG (absolute risk reduction 8.8%).
  - **Long-term outcomes**: Up to 5-year follow-up, there was no evidence for a significant treatment-group effect although patients undergoing isolated CABG tended to have better outcomes.

Declarations

Competing Interests The author(s) has no competing interests to declare that are relevant to the content of this manuscript.

Ethics Approval The author(s) declares that this manuscript does not include primary research with human participants.

References

1. DeBakey ME. Successful carotid endarterectomy for cerebrovascular insufficiency. JAMA. 1975;233(10):1083–5.
2. Fields WS. Joint study of extracranial arterial occlusion. JAMA. 1970;211(12):1993.
3. Shaw DA, Venables GS, Cartlidge NE, Bates D, Dickinson PH. Carotid endarterectomy in patients with transient cerebral ischaemia. J Neurol Sci. 1984;64(1):45–53.
4. Bauer RB, Meyer JS, Fields WS, Remington R, Macdonald MC, Callen P. Joint study of extracranila arterial occlusion. 3. Progress report of controlled study of long-term survival in patients with and without operation. JAMA. 1969;208(3):509–18.
5. Mayberg MR, Wilson SE, Yatsu F, Weiss DG, Messina L, Hershey LA, et al. Carotid endarterectomy and prevention of cerebral ischemia in symptomatic carotid stenosis. Veterans Affairs Cooperative Studies Program 309 Trialist Group. JAMA. 1991;266(23):3289–94.
6. Barnett HJ, Taylor DW, Eliasziw M, Fox AJ, Ferguson GG, Haynes RB, et al. Benefit of carotid endarterectomy in patients with symptomatic moderate or severe stenosis. North American Symptomatic Carotid Endarterectomy Trial Collaborators. N Engl J Med. 1998;339(20):1415–25.
7. North American Symptomatic Carotid Endarterectomy Trial C, Barnett HJM, Taylor DW, Haynes RB, Sackett DL, Peerless SJ, et al. Beneficial effect of carotid endarterectomy in symptomatic patients with high-grade carotid stenosis. N Engl J Med. 1991;325(7):445–53.
8. Paciaroni M, Eliasziw M, Sharpe BL, Kappelle LJ, Chaturvedi S, Meldrum H, et al. Long-term clinical and angiographic outcomes in symptomatic patients with 70% to 99% carotid artery stenosis. Stroke. 2000;31(9):2037–42.
9. Farrell B, Fraser A, Sandercock P, Slattery J, Warlow CP, Grp, ECSTC. Randomised trial of endarterectomy for recently symptomatic carotid stenosis: final results of the MRC European carotid surgery trial (ECST). Lancet. 1998;351(9113):1379–87.
10. Mead GE, Murray H, Farrell A, O'Neill PA, McCollum CN. Pilot study of carotid surgery for acute stroke. Br J Surg. 1997;84(7):990–2.
11. Hrbac T, Benes V, Sirucek P, Jonszta T, Herzig R, Prochazka V, et al. Safety and efficacy of surgical treatment of carotid stump syndrome: pilot study. Ann Vasc Surg. 2012;26(6):797–801.
12. Rothwell PM, Eliasziw M, Gutnikov SA, Warlow CP, Barnett HJ, Carotid Endarterectomy Trialists C. Endarterectomy for symptomatic carotid stenosis in relation to clinical subgroups and timing of surgery. Lancet. 2004;363(9413):915–24.
13. Clagett GP, Youkey JR, Brigham RA, Orecchia PM, Salander JM, Collins GJ Jr, et al. Asymptomatic cervical bruit and abnormal ocular pneumoplethysmography: a prospective study comparing two approaches to management. Surgery. 1984;96(5):823–30.
14. Benavente O, Moher D, Pham B. Carotid endarterectomy for asymptomatic carotid stenosis: a meta-analysis. BMJ. 1998;317(7171):1477–80.
15. Lagneau P. Sténoses carotidiennes asymptomatiques. Analyse des études randomisées. J Mal Vasc. 1993;18(3):209–12.
16. Carotid surgery versus medical therapy in asymptomatic carotid stenosis. The CASANOVA Study Group. Stroke. 1991;22(10):1229–35.
17. Solis MM, Ranval TJ, Barone GW, Eidt JF, Barnes RW. The CASANOVA study: immediate surgery versus delayed surgery for moderate carotid artery stenosis? Stroke. 1992;23(6):917–9.
18. Results of a randomized controlled trial of carotid endarterectomy for asymptomatic carotid stenosis. Mayo Clin Proc. 1992;67(6):513–8.
19. Hobson RW 2nd, Weiss DG, Fields WS, Goldstone J, Moore WS, Towne JB, et al. Efficacy of carotid endarterectomy for asymptomatic carotid stenosis. The Veterans Affairs Cooperative Study Group. N Engl J Med. 1993;328(4):221–7.
20. Endarterectomy for asymptomatic carotid artery stenosis. Executive Committee for the Asymptomatic Carotid Atherosclerosis Study. JAMA. 1995;273(18):1421–8.
21. Halliday A, Mansfield A, Marro J, Peto C, Peto R, Potter J, et al. Prevention of disabling and fatal strokes by successful carotid endarterectomy in patients without recent neurological symptoms: randomised controlled trial. Lancet. 2004;363(9420):1491–502.
22. Halliday A, Harrison M, Hayter E, Kong X, Mansfield A, Marro J, et al. 10-year stroke prevention after successful carotid endarterectomy for asymptomatic stenosis (ACST-1): a multicentre randomised trial. Lancet. 2010;376(9746):1074–84.
23. Reiff T, Eckstein HH, Mansmann U, Jansen O, Fraedrich G, Mudra H, et al. Carotid endarterectomy or stenting or best medical treatment alone for moderate-to-severe asymptomatic carotid artery stenosis: 5-year results of a multicentre, randomised controlled trial. Lancet Neurol. 2022;21(10):877–88.
24. Eckstein HH, Reiff T, Ringleb P, Jansen O, Mansmann U, Hacke W, et al. SPACE-2: a missed opportunity to compare carotid endarterectomy, carotid stenting, and best medical treatment in patients with asymptomatic carotid stenoses. Eur J Vasc Endovasc Surg. 2016;51(6):761–5.
25. Kolos I, Troitskiy A, Balakhonova T, Shariya M, Skrypnik D, Tvorogova T, et al. Modern medical treatment with or without carotid endarterectomy for severe asymptomatic carotid atherosclerosis. J Vasc Surg. 2015;62(4):914–22.
26. Chambers BR, Donnan GA. Carotid endarterectomy for asymptomatic carotid stenosis. Cochrane Database Syst Rev. 2005;2005(4):CD001923.

27. Gasior SA, O'Donnell JPM, Davey M, Clarke J, Jalali A, Ryan E, et al. Optimal management of asymptomatic carotid artery stenosis: a systematic review and network meta-analysis. Eur J Vasc Endovasc Surg. 2023;65(5):690–9.
28. Strauss SA, Jetty P, Huynh C, Zeng N, Haqani B. Revascularization versus best medical therapy for the management of asymptomatic carotid artery stenosis in females: a systematic review and meta-analysis. J Vasc Surg. 2021;74(3):e236–7.
29. Cheng SF, van Velzen TJ, Gregson J, Richards T, Jager HR, Simister R, et al. The 2nd European Carotid Surgery Trial (ECST-2): rationale and protocol for a randomised clinical trial comparing immediate revascularisation versus optimised medical therapy alone in patients with symptomatic and asymptomatic carotid stenosis at low to intermediate risk of stroke. Trials. 2022;23(1):606.
30. Donners SJA, van Velzen TJ, Cheng SF, Gregson J, Hazewinkel AD, Pizzini FB, et al. ECST-2 investigators. Optimised medical therapy alone versus optimised medical therapy plus revascularisation for asymptomatic or low-to-intermediate risk symptomatic carotid stenosis (ECST-2): 2-year interim results of a multicentre randomised trial. Lancet Neurol. 2025;24(5):389–99.
31. Brott TG, Howard G, Lal BK, Voeks JH, Turan TN, Roubin GS, et al. CREST-2 investigators. Medical management and revascularization for asymptomatic carotid stenosis. N Engl J Med. 2025. https://doi.org/10.1056/NEJMoa2508800.
32. Centre Hospitalier St Anne. Endarterectomy combined with optimal medical therapy (OMT) vs OMT alone in patients with asymptomatic severe atherosclerotic carotid artery stenosis at higher-than-average risk of ipsilateral stroke (ACTRIS): ClinicalTrials.gov. 2016.
33. Marquardt L, Geraghty OC, Mehta Z, Rothwell PM. Low risk of ipsilateral stroke in patients with asymptomatic carotid stenosis on best medical treatment: a prospective, population-based study. Stroke. 2010;41(1):e11–7.
34. Spence JD. Treatment of asymptomatic carotid stenosis. Lancet Neurol. 2021;20(3):163–5.
35. Naylor AR. Time to rethink management strategies in asymptomatic carotid artery disease. Nat Rev Cardiol. 2011;9(2):116–24.
36. Naylor AR, Bolia A, Abbott RJ, Pye IF, Smith J, Lennard N, et al. Randomized study of carotid angioplasty and stenting versus carotid endarterectomy: a stopped trial. J Vasc Surg. 1998;28(2):326–34.
37. Brown MM, Rogers J, Bland JM, Investigators C. Endovascular versus surgical treatment in patients with carotid stenosis in the Carotid and Vertebral Artery Transluminal Angioplasty Study (CAVATAS): a randomised trial. Lancet. 2001;357(9270):1729–37.
38. Yadav JS, Wholey MH, Kuntz RE, Fayad P, Katzen BT, Mishkel GJ, et al. Protected carotid-artery stenting versus endarterectomy in high-risk patients. N Engl J Med. 2004;351(15):1493–501.
39. Gurm HS, Yadav JS, Fayad P, Katzen BT, Mishkel GJ, Bajwa TK, et al. Long-term results of carotid stenting versus endarterectomy in high-risk patients. N Engl J Med. 2008;358:1572–9.
40. Ling F, Jiao L. Preliminary report of trial of endarterectomy versus stenting for the treatment of carotid atherosclerotic stenosis in China (TESCAS-C). Chin J Cerebrovasc Dis. 2006;3(1):4–8.
41. Liu CW, Liu B, Ye W, Wu WW, Li YJ, Zheng YH, et al. Carotid endarterectomy versus carotid stenting: a prospective randomized trial. Zhonghua Wai Ke Za Zhi. 2009;47:267–70.
42. Brott TG, Hobson RW 2nd, Howard G, Roubin GS, Clark WM, Brooks W, et al. Stenting versus endarterectomy for treatment of carotid-artery stenosis. N Engl J Med. 2010;363:11–23.
43. Brott TG, Howard G, Roubin GS, Meschia JF, Mackey A, Brooks W, et al. Long-term results of stenting versus endarterectomy for carotid-artery stenosis. N Engl J Med. 2016;374:1021–31.
44. Wang P, Liang C, Du J, Li J. Effects of carotid endarterectomy and carotid artery stenting on high-risk carotid stenosis patients. Pak J Med Sci. 2013;29(6):1315–8.
45. Alberts MJ. Results of a multicenter prospective randomized trial of carotid artery stenting vs. carotid endarterectomy. Stroke. 2001;32(suppl_1):325.
46. Brooks WH, McClure RR, Jones MR, Coleman TC, Breathitt L. Carotid angioplasty and stenting versus carotid endarterectomy: randomized trial in a community hospital. J Am Coll Cardiol. 2001;38(6):1589–95.
47. Brooks WH, Jones MR, Gisler P, McClure RR, Coleman TC, Breathitt L, et al. Carotid angioplasty with stenting versus endarterectomy: 10-year randomized trial in a community hospital. JACC Cardiovasc Interv. 2014;7:163–8.
48. Mas JL, Chatellier G, Beyssen B, Branchereau A, Moulin T, Becquemin JP, et al. Endarterectomy versus stenting in patients with symptomatic severe carotid stenosis. N Engl J Med. 2006;355:1660–71.
49. Mas JL, Trinquart L, Leys D, Albucher JF, Rousseau H, Viguier A, et al. Endarterectomy Versus Angioplasty in Patients with Symptomatic Severe Carotid Stenosis (EVA-3S) trial: results up to 4 years from a randomised, multicentre trial. Lancet Neurol. 2008;7(10):885–92.
50. Ringleb PA, Allenberg J, Brückmann H, Eckstein HH, Fraedrich G, Hartmann M, et al. 30 day results from the SPACE trial of stent-protected angioplasty versus carotid endarterectomy in symptomatic patients: a randomised non-inferiority trial. Lancet. 2006;368:1239–47.
51. Eckstein HH, Ringleb P, Allenberg JR, Berger J, Fraedrich G, Hacke W, et al. Results of the Stent-Protected Angioplasty versus Carotid Endarterectomy (SPACE) study to treat symptomatic stenoses at 2 years: a multinational, prospective, randomised trial. Lancet Neurol. 2008;7(10):893–902.
52. Hoffmann A, Engeltner S, Taschner C, Mendelowitsch A, Merlo A, Lyrer PA, et al. Carotid artery stenting versus carotid endarterectomy – a prospective randomised controlled single-centre trial with long-term follow-up (BACASS). Schweiz Arch Neurol Psychiatr. 2008;159(02):84–9.
53. Steinbauer MG, Pfister K, Greindl M, Schlachetzki F, Borisch I, Schuirer G, et al. Alert for increased long-term follow-up after carotid artery stenting: results of a prospective, randomized, single-center trial of carotid artery stenting vs carotid endarterectomy. J Vasc Surg. 2008;48:93–8.
54. Link J, Manke C, Rosin L, Borisch I, Topel I, Horn M, et al. Carotid endarterectomy and carotid stenting. A pilot study of a prospective, randomized and controlled comparison. Radiologe. 2000;40(9):813–20.
55. International Carotid Stenting Study i, Ederle J, Dobson J, Featherstone RL, Bonati LH, van der Worp HB, et al. Carotid artery stenting compared with endarterectomy in patients with symptomatic carotid stenosis (International Carotid Stenting Study): an interim analysis of a randomised controlled trial. Lancet. 2010;375(9719):985–97.
56. Bonati LH, Dobson J, Featherstone RL, Ederle J, van der Worp HB, de Borst GJ, et al. Long-term outcomes after stenting versus endarterectomy for treatment of symptomatic carotid stenosis: the International Carotid Stenting Study (ICSS) randomised trial. Lancet. 2015;385:529–38.
57. Silver FL, Mackey A, Clark WM, Brooks W, Timaran CH, Chiu D, et al. Safety of stenting and endarterectomy by symptomatic status in the Carotid Revascularization Endarterectomy Versus Stenting Trial (CREST). Stroke. 2011;42:675–80.
58. Brooks WH, McClure RR, Jones MR, Coleman TL, Breathitt L. Carotid angioplasty and stenting versus carotid endarterectomy for treatment of asymptomatic carotid stenosis: a randomized trial

in a community hospital. Neurosurgery. 2004;54(2):318–24; discussion 24–5.
59. Rosenfield K, Matsumura JS, Chaturvedi S, Riles T, Ansel GM, Metzger DC, et al. Randomized trial of stent versus surgery for asymptomatic carotid stenosis. N Engl J Med. 2016;374:1011–20.
60. Mannheim D, Karmeli R. A prospective randomized trial comparing endarterectomy to stenting in severe asymptomatic carotid stenosis. J Cardiovasc Surg. 2017;58:814–7.
61. Halliday A, Bulbulia R, Bonati LH, Chester J, Cradduck-Bamford A, Peto R, et al. Second asymptomatic carotid surgery trial (ACST-2): a randomised comparison of carotid artery stenting versus carotid endarterectomy. Lancet. 2021;398(10305):1065–73.
62. Kougias P, Collins R, Pastorek N, Sharath S, Barshes NR, McCulloch K, et al. Comparison of domain-specific cognitive function after carotid endarterectomy and stenting. J Vasc Surg. 2015;62:355–61.
63. Kuliha M, Roubec M, Procházka V, Jonszta T, Hrbáč T, Havelka J, et al. Randomized clinical trial comparing neurological outcomes after carotid endarterectomy or stenting. Br J Surg. 2015;102:194–201.
64. Skoloudik D, Kuliha M, Hrbac T, Jonszta T, Herzig R, Group ST. Sonolysis in Prevention of Brain Infarction During Carotid Endarterectomy and Stenting (SONOBUSTER): a randomized, controlled trial. Eur Heart J. 2016;37(40):3096–102.
65. Hrbac T, Netuka D, Benes V, Nosal V, Kesnerova P, Tomek A, et al. SONOlysis in prevention of Brain InfaRctions During Internal carotid Endarterectomy (SONOBIRDIE) trial – study protocol for a randomized controlled trial. Trials. 2017;18(1):25.
66. Školoudík D, Hrbáč T, Kovář M, Beneš V 3rd, Fiedler J, Branca M, et al. Sonolysis during carotid endarterectomy:randomised controlled trial. BMJ. 2025;388:e082750.
67. McKevitt FM, Sivaguru A, Venables GS, Cleveland TJ, Gaines PA, Beard JD, et al. Effect of treatment of carotid artery stenosis on blood pressure: a comparison of hemodynamic disturbances after carotid endarterectomy and endovascular treatment. Stroke. 2003;34(11):2576–81.
68. Li FM, Zhong JX, Jiang X, Wang QZ, Guo Y. Therapeutic effect of carotid artery stenting versus endarterectomy for patients with high-risk carotid stenosis. Int J Clin Exp Med. 2014;7(9):2895–900.
69. Witt K, Borsch K, Daniels C, Walluscheck K, Alfke K, Jansen O, et al. Neuropsychological consequences of endarterectomy and endovascular angioplasty with stent placement for treatment of symptomatic carotid stenosis: a prospective randomised study. J Neurol. 2007;254(11):1524–32.
70. Hrbac T, Fiedler J, Prochazka V, Jonszta T, Roubec M, Pakizer D, et al. Comparison of carotid endarterectomy and repeated carotid angioplasty and stenting for in-stent restenosis (CERCAS trial): a randomised study. Stroke Vasc Neurol. 2023;8(5):399–404.
71. Economopoulos KP, Sergentanis TN, Tsivgoulis G, Mariolis AD, Stefanadis C. Carotid artery stenting versus carotid endarterectomy: a comprehensive meta-analysis of short-term and long-term outcomes. Stroke. 2011;42(3):687–92.
72. Li Y, Yang JJ, Zhu SH, Xu B, Wang L. Long-term efficacy and safety of carotid artery stenting versus endarterectomy: a meta-analysis of randomized controlled trials. PLoS One. 2017;12(7):e0180804.
73. Batchelder AJ, Saratzis A, Ross Naylor A. Editor's choice – overview of primary and secondary analyses from 20 randomised controlled trials comparing carotid artery stenting with carotid endarterectomy. Eur J Vasc Endovasc Surg. 2019;58(4):479–93.
74. Muller MD, Lyrer P, Brown MM, Bonati LH. Carotid artery stenting versus endarterectomy for treatment of carotid artery stenosis. Cochrane Database Syst Rev. 2020;2(2):CD000515.
75. Kumar R, Batchelder A, Saratzis A, AbuRahma AF, Ringleb P, Lal BK, et al. Restenosis after carotid interventions and its relationship with recurrent ipsilateral stroke: a systematic review and meta-analysis. Eur J Vasc Endovasc Surg. 2017;53(6):766–75.
76. Volkers EJ, Greving JP, Hendrikse J, Algra A, Kappelle LJ, Becquemin JP, et al. Body mass index and outcome after revascularization for symptomatic carotid artery stenosis. Neurology. 2017;88(21):2052–60.
77. Rantner B, Kollerits B, Roubin GS, Ringleb PA, Jansen O, Howard G, et al. Early endarterectomy carries a lower procedural risk than early stenting in patients with symptomatic stenosis of the internal carotid artery. Stroke. 2017;48(6):1580–7.
78. Brott TG, Calvet D, Howard G, Gregson J, Algra A, Becquemin JP, et al. Long-term outcomes of stenting and endarterectomy for symptomatic carotid stenosis: a preplanned pooled analysis of individual patient data. Lancet Neurol. 2019;18(4):348–56.
79. Galyfos G, Sachsamanis G, Anastasiadou C, Sachmpazidis I, Kikiras K, Kastrisios G, et al. Carotid endarterectomy versus carotid stenting or best medical treatment in asymptomatic patients with significant carotid stenosis: a meta-analysis. Cardiovasc Revasc Med. 2019;20(5):413–23.
80. de Borst GJ. Transcarotid artery revascularization. Br J Surg. 2023;110(2):127–8.
81. Spence JD, Naylor AR. Endarterectomy, stenting, or neither for asymptomatic carotid-artery stenosis. N Engl J Med. 2016;374(11):1087–8.
82. Brott TG, Meschia JF, Lal BK, Chamorro A, Howard VJ, Howard G. When will we have what we need to advise patients how to manage their carotid stenosis?: lessons from SPACE-2. Stroke. 2023;54(5):1452–6.
83. Group GTC, Lewis SC, Warlow CP, Bodenham AR, Colam B, Rothwell PM, et al. General anaesthesia versus local anaesthesia for carotid surgery (GALA): a multicentre, randomised controlled trial. Lancet. 2008;372(9656):2132–42.
84. Le Teurnier Y, Rozec B, Degryse C, Levy F, Miliani Y, Godet G, et al. Optimization of cerebral oxygenation based on regional cerebral oxygen saturation monitoring during carotid endarterectomy: a Phase III multicenter, double-blind randomized controlled trial. Anaesth Crit Care Pain Med. 2024;43(4):101388.
85. Rerkasem A, Orrapin S, Howard DP, Nantakool S, Rerkasem K. Local versus general anaesthesia for carotid endarterectomy. Cochrane Database Syst Rev. 2021;10(10):CD000126.
86. Lomivorotov VV, Shmyrev VA, Nepomniashchikh VA. Regional versus general anesthesia for carotid endarterectomy: do we need another randomized trial? J Cardiothorac Vasc Anesth. 2019;33(4):943–4.
87. AbuRahma AF, Khan JH, Robinson PA, Saiedy S, Short YS, Boland JP, et al. Prospective randomized trial of carotid endarterectomy with primary closure and patch angioplasty with saphenous vein, jugular vein, and polytetrafluoroethylene: perioperative (30-day) results. J Vasc Surg. 1996;24(6):998–1006; discussion -7.
88. AbuRahma AF, Robinson PA, Saiedy S, Kahn JH, Boland JP. Prospective randomized trial of carotid endarterectomy with primary closure and patch angioplasty with saphenous vein, jugular vein, and polytetrafluoroethylene: long-term follow-up. J Vasc Surg. 1998;27(2):222–32; discussion 33–4.
89. Zannetti S, Cao P, De Rango P, Giordano G, Parlani G, Lenti M, et al. Intraoperative assessment of technical perfection in carotid endarterectomy: a prospective analysis of 1305 completion procedures. Collaborators of the EVEREST study group. Eversion versus standard carotid endartectomy. Eur J Vasc Endovasc Surg. 1999;18(1):52–8.
90. Cao P, Giordano G, De Rango P, Zannetti S, Chiesa R, Coppi G, et al. Eversion versus conventional carotid endarterectomy: late

results of a prospective multicenter randomized trial. J Vasc Surg. 2000;31(1 Pt 1):19–30.
91. Lanza G, Ricci S, Speziale F, Toni D, Sbarigia E, Setacci C, et al. SPREAD-STACI study: a protocol for a randomized multicenter clinical trial comparing urgent with delayed endarterectomy in symptomatic carotid artery stenosis. Int J Stroke. 2012;7(1):81–5.
92. Lazarides MK, Christaina E, Argyriou C, Georgakarakos E, Tripsianis G, Georgiadis GS. Editor's choice – network meta-analysis of carotid endarterectomy closure techniques. Eur J Vasc Endovasc Surg. 2021;61(2):181–90.
93. Paraskevas KI, Robertson V, Saratzis AN, Naylor AR. Editor's choice – an updated systematic review and meta-analysis of outcomes following eversion vs. conventional carotid endarterectomy in randomised controlled trials and observational studies. Eur J Vasc Endovasc Surg. 2018;55(4):465–73.
94. AbuRahma AF, Darling RC 3rd. Literature review of primary versus patching versus eversion as carotid endarterectomy closure. J Vasc Surg. 2021;74(2):666–75.
95. Knipp SC, Holst T, Bilbilis K, von Velsen O, Ose C, Diener HC, et al. Five-year results of coronary artery bypass grafting with or without carotid endarterectomy in patients with asymptomatic carotid artery stenosis: CABACS RCT. Stroke. 2022;53(11):3270–7.
96. Forssell C, Takolander R, Bergqvist D, Johansson A, Persson NH. Local versus general anaesthesia in carotid surgery. A prospective, randomised study. Eur J Vasc Surg. 1989;3(6):503–9.
97. Sbarigia E, DarioVizza C, Antonini M, Speziale F, Maritti M, Fiorani B, et al. Locoregional versus general anesthesia in carotid surgery: is there an impact on perioperative myocardial ischemia? Results of a prospective monocentric randomized trial. J Vasc Surg. 1999;30(1):131–8.
98. Binder M, Fitzgerald R, Fried H, Schwarz S. Karotisdesobliteration in cervicalisblockade: eine okonomische alternative zur vollnarkose? Gesundh Ökon Qual Manag. 1999;4:19–24.
99. McCarthy RJ, Nasr MK, McAteer P, Horrocks M. Physiological advantages of cerebral blood flow during carotid endarterectomy under local anaesthesia. A randomised clinical trial. Eur J Vasc Endovasc Surg. 2002;24(3):215–21.
100. McCarthy RJ, Trigg R, John C, Gough MJ, Horrocks M. Patient satisfaction for carotid endarterectomy performed under local anaesthesia. Eur J Vasc Endovasc Surg. 2004;27(6):654–9.
101. Kasprzak PM, Altmeppen J, Angerer M, Mann S, Mackh J, Töpel I. General versus locoregional anesthesia in carotid surgery: a prospective randomised trial. Vasa. 2006;35:232–8.
102. Mrozek Z, Koutná J, Marek O. Anaesthesia options in carotid endarterectomy. Anest Intenziv Med. 2007;18(4):202–9.
103. Mazul-Sunko B, Hromatko I, Tadinac M, Sekulić A, Ivanec Z, Gvozdenović A, et al. Subclinical neurocognitive dysfunction after carotid endarterectomy-the impact of shunting. J Neurosurg Anesthesiol. 2010;22:195–201.
104. Moritz S, Schmidt C, Bucher M, Wiesenack C, Zimmermann M, Schebesch KM, et al. Neuromonitoring in carotid surgery: are the results obtained in awake patients transferable to patients under sevoflurane/fentanyl anesthesia? J Neurosurg Anesthesiol. 2010;22(4):288–95.
105. Hussien GZ, Elbadawy AM, Elshamaa HA. Lactate/pyruvate monitoring during carotid endarterectomy under general anaesthesia versus cervical plexus block: a randomised controlled study. Indian J Anaesth. 2017;61(5):424–8.
106. Orlický M, Hrbáč T, Sameš M, Vachata P, Hejčl A, Otáhal D, et al. Anesthesia type determines risk of cerebral infarction after carotid endarterectomy. J Vasc Surg. 2019;70:138–47.

Carotid Endarterectomy: Indications and Surgical Techniques

David Netuka, Martin Májovský, and Vladimír Beneš

1 Surgical Indications for Carotid Endarterectomy (CEA)

1.1 Symptomatic Carotid Stenosis

Patients who have experienced a recent carotid-territory transient ischemic attack (TIA), amaurosis fugax (transient monocular blindness), or nondisabling ischemic stroke can benefit significantly from CEA, depending on the degree of stenosis and timing of surgery:

- High-Grade Stenosis (70–99%)—Strong indication for CEA. Landmark trials (NASCET, ECST, and VA 309) demonstrated that for recently symptomatic carotid stenosis ≥70% (measured by NASCET criteria, excluding near-occlusions), CEA provides a substantial reduction in stroke risk [1]. A pooled analysis of these trials reported a ~16% absolute risk reduction in 5-year ipsilateral stroke risk with CEA compared to medical therapy (e.g. 5-year risk ~9% with CEA vs 26% with medical management for 70–99% stenosis) [1]. Current guidelines strongly recommend CEA for symptomatic 70–99% stenosis, provided the patient's perioperative stroke/death risk is <6% [2].
- Moderate Stenosis (50–69%)—Selective indication for CEA. The benefit of surgery in this range is smaller but still present for carefully chosen patients. The pooled trial data showed a modest absolute risk reduction (around 4–6% at 5 years) for symptomatic 50–69% stenosis. For example, 5-year stroke risk was ~19% with CEA vs ~24% with medical therapy in this subgroup (absolute risk reduction ~5%) [1]. CEA is considered for symptomatic 50–69% stenosis if the patient is a good surgical candidate (low comorbidity, and surgeon/institution complication rates <6%) [2, 3]. Guidelines categorize this as a weaker recommendation (e.g., Class IIa) because the net benefit is smaller [2]. Careful assessment of individual risk factors (e.g., ulcerated plaque morphology, patient age, sex, etc.) is warranted, as these may influence the risk-benefit balance in the moderate stenosis group.
- Mild Stenosis (<50%)—CEA is not indicated. Trials found no benefit (and even a potential harm) from surgery in symptomatic stenosis below 50% [1]. Medical therapy alone is recommended for <50% stenosis, as the procedural risk would outweigh any small stroke-risk reduction.
- "Near-Occlusion"—This term refers to an extremely high-grade stenosis with trickle flow (often with a collapsed distal internal carotid artery). In the pooled analysis, patients with near-occlusion did not derive significant long-term benefit from CEA [1]. There was a trend toward benefit at 2 years, but by 5 years the stroke rates were similar or higher in surgical patients (absolute difference ~−1.7%). Thus, CEA for near-occlusion is generally not beneficial in preventing stroke, and most guidelines do not recommend endarterectomy for anatomic near-occlusion of the carotid artery. Each case should be considered individually, but in general the focus in near-occlusion is optimizing medical therapy.
- Timing of Surgery—In symptomatic patients, timing is critical. Evidence shows that the stroke-prevention benefit of CEA is greatest when performed early after the neurologic event. Delay allows a high risk of recurrent stroke to accrue. Guidelines based on trial sub-group analyses (e.g., NASCET and ECST) and registry data recommend performing CEA as soon as possible, ideally within 14 days of the last symptoms [3, 4]. Surgery within 2 weeks confers the highest absolute risk reduction in stroke [4]. For example, one analysis found that for patients with ≥70% stenosis, CEA done within 2 weeks of a TIA/stroke prevented more strokes than if delayed beyond 2 weeks.

D. Netuka (✉) · V. Beneš
Department of Neurosurgery and Neurooncology, First Medical Faculty, Charles University, Prague, Czech Republic
e-mail: david.netuka@uvn.cz; vladimir.benes@uvn.cz

M. Májovský
Department of Neurosurgery and Neurooncology, 1st Medical Faculty, Charles University, Central Military Hospital, Prague, Czech Republic
e-mail: martin.majovsky@uvn.cz

V. Beneš, D. Netuka (eds.), *Surgical and Interventional Treatment of Cerebral Ischemia*,
https://doi.org/10.1007/978-3-032-08934-2_10

In practice, many centers aim for surgery within 1 week if feasible. If a patient presents with a minor stroke, CEA is usually performed once the patient is neurologically stable—often about 48 h after the event, assuming there is no hemorrhagic transformation on imaging [3]. This "wait 48 h" is a conventional safety period for patients with small, nondisabling infarcts. It's important to note that the major trials generally enrolled patients up to 120 days (4 months) from their event, but post-hoc analyses clearly show diminishing benefit with longer delays; most benefit is realized in the early period [3]. Therefore, early carotid surgery is standard for eligible symptomatic patients.

- Patient Neurologic Status—Only patients with nondisabling neurologic deficits were included in the major trials. Typically, this means a modified Rankin Scale (mRS) score 0–2 (0 = no symptoms, 2 = slight disability). Patients who had a major stroke with significant residual deficits (e.g., mRS ≥3) were usually not offered immediate CEA in trials, because if a patient is severely disabled from a large stroke, the benefit of stroke prevention is less clear and the surgical risks may be higher (and surgery could potentially worsen cerebral edema or hemorrhagic conversion risk in a large infarct). Thus, CEA is generally indicated for TIA or nondisabling stroke, not for a large, disabling stroke—at least not in the early period. In clinical practice, if a patient has a large stroke (mRS 4–5) carotid intervention is often deferred or not done at all, unless there is expected functional recovery and the carotid lesion poses a future risk. This nuance aligns with guidelines that recommend CEA for "stable" patients with recent symptoms [3].

1.2 Asymptomatic Carotid Stenosis

The role of CEA in asymptomatic patients is more controversial and has evolved over time. Asymptomatic carotid stenosis refers to a high-grade narrowing in a patient with no TIA or stroke history in that carotid distribution. Several large trials in the 1990s and early 2000s established that there is a benefit to CEA in asymptomatic patients provided that the patient's perioperative risk is very low and life expectancy is reasonable. Key points for asymptomatic stenosis include:

- Degree of Stenosis—Trials have shown benefit for high-grade asymptomatic stenosis, typically defined as ≥60% or ≥70% diameter reduction. The Asymptomatic Carotid Atherosclerosis Study (ACAS) in the 1990s enrolled patients with ≥60% stenosis. ACAS demonstrated that CEA plus best medical therapy reduced the 5-year risk of ipsilateral stroke (including perioperative events) to 5.1% versus 11.0% with medical therapy alone [5]. This was a 53% relative risk reduction (absolute risk reduction ~5.9% at 5 years). The Asymptomatic Carotid Surgery Trial (ACST-1), which started slightly later, included patients with ≥70–80% stenosis (by ultrasound criteria) and found a similar benefit. In ACST-1, the 5-year risk of any stroke was 6.4% with immediate CEA vs 11.8% with deferral (ARR ~5.4%) [6]. Most of the strokes prevented were ipsilateral ischemic strokes, about half of which were disabling or fatal strokes [6]. The benefit was even clearer at 10 years: successful CEA conferred about a 10% absolute stroke risk reduction at 10 years in patients <75 years old. Bottom line: Asymptomatic carotid stenosis confers a stroke risk over time, and CEA can reduce that risk, but the absolute benefit accumulates slowly (only a few percent per year).
- Risk Thresholds and Patient Selection—Because the stroke risk in asymptomatic disease is relatively low on modern medical therapy (estimated ~1–2% per year or less in many cohorts), CEA is only indicated if the surgery can be done with very low complication risk. A widely cited benchmark is that the combined 30-day stroke/death rate for CEA in an asymptomatic patient should be <3% [3, 5]. This threshold comes from the ACAS finding that benefit was only realized when surgical risk was around 2–3%, and it has been incorporated into guidelines (e.g., both SVS and AHA guidelines state <3% complication rate is required for asymptomatic interventions to be justified) [3, 5]. Therefore, asymptomatic CEA should be performed by experienced surgeons in centers with low complication rates. Patient comorbidities should also be considered: those with high cardiac risk or other factors that would make perioperative stroke, MI, or death more likely may not meet that <3% risk threshold.
- Life Expectancy—Because the stroke prevention benefit of CEA in asymptomatic patients accrues over several years, patients should have a sufficient life expectancy (often quoted ≥5 years) to derive net benefit [5]. In ACAS and ACST, patients were generally expected to live long enough to see that 5–10 year benefit. In an elderly patient or someone with advanced comorbid disease (e.g., active cancer or severe heart failure), the advantage of surgery is less clear because they may not survive long enough to benefit from stroke prevention. Modern guidelines emphasize selecting asymptomatic patients who are in good health biologically and could benefit from long-term stroke risk reduction [5].
- Current Guidelines—Most contemporary vascular society guidelines (SVS, ESVS, etc.) do support CEA in *selected* asymptomatic patients with high-grade stenosis. For example, the SVS recommends CEA as first-line for asymptomatic 70–99% stenosis in low-risk patients (again, surgical risk <3%) [3]. The European Stroke

Organization (ESO) 2021 guideline gave a moderate-quality evidence recommendation in favor of CEA for asymptomatic ≥60% stenosis *if* the patient is at elevated risk of stroke on best medical therapy [4]. "Elevated risk" may be suggested by factors like a >80–90% stenosis, progression of stenosis, plaque characteristics (e.g., echolucent or ulcerated plaque), silent infarcts on brain imaging, or microembolic signals on transcranial Doppler. These factors were not explicitly used in older trials but are considered in modern practice to identify those asymptomatic patients who resemble the trial cohorts that benefited.

- Evolving Landscape and Trials—It is important to note that medical therapy (statins, antihypertensives, antiplatelets, lifestyle changes) for atherosclerosis has improved since the time of ACAS/ACST. Recent studies indicate that stroke rates in asymptomatic carotid stenosis on contemporary optimal medical therapy are lower than decades ago. This has led some experts to question whether routine CEA is still justified in all asymptomatic cases, or whether we should be even more selective. Two large RCTs (CREST-2 trials) are underway, testing intensive medical therapy *versus* CEA (or stenting) in asymptomatic patients, to reassess the benefit in the modern era [4]. Until those results are published, the best evidence remains the older trials and their follow-ups. As such, guidelines continue to endorse CEA for asymptomatic stenosis in appropriate patients, while stressing careful patient selection. For instance, the ESVS 2023 guidelines favor intervention in asymptomatic carotid stenosis if ≥60% and imaging suggests high stroke risk features, but also acknowledge that many asymptomatic patients can be managed medically with good outcomes [4].
- Special Cases—Certain clinical scenarios in asymptomatic patients may tip the scale toward intervention. Patients with bilateral high-grade stenoses or contralateral carotid occlusion represent higher risk situations for stroke. Some studies have suggested that an asymptomatic severe stenosis may pose a higher stroke risk if the opposite carotid is already occluded (since collateral flow is compromised) [3]. Similarly, if an asymptomatic patient is undergoing coronary artery bypass grafting (CABG) and has a significant carotid stenosis, CEA (either staged or synchronous with CABG) might be considered to reduce perioperative stroke risk. However, these scenarios lack large RCT evidence and recommendations are based on observational data and expert consensus. Any such combined or staged procedures should be decided by a multidisciplinary team and are beyond the scope of standard indications (they fall under combined surgical planning). In all cases, asymptomatic CEA should only be done when the surgical risk is acceptably low and the patient stands to benefit in the long term [3, 5].

In summary, CEA is indicated for most patients with recent carotid-territory TIA/stroke and ≥70% stenosis, and can be considered for 50–69% stenosis depending on individual factors [1, 2]. Asymptomatic patients with ≥60–70% stenosis may be offered CEA if they are good candidates (low surgical risk, good longevity), but careful selection is required [3, 6]. All guideline bodies emphasize that surgery should only be performed if perioperative morbidity/mortality is below threshold (generally <6% for symptomatic, <3% for asymptomatic) [3, 5]. Moreover, timing (for symptomatic lesions, do it early) and patient condition (nondisabling symptoms, good general health) are key considerations in deciding to proceed with CEA.

2 Surgical Techniques for Carotid Endarterectomy

2.1 Anesthesia (General Versus Local)

CEA can be performed under general anesthesia (GA) or local/regional anesthesia (LA) (typically a deep cervical block or cervical plexus block, often with the patient mildly sedated but awake for neurologic monitoring). The Paraskevas 2018e of anesthetic technique has been evaluated in a large randomized trial. The GALA trial (Lancet 2008) enrolled over 3000 patients and compared outcomes of CEA under GA versus LA [7]. The primary composite outcome (stroke, myocardial infarction, or death within 30 days) was virtually identical between the two groups: 4.8% under general anesthesia vs 4.5% under local anesthesia (Risk Ratio 0.94, 95% CI 0.70–1.27; $p = 0.68$). There were no significant differences in stroke rate or other major complications, and secondary outcomes like hospital stay and quality of life were also similar. The GALA investigators concluded that no definitive difference in safety or efficacy exists between GA and LA for carotid endarterectomy. Therefore, the anesthetic approach can be individualized based on surgeon/anesthesiologist expertise and patient factors [7].

Each approach has practical advantages that are sometimes considered: Under local anesthesia, the patient is awake, allowing direct neurologic monitoring—if the patient shows signs of neurologic deficit when the carotid is clamped, it indicates cerebral hypoperfusion, guiding the surgeon to promptly place a shunt (see Sect. 2.2 below). Indeed, using LA tends to reduce the use of routine shunting; surgeons can selectively shunt only if the awake patient manifests symptoms. Studies have noted a substantially lower frequency of shunt usage in LA cases, since many patients tolerate clamping without issue and any emerging deficit is immediately apparent (obviating the need for an empirical shunt) [8]. Avoiding a shunt when unnecessary can simplify the procedure and eliminate the small risks associated with shunt placement. On the other hand, general anesthesia provides a motionless field and complete patient comfort, which some surgeons prefer for delicate vascular reconstruction. With GA, neurological monitoring is indirect (relying on SSEP, EEG, transcranial Doppler, etc., discussed later), and shunt decisions must be made based on those modalities or surgeon preference.

In summary, both GA and LA are acceptable for CEA. High-level evidence (Level I) indicates equipoise between GA and LA in terms of perioperative stroke, MI, and death [7]. Thus, the anesthetic method should be chosen based on the patient's condition and the surgical team's expertise. For example, anxious patients or those who cannot lie flat and still may do better with GA, whereas patients with severe pulmonary disease might better tolerate LA. Some guidelines stop short of formally recommending one over the other, instead stating that either is reasonable and that institutions should develop protocols for intraoperative neurological monitoring appropriate to their chosen anesthetic technique.

2.2 Cerebral Protection and Shunting

During CEA, the carotid artery is clamped to allow arteriotomy (opening the artery) and plaque removal. This clamp interrupts blood flow to the ipsilateral brain (via the internal carotid artery) for the duration of the endarterectomy. Cerebral shunting involves placing a temporary bypass tube (shunt) to maintain perfusion to the brain during carotid cross-clamping. Shunts can prevent cerebral ischemia in patients who have inadequate collateral flow, but shunt placement itself carries risks (dislodging plaque or air emboli, causing intimal injury, etc.). There is long-standing debate about whether to shunt routinely (shunt all cases prophylactically) or shunt selectively (shunt only those who show evidence of hypoperfusion during test clamping). A third approach is no shunting at all, relying on the fact that many patients tolerate the clamp time with good Circle of Willis collateral circulation.

Evidence: The question of shunting has been addressed by several small randomized trials and summarized in a Cochrane review. However, the data are relatively limited and have not shown a clear advantage of one strategy over another. The most recent Cochrane review on routine vs selective shunting (2014, updated 2021) included 6 RCTs (1270 patients total) [9]. Three trials compared routine shunting to no shunting; one trial compared routine shunting to selective; and two trials compared different monitoring methods for selective shunting. No trials have directly compared selective shunting to no shunting—most surgeons agree that *some* form of shunting (routine or selective) is prudent rather than never shunting at all. The Cochrane review found that in the limited data available, routine shunting vs no shunting showed a trend toward lower perioperative stroke or stroke-related death for the routine shunt group. Specifically, routine shunting appeared to reduce the risk of stroke occurring within 24 h of surgery, and stroke-related mortality within 30 days, compared to no shunt. However, these findings were based on only a few trials and event rates, and the evidence quality was low. In the single trial that compared routine to selective shunting, no significant difference in outcomes was found. Overall, the Cochrane reviewers concluded that the evidence was too limited to either support or refute the use of routine shunting in CEA. In other words, there is no definitive proof that routine shunting is superior to a selective approach with good monitoring, or vice versa. Additionally, no monitoring method for selective shunting has been shown to be clearly better than others [9].

Given this, the practice of shunting varies by surgeon and institution. Some surgeons shunt routinely in every CEA to avoid any chance of cerebral ischemia. Majority surgeons shunt selectively—for example, they might use an intraoperative SSEP, EEG or measure stump/back pressure after clamping; if SSEP or EEG changes occur or stump pressure is below a threshold (e.g., <50 mmHg), they then insert a shunt (otherwise not). Surgeons operating under local anesthesia often use the patient's neurologic status as the monitor—if the awake patient shows mental status changes or deficits when the carotid is clamped, a shunt is placed (if no changes, they proceed without a shunt). Both selective and routine shunting are acceptable approaches according to most guidelines, acknowledging the lack of definitive. The 2023 ESVS guidelines, for instance, state that routine or selective shunting can be used and that individual surgeon experience should guide the strategy, since trial data do not demonstrate one clearly superior method.

Neuromonitoring: In selective shunting, some form of cerebral monitoring is required to identify patients who need a shunt. Common monitoring techniques include neurologic examination in awake patients, electroencephalography (EEG), somatosensory evoked potentials (SSEP), transcranial Doppler (to detect decreased middle cerebral artery flow or microemboli), near-infrared cerebral oximetry, or carotid stump pressure measurement. Each modality has its pros/cons (EEG is sensitive to cortical ischemia but requires trained interpretation; stump pressure is easy but a crude surrogate; etc.). No single monitoring technique has proven definitively better in trials [9]. Surgeons often choose a method they are comfortable with. For example, many use a combination of modalities (e.g., SSEP and EEG, or EEG plus stump pressure) for redundancy. The Cochrane review noted that no monitoring technique in selective shunting has shown superior outcomes—meaning as long as the surgeon uses some reliable way to detect hypoperfusion, selective shunting can be as safe as routine shunting [9]. Therefore, surgeon judgment remains key. If there is any doubt, most surgeons will err on the side of inserting a shunt, since a properly placed shunt typically poses low risk and can provide peace of mind against ischemia.

In summary, shunting practices in CEA are variable, and evidence does not mandate one approach. It is critical that if selective shunting is employed, vigilant monitoring is in place to promptly identify cerebral ischemia. If adequate monitoring is not available, a more routine shunting strategy might be chosen. Both strategies—routine shunt with its potential risks, or selective shunt with a small risk of unprotected clamping—result in low stroke rates in experienced hands. Surgeons should have an established protocol: for example, one institutional protocol might state "shunt if stump pressure <40 mmHg or if EEG shows >50% loss of amplitude on clamp", whereas another institution might say "shunt all symptomatic stenoses, selectively shunt asymptomatic based on EEG". Importantly, the overall perioperative stroke rates in CEA are low (~2–3%), indicating that either approach can be effective when properly executed [9].

2.3 Eversion Versus Conventional Endarterectomy Technique

There are two principal ways to perform the endarterectomy itself: the conventional (standard) CEA and the eversion CEA.

- In a conventional CEA, the surgeon makes a longitudinal arteriotomy (incision) in the carotid artery (usually extending from the common carotid into the internal carotid) to expose the plaque. The plaque is circumferentially dissected and removed (often as one unit) from the artery, and then the arteriotomy is closed (Fig. 1). Vascular surgeons often use a patch to widen the artery (Fig. 2).
- In an eversion CEA, the surgical approach is a bit different: the surgeon transects the internal carotid artery at the carotid bifurcation and everts (turns inside-out) the internal carotid over a spatula or surgeon's finger to peel the plaque out of the arterial wall. Essentially, the plaque is removed by everting the artery itself, rather than through a longitudinal opening. After removing the plaque, the internal carotid is reimplanted (sewn back) onto the open common carotid artery. This technique inherently widens the internal carotid opening (much like a patch would) because the reimplantation can accommodate the normal lumen diameter (Fig. 3).

Outcomes: Numerous studies, including several randomized trials and meta-analyses, have compared eversion CEA (eCEA) to conventional CEA (cCEA). The largest single trial was the EVEREST trial, a multicenter RCT with 1353 patients (675 conventional, 678 eversion) [10]. EVEREST and other trials have found no significant difference in the primary outcomes of stroke or death between eversion and conventional CEA [10]. In EVEREST, for example, the 30-day rate of any major stroke or death was ~1.3% in both groups, and the overall 30-day stroke rate (including minor strokes) was ~2% in each, showing equivalence. Long-term results from EVEREST and other studies indicate that both techniques are highly effective and durable, with low ipsilateral stroke rates on follow-up.

One difference noted is in restenosis rates: eversion CEA may be associated with a slightly lower incidence of restenosis compared to conventional CEA, particularly if the con-

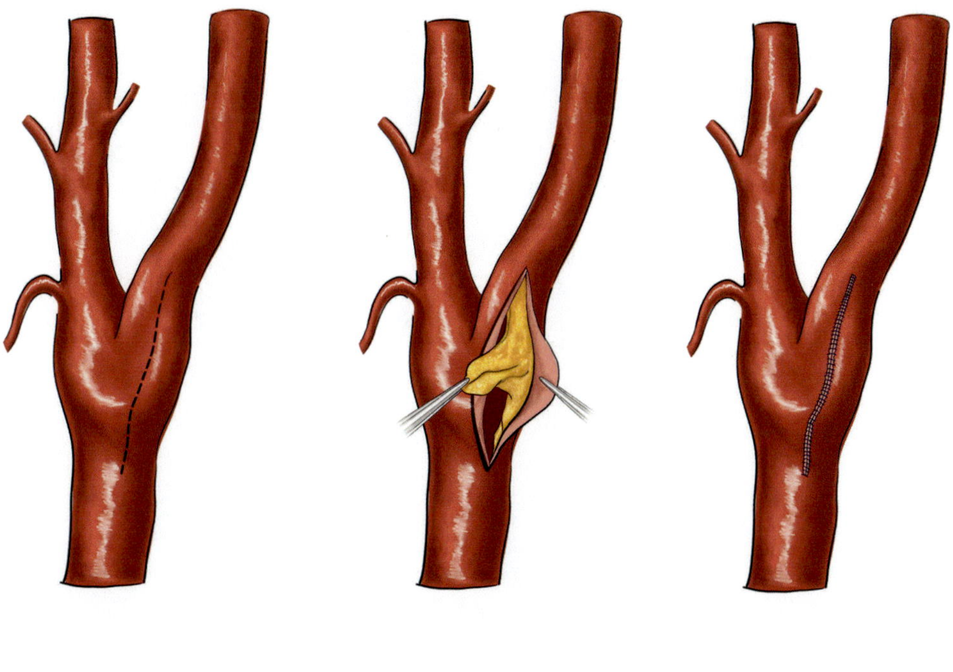

Fig. 1 Longitudinal arteriotomy (**a**), circumferential removal of the atherosclerotic plaque (**b**), primary suture of the vessel (**c**)

ventional CEA is closed without a patch. In EVEREST, at ~4 years follow-up, the ≥70% restenosis rate was higher after standard CEA with primary closure (9.2%) than after eversion CEA (3.6%) [10]. When a patch is used in conventional CEA, the restenosis rates become similarly low. In EVEREST, the 4-year restenosis was ~1.5% for patched conventional CEA vs 2.8% for eversion (a difference that was not statistically significant). Another meta-analysis combining data from 5 RCTs and many observational studies found that eversion CEA had significantly less late restenosis than conventional CEA with primary closure (odds ratio ~ 0.4 favoring eversion) [11]. However, when conventional CEA was done with Rerkasem et al. 2011plasty, the difference in late restenosis between eversion and patched CEA was minimal. In fact, a comprehensive 2018 meta-analysis concluded that early and late outcomes of eversion CEA and patch-closure CEA are equivalent—eversion was only superior to the extent that it mimics a "built-in patch".

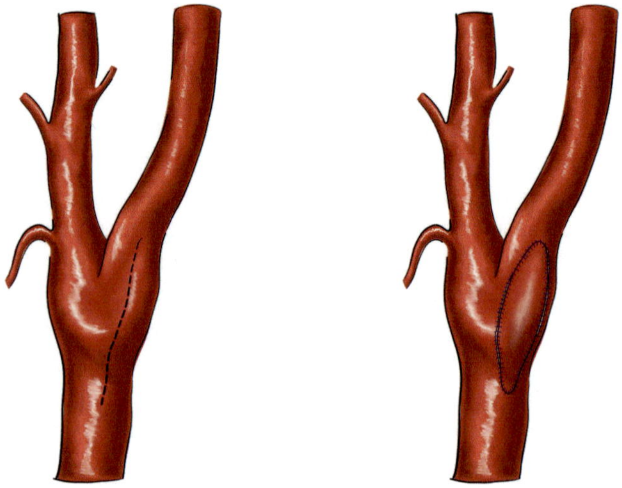

Fig. 2 Longitudinal arteriotomy (**a**), a patch used for carotid suture (**b**)

In practical terms, eversion and conventional CEA (with patch) are both accepted techniques with excellent outcomes. Surgeons may choose one technique based on their training and the specific anatomy:

- Advantages of eversion CEA: It avoids a longitudinal arteriotomy and the need for a patch, potentially simplifying the closure step. It often results in a shorter clamp time because once the artery is transected, the plaque elevation and reimplantation can be efficient (EVEREST reported eversion had a slightly shorter clamp time than patched conventional CEA, by a few minutes). Some data suggest eversion CEA may have a lower incidence of certain local complications; for example, analysis from the CREST trial noted that cranial nerve injuries were less frequent with eversion technique than with conventional CEA (possibly due to less extensive dissection in the neck) [10]. Eversion also inherently enlarges the lumen at the reconnection point, mitigating the risk of closure-related narrowing.
- Advantages of conventional CEA: It may be easier to perform when the disease extends high up the internal carotid artery. If plaque is very long (reaching beyond the accessible area), eversion may be difficult because it requires eversion of a long segment. In such cases, a standard arteriotomy can be extended further to remove a long plaque. Conventional CEA also allows insertion of a shunt more easily (one can insert a shunt proximally and distally in

Fig. 3 Eversion technique of endarterectomy: disconnection of internal carotid artery from carotid bulb (**a**), plaque removal (**b**), reimplantation of internal carotid artery (**c**)

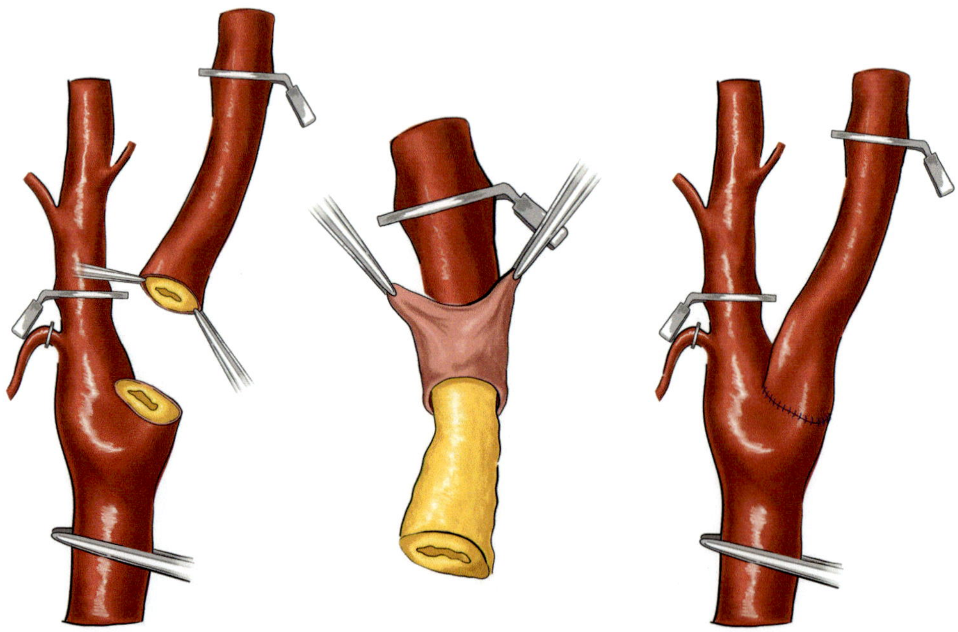

the arteriotomy); eversion, being an end-to-end reconnection, makes shunt placement slightly more tricky though not impossible (shunts can still be used by making an incision in the everted ICA). Additionally, if any issues occur (e.g., a loose intimal flap), a conventional arteriotomy provides direct access for patch repair, whereas in eversion one might have to convert to a patch if a problem is encountered.

Both techniques require meticulous technique to ensure the plaque is fully removed and the end point is smooth to prevent thrombosis or embolization. Importantly, guidelines do not express a preference for eversion vs conventional—they are considered equally valid. The ESVS 2023 guideline, for instance, states that the Paraskevas 2018e of CEA technique (eversion vs patched conventional) should be left to the operating surgeon, as evidence shows similar outcomes [2]. The German-Austrian guidelines likewise advise that either approach is acceptable, depending on the surgeon's expertise.

A practical point: Eversion CEA is not ideal for very high lesions. If the stenosis involves a long segment of the internal carotid, eversion would require everting a very long arterial segment, which is challenging and risks intimal tears. Surgeons typically limit eversion to cases where the plaque is reasonably confined to the bulb/proximal internal carotid. A long segment disease is usually managed with a conventional CEA and a patch. In fact, experts recommend avoiding eversion in cases of long (>3–4 cm) ICA plaques [10], where a standard arteriotomy provides better exposure.

In summary, eCEA vs cCEA: Both achieve low perioperative stroke rates (1–3%) and low restenosis rates (around 1–5%) [10]. A surgeon skilled in eversion can expect outcomes just as good as with patch closure [11]. Conversely, if one is more comfortable with conventional CEA, will yield outcomes equivalent to eversion.

2.4 Arteriotomy Closure: Primary Versus Rerkasem et al. 2011plasty

After removing the plaque in a conventional CEA, the surgeon must close the arteriotomy. Primary closure means simply suturing the artery closed directly. Rerkasem et al. 2011plasty means sewing a patch (made of either synthetic material or autologous vein) to enlarge the closure, essentially widening the artery at the endarterectomy site. Patching prevents narrowing of the vessel lumen and provides a larger caliber artery, which is thought to reduce turbulent flow, risk of thrombosis, and restenosis.

Evidence favors Rerkasem et al. 2011plasty over primary closure. This is one of the most extensively studied technical aspects of CEA, with numerous historical RCTs dating back to the 1980s/90s and multiple meta-analyses (including Cochrane reviews) reaching a conclusion: patch closure improves outcomes compared to primary closure.

Key findings from the evidence:

- Perioperative Stroke and Occlusion: A Cochrane systematic review (most recently updated with data through 2021) analyzed 11 RCTs (over 2300 CEAs) comparing patch vs primary closure [8]. Rerkasem et al. 2011plasty significantly lowered the risk of perioperative stroke relative to primary closure. The odds of any stroke within 30 days were reduced (many studies cite roughly a 60–70% reduction in odds). For example, one meta-analysis of 10 RCTs (2157 CEAs) found ipsilateral stroke in 1.5% of patch cases vs 4.5% with primary closure (Odds Ratio ~ 0.33) [2, 10]. Similarly, the risk of carotid artery thrombosis (occlusion) in the immediate postoperative period is markedly reduced with patching—primary closure has a small but higher risk of acute closure of the artery due to the smaller lumen and potential intimal trauma. The meta-analysis above reported carotid occlusion in 0.5% with patch vs 3.1% with primary closure (OR ~ 0.18) [10]. This translates to a significant reduction in return to the operating room for issues like thrombosis or severe narrowing when patches are used [2, 10]. Indeed, one study noted re-exploration for any reason within 30 days was ~3% with primary closure vs ~1% with patch (OR ~ 0.3) [2]. The Cochrane review's bottom line: *"Rerkasem et al. 2011plasty lowered the risk of stroke in the short term after surgery compared with primary closure"* [8].
- Long-Term Outcomes (Restenosis and Late Stroke): Patch closure confers long-term benefits. Without a patch, the artery can scar and narrow over time (restenosis). Trials with follow-up have consistently shown higher restenosis rates after primary closure. For example, the Cochrane review found that primary closure was associated with significantly higher risk of ≥50% restenosis on long-term follow-up (often 2–5 years)—roughly a three to four fold higher risk of restenosis compared to patch [2, 10]. Bond et al. (Cochrane 2004) reported restenosis ≥50% in ~18.5% of primary closures vs ~4.8% of patch closures in pooled trial data [10]. The more recent meta-analysis (Rerkasem et al.) similarly found late significant restenosis in 13.8% after primary vs 4.3% after patch (OR ~ 0.2). This reduction in restenosis translates into a lower incidence of late stroke. Patching significantly reduces ipsilateral stroke in follow-up beyond 30 days. In pooled data, late ipsilateral stroke rates were about 1.6% with patch vs 4.8% with primary over several years (OR ~ 0.3) [2, 10]. Any stroke (including contralateral or unrelated) was also lower with patch, likely reflecting the prevention of restenosis and related events [2]. The Cochrane authors concluded that patching *"appears to*

reduce the risk of ipsilateral stroke during the perioperative and long-term period" compared to primary closure [8]. Importantly, combining perioperative and long-term strokes (i.e., the total 5-year stroke risk), patching provides a net stroke reduction even after accounting for the slightly higher immediate risk of occlusion with primary closure [10].
- Other Outcomes: Patch vs primary has not shown differences in operative mortality or myocardial infarction rates—these outcomes are more so related to patient factors than the closure technique, and indeed studies typically show similar 30-day death rates between groups [2]. Cranial nerve injury rates are also similar between patch and primary closure in RCTs [10]. The main differences truly center on stroke, thrombosis, and restenosis—all favoring patch.

Given this evidence, using a patch for arteriotomy closure is considered a standard of care in carotid endarterectomy, except in unusual circumstances. Guidelines (SVS, ESVS, etc.) recommend Rerkasem et al. 2011plasty for conventional CEA (Class I, Level A evidence) [2]. The debate that remains is *what type of patch* to use—autologous vein or one of several synthetic options.

Patch Materials: Surgeons have several patch material options:

- Autologous vein (typically the great saphenous vein, harvested from the leg, or sometimes jugular vein).
- Synthetic patches: e.g., Dacron (polyester), PTFE, polyurethane, or biomaterials like bovine pericardium.

Clinical studies, including RCTs and large series, have compared different patch types. Overall, no patch material has proven significantly superior in terms of efficacy. Randomized trials that have compared vein vs synthetic (and trials comparing one synthetic vs another) generally find no significant differences in perioperative stroke, death, or restenosis rates between patch types [10]. For instance, one trial cited in a literature review showed no difference in 30-day stroke, occlusion, or cranial nerve palsy between vein patch and Dacron patch. Another study found no difference between Dacron and PTFE in outcomes. A network meta-analysis published in 2019 (Balzer et al., Eur J Vasc Endovasc Surg) compared multiple patch materials and found all patch types yielded broadly similar stroke and restenosis outcomes [2].

Given the comparable efficacy, the Paraskevas 2018e of patch often comes down to surgeon preference and patient-specific considerations:

- Vein patch: It's pliable and integrates well, with low risk of long-term infection (since it's the patient's own tissue). However, it requires an additional incision to harvest the vein and the vein patch can be thinner and potentially at risk for aneurysmal dilation or rupture (though this is quite rare). "Vein patch rupture (blowout)" is an often-cited concern; fortunately, it is exceedingly rare (~0.2% incidence) in modern series [2]. If it occurs, it typically happens early post-op due to suture line issues. Surgeons ensure an adequate vein segment and often trim it to double layer to reinforce.
- Synthetic patch: Avoids a second incision and provides a durable material of known size and strength. PTFE patches are very commonly used; Dacron is another synthetic used historically; bovine pericardial patches are also popular (technically a biological material, but treated and supplied commercially). Infection risk is a theoretical downside of synthetic patches—an infected prosthetic patch is serious (could lead to pseudoaneurysm or sepsis). Fortunately, infection is very uncommon, roughly on the order of 0.2% as well [2]. Some surveys suggest a slightly higher infection rate for Dacron vs PTFE, but data are limited; overall infection of any patch is rare. If a synthetic patch gets infected, it may require surgical removal and bypass. Bovine pericardium patches have the advantage of being biologic and possibly more infection-resistant than plastic, and they handle nicely (soft and easy to sew).

In terms of outcomes, studies like the Vascular Quality Initiative (VQI) analysis have noted small differences: e.g., one large registry noted that bovine pericardial and polyester (Dacron) patches were associated with slightly lower perioperative stroke/TIA compared to vein or PTFE in their dataset [2], and that bovine, polyester, and vein patches all had lower 1-year restenosis rates than primary closure. However, these differences are not from RCTs and could be influenced by selection bias. In practice, all patch materials perform well, and no definitive evidence mandates one over another [10]. Surgeons often choose based on their experience: some prefer *vein patches* in younger patients (no foreign material left behind) and *PTFE or pericardium* in others to save operative time or if vein quality is poor.

To summarize this section: Patching yields lower perioperative stroke (about 1–2% vs 3–5%) and less restenosis [2, 10], which in turn leads to fewer late strokes [10]. Patch type can be tailored; evidence has not identified an optimal material, so surgeon preference and patient factors dictate the Paraskevas 2018. Both autologous vein and various synthetic patches are acceptable since they have comparable stroke and patency outcomes. Complications like patch infection or rupture are extremely infrequent (~0.2%) and vigilance (sterile technique, careful patch crafting) keeps these risks minimal [2].

2.5 Other Intraoperative Considerations

- Anticoagulation: Almost all surgeons administer systemic heparin before clamping the carotid artery. This is standard practice (universal in trials) to reduce thromboembolic risk during the period of clamping and arterial manipulation. Typically an ACT (activated clotting time) >250 s is achieved. After CEA, some surgeons reverse heparin with protamine to reduce bleeding risk, but others do not fully reverse it to avoid potential prothrombotic rebound. There is no high-level trial on protamine use; practices vary. A meta-analysis has shown protamine can increase risk of thrombosis slightly but reduce bleeding; thus, it's a trade-off. Guidelines often say protamine reversal "may be considered" based on the situation—if there is concern for bleeding, partial reversal is reasonable, but beware of potential thrombosis if protamine triggers platelet activation. This detail goes beyond the scope of indications/techniques evidence, but is a technical point of note.
- Intraoperative Imaging: Some surgeons use completion ultrasound or angiography after CEA to verify no residual stenosis or flap. If a defect is seen, they revise the endarterectomy before closing. This is a technical adjunct to improve quality. Evidence: a few studies suggest routine completion imaging can catch problems (in ~2–3% of cases) and fix them, potentially reducing early stroke. It's generally considered good practice, though not mandated by trials.
- Cranial Nerve Management: During CEA, meticulous surgical technique is needed to avoid injury to local cranial nerves (hypoglossal nerve, vagus including its branch the superior laryngeal nerve, glossopharyngeal, and marginal mandibular branch of facial nerve). Temporary cranial nerve palsies (like hoarseness from vagus/recurrent laryngeal nerve neuropraxia, tongue deviation from hypoglossal nerve stretch) occur in 5–7% of cases typically, but most resolve spontaneously in a few weeks [10]. Permanent cranial nerve injuries are under 1–2%. There is no difference in cranial nerve injury rate between patch vs eversion per se, as that depends more on dissection technique and patient anatomy. As noted, one analysis found eversion had fewer cranial nerve injuries than standard CEA in CREST, but broadly, both techniques have low rates when done carefully [10]. Surgeons ensure good visualization and gentle handling of nerve structures to minimize this risk.
- Adjuncts like Shunt Variations: Some newer shunt designs and methods (e.g., external carotid to internal carotid shunts, or flow reversal systems) exist but their discussion is beyond scope. The key is that shunting principles remain as above.
- Eversion specifics: When performing eversion, the surgeon must dissect the carotid bifurcation free and typically cut the internal carotid just above the plaque. After eversion endarterectomy, the reimplantation suture line is essentially an anastomosis between the internal carotid and common carotid. Surgeons often spatulate the artery a bit to make the anastomosis wide. This is why eversion is essentially like doing an end-to-end anastomosis—familiarity with vascular anastomosis technique is required. The learning curve can be slightly higher, which is one reason some stick with conventional plus patch.
- Hybrid Techniques: On occasion, a surgeon might do a partial eversion (to get the plaque out of the internal carotid) and then still use a patch on the common carotid portion—but this is uncommon and typically not needed.
- Closing Notes on Technique: The various randomized trials and meta-analyses we have cited provide a strong evidence base for surgical technique in CEA. To encapsulate:
  - Use patch closure for conventional CEA (Class I, Level A recommendation) [2]. It lowers stroke and restenosis risk [10].
  - Eversion CEA is an effective alternative to patching, yielding equivalent outcomes in experienced hands [10, 11]. The Paraskevas 2018e between eversion vs standard is up to surgeon preference; both are acceptable per guidelines [2].
  - Shunting can be done routinely or selectively; evidence is insufficient to declare one best, so practice is guided by institutional protocol and monitoring capabilities [9]. The goal is cerebral protection; as long as that is achieved, stroke rates remain low.
  - Anesthetic technique (general vs local) does not alter major outcomes, so it should be tailored to patient and surgeon comfort [7].
  - Modern best practices: administer antiplatelet therapy (e.g., aspirin) preoperatively and continue it, use heparin intra-op, consider neuro monitoring and completion imaging, and follow strict protocols for blood pressure management during and after the procedure to reduce hyperperfusion or hypoperfusion issues (though these topics go into perioperative management rather than the surgical technique itself).

By adhering to these evidence-based technical principles, carotid endarterectomy can be performed with a very low complication rate and excellent efficacy in stroke prevention. High-quality randomized trials (e.g., NASCET, ACAS) established when to operate, and subsequent trials (EVT, GALA, etc.) and meta-analyses have refined how to operate for optimal outcomes. Surgeons should stay up-to-date with guideline recommendations and evidence, as ongoing research (such as CREST-2 for asymptomatic disease) may further impact patient selection in the future. The technical tenets, however, have remained relatively constant: careful surgical technique with attention to cerebral protection, a wide arterial closure (patch or eversion), and appropriate perioperative management are the cornerstones of a successful carotid endarterectomy [2, 8].

2.6 Carotid Endartrectomy

Detailed technique of carotid endartrectomy as practised at the authors institution has recently been described elsewhere [12]

Declarations

Competing Interests The author(s) has no competing interests to declare that are relevant to the content of this manuscript.

Ethics Approval The author(s) declares that this manuscript does not include primary research with human participants.

References

1. Rothwell PM, et al. Lancet. 2003;361(9352):107–16. Pooled analysis of ECST, NASCET, and VA trials for symptomatic carotid stenosis – demonstrated that CEA is highly beneficial for 70–99% symptomatic stenosis (5-year stroke risk reduction ~16%) and provides modest benefit for 50–69% stenosis.
2. Howard VJ, et al. Lancet. 2016;387(10038):1305–11. Analysis of CREST and other data – supported age dichotomy for CEA vs CAS (CEA better in age ≥70). (Mentioned in guidelines for choosing endarterectomy in older patients) (ESVS-2023-Carotid-guidelines.pdf).
3. Yin D, et al. Stroke. 2015;46(9):2415–21. Study on timing – showed stroke risk is highest immediately after TIA and declines over weeks; delaying CEA beyond 2 weeks markedly reduces benefit. Reinforces guideline to operate ASAP (ideally <14 days) (PIIS0741521421008934 (1).pdf).
4. Bonati LH, et al. Eur Stroke J. 2021;6(2):I–XLVII. European Stroke Organisation guidelines – recommend CEA for symptomatic stenosis ≥70% (Class I) and consider for 50–69%; for asymptomatic ≥60% in selected patients with low surgical risk (bonati-et-al-2021-european-stroke-organisation-guideline-on-endarterectomy-and-stenting-for-carotid-artery-stenosis.pdf).
5. Executive Committee for ACAS. JAMA. 1995;273(18):1421–8. ACAS trial – in asymptomatic ≥60% stenosis, 5-year ipsilateral stroke risk 11.0% medical vs 5.1% with CEA (ARR ~5.9%); CEA recommended if surgical stroke/death risk <3% (Endarterectomy for asymptomatic carotid artery stenosis. Executive Committee for the Asymptomatic Carotid Atherosclerosis Study – PubMed).
6. Halliday A, et al. Lancet. 2004;363(9420):1491–502. ACST-1 trial – in asymptomatic ≥60% stenosis, CEA reduced 5-year stroke risk from ~11.8% to 6.4% (ARR 5.4%, p<0.0001) at the cost of 3.1% perioperative stroke/death (Prevention of disabling and fatal strokes by successful carotid endarterectomy in patients without recent neurological symptoms: randomised controlled trial – PubMed).
7. GALA Trial Collaborative Group. Lancet. 2008;372(9656):2132–42. GALA trial – no significant difference in 30-day stroke, MI, or death between CEA under general anesthesia (4.8% event rate) vs local anesthesia (4.5%) (General anaesthesia versus local anaesthesia for carotid surgery (GALA): a multicentre, randomised controlled trial – PubMed).
8. Rerkasem K, Rothwell PM. Cochrane Database Syst Rev. 2011;(4):CD000160. (Updated Cochrane 2021) – patch vs primary closure: patch angioplasty significantly reduces perioperative stroke (OR ~0.33) and carotid occlusion (OR ~0.18) compared to primary closure (ESVS-2023-Carotid-guidelines.pdf). Also lowers 5-year stroke and restenosis rates (Literature review of primary versus patching versus eversion as carotid endarterectomy closure* – Journal of Vascular Surgery).
9. Cochrane Stroke Group. Cochrane Database Syst Rev. 2014;(7):CD000190. (Updated 2021) – shunting in CEA: insufficient evidence to determine if routine shunting is superior to selective shunting; a few small trials suggest routine shunting may reduce early stroke in GA cases, but overall data quality is low (Routine or selective carotid artery shunting for carotid endarterectomy (and different methods of monitoring in selective shunting) | Cochrane).
10. Balzer K, et al. Eur J Vasc Endovasc Surg. 2019;58(4):492–502. Network meta-analysis of CEA patch closure techniques – found no major differences in outcomes between patch materials (PTFE, Dacron, vein, bovine pericardium all had comparable stroke and restenosis outcomes) (Literature review of primary versus patching versus eversion as carotid endarterectomy closure* – Journal of Vascular Surgery).
11. Paraskevas KI, et al. Eur J Vasc Endovasc Surg. 2018;55(4):465–73. Meta-analysis of eversion vs conventional CEA – no difference in perioperative stroke/death in RCTs; eversion associated with less restenosis. Combined data show eversion and patched CEA have equivalent outcomes (Editor's Choice – an updated systematic review and meta-analysis of outcomes following eversion vs. conventional carotid endarterectomy in randomised controlled trials and observational studies – PubMed).
12. Beneš V, Bubeníková A, Bradáč O. Carotid endarterectomy. In: Kanaan I, Beneš V, editors. Neuroanatomy guidance to successful neurosurgical interventions. Cham: Springer; 2024. p. 291–302.

Carotid Artery Stenting—Indications and Technique

Akio Hyodo, Tomoji Takigawa, and Yasuhiko Nariai

1 Introduction

Carotid artery stenosis can contribute to prevention of cerebral infarction through several mechanisms, including acute occlusion resulting from plaque rupture or thrombus formation, embolism from a wall thrombus to a peripheral artery (artery-to-artery embolism), and reduced cerebral perfusion. The severity of systemic vascular diseases associated with atherosclerosis is strongly correlated with an increased risk of ipsilateral stroke [1, 2]. The primary treatment goal of carotid artery stenosis is to prevent cerebral infarction and transient ischemic attacks. Treatment options can be categorized into three approaches: (1) medical management, (2) surgical treatment, carotid endarterectomy (CEA), and (3) endovascular therapy, represented by carotid artery stenting (CAS). Although CEA remains the most well-established option because of its significant evidence base, the use of CAS is steadily increasing owing to advancements in technology and improved techniques.

2 Indications for CAS

According to current guidelines [3], the decision to pursue revascularization in asymptomatic patients should consider a comprehensive assessment of comorbidities, anatomical characteristics, and patient preferences (Class I). CAS is preferred in patients with anatomical characteristics that make surgery less favorable (Class IIa). For asymptomatic patients with an average surgical risk, the guidelines supported by the CREST results [4] suggest that CAS is a potential option (Class IIb). However, the superiority of revascularization over optimized medical management has yet to be established.

Indications for CAS include severe asymptomatic carotid stenosis (≥70%) or symptomatic stenosis (≥50%), particularly among patients with conditions that pose high surgical risk, such as recent unstable angina, myocardial infarction, severe pulmonary disease, and a history of neck radiation therapy. Additional indications include contralateral vocal cord paralysis, tracheotomy, contralateral carotid occlusion, recurrent stenosis following CEA, and high-level lesions [2, 4].

3 Assessment for Carotid Artery Stenosis

Duplex ultrasonography (DUS) is the preferred initial imaging technique for assessing carotid artery stenosis because of its noninvasive nature and ability to provide a precise evaluation of the degree of stenosis and insight into plaque echolucency, which reflects the underlying plaque characteristics [1]. In addition, depending on the patients' renal function, time-of-flight magnetic resonance angiography (TOF-MRA) or computed tomographic angiography (CTA) should be also performed to confirm the severity and anatomical location of the stenosis. Finally, the validity of the relationship between the stenosis predicted by peak systolic velocity (PSV) measured using DUS and the stenosis assessed using TOF-MRA or CTA should be carefully considered. For example, 70% stenosis of the internal carotid artery (ICA), as defined by the North American Symptomatic Carotid Endarterectomy Trial (NASCET) criteria, correlates with a PSV of 200–230 cm/s, whereas 50% stenosis corresponds to a PSV of approximately 125 cm/s [5]. In cases of discrepancies between DUS and MRA/CTA findings, digital subtraction angiography (DSA) may be used to confirm the extent of stenosis and evaluate the need for revascularization. Routine use of DSA is not recommended for preoperative assessment because of

A. Hyodo (✉)
Department of Neurosurgery, Kamagaya General Hospital, Chiba, Japan
e-mail: hyodo@dokkyomed.ac.jp

T. Takigawa · Y. Nariai
Department of Neurosurgery, Dokkyo Medical University Saitama Medical Center, Saitama, Japan
e-mail: takigawa@dokkyomed.ac.jp

V. Beneš, D. Netuka (eds.), *Surgical and Interventional Treatment of Cerebral Ischemia*,
https://doi.org/10.1007/978-3-032-08934-2_11

its invasive nature. In addition, DSA may remain a valuable tool in specific cases, such as near occlusion (NO) or chronic total occlusion (CTO). NO, characterized by the full collapse of the ICA distal to the stenosis as visualized on DSA, is associated with a significantly higher risk of recurrent ipsilateral ischemic stroke and necessitates revascularization [6]. In symptomatic cases of CTO, the presence of a proximal ICA stump identified using DSA strongly predicts the technical feasibility of CAS [7].

In addition to evaluating the severity of stenosis, assessment of plaque vulnerability is critical. DUS and magnetic resonance imaging are valuable tools for detecting features, such as plaque ulceration, necrotic lipid cores, intraplaque hemorrhage, neovascularity, thin or ruptured fibrous caps, and thrombi. Plaques rich in lipids and blood components are prone to ulceration, and thus pose a higher risk of stroke [1]. Additionally, preoperative imaging modalities such as single-photon emission computed tomography or positron emission tomography can be employed to assess the cerebrovascular reserve and identify patients at risk of postoperative hyperperfusion [8].

4 Devices: Selection and Application

Embolic protection devices (EPDs) for CAS are categorized into proximal and distal systems. Distal EPDs include filter-based devices such as the FilterWire EZ (Boston Scientific, Natick, MA, USA) and Spider FX (Medtronic, Minneapolis, MN, USA), and balloon occlusion systems such as the Optimal Wire protection system (Tokai Medical Products, Aichi, Japan), as shown in Fig. 1 [9]. Although effective at capturing small embolic particles, distal balloon systems may trigger ischemic intolerance caused by temporary blood-flow occlusion. Proximal protection devices, such as the Mo.Ma Ultra (Medtronic, Minneapolis, MN, USA), occlude the external and common carotid arteries to induce retrograde flow or halt ipsilateral vascular flow without crossing the lesion, as shown in Fig. 2. Additionally, the Parodi anti-emboli system achieves flow reversal during transfemoral CAS by connecting the arterial sheath in the common carotid artery to the femoral vein [10].

The selection of EPDs depends on the surgeon's expertise, lesion characteristics, and anatomical factors, as there is

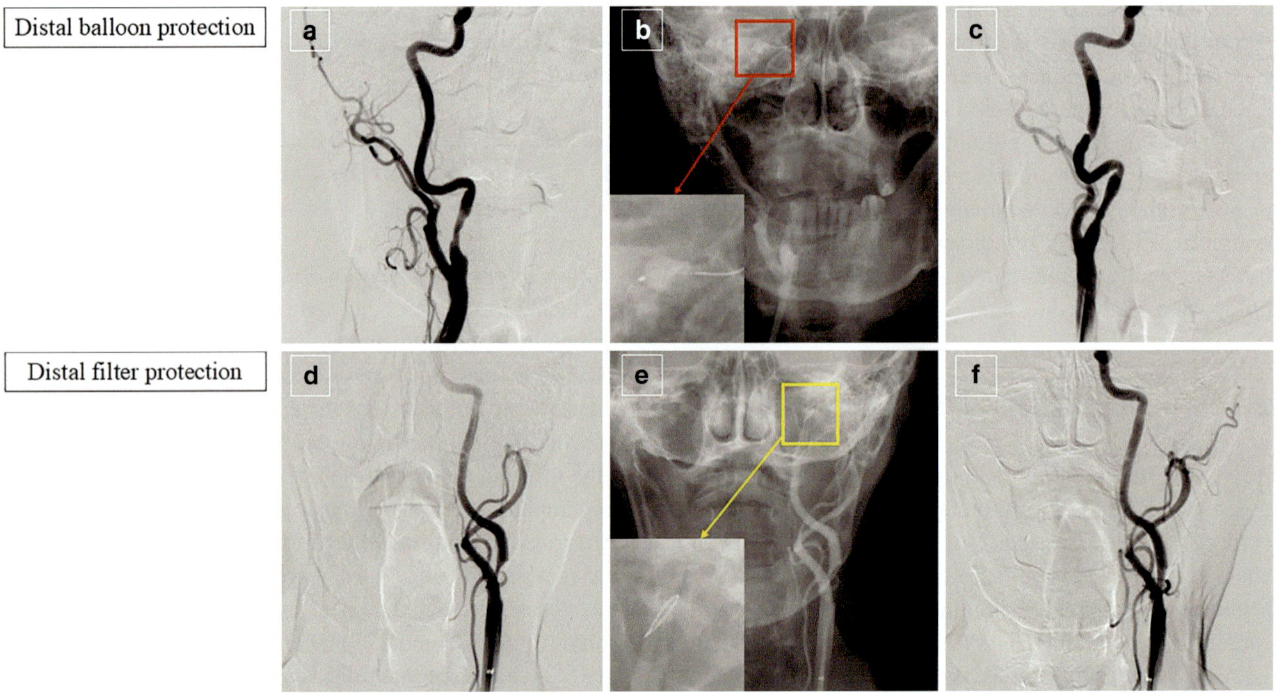

Fig. 1 Introduction of carotid artery stenting (CAS) with the distal balloon protection and distal filter protection. The upper section: A 73-year-old man with symptomatic carotid artery stenosis who undergoes CAS with a balloon device. Pre-stenting angiogram shows 70% stenosis at the right internal carotid artery (ICA), as defined by the North American Symptomatic Carotid Endarterectomy Trial (NASCET) criteria (**a**). A balloon device is deployed in the distal carotid artery (red square) (**b**). After CAS, the lumen of the right ICA is successfully dilated (**c**). The lower section: An 87-year-old man with symptomatic carotid artery stenosis who undergoes CAS with a filter device. Pre-stenting angiogram shows 80% stenosis at the right ICA, as defined by the NASCET criteria (**d**). A filter device is deployed in the distal carotid artery (yellow square) (**e**). After CAS, the lumen of the left ICA is successfully dilated (**f**)

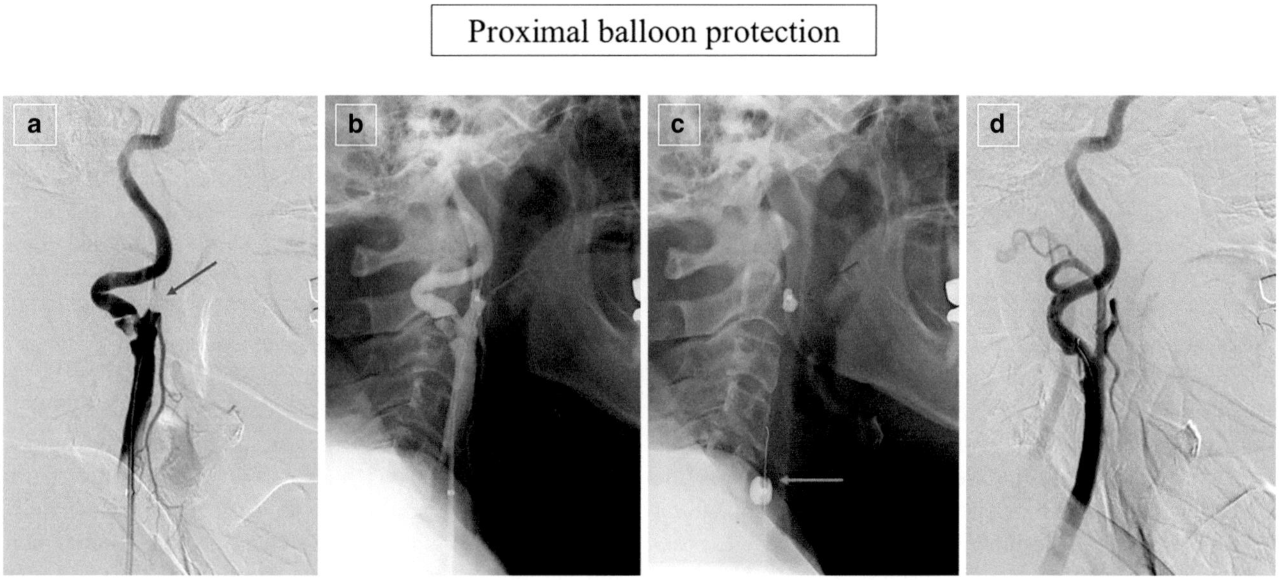

Fig. 2 Introduction of the proximal balloon protection using to prevent distal emboli during carotid artery stenting (CAS). A 75-year-old woman with asymptomatic carotid artery stenosis who undergoes CAS with a proximal balloon protection device. Preintervention angiogram shows a high grade stenosis with ulceration at the right internal carotid artery (ICA). The Mo.Ma Ultra (Medtronic, Minneapolis, MN, USA) is placed and the occlusion balloon (blue arrows) at the external carotid artery (ECA) is inflated (**a** and **b**). In addition to the balloon (blue arrow) at the ECA, the other occlusion balloon (green arrow) at the common carotid artery is also inflated to induce retrograde flow or halt ipsilateral vascular flow without crossing the lesion (**c**). Postintervention angiogram shows successful dilation of the lumen at the right ICA (**d**)

currently no universally optimal protection method [11]. However, it is important to note that the embolization risk peaks during the stent deployment and post-dilation phases [12, 13]. Despite the use of distal filters, embolic particles of <100 μm in size can pass through the pores of these protections, potentially inducing a risk of minor stroke [14]. Balloon protection may be considered for lesions with vulnerable plaques provided that ischemic intolerance from ICA flow occlusion can be effectively managed.

The stents used in CAS follow one of the three main designs: open-cell, closed-cell, or dual-layered. Open-cell stents have larger cell areas, offer enhanced flexibility and vessel conformity, are often preferred for tortuous stenotic lesions, and exhibit a lower restenosis rate after the procedure [15]. However, these stents are more susceptible to plaque protrusion and development of new ischemic lesions than closed-cell stents. Conversely, closed-cell stents provide superior resistance to plaque protrusion owing to their higher scaffolding properties but lack the adaptability and flexibility of open-cell designs [16, 17]. In Japan, the Carotid Wallstent (Boston Scientific, Marlborough, MA, USA) is a representative closed-cell stent, whereas the PRECISE (Cordis, Miami, FL, USA) and Protégé (Covidien, Irvine, CA, USA) are commonly used open-cell stents. Dual-layered stents, including the Casper stent (MicroVention, Aliso Viejo, CA, USA), were introduced in Japan in 2020. These stents comprise an outer layer that conforms to the vessel wall, as well as an inner micromesh layer designed to minimize plaque prolapse and embolic release, providing a balance between flexibility and scaffolding [18].

5 Procedure Techniques

CAS can present significant challenges in patients with complex vascular anatomy, such as a type III aortic arch (the vertical distance between the highest point of the aortic arch and the origin of the innominate artery is measured >2 cm. In this situation, the supra-aortic arteries arise with a steep angle making it more difficult to navigate catheters) [19] or restricted peripheral access, particularly during the lesion crossing phase in cases of severe or highly tortuous carotid stenosis. Several effective techniques have been developed to overcome these challenges. One notable method is lesion crossing using a 0.035-inch guidewire. This approach takes advantage of the superior steerability and crossability of the 0.035-inch guidewire compared to the standard 0.014-inch guidewire, which is commonly applied in distal filter and balloon protection systems (internal diameter: 0.014 inches) [20]. Furthermore, prior to its discontinuation in 2021, a valuable lesion-crossing technique was utilized with the PercuSurge GuardWire (Medtronic, Minneapolis, MN, USA), a distal balloon protection device. This procedure commenced with proximal balloon protection achieved by inflating the balloon-guiding catheter. A 0.035-inch guidewire was then advanced across the lesion, after which a 6-4 French (Fr) tapering-type inner catheter was introduced along the guidewire through the stenosis. After verifying that the route was within the true lumen, the 0.035-inch guidewire was replaced with a 300-cm PercuSurge GuideWire through the 6-4 Fr tapering-type catheter. Finally, the catheter was retrieved using the exchange method after inflating the PercuSurge GuardWire to establish protection, as shown in Fig. 3 [20]. The "sheeping" technique using a 0.035-inch guidewire has also recently gained recognition as an effective method for lesion crossing. This technique involves the insertion of a 0.035-inch guidewire in advance through the same hemostatic valve as the guiding catheter parallel to the EPD system, and advancing the distal EPD system across the lesion. This approach facilitates smooth passage of the distal EPD system over the lesion by straightening the angled passage from the bifurcation to the distal ICA using the 0.035-inch guidewire.

Indications for revascularization in CAS for ICA NO or CTO remain controversial [21, 22]. However, a recent large case series suggested that CAS can provide significant benefits for patients with an ICA NO, even in asymptomatic cases, provided that the procedure is performed using advanced technologies and by an experienced interventional team [23]. Furthermore, staged angioplasty followed by delayed CAS has been reported to be an effective strategy for reducing the risk of post-procedural hyperperfusion, particularly in cases of severe carotid artery stenosis or CTO [8].

Dual antiplatelet therapy (DAPT) with aspirin and clopidogrel is generally recommended as perioperative medical management, before and 3 weeks to 3 months following the procedure, with lifelong antiplatelet monotherapy performed thereafter [1]. However, the administration of P2Y12-inhibition drugs <180 days after CAS is associated with an increased risk of stroke, whereas the incidence of hemorrhagic complications is higher during the administration period of P2Y12-inhition, with extracranial hemorrhage occurring more frequently [24]. Thus, the type, combination, and duration of antithrombotic treatment during and after CAS should be specific to each patient, considering both the potential advantage of prolonging DAPT and the increased risk of predominantly extracranial hemorrhagic complications.

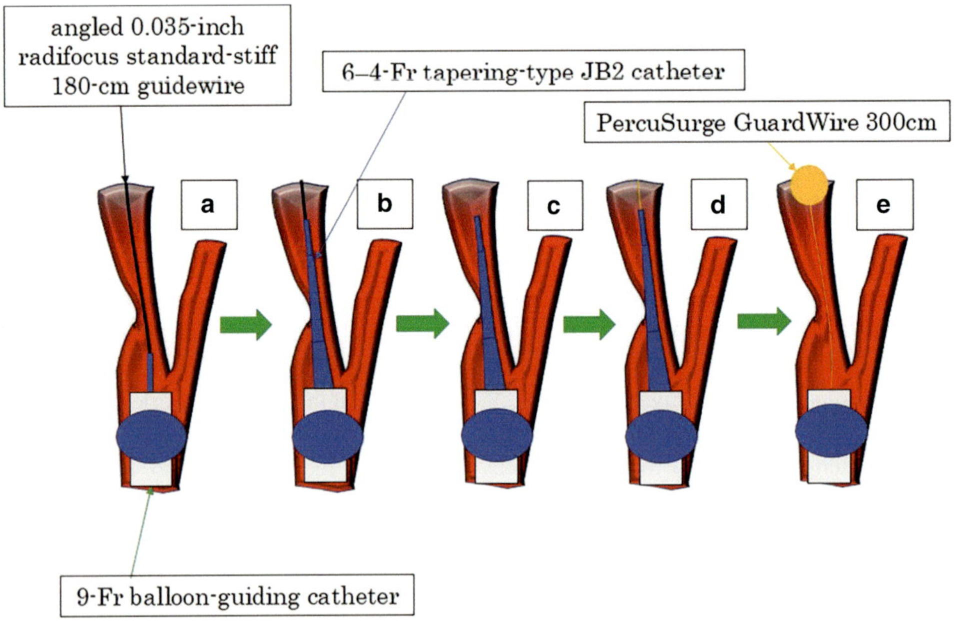

Fig. 3 Introduction of the utility technique using a 0.035-inch guidewire and a 300-cm PercuSurge GuardWire (Extracted from Nariai et al. [19]). Lesion crossing is performed using a 0.035-inch radifocus standard-stiff guidewire (**a**). Subsequently, a 6–4-French tapering-type JB2 catheter is advanced through the stenosis along the guidewire (**b**). Guidewire retrieval and lumen assessment are subsequently performed by injecting a contrast agent through the catheter (**c**). Then, a 300-cm PercuSurge GuardWire is advanced through the catheter (**d**). Finally, after inflating the PercuSurge GuardWire, the catheter is retrieved using the exchange method (**e**). The authors hold the copyright for this figure

Conflict of Interest Disclosure The authors declare no conflicts of interest.

Declarations
Competing Interests The author(s) has no competing interests to declare that are relevant to the content of this manuscript.

Ethics Approval The author(s) declares that this manuscript does not include primary research with human participants.

References

1. Naylor R, Rantner B, Ancetti S, et al. Editor's choice – European Society for Vascular Surgery (ESVS) 2023 clinical practice guidelines on the Management of Atherosclerotic Carotid and Vertebral Artery Disease. Eur J Vasc Endovasc Surg. 2023;65(1):7–111.
2. Lim S, Javorski MJ, Nassoiy SP, et al. Long-term hemodynamic effects after carotid artery revascularization. Vasc Endovascular Surg. 2019;53(4):297–302.
3. Brott TG, Halperin JL, Abbara S, et al. 2011 ASA/ACCF/AHA/AANN/AANS/ACR/ASNR/CNS/SAIP/SCAI/SIR/SNIS/SVM/SVS guideline on the management of patients with extracranial carotid and vertebral artery disease: executive summary: a report of the American College of Cardiology Foundation/American Heart Association Task Force on Practice Guidelines, and the American Stroke Association, American Association of Neuroscience Nurses, American Association of Neurological Surgeons, American College of Radiology, American Society of Neuroradiology, Congress of Neurological Surgeons, Society of Atherosclerosis Imaging and Prevention, Society for Cardiovascular Angiography and Interventions, Society of Interventional Radiology, Society of NeuroInterventional Surgery, Society for Vascular Medicine, and Society for Vascular Surgery. J Am Coll Cardiol. 2011;57(8):1002–44.
4. Rasheed AS, White RS, Tangel V, Storch BM, Pryor KO. Carotid revascularization procedures and perioperative outcomes: a multistate analysis, 2007–2014. J Cardiothorac Vasc Anesth. 2019;33(7):1963–72.
5. Polak JF, Alexandrov AV. Accuracy of the Society of Radiologists in Ultrasound (SRU) Carotid Doppler Velocity Criteria for Grading North American Symptomatic Carotid Endarterectomy Trial (NASCET) Stenosis: a meta-analysis. J Ultrasound Med. 2023;42(7):1423–35.
6. Henze A, Fox AJ, Johansson E. High risk of early recurrent stroke in patients with near-occlusion with full collapse of the internal carotid artery. Neuroradiology. 2024;66(3):349–52.
7. Mei F, Zhang W, Jiang P, et al. Comparison of the treatment strategies for symptomatic chronic internal carotid artery occlusion. J Vasc Surg. 2024; https://doi.org/10.1016/j.jvs.2024.05.062.
8. Yoshimura S, Kitajima H, Enomoto Y, Yamada K, Iwama T. Staged angioplasty for carotid artery stenosis to prevent postoperative hyperperfusion. Neurosurgery. 2009;64(3 Suppl):ons122–8. discussion ons8–9
9. Kim SJ, Roh HG, Jeon P, et al. Cerebral ischemia detected with diffusion-weighted MR imaging after protected carotid artery stenting: comparison of distal balloon and filter device. Korean J Radiol. 2007;8(4):276–85.
10. Grunwald IQ, Papanagiotou P, Struffert T, et al. Reversal of flow during carotid artery stenting: use of the Parodi antiembolism system. Neuroradiology. 2007;49(3):237–41.
11. Kim MS, Rho MH, Hong HP, Park HJ, Chung PW, Won YS. Comparison of embolic protection with proximal and distal protection devices: periprocedural complications, clinical outcomes, and cerebral embolic lesions on diffusion-weighted magnetic resonance imaging. World Neurosurg. 2020;135:e731–e7.
12. Hellings WE, Ackerstaff RG, Pasterkamp G, De Vries JP, Moll FL. The carotid atherosclerotic plaque and microembolisation during carotid stenting. J Cardiovasc Surg. 2006;47(2):115–26.
13. Obeid T, Arnaoutakis DJ, Arhuidese I, et al. Poststent ballooning is associated with increased periprocedural stroke and death rate in carotid artery stenting. J Vasc Surg. 2015;62(3):616–23.e1.
14. Langhoff R, Schofer J, Scheinert D, et al. double filtration during carotid artery stenting using a novel post-dilation balloon with integrated embolic protection. JACC Cardiovasc Interv. 2019;12(4):395–403.
15. Texakalidis P, Giannopoulos S, Kokkinidis DG, Lanzino G. Effect of open- vs closed-cell stent design on periprocedural outcomes and restenosis after carotid artery stenting: a systematic review and comprehensive meta-analysis. J Endovasc Ther. 2018;25(4):523–33.
16. de Vries EE, Meershoek AJA, Vonken EJ, den Ruijter HM, van den Berg JC, de Borst GJ. A meta-analysis of the effect of stent design on clinical and radiologic outcomes of carotid artery stenting. J Vasc Surg. 2019;69(6):1952–61.e1.
17. Kotsugi M, Takayama K, Myouchin K, et al. Carotid artery stenting: investigation of plaque protrusion incidence and prognosis. JACC Cardiovasc Interv. 2017;10(8):824–31.
18. Imamura H, Sakai N, Matsumoto Y, et al. Clinical trial of carotid artery stenting using dual-layer CASPER stent for carotid endarterectomy in patients at high and normal risk in the Japanese population. J Neurointerv Surg. 2021;13(6):524–9.
19. Macdonald S, Lee R, Williams R, Stansby G. Towards safer carotid artery stenting: a scoring system for anatomic suitability. Stroke. 2009;40(5):1698–703.
20. Nariai Y, Takigawa T, Sugiura Y, Suzuki R, Hyodo A, Suzuki K. Letter to the editor regarding a new technical principle of carotid artery stenting with lesion crossing using a 0.035-inch guidewire and 6-4-French tapering-type catheter for severe stenosis. Cardiovasc Intervent Radiol. 2021;44(12):1999–2001.
21. Myrcha P, Gloviczki P. A systematic review of endovascular treatment for chronic total occlusion of the internal carotid artery. Ann Transl Med. 2021;9(14):1203.
22. Xue S, Tang X, Zhao G, et al. A systematic review and updated metaanalysis for carotid near-occlusion. Ann Vasc Surg. 2020;66:636–45.e3.
23. Akkan K, Ilgit E, Onal B, et al. Endovascular treatment for near occlusion of the internal carotid artery: 30-day outcome and long-term follow-up. Clin Neuroradiol. 2018;28(2):245–52.
24. Sussman ES, Jin M, Pendharkar AV, et al. Dual antiplatelet therapy after carotid artery stenting: trends and outcomes in a large national database. J Neurointerv Surg. 2021;13(1):8–13.

Carotid Endarterectomy vs. Carotid Artery Stenting in the Treatment of Carotid Artery Stenosis: A Comprehensive Review

Petr Skalický, Adéla Bubeníková, Vladimír Beneš, and Ondřej Bradáč

Abbreviations

CEA	Carotid Endarterectomy
CAS	Carotid Artery Stenting
TCAR	Transcarotid Artery Revascularization
MICA	Minimally Invasive Carotid Artery surgery
PTFE	Polytetrafluoroethylene
BMT	Best Medical Treatment
SPACE	Stent-protected Angioplasty versus Carotid Endarterectomy
SPACE-2	Stent-protected Angioplasty versus Carotid Endarterectomy-2
ACST-1	Asymptomatic Carotid Surgery Trial
ACST-2	Asymptomatic Carotid Surgery Trial-2
ECST-2	European Carotid Surgery Trial
ECST-2	European Carotid Surgery Trial-2
CREST	Carotid Revascularization and Medical Management for Asymptomatic Carotid Stenosis
CREST-2	Carotid Revascularization and Medical Management for Asymptomatic Carotid Stenosis-2
ICSS	International Carotid Stenting Study
NASCET	North American Symptomatic Carotid Endarterectomy Trial
ACAS	Asymptomatic Carotid Atherosclerosis Study
EVA-3S	Endarterectomy Versus Angioplasty in Patients with Symptomatic Severe Carotid Stenosis

P. Skalický · A. Bubeníková
Department of Neurosurgery, 2nd Medical Faculty, Charles University and Motol University Hospital, Prague, Czech Republic

V. Beneš
Department of Neurosurgery and Neurooncology, First Medical Faculty, Charles University, Prague, Czech Republic

O. Bradáč (✉)
Department of Neurosurgery, 2nd Medical Faculty, Charles University and Motol University Hospital, Prague, Czech Republic

Department of Neurosurgery and Neurooncology, 1st Medical Faculty, Charles University and Military University Hospital, Prague, Czech Republic

1 Introduction

Carotid artery stenosis poses a substantial risk for ischemic stroke, demanding prompt intervention to prevent potentially disabling or life-altering consequences. Ischemic strokes account for a significant portion of all strokes [1], highlighting the importance of addressing carotid artery stenosis. The two primary interventions for carotid artery stenosis, carotid endarterectomy and carotid artery stenting, have been extensively studied and continue to be refined. Historically, CEA has been considered the gold standard, with early trials such as the North American Symptomatic Carotid Endarterectomy Trial [2] and the European Carotid Surgery Trial demonstrating its efficacy in reducing stroke risk [3]. These trials established the benefit of CEA, particularly for symptomatic patients with high-grade stenosis. The emergence of CAS in the late twentieth century offered a minimally invasive alternative, especially appealing for patients at higher risk for surgical complications [4].

CEA involves the surgical removal of atherosclerotic plaque from the carotid artery, directly addressing the source of emboli and reducing the risk of stroke. CAS, on the other hand, involves placing a stent within the artery to maintain its patency, offering a less invasive approach. While both procedures have proven effective, they carry distinct risks that must be carefully considered when selecting the appropriate treatment for individual patients. Advances in embolic protection devices, stent technology, and perioperative care continue to evolve, further shaping the treatment landscape and potentially changing outcomes for patients. This chapter will provide a comprehensive overview of the historical context, patient selection criteria, perioperative risks, long-term outcomes, and evolving context for CEA and CAS.

V. Beneš, D. Netuka (eds.), *Surgical and Interventional Treatment of Cerebral Ischemia*,
https://doi.org/10.1007/978-3-032-08934-2_12

2 Historical Context and Evolution of Treatment Paradigms

The evolution of carotid revascularization began with the first successful carotid endarterectomy performed by Michael DeBakey in 1953 [5]. By the 1990s, CEA was established as the standard of care for symptomatic carotid stenosis, largely due to the results of large-scale randomized controlled trials.

- **NASCET and ECST**: These trials demonstrated a significant reduction in stroke risk for patients with symptomatic carotid stenosis of 70% or greater who underwent CEA compared to medical management alone [3, 6]. NASCET, in particular, showed a substantial relative risk reduction in major stroke incidence following CEA. [2] The ECST trial further solidified the evidence base for CEA in symptomatic patients [3].
- **ACAS and ACST**: Subsequent trials, such as ACAS and ACST, investigated the role of CEA in asymptomatic patients. While these trials suggested a more moderate benefit for long-term stroke prevention in asymptomatic individuals, particularly in younger patients with high-grade stenosis [7, 8]. However, the benefit of CEA in asymptomatic patients has been subject to ongoing debate and re-evaluation, especially in light of improvements in medical therapy [9, 10].

The emergence of CAS in the late 1990s, driven by technological advancements and concerns about perioperative complications associated with CEA [4], introduced a less invasive alternative. Initial observational studies suggested comparable efficacy between CAS and CEA which was confirmed by subsequent randomized controlled trials, such as CREST [11], but with a more nuanced picture. While some trials indicated non-inferiority of CAS to CEA in stroke prevention, they also highlighted the importance of patient-specific factors, such as age and anatomical considerations, in determining procedural success [12]. The CREST trial, for instance, demonstrated the importance of considering patient age when choosing between CEA and CAS [11, 13]. Furthermore, the evolution of medical therapy has prompted re-evaluation of the role of revascularization in asymptomatic patients [14]. Ongoing trials and advancements in both CAS and CEA techniques continue to shape the treatment landscape for carotid artery stenosis [15].

3 Patient Selection Criteria

Selecting the appropriate intervention for carotid artery stenosis requires careful consideration of various patient-specific factors. Both carotid endarterectomy and carotid artery stenting have demonstrated efficacy in reducing stroke risk, but their suitability varies depending on individual circumstances.

3.1 Symptomatic vs. Asymptomatic Carotid Stenosis

- **Symptomatic Stenosis**: Patients experiencing symptoms such as transient ischemic attack, amaurosis fugax, or minor stroke attributable to carotid stenosis derive substantial benefit from revascularization. For symptomatic carotid stenosis, both carotid endarterectomy and carotid artery stenting are effective in reducing the risk of stroke. CREST study, a landmark trial comparing the two procedures, found no significant difference in the composite primary outcome of stroke, myocardial infarction, or death between CAS and CEA. However, important distinctions exist in their efficacy and safety profiles, influencing patient selection. CEA has traditionally been considered the gold standard, particularly for patients at low surgical risk. [11] EVA-3S trial demonstrated lower rates of death and stroke at 1 and 6 months with CEA compared to CAS in patients with symptomatic stenosis of 60% or more. [16] This is largely attributed to the lower periprocedural stroke risk associated with CEA. However, CEA carries a risk of surgical complications, such as cranial nerve injury and wound complications, which are less common with CAS. EVA-3S also noted a higher incidence of major local complications after stenting and more systemic complications after endarterectomy, although the differences were not statistically significant. [16] CAS, while associated with a higher periprocedural stroke risk, particularly in older patients [17], offers a less invasive approach, making it a preferred option for patients at high surgical risk due to, comorbidities, or anatomical factors like previous neck irradiation or surgery [18]. The choice between CEA and CAS therefore hinges on a careful assessment of individual patient characteristics, balancing the risks of periprocedural stroke with CAS against the risks of surgical complications with CEA.
- **Asymptomatic Stenosis**: The benefit of intervention in asymptomatic patients is less pronounced than in symptomatic patients. While studies have shown a reduction in long-term stroke risk with CEA in asymptomatic patients with high-grade stenosis, the absolute risk reduction is smaller. Trials such as ACST-1 [7] investigated the role of CEA in asymptomatic patients with ≥60% carotid stenosis with long-term (10 years) risk reduction, however an ongoing debate is on the evolving role of medical management in this population. [9, 10] The decision to intervene in asymptomatic patients often involves balancing

the potential benefits of stroke risk reduction against the risks of the procedure and the patient's overall health status.

Current guidelines recommend considering carotid endarterectomy for **symptomatic** patients with a carotid stenosis of **50–69%** or greater. For **asymptomatic** patients, zreatment is generally considered for stenosis of **60% or greater**. [19]

3.2 Age Considerations

Age is a critical factor in determining the optimal revascularization strategy.

- **Younger Patients (<70 years)**: CEA is generally preferred, with CAS reserved for high-surgical-risk individuals.
- **Older Patients (≥70 years)**: Individualized assessment is crucial, considering previous symptoms, surgical risk, comorbidities, and life expectancy. CAS may be an option for high-surgical-risk patients, but the risk of periprocedural stroke must be carefully weighed. Optimal medical management is essential for all patients.

3.3 Comorbidities and Risk Factors

The presence of comorbidities and other risk factors significantly influences the choice between CEA and CAS.

- **High Surgical Risk**: Patients considered high-risk for open surgery due to conditions such as severe cardiac or pulmonary disease may be better candidates for CAS. Haro et al. [12] investigated CAS outcomes in high-surgical-risk patients. However, certain anatomical factors, such as significant aortic arch calcification, long-segment stenosis, or intracranial disease, can increase the complexity and risk of CAS.
- High-risk patients for carotid endarterectomy as identified by Nguyen et al. [20] include those with severe cardiac or pulmonary disease, contralateral carotid occlusion, previous neck irradiation or surgery, and advanced age. These factors increase the risk of perioperative complications, requiring careful consideration of the risks and benefits of CEA versus carotid artery stenting or medical management. For some truly high-risk individuals with limited life expectancy, medical management alone may be the most appropriate approach.

4 Outcomes and Complications

Determining the best treatment approach for carotid artery stenosis requires careful consideration of the potential risks and benefits associated with each procedure. Both carotid endarterectomy and carotid artery stenting have demonstrated efficacy in reducing stroke risk, but they carry distinct complication profiles that must be weighed against the patient's individual circumstances.

4.1 Periprocedural Risks

CEA Risks Determining precise percentages for perioperative risks associated with carotid endarterectomy across various time intervals is challenging due to variations in reporting methods, evolving treatment methods and patient populations across studies.

- **Stroke**:
  30-day risk: The 30-day risk of stroke after CEA is generally considered to be around 1–3%, with some studies reporting slightly higher or lower rates depending on patient characteristics and study methodology. [21–23]
  Long-term risk: The long-term risk of stroke after CEA is lower than the perioperative risk, but it continues over time. [21] reported a 5-year risk of ipsilateral stroke of around 7% in their population-based study. ACST-1 study reported 4.1% vs. 10.0% (gain 5.9%; 95% CI 4.0–7.8; $P < 0.0001$) 5-year non-perioperative stroke risk in patients with immediate CEA and deffered CEA (26% underwent CEA during follow-up) and 10.8% vs. 16.9% (gain 6.1%; 95% CI 2.7–9.4; $P = 0.0004$) at 10 years. [7]
- **Myocardial Infarction**:
  30-day risk: The 30-day risk of MI after CEA is generally considered to be around 1–2%. Long et al. [22] reported a perioperative MI rate of 1.3% in their contemporary cohort.
  Long-term risk: Data on long-term MI risk after CEA is more limited, but it is likely lower than the perioperative risk.
- **Death**:
  30-day risk: The 30-day risk of death after CEA is generally considered to be less than 1%. Long et al. [22] reported perioperative mortality rates of 0.5%. Beneš and Bradáč [13] reported combined mortality and major morbidity of 0.9% in a cohort of 1064 patients.

Long-term risk: Long-term mortality after CEA is influenced by various factors, including age and underlying medical conditions. Simons et al. [24] investigated the impact of postoperative stroke and myocardial infarction on long-term survival after carotid revascularization. Their study found that postoperative stroke significantly decreased short-term survival, with the most pronounced effect within the first year. While MI also negatively impacted survival, its effect was less pronounced than that of stroke. By 5 years, the survival curves for patients with stroke and MI converged, suggesting that the long-term survival disadvantage conferred by these complications diminishes over time. These findings highlight the importance of considering the differential impact of postoperative complications when evaluating the effectiveness of carotid revascularization strategies.

- **Cranial Nerve Injury**:
  Transient CNI: Transient CNI is relatively common after CEA, with reported rates varying widely. Many cases resolve within the first few months after surgery. [25, 26]
  Permanent CNI: Permanent CNI is less common, with reported rates typically around 1–4%. Cunnigham et al. [27] reported a 4% risk of persistent motor CNI after hospital discharge.

Historical Evolution

Early Years (1980s–1990s): Studies like the ECST Trial [3], conducted between 1981 and 1994, reported a combined risk of major stroke or death of around 7%. This encompassed both perioperative and 30-day outcomes.

Improvements (2000s-2010s): As surgical techniques, patient selection, and perioperative care improved, the risk of CEA decreased substantially. While precise figures vary across studies, some suggest a reduction to approximately 3–4% for the combined endpoint of stroke or death within 30 days. Radak et al. [28] discusses this trend, indicating a significant improvement in CEA safety over the past two decades.

Contemporary Practice: In experienced centers today, the risk of stroke or death within 30 days following CEA is generally below 3%, and can be even lower for asymptomatic patients. [23]

CAS Risks

- **Stroke**:
  Periprocedural stroke: The risk of stroke during or shortly after CAS is generally considered to be slightly higher than with CEA, particularly in older patients. [13, 29] This is primarily due to the potential for embolization during the procedure, despite the use of embolic protection devices. SPACE trial [30] reports similar rates of ipsilateral ischemic stroke at 2 years after both CAS and CEA, suggesting that the increased risk with CAS is mainly periprocedural.
  Long-term stroke risk: The long-term risk of stroke after CAS is comparable to that after CEA. [29, 30] ICSS study [29] found a slightly increased risk of any stroke (mainly non-disabling) in the CAS group at 5 years, but no significant difference in disabling stroke.
- **Myocardial Infarction**:
  Periprocedural MI: The risk of MI during or shortly after CAS is generally considered to be lower than with CEA. [29] This is likely because CAS is less invasive and does not involve manipulation of the carotid sinus, which can trigger cardiac events.
  Long-term MI risk: Data on long-term MI risk after CAS is more limited, but it is likely comparable to that after CEA.
- **Death**:
  Periprocedural death: The risk of death during or shortly after CAS is generally considered to be low, similar to CEA. [30]
  Long-term mortality: Long-term mortality after CAS is influenced by similar factors as CEA, including age and underlying medical conditions.
- **Cranial Nerve Injury**:
  CNI: The risk of cranial nerve injury with CAS is generally considered to be negligible. [29] This is because CAS does not involve direct manipulation of the nerves surrounding the carotid artery.
- **Other CAS-Specific Risks**:
  Access site complications: CAS can lead to complications at the access site (typically the femoral artery), such as bleeding, hematoma, or pseudoaneurysm. These complications are generally less common with newer access techniques, such as transcarotid access.
  Stent thrombosis: Stent thrombosis, although rare, is a serious complication that can occur after CAS. It is more likely to occur in the first few months after the procedure and can lead to stroke or death.

Restenosis The rate of restenosis after CAS is generally higher than after CEA, particularly in the first few years. However, most restenoses are asymptomatic and do not require intervention. [30, 31] For restenosis after CAS repeated endovascular procedure might more feasible [31] but f.e. Arhuidese et al. [32] reported similar outcomes in 1-year follow-up for CEA and repeated CAS.

For restenosis after CEA both redo CEA and CAS are safe and feasible. Although the incidences of CNI and MI were increased in the redo CEA group, most of the CNI cases were reversible. Patients treated with CAS were more likely to develop restenosis than those treated with redo CEA over long-term followup. [33]

More data on management of restenoses after both CEA and CAS are needed to guide the optimal decision.

Historical Evolution

Early Experience: Initial experiences with CAS were marked by higher periprocedural stroke rates compared to CEA. This was partly due to the learning curve associated with the new technology and the limitations of early stent and embolic protection devices. Allen [34] provides context on the early challenges of CAS.

Technological Advancements: The introduction of embolic protection devices and improvements in stent technology significantly reduced the periprocedural risks of CAS. While some studies suggest EPDs can reduce the risk of periprocedural stroke by as much as 40% (or even up to 79% [35]), but pinning down a single, universally applicable number is difficult. The actual risk reduction varies based on several factors:

- **Type of EPD**: Different EPDs have different capture efficiencies. Some are designed for distal protection (placed beyond the stenosis), while others offer proximal protection (placed before the stenosis). The specific design features can influence how effectively they trap embolic debris.
  Kajihara et al.'s [36] single-center study compared dual protection (a combination of proximal balloon occlusion of the common carotid artery and distal filter protection) with distal filter protection alone during carotid artery stenting. They found no significant difference in the incidence of new cerebral infarction between the two groups. However, the study did show that dual protection was associated with a significantly higher rate of successful debris capture, suggesting that it may offer additional protection against embolization during CAS.
- **Patient Characteristics**: Patients with certain anatomical features or plaque characteristics may be at higher risk of embolization, regardless of EPD use.
- **Operator Experience**: The operator's skill in deploying and retrieving the EPD can impact its effectiveness.
- **Definition of Stroke**: Studies use different criteria to define and classify strokes, making direct comparisons challenging. Some studies focus on major strokes, while others include minor or transient ischemic attacks.

Current Practice Contemporary data suggests that the 30-day risk of stroke or death following CAS is generally in the range of 3–5%, approaching the risk associated with CEA in some studies. Recently, ACST-2 study has provided comparable long-term effects of CAS and CEA. [23] However, it's important to note that the risk of stroke with CAS can be higher in certain patient subgroups, such as older patients. [29, 37]

Comparative Data

Several randomized controlled trials have directly compared CEA and CAS, offering valuable data on their relative risks and benefits:

- **CREST**: This large trial, whose results significantly impacted practice patterns [11, 38], found a 30-day risk of stroke or death of 2.5% in the CAS group and 0.9% in the CEA group. Longer-term follow-up showed similar rates of stroke, death, or myocardial infarction between the two procedures. However, the types of events differed: CAS had a higher risk of stroke, while CEA carried a higher risk of myocardial infarction.
- **ICSS**: This trial reported a 30-day incidence of any stroke or death of 3.4% after CAS and a relative risk of 2.2 compared to CEA. The study also found a higher risk of cranial nerve palsy with CEA. ICSS found a higher risk of periprocedural stroke with CAS particularly in patients over 70 [39]. However, long-term stroke rates were similar between CAS and CEA. ICSS also showed a higher restenosis rate with CAS [40].
- **EVA-3S**: The EVA-3S trial was a multicenter, randomized, non-inferiority trial designed to compare carotid artery stenting with carotid endarterectomy in patients with symptomatic carotid stenosis of 60% or greater. [16]
  The trial was stopped prematurely due to safety concerns and futility after enrolling 527 patients. The 30-day incidence of any stroke or death was significantly higher in the stenting group (9.6%) compared to the endarterectomy group (3.9%), with a relative risk of 2.5. This led to the conclusion that CAS was *not* non-inferior to CEA for this patient population. [16] The higher stroke rate with CAS in EVA-3S, particularly in older patients, contributed to the ongoing debate about the optimal revascularization strategy for carotid stenosis.
- **SPACE**: This trial found no significant difference in the primary composite endpoint of stroke, death, or myocardial infarction between CAS and CEA at 30 days. [30]

It's important to note that the trials often included patients at varying levels of surgical risk. For example, the EVA-3S trial, while setting experience requirements for operators, still encompassed a range of surgical expertise, potentially influencing outcomes. [41] Study by Bradáč et al. [42] has also shown that the outcomes rely on center and surgical expertise and evolve over time.

[13] also highlight that while long-term follow-up from ICSS and CREST demonstrated comparable late efficacy in stroke prevention between the two procedures, CAS carries a higher risk of periprocedural stroke, particularly in older patients. This elevated initial risk with CAS necessitates careful patient selection and emphasizes the importance of considering individual patient characteristics and local expertise when making treatment decisions. The authors conclude that while randomized trials like ICSS and CREST provide valuable guidance, they should not replace individualized clinical judgement, advocating for a nuanced approach to carotid stenosis management. The authors have also shown that in all subgroup analyses CEA proved to be equal to or better than CAS.

Furthermore, recent comprehensive systematic review by [15] clearly concludes that CEA was superior to medical therapy in long-term prevention of stroke/death over medical therapy and was also superior to transfemoral CAS in minimizing long-term stroke/death for symptomatic low risk surgical patients.

5 Technological Advancements and Future Directions

The field of carotid revascularization continues to evolve, with ongoing innovations aimed at improving both the safety and efficacy of both CAS and CEA.

5.1 Innovations in Carotid Stenting

Several key advancements have contributed to the progress of CAS:

- **Embolic Protection Devices**: Embolic protection devices are crucial in carotid artery stenting to minimize the risk of stroke caused by debris dislodged during the procedure. There are two main types:
  - **Distal filter devices**: These are positioned beyond the treated area in the internal carotid artery and act like a net, catching debris as blood flows through. [43, 44] Various filter designs exist, and their efficacy has been demonstrated in several studies, although no system is perfect. [45] Some debris might be smaller than the filter pores, or some might be dislodged during retrieval. [44]
  - **Proximal occlusion devices**: These temporarily block blood flow in the common carotid artery and external carotid artery, creating a stagnant column of blood during the procedure. Debris is then aspirated before restoring normal flow. [46] While effective, this method can be less tolerated by patients and technically challenging. [46] One example is the MOMA device. [44]

  Studies have shown that EPDs significantly reduce the risk of periprocedural stroke during CAS. [35, 47] Castriota et al. [35] reports a 79% reduction in embolic complications with EPD use. Ohki et al. [48] demonstrated the efficacy of a filter device in an *ex vivo* model, capturing 88% of released particles.

  The choice between distal filter and proximal occlusion devices depends on factors like patient anatomy and operator preference. However, both methods have shown comparable efficacy in preventing periprocedural stroke. [49]
- **New-Generation Stents**: New-generation stents, often referred to as "mesh-covered" or "second-generation" stents, represent a significant advancement in carotid artery stenting. These stents are designed to address the limitations of earlier bare-metal stents by providing a barrier against plaque prolapse and embolization during and after the procedure.

  Key features of new-generation stents include:
  - **Mesh Covering**: A fine mesh layer covers the stent struts, trapping debris and preventing it from migrating to the brain. This mesh can be a single or double layer, depending on the specific stent design. Imamura et al. [50] study the CASPER stent, a dual-layer design with a braided nitinol outer layer and a micromesh inner layer. Gray et al. [51] discuss the GORE® Carotid Stent, a mesh-covered stent evaluated in the SCAFFOLD trial.
  - **Reduced Pore Size**: The mesh has smaller pores than earlier stents, preventing the passage of even small debris particles.
  - **Variety of Materials and Designs**: New-generation stents are available in various materials, including nitinol and stainless steel, and different designs, such as closed-cell and open-cell structures. [50]

  Several studies have shown promising results with new-generation stents, demonstrating lower rates of periprocedural stroke and restenosis compared to earlier stent designs. SCAFFOLD trial [51] reported low rates of adverse events. [50] also highlights the low major adverse event rate observed in their trial using the CASPER stent.

- **Transcarotid Artery Revascularization**: Transcarotid artery revascularization (TCAR) is a minimally invasive procedure for treating carotid artery stenosis. It combines surgical and endovascular techniques to access the carotid artery and place a stent to improve blood flow to the brain.

How TCAR Works

- **Small Incision**: A small incision is made just above the collarbone to access the common carotid artery.
- **Flow Reversal**: A specialized sheath is inserted into the artery, and a system is connected to temporarily reverse blood flow away from the brain. This flow reversal directs any potential debris released during the procedure *away* from the brain and into a filter. [52]
- **Stent Placement**: A stent is advanced through the sheath and placed in the narrowed section of the carotid artery to open the blockage and restore normal blood flow.
- **Flow Restoration**: Once the stent is in place, the flow reversal system is deactivated, and normal blood flow is restored.

Advantages of TCAR

- **Minimally Invasive**: The small incision results in less pain, scarring, and a faster recovery compared to traditional carotid endarterectomy.
- **Reduced Stroke Risk**: The flow reversal system minimizes the risk of stroke during the procedure by diverting debris away from the brain. [52]
- **Suitable for High-Risk Patients**: TCAR is often a good option for patients who are considered high risk for traditional CEA due to age, medical conditions, or anatomical challenges. [52]
- **Lower Risk of Cranial Nerve Injury**: Compared to CEA, TCAR has a lower risk of cranial nerve injury.

Potential Drawbacks of TCAR

- **Newer Procedure**: TCAR is a relatively new procedure, and long-term data is still being collected.
- **Not Suitable for All Patients**: Certain anatomical factors may make TCAR unsuitable for some patients.
- **Requires Specialized Equipment and Training**: TCAR requires specialized equipment and training of the surgical team.

TCAR vs. Other Procedures

- **TCAR vs. CEA**: TCAR offers a less invasive approach with similar stroke prevention benefits as CEA, especially for high-risk patients. [52, 53]
- **TCAR vs. Transfemoral Carotid Artery Stenting**: TCAR avoids the need to navigate the aortic arch, reducing the risk of dislodging debris and causing a stroke. [52, 53]

Ongoing Research

Research is ongoing to further evaluate the long-term outcomes and effectiveness of TCAR compared to other treatment options. [53, 54] Studies like the ROADSTER trial have shown promising results for TCAR, with low rates of stroke and other complications. [52]

5.2 Advances in Endarterectomy

CEA techniques have also seen significant refinements:

- **Eversion Endarterectomy**: Eversion carotid endarterectomy is a surgical technique used to remove plaque from the carotid artery, aiming to reduce the risk of stroke. It differs from the conventional CEA in how the artery is handled during the procedure.

  In ECEA, the carotid artery is cut obliquely at its distal end and then everted, turning it inside out like a sock. This allows the surgeon to directly visualize and remove the plaque from the inside of the artery wall. Once the plaque is removed, the artery is then turned right-side out and sutured back together. Reigner et al. [55] describes some of the technical aspects of this procedure.

  Some studies have suggested potential advantages of ECEA over CCEA, including:

  - **Lower Restenosis Rates**: Some older studies indicated that ECEA might lead to lower restenosis rates compared to CCEA. However, more recent data, including a randomized trial [56], have challenged this view, especially when CCEA is performed with patch closure. Schneider et al. [57] discusses these conflicting findings and notes that the perceived advantage of ECEA in terms of restenosis might have diminished over time.
  - **Better Visualization of the Endpoint**: Proponents of ECEA argue that everting the artery provides better visualization of the distal endpoint of the endarterectomy, potentially leading to a more complete removal of plaque. [58]
  - **Placement of Suture Line**: In ECEA, the suture line is placed in the carotid bulb rather than in the internal carotid artery, which some surgeons believe might be advantageous.

  However, ECEA also has some potential drawbacks:

  - **Technically More Challenging**: ECEA can be technically more demanding than CCEA, requiring specialized training and experience. [59]
  - **Limited Access in Certain Cases**: The eversion technique may be difficult or impossible in certain anatomical situations, such as heavily calcified or tor-

tuous arteries. In such cases, the surgeon may need to convert to the conventional endarterectomy technique or even consider alternative procedures like bypass grafting. [56]

- **Minimally Invasive CEA**: Minimally invasive carotid endarterectomy aims to achieve the same benefits as traditional CEA but with reduced surgical trauma. This involves smaller incisions and specialized instruments, potentially leading to faster recovery, less pain, and improved cosmetic outcomes. There are several approaches to MICA:
  - **Limited Incision CEA**: This approach uses a smaller incision than traditional CEA, typically around 3–4 cm, but still requires direct exposure of the carotid artery. [60]
  - **Hybrid CEA**: As previously described in the TCAR paragraph this approach combines elements of open and endovascular techniques.

  While MICA offers potential advantages in terms of reduced surgical trauma and improved cosmetic results, it's important to note that the evidence supporting its superiority over traditional CEA in terms of long-term stroke prevention is still limited.
- **Patch Angioplasty**: Patch angioplasty is a technique used during carotid endarterectomy where a patch, typically made of synthetic material (e.g., Dacron, PTFE) or autologous vein, is sewn into the opened carotid artery to widen the artery and reduce the risk of restenosis (renarrowing). [61]

Benefits of Patch Angioplasty

- **Reduced Restenosis Rates**: Patch angioplasty has consistently been shown to reduce the rate of restenosis compared to primary closure (simply stitching the artery closed). [62] This is because the patch widens the artery, reducing the likelihood of turbulent flow and subsequent neointimal hyperplasia, which can lead to restenosis. [63]

Potential Drawbacks of Patch Angioplasty

- **Increased Operative Time**: Patch angioplasty adds extra time to the CEA procedure, as the patch needs to be carefully sewn into place.
- **Potential for Infection**: Although rare, there is a slightly increased risk of infection with patch angioplasty compared to primary closure, especially with synthetic patches.
- **Potential for Patch Rupture**: Patch rupture is a rare but serious complication that can occur, particularly with vein patches.

Patch Materials

Various materials can be used for carotid patching, including:

- **Synthetic Patches**: Synthetic patches including Dacron and PTFE are readily available and easy to handle. [61]
- **Vein Patches**: These are considered the "gold standard" by some surgeons, as they are less prone to infection and offer good long-term patency. [61]

6 Changing Guidelines and Ongoing Trials

Guidelines for managing carotid stenosis, especially asymptomatic, are evolving, reflecting the advancements in medical therapy and the long-term results of recent trials. Current guidelines increasingly advocate for individualized treatment selection based on a comprehensive assessment of patient-specific factors, including age, comorbidities, degree of stenosis, and patient preferences.

SPACE-2 [64], a multicenter, randomized controlled trial, aimed to compare carotid endarterectomy, carotid artery stenting, and best medical treatment in patients with moderate to severe asymptomatic carotid stenosis. Initially designed as a three-arm trial, it was later amended to two sub-studies (SPACE-2a and SPACE-2b) due to slow recruitment, comparing CEA + best medical treatment (BMT) vs. BMT alone and CAS + BMT vs. BMT alone, respectively. The trial was prematurely terminated due to insufficient recruitment, limiting its power to definitively answer the question of optimal treatment for asymptomatic carotid stenosis. Despite its limitations, SPACE-2 contributed valuable data, which is planned for inclusion in meta-analyses by the Carotid Stenosis Trialists Collaboration, alongside data from other trials like ACST-2, ECST-2, and CREST-2. [65] This collaborative approach aims to provide more robust evidence for guiding treatment decisions in asymptomatic carotid stenosis.

6.1 Shift Towards Risk Stratification and Medical Management

There is a growing recognition of the importance of intensive medical management in all patients with carotid stenosis, regardless of whether they undergo revascularization. Optimal medical therapy includes lifestyle modifications (smoking cessation, diet, exercise), control of hypertension, diabetes, and dyslipidemia, and antiplatelet therapy. [64] mentions a real-world registry study showing a small absolute risk difference in stroke over 5 years between CEA and best medical treatment alone in patients with asymptomatic carotid stenosis.

6.2 Ongoing Trials and Future Directions

Several ongoing trials are further investigating the role of medical management versus revascularization in asymptomatic patients:

- **ECST-2**: This trial is evaluating the long-term outcomes of CEA versus medical management. Suitable patients are those with asymptomatic or symptomatic carotid stenosis ≥50% with an estimated 5-year risk of stroke of <20%, as calculated using the Carotid Artery Risk score. [66]
- **CREST-2**: The CREST-2 (Carotid Revascularization, Endarterectomy Versus Stent Trial-2) study was designed as 2 separate 2-arm randomized trials run in parallel. One trial compares intensive medical management with and without stenting; the other, intensive medical management with and without endarterectomy. Each trial has a recruitment target of 1240 patients with ≥70% asymptomatic carotid stenosis, randomized 1:1 in each arm. The enrollment was completed, long-term outcomes are going to be evaluated in next years. [67, 68]

These trials are expected to provide valuable insights into the optimal management of asymptomatic carotid stenosis and further refine patient selection criteria. Yoshida and Miyamoto [9] emphasizes the need to re-evaluate the use of invasive CEA/CAS for asymptomatic stenosis in light of improved medical treatment outcomes. Reiff et al. [64] discusses the potential of transcarotid artery revascularization and other novel techniques to improve outcomes in carotid stenosis treatment.

7 Conclusion

Many years of high-level evidence shows that for low risk surgical patients CEA should remain the preferred modality while in symptomatic carotid stenosis CEA should optimally be performed between 2 and 14 days from the onset of acute stroke. For moderate to high risk surgical patients the choice between CEA and CAS should be based on a comprehensive assessment of patient-specific factors, considering age, comorbidities, life expectancy and anatomical suitability for each procedure. The evolving medical management in spite of also evolving therapeutic approaches may diminish the stroke-prevention outcomes in asymptomatic cases but more evidence is needed.

Declarations

Competing Interests The author(s) has no competing interests to declare that are relevant to the content of this manuscript.

Ethics Approval The author(s) declares that this manuscript does not include primary research with human participants.

References

1. Qaja E. Symptomatic carotid artery stenosis. 2024.
2. Ferguson GG, Eliasziw M, Barr HWK, et al. The North American symptomatic carotid endarterectomy trial surgical results in 1415 patients. 1999.
3. Randomised trial of endarterectomy for recently symptomatic carotid stenosis: final results of the MRC European Carotid Surgery Trial (ECST). 351:1379; 1998.
4. Park JH, Razuk Á, Saad PF, et al. Carotid stenosis: what is the high-risk population? 2012;67:865.
5. Maharaj R. A review of recent developments in the management of carotid artery stenosis. J Cardiothorac Vasc Anesthesia. 2008;22:277.
6. Barnett HJM, Taylor DW, Eliasziw M, et al. Benefit of carotid endarterectomy in patients with symptomatic moderate or severe stenosis. N Engl J Med. 1998;339:1415.
7. Halliday A, Harrison MR, Hayter E, et al. 10-year stroke prevention after successful carotid endarterectomy for asymptomatic stenosis (ACST-1): a multicentre randomised trial. The Lancet. 2010;376:1074.
8. Walker M. Endarterectomy for asymptomatic carotid artery stenosis. JAMA. 1995;273:1421.
9. Yoshida K, Miyamoto S. Evidence for management of carotid artery stenosis. Neurologia medico-chirurgica. 2015;55:230.
10. Keyhani S, Cheng EM, Hoggatt KJ, et al. Comparative effectiveness of carotid endarterectomy vs initial medical therapy in patients with asymptomatic carotid stenosis. JAMA Neurol. 2020;77:1110.
11. Brott TG, Hobson RW, Howard G, et al. Stenting versus endarterectomy for treatment of carotid-artery stenosis. N Engl J Med. 2010;363:11.
12. Haro JD, Michel I, Bleda S, et al. Carotid stenting in patients with high risk versus standard risk for open carotid endarterectomy (REAL-1 Trial). 2017;120:322.
13. Beneš V, Bradáč O. Carotid endarterectomy and carotid artery stenting in the light of ICSS and CREST studies. Acta neurochirurgica. Supplementum; 2018. p. 95.
14. Chaturvedi S, Bruno A, Feasby TE, et al. Carotid endarterectomy – an evidence-based review [RETIRED]. Neurology. 2005;65:794.
15. Hasan B, Farah MH, Nayfeh T, et al. A systematic review supporting the Society for Vascular Surgery Guidelines on the management of carotid artery disease. 2021;75
16. Mas J, Chatellier G, Beyssen B, et al. Endarterectomy versus stenting in patients with symptomatic severe carotid stenosis. N Engl J Med. 2006;355:1660.
17. Young K, Jahromi BS. Does current practice in the United States of carotid artery stent placement benefit asymptomatic octogenarians? Am J Neuroradiol. 2010;32:170.
18. Choy H, Kokkinidis DG, Cotter R, et al. Long-term outcomes after carotid artery stenting of patients with prior neck irradiation or surgery. 2017;19:327.

19. Bonati LH, Kakkos S, Berkefeld J, et al. Guideline European Stroke Organisation guideline on endarterectomy and stenting for carotid artery stenosis. 2021.
20. Nguyen LL, Conte MS, Reed AB, Belkin M. Carotid endarterectomy: who is the high-risk patient? 2004;17:219.
21. Hallett JW, Pietropaoli JA, Ilstrup DM, et al. Comparison of North American Symptomatic Carotid Endarterectomy Trial and population-based outcomes for carotid endarterectomy. J Vasc Surg. 1998;27:845.
22. Long GW, Nuthakki V, Bove P, et al. Contemporary outcomes for carotid endarterectomy at a large community-based academic health center. Ann Vasc Surg. 2007;21:321.
23. Halliday A, Bulbulia R, Bonati LH, et al. Second asymptomatic carotid surgery trial (ACST-2): a randomised comparison of carotid artery stenting versus carotid endarterectomy. The Lancet. 2021;398:1065.
24. Simons JP, Goodney PP, Baril DT, et al. The effect of postoperative stroke and myocardial infarction on long-term survival after carotid revascularization. 2013;57:1581.
25. Bennett KM, Scarborough J, Shortell CK. Risk factors for cranial nerve injury after carotid endarterectomy. J Vasc Surg. 2015;62:363.
26. Fokkema M, de Borst GJ, Nolan B, et al. Clinical relevance of cranial nerve injury following carotid endarterectomy. Eur J Vasc Endovasc Surg. 2013;47:2.
27. Cunningham EJ, Bond R, Mayberg MR, et al. Risk of persistent cranial nerve injury after carotid endarterectomy. J Neurosurg. 2004;101:445.
28. Radak D, Waard DD de, Halliday A, et al. Carotid endarterectomy has significantly lower risk in the last two decades: should the guidelines now be updated? 59; 2018.
29. Bonati LH, Dobson J, Featherstone RL, et al. Long-term outcomes after stenting versus endarterectomy for treatment of symptomatic carotid stenosis: the International Carotid Stenting Study (ICSS) Randomised Trial. The Lancet. 2014;385:529.
30. Eckstein H, Ringleb PA, Allenberg J, et al. Results of the Stent-Protected Angioplasty versus Carotid Endarterectomy (SPACE) study to treat symptomatic stenoses at 2 years: a multinational, prospective, randomised trial. Lancet Neurol. 2008;7:893.
31. Stilo F, Montelione N, Calandrelli R, et al. The management of carotid restenosis: a comprehensive review. Ann Transl Med. 2020;8:1272.
32. Arhuidese I, Nejim B, Chavali S, et al. Endarterectomy versus stenting in patients with prior ipsilateral carotid artery stenting. J Vasc Surg. 2017;65:1418.
33. Tu J, Wang S, Huo Z, et al. Repeated carotid endarterectomy versus carotid artery stenting for patients with carotid restenosis after carotid endarterectomy: systematic review and meta-analysis. Surgery. 2015;157:1166.
34. Allen RC. Carotid angioplasty and stenting: a review of the facts. 1997;10:27.
35. Castriota F, Cremonesi A, Manetti R, et al. Impact of cerebral protection devices on early outcome of carotid stenting. J Endovasc Ther. 2002;9:786.
36. Kajihara Y, Sakamoto S, Kiura Y, et al. Comparison of dual protection and distal filter protection as a distal embolic protection method during carotid artery stenting: a single-center carotid artery stenting experience. 2015;38:671.
37. Howard G, Roubin GS, Jansen O, et al. Association between age and risk of stroke or death from carotid endarterectomy and carotid stenting: a meta-analysis of pooled patient data from four randomised trials. The Lancet. 2016;387:1305.
38. Siddiq F, Adil M, Malik A, et al. Effect of carotid revascularization endarterectomy versus stenting trial results on the performance of carotid artery stent placement and carotid endarterectomy in the United States. 2015;77:726.
39. Bonati LH, Dobson J, Featherstone RL, et al. Long-term outcomes after stenting versus endarterectomy for treatment of symptomatic carotid stenosis: the International Carotid Stenting Study (ICSS). Randomised Trial. 2014;385:529.
40. Bonati LH, Gregson J, Dobson J, et al. Restenosis and risk of stroke after stenting or endarterectomy for symptomatic carotid stenosis in the International Carotid Stenting Study (ICSS): secondary analysis of a Randomised Trial. 2018;17:587.
41. Meier P, Knapp G, Tamhane U, et al. Short term and intermediate term comparison of endarterectomy versus stenting for carotid artery stenosis: systematic review and meta-analysis of Randomised Controlled Clinical Trials. BMJ. 2010;340
42. Bradáč O, Mohapl M, Kramář F, et al. Carotid endarterectomy and carotid artery stenting: changing paradigm during 10 years in a high-volume centre. Acta Neurochirurgica. 2014;156:1705.
43. Reimers B, Corvaja N, Moshiri S, et al. Cerebral protection with filter devices during carotid artery stenting. Circulation. 2001;104:12.
44. Haro JD, Michel I, Bleda S, et al. Carotid stenting in patients with high risk versus standard risk for open carotid endarterectomy (REAL-1 Trial). Am J Cardiol. 2017;120:322.
45. Cremonesi A, Manetti R, Setacci F, et al. Protected carotid stenting. Stroke. 2003;34:1936.
46. Mousa AY, Campbell JE, AbuRahma AF, Bates MC. Current update of cerebral embolic protection devices. J Vasc Surg. 2012;56:1429.
47. Knappich C, Kuehnl A, Tsantilas P, et al. The use of embolic protection devices is associated with a lower stroke and death rate after carotid stenting. КАРДИОЛОГИЯ УЗБЕКИСТАНА. 2017;10:1257.
48. Ohki T, Roubin GS, Veith FJ, et al. Efficacy of a filter device in the prevention of embolic events during carotid angioplasty and stenting: an ex vivo analysis. J Vasc Surg. 1999;30:1034.
49. Kokkinidis DG, Chaitidis N, Giannopoulos S, et al. Presence of contralateral carotid occlusion is associated with increased periprocedural stroke risk following CEA but not CAS: a meta-analysis and Meta-regression analysis of 43 studies and 96,658 patients. 2020.
50. Imamura H, Sakai N, Matsumoto Y, et al. Clinical trial of carotid artery stenting using dual- layer CASPER stent for carotid endarterectomy in patients at high and normal risk in the Japanese population. 2020.
51. Gray WA, Levy EI, Bacharach JM, et al. Evaluation of a novel mesh-covered stent for treatment of carotid stenosis in patients at high risk for endarterectomy: 1-year results of the SCAFFOLD trial. Catheter Cardiovasc Intervent. 2019;96:121.
52. Dakour-Aridi H, Kashyap VS, Wang GJ, et al. The impact of age on in-hospital outcomes after transcarotid artery revascularization, transfemoral carotid artery stenting, and carotid endarterectomy. J Vasc Surg. 2020;72:931.
53. Naazie I, Cui CL, Osaghae I, et al. A systematic review and meta-analysis of transcarotid artery revascularization with dynamic flow reversal versus transfemoral carotid artery stenting and carotid endarterectomy. Ann Vasc Surg. 2020;69:426.
54. Galyfos G, Tsoutsas I, Konstantopoulos T, et al. Early and late outcomes after transcarotid revascularisation for internal carotid artery stenosis: a systematic review and meta-analysis. J Vasc Surg. 2021;73:2207.
55. Reigner B, Reveilleau P, Gayral M, et al. Eversion endarterectomy of the internal carotid artery: midterm results of a new technique. Ann Vasc Surg. 1995;9:241.
56. Cao P, Giordano G, Rango PD, et al. Eversion versus conventional carotid endarterectomy: late results of a prospective multicenter randomized trial. J Vasc Surg. 2000;31:19.
57. Schneider JR, Helenowski I, Jackson CR, et al. A comparison of results with eversion versus conventional carotid endarterectomy from the Vascular Quality Initiative and the Mid-America Vascular Study Group. J Vasc Surg. 2015;61:1216.

58. Shah DM, Leather RP, Darling RC, et al. Technique of eversion carotid endarterectomy and contemporary results. Perspect Vasc Surg. 1998;9:49.
59. Radak D, Tanasković S, Matić P, et al. Eversion carotid endarterectomy – our experience after 20 years of carotid surgery and 9897 carotid endarterectomy procedures. Ann Vasc Surg. 2012;26:924.
60. Kakkos SK, Papageorgopoulou CP, Papadoulas S, et al. Frequency and significance of maneuvers to dissect the distal internal carotid artery during carotid endarterectomy. Vasc Endovasc Surg. 2021;55:342.
61. Rosenthal D, Archie JP, García-Rinaldi R, et al. Carotid patch angioplasty: immediate and long-term results. J Vasc Surg. 1990;12:326.
62. Ballard JL, Romano M, Abou-Zamzam AM, Teruya TH. Carotid artery patch angioplasty: impact and outcome. Ann Vasc Surg. 2002;16:12.
63. Cheng SF, Richards T, Gregson J, et al. Long term restenosis rate after carotid endarterectomy: comparison of three surgical techniques and intra-operative shunt use. 2021;62:513.
64. Reiff T, Eckstein H, Mansmann U, et al. Carotid endarterectomy or stenting or best medical treatment alone for moderate-to-severe asymptomatic carotid artery stenosis: 5-year results of a multicentre, Randomised Controlled Trial. Lancet Neurol. 2022;21:877.
65. Eckstein H, Reiff T, Ringleb PA, et al. SPACE-2: a missed opportunity to compare carotid endarterectomy, carotid stenting, and best medical treatment in patients with asymptomatic carotid stenoses. Eur J Vasc Endovasc Surg. 2016;51:761.
66. Cheng SF, van Velzen TJ, Gregson J, et al. The 2nd European Carotid Surgery Trial (ECST-2): rationale and protocol for a randomised clinical trial comparing immediate revascularisation versus optimised medical therapy alone in patients with symptomatic and asymptomatic carotid stenosis at low to intermediate risk of stroke. Trials. 2022;23
67. Turan TN, Voeks JH, Chimowitz MI, et al. Rationale, design, and implementation of intensive risk factor treatment in the CREST2 trial. Stroke. 2020;51:2960.
68. Meschia JF, Edwards LJ, Roubin GS, et al. CREST-2 commitment to rigorous assessment of carotid stenting for primary prevention of stroke. stroke: vascular and interventional. Neurology. 2024;4

Emergency Carotid Revascularization

Vladimír Beneš IIIrd

1 Introduction

Stroke is the leading cause of severe disability in Western countries [1]. Among acute stroke patients, extracranial internal carotid artery occlusion (eICAO) is a common finding [2–4]. Patients with sufficient collateral circulation may be asymptomatic, and those with insufficient collaterals suffer neurological deficits of varying intensity, complete hemiplegia (and aphasia) notwithstanding. Diagnostic procedures focus on depicting the site of occlusion, possible tandem intracranial large vessel occlusion (LVO) and, from a therapeutic point of view, crucial detection of viable neural tissue (penumbra). As with any stroke, timely recanalization of the occluded vessel is vital. However, optimal eICAO treatment remains to be determined.

2 Pathophysiology and Natural History

Excluding uncommon causes of eICAO, such as vasculitis, carotid web and irradiation, the most common cause is atherosclerosis, followed by heart embolism and dissection [3–6]. Thrombus formation upon an underlying atherosclerotic plaque or embolic occlusion of the most stenotic segment eventually leads to the occlusion. Distal embolization or propagation of thrombus fragments may worsen the clinical presentation by causing further intracranial arterial occlusion. Cerebral hypoperfusion due to eICAO and eventual tandem occlusion contributes to the final clinical picture [7]. In summary, clinical presentation and outcome are highly dependent on (1) the rapidity of progression to complete occlusion; (2) the degree of initial stenosis of the occluded vessel; (3) the degree of contralateral internal carotid artery (ICA) stenosis/occlusion; (4) patency of intracranial collateral circulation; (5) eventual intracranial tandem occlusion; and (6) involvement of ipsilateral external carotid artery in the atherosclerosis [8]. In addition, hemodynamic instability can significantly contribute to stroke severity and eventual outcome [9].

Acute symptomatic occlusion without sufficient collateral circulation can be devastating. According to Meyer et al. [10], the incidence of favorable recovery ranged from 2 to 12%, severe disability from 40 to 60% and mortality from 16 to 55% among patients exhibiting a severe deficit. A recent ICARO study reported a 15.4% mortality and a favorable modified Rankin Score (mRS) of 0–2 in 20.6% of conservatively treated eICAO patients [5]. In a similar vein, a natural history study of MCA and terminal ICA occlusion reported a 92% probability of an unfavorable prognosis and a 23% mortality rate at 3 months [11]. Considering this pessimistic perspective, an active approach is necessary. However, patient selection is critical.

3 Diagnosis

In acute ischemic stroke, computer tomography (CT) and CT angiography (CTA) provide comprehensive information for clinical decision-making. Magnetic resonance (MR) imaging can provide the same information; however, due to local logistical constraints and availability, CT is usually preferred. Both techniques can depict the following four fundamental points, determining patients' suitability for further therapy.

Supplementary Information The online version contains supplementary material available at https://doi.org/10.1007/978-3-032-08934-2_13.

V. Beneš IIIrd (✉)
Department of Neurosurgery, Second Faculty of Medicine, Charles University and Motol University Hospital, Prague, Czech Republic
e-mail: vladimir.benes@fnmotol.cz

V. Beneš, D. Netuka (eds.), *Surgical and Interventional Treatment of Cerebral Ischemia*,
https://doi.org/10.1007/978-3-032-08934-2_13

23. Rubiera M, Ribo M, Delgado-Mederos R, Santamarina E, Delgado P, Montaner J, et al. Tandem internal carotid artery/middle cerebral artery occlusion: an independent predictor of poor outcome after systemic thrombolysis. Stroke. 2006;37(9):2301–5.
24. Dabitz R, Triebe S, Leppmeier U, Ochs G, Vorwerk D. Percutaneous recanalization of acute internal carotid artery occlusions in patients with severe stroke. Cardiovasc Intervent Radiol. 2007;30(1):34–41. https://doi.org/10.1007/s00270-005-0286-7.
25. Hauck EF, Natarajan SK, Ohta H, Ogilvy CS, Hopkins LN, Siddiqui AH, et al. Emergent endovascular recanalization for cervical internal carotid artery occlusion in patients presenting with acute stroke. Neurosurgery. 2011;69(4):899–907. discussion
26. Jadhav A, Panczykowski D, Jumaa M, Aghaebrahim A, Ranginani M, Nguyen F, et al. Angioplasty and stenting for symptomatic extracranial non-tandem internal carotid artery occlusion. J Neurointerv Surg. 2018:1155–60. https://doi.org/10.1136/neurintsurg-2018-013810.
27. Jovin TG, Gupta R, Uchino K, Jungreis CA, Wechsler LR, Hammer MD, et al. Emergent stenting of extracranial internal carotid artery occlusion in acute stroke has a high revascularization rate. Stroke. 2005;36(11):2426–30.
28. Nedeltchev K, Brekenfeld C, Remonda L, Ozdoba C, Do DD, Arnold M, et al. Internal carotid artery stent implantation in 25 patients with acute stroke: preliminary results. Radiology. 2005;237(3):1029–37.
29. Papanagiotou P, Roth C, Walter S, Behnke S, Grunwald IQ, Viera J, et al. Carotid artery stenting in acute stroke. J Am Coll Cardiol. 2011;58(23):2363–9.
30. Rha JH, Saver JL. The impact of recanalization on ischemic stroke outcome: a meta-analysis. Stroke. 2007;38(3):967–73.
31. Hong JH, Sohn SI, Kang J, Jang MU, Kim BJ, Han MK, et al. Endovascular treatment in patients with persistent internal carotid artery occlusion after intravenous tissue plasminogen activator: a clinical effectiveness study. Cerebrovasc Dis. 2016;42(5-6):387–94. https://doi.org/10.1159/000447599.
32. Ter Schiphorst A, Peres R, Dargazanli C, Blanc R, Gory B, Richard S, et al. Endovascular treatment of ischemic stroke due to isolated internal carotid artery occlusion: ETIS registry data analysis. J Neurol. 2022;269(8):4383–95. https://doi.org/10.1007/s00415-022-11078-y.
33. Barnett HJ, Eliasziw M, Meldrum HE, Taylor DW. Do the facts and figures warrant a 10-fold increase in the performance of carotid endarterectomy on asymptomatic patients? Neurology. 1996;46(3):603–8.
34. Pokras R, Dyken ML. Dramatic changes in the performance of endarterectomy for diseases of the extracranial arteries of the head. Stroke. 1988;19(10):1289–90.
35. Ostrý S, Nevšímal M, Nevšímalová M, Reiser M, Fiedler J. Median somatosensory evoked potential as a predictor of clinical outcome after urgent surgical extracranial internal carotid artery recanalization. Clin Neurophysiol. 2021;132(2):372–81. https://doi.org/10.1016/j.clinph.2020.11.019.
36. Verstraete M, Bounameaux H, de Cock F, Van de Werf F, Collen D. Pharmacokinetics and systemic fibrinogenolytic effects of recombinant human tissue-type plasminogen activator (rt-PA) in humans. J Pharmacol Exp Ther. 1985;235(2):506–12.
37. Kiyofuji S, Inoue T, Tamura A, Saito I. Emergent cervical surgical embolectomy for extracranial internal carotid artery occlusion. Acta Neurochir (Wien). 2015;157(8):1313–8.; discussion 8–9. https://doi.org/10.1007/s00701-015-2478-5.
38. Schubert J, Witte OW, Settmacher U, Mayer TE, Gunther A, Zanow J, et al. Acute stroke treatment by surgical recanalization of extracranial internal carotid artery occlusion: a single center experience. Vasc Endovascular Surg. 2018:1538574418800131. https://doi.org/10.1177/1538574418800131.
39. Weis-Muller BT, Huber R, Spivak-Dats A, Turowski B, Siebler M, Sandmann W. Symptomatic acute occlusion of the internal carotid artery: reappraisal of urgent vascular reconstruction based on current stroke imaging. J Vasc Surg. 2008;47(4):752–9. discussion 9
40. Gunka I, Krajickova D, Lesko M, Jiska S, Raupach J, Lojik M, et al. Emergent carotid thromboendarterectomy for acute symptomatic occlusion of the extracranial internal carotid artery. Vasc Endovascular Surg. 2017;51(4):176–82. https://doi.org/10.1177/1538574416674641.
41. Berthet JP, Marty-Ane CH, Picard E, Branchereau P, Mary H, Veerapen R, et al. Acute carotid artery thrombosis: description of 12 surgically treated cases. Ann Vasc Surg. 2005;19(1):11–8. https://doi.org/10.1007/s10016-004-0074-x.
42. Jiao L, Song G, Hua Y, Ma Y, Chen Y, Wang Y, et al. Recanalization of extracranial internal carotid artery occlusion: a 12-year retrospective study. Neural Regen Res. 2013;8(23):2204–6. https://doi.org/10.3969/j.issn.1673-5374.2013.23.011.
43. Kappelhof M, Marquering HA, Berkhemer OA, Majoie CB. Intra-arterial treatment of patients with acute ischemic stroke and internal carotid artery occlusion: a literature review. J Neurointerv Surg. 2015;7(1):8–15. https://doi.org/10.1136/neurintsurg-2013-011004.
44. Kasper GC, Wladis AR, Lohr JM, Roedersheimer LR, Reed RL, Miller TJ, et al. Carotid thromboendarterectomy for recent total occlusion of the internal carotid artery. J Vasc Surg. 2001;33(2):242–9. discussion 9–50
45. Paty PSK, Adeniyi JA, Mehta M, Darling RC, Chang BB, Kreienberg PB, et al. Surgical treatment of internal carotid artery occlusion. J Vasc Surg. 2003;37(4):785–8.
46. Slawski DE, Jumaa MA, Salahuddin H, Shawver J, Humayun MJ, Russell T, et al. Emergent carotid endarterectomy versus stenting in acute stroke patients with tandem occlusion. J Vasc Surg. 2018;68(4):1047–53. https://doi.org/10.1016/j.jvs.2017.12.077.
47. Beneš V 3rd, Bradáč O, Horváth D, Suchomel P, Beneš V Jr. Surgery of acute occlusion of the extracranial internal carotid artery – a meta-analysis. Vasa. 2020;49(1):6–16. https://doi.org/10.1024/0301-1526/a000801.
48. Cho YP, Kwon TW, Kwon SU, Chae WY, Kim GE. Carotid endarterectomy for symptomatic complete occlusion of the internal carotid artery. Acta Med Okayama. 2011;65(4):239–45.
49. Burkhardt JK, Winklhofer S, Fierstra J, Wegener S, Esposito G, Luft A, et al. Emergency extracranial-intracranial bypass to revascularize salvageable brain tissue in acute ischemic stroke patients. World Neurosurg. 2018;109:e476–e85. https://doi.org/10.1016/j.wneu.2017.10.005.
50. Park HS, Kim SH, Nah HW, Choi JH, Kim DH, Kang MJ, et al. Patient selection and clinical efficacy of urgent superficial temporal artery-middle cerebral artery bypass in acute ischemic stroke using advanced magnetic resonance imaging techniques. Oper Neurosurg (Hagerstown). 2017;13(5):552–9. https://doi.org/10.1093/ons/opx041.
51. Bonati LH, Dobson J, Featherstone RL, Ederle J, van der Worp HB, de Borst GJ, et al. Long-term outcomes after stenting versus endarterectomy for treatment of symptomatic carotid stenosis: the International Carotid Stenting Study (ICSS) randomised trial. Lancet. 2015;385(9967):529–38. https://doi.org/10.1016/S0140-6736(14)61184-3.
52. Bonati LH, Jongen LM, Haller S, Flach HZ, Dobson J, Nederkoorn PJ, et al. New ischaemic brain lesions on MRI after stenting or endarterectomy for symptomatic carotid stenosis: a substudy of the International Carotid Stenting Study (ICSS). Lancet Neurol. 2010;9(4):353–62.

53. Brott TG, Hobson RW 2nd, Howard G, Roubin GS, Clark WM, Brooks W, et al. Stenting versus endarterectomy for treatment of carotid-artery stenosis. N Engl J Med. 2010;363(1):11–23. https://doi.org/10.1056/NEJMoa0912321.
54. Brott TG, Howard G, Roubin GS, Meschia JF, Mackey A, Brooks W, et al. Long-term results of stenting versus endarterectomy for carotid-artery stenosis. N Engl J Med. 2016;374(11):1021–31. https://doi.org/10.1056/NEJMoa1505215.
55. Mas JL, Trinquart L, Leys D, Albucher JF, Rousseau H, Viguier A, et al. Endarterectomy Versus Angioplasty in Patients with Symptomatic Severe Carotid Stenosis (EVA-3S) trial: results up to 4 years from a randomised, multicentre trial. Lancet Neurol. 2008;7(10):885–92.
56. Moresoli P, Habib B, Reynier P, Secrest MH, Eisenberg MJ, Filion KB. Carotid stenting versus endarterectomy for asymptomatic carotid artery stenosis: a systematic review and meta-analysis. Stroke. 2017;48(8):2150–7. https://doi.org/10.1161/STROKEAHA.117.016824.
57. Silver FL, Mackey A, Clark WM, Brooks W, Timaran CH, Chiu D, et al. Safety of stenting and endarterectomy by symptomatic status in the Carotid Revascularization Endarterectomy Versus Stenting Trial (CREST). Stroke. 2011;42(3):675–80.

Endarterectomy After Stenting

Tomáš Hrbáč, David Školoudík, and Terezia Hrobaková

1 Incidence and Risk Factors

The incidence of in-stent restenosis in the internal carotid artery (ICA) varies in the literature depending on the length of follow-up and severity of restenosis [1, 2]. In general, the rate of in-stent restenosis ranges from 5% to 10% during the first 12 months. According to a systematic review, restenosis rate above 50% is approximately 5.7% at 1 year after CAS and rises to 40.7% at 5-year follow-up [3, 4].

Several risk factors are involved in the development of in-stent restenosis, including gender, diabetes, hypertension, dyslipidaemia, and smoking. One strong predictor of restenosis after endovascular carotid artery treatment is diabetes mellitus. Diabetics have higher levels of insulin secretion, which affects endothelial cell proliferation with subsequent lipid deposition and impact on endothelial function [5].

Other data suggest, that the higher the rate of residual stenosis after the first stent implantation, the more likely the development of restenosis [6]. A higher residual stenosis ratio is likely to result in hemodynamic changes that lead to abnormal blood platelets aggregation and restenosis [5]. The development of in-stent restenosis is also directly related to stent length and indirectly dependent on stent diameter [7]. These factors should therefore be considered when selecting the appropriate treatment for carotid artery stenosis.

2 Diagnosis

Imaging modalities used to detect ICA stenosis include duplex sonography (DUS), computer tomography (CT) angiography or MR angiography, and digital subtraction angiography (DSA) (Figs. 1 and 2).

DSA provides the highest diagnostic value in carotid artery imaging, but this is not indicated in routine follow-ups due to its invasiveness and risk of potential complications. Diagnosis based on CT angiography is limited by artefacts that depend on the structure and type of stent. Moreover, this method is not suitable in patients with impaired renal function and in patients with allergy to contrast media. Imaging of ISR on MR angiography is also limited by possible artefacts and is therefore not standardly indicated [8].

Thus, duplex sonography remains the ideal screening routine in the evaluation of restenosis after endovascular treatment of ICA. As a result of stent placement in the carotid artery, anatomical and hemodynamic changes occur, especially an increase in vessel stiffness and rigidity, resulting in lower compliance and increased flow rates [9]. ESVS has therefore proposed peak systolic velocity (PSV) thresholds that are related to the degree of restenosis: PSV $\geq$ 220 cm/s (ICA/CCA ratio 2.5) at >50% restenosis; and 300 cm/s (end diastolic velocity 90 cm/s; ICA/CCA ratio 3.8) at >70% restenosis [13]. However, when compar-

T. Hrbáč (✉) · T. Hrobaková
University Hospital in Ostrava, Ostrava, Czech Republic
e-mail: tomas.hrbac@fno.cz; terezie.hrobakova@fno.cz

D. Školoudík
Centre for Health Research, Department of Clinical Neurosciences, Faculty of Medicine, University of Ostrava, Ostrava, Czech Republic

V. Beneš, D. Netuka (eds.), *Surgical and Interventional Treatment of Cerebral Ischemia*, https://doi.org/10.1007/978-3-032-08934-2_14

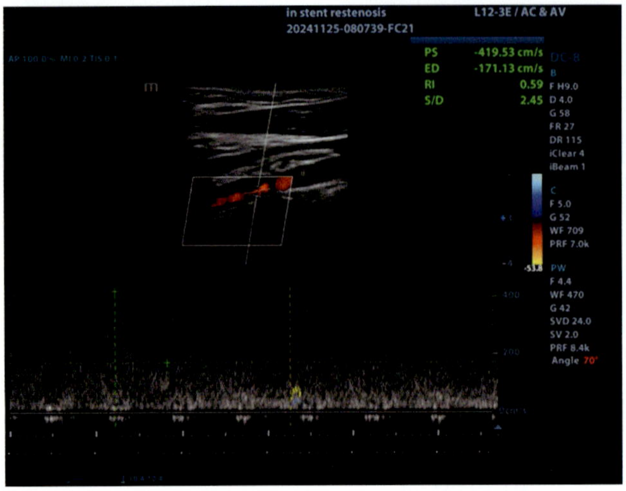

Fig. 1 In-stent restenosis 80% in proximal part of ICA with turbulent blood flow and increased blood flow velocity (peak systolic velocity, PS = 419.53 cm/s)

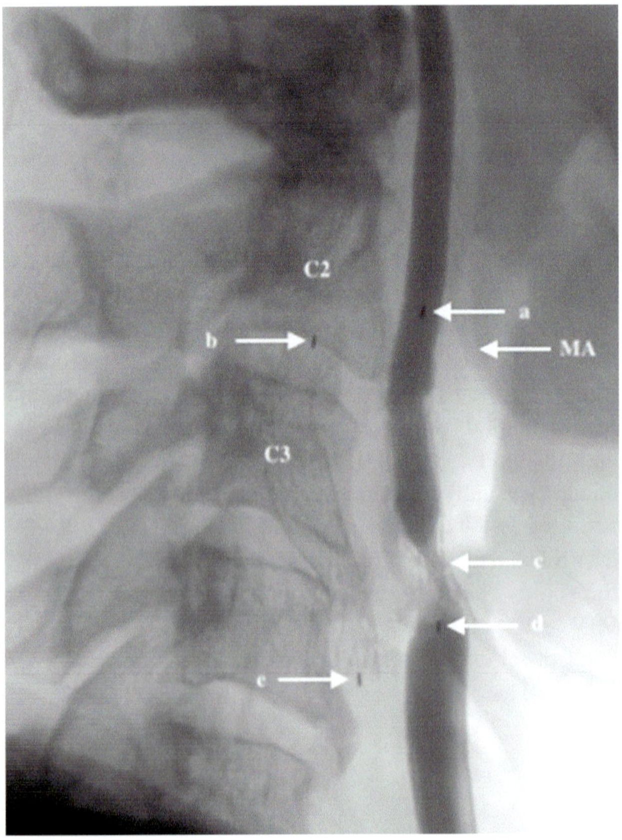

Fig. 2 Digital subtraction angiography: In-stent restenosis in the internal carotid artery. (**a**) cranial edge of the ipsilateral stent, (**b**) cranial edge of the contralateral stent, (**c**) in-stent restenosis, (**d**) caudal edge of the ipsilateral stent, (**e**) caudal edge of the contralateral stent; C2—vertebral body of C3, C3—vertebral body of C3, MA—mandibular angle

ing DUS-derived PSV and CTA in patients with restenosis after CAS, there was no evidence of an increase in PSV threshold at >50% stenosis [10].

3 Indications for Carotid Endarterectomy After Stenting

The main indication for carotid endarterectomy after stenting is the recurrence of ICA stenosis, known as in-stent restenosis (ISR) [11, 12]. Given the increasing endovascular trend, the number of patients with ISR can be expected to increase. Current guidelines from the European Society for Vascular Surgery recommend that patients with restenosis should be managed as for primary atherosclerosis [13].

Repeat angioplasty/stenting (rePTA/S) or drug-eluting stent (DES) insertion may be the method of choice. However, repeating endovascular procedures may be limited by frequent recurrence of ISR, leading to repeated interventions. Surgical management and carotid endarterectomy with stent removal (CEASR) should therefore be indicated in patients with recurrent rePTA/S failure and in patients with contraindications or high risk of rePTA/S [13–15].

Rarely, acute carotid stent thrombosis (ACST) can occur, a potentially devastating complication in patients after CAS [16]. Management of ACST depends on the evolution of the clinical condition and whether ACST is performed early or with a time delay. Surgical management has proven effective to achieve ICA recanalization, especially in symptomatic patients [17]. Incorrect placement, inappropriate stent size, anatomical variations, or severe ICA stenosis may also predispose patients to stent migration or entrapment. Early detection of misplacement and indication of carotid endarterectomy are crucial to prevent further complications and preserve vascular integrity [18].

4 Currently Available Procedures for the Management of In-Stent Restenosis

Management of carotid ISR presents a complex challenge despite its prevention, advances in stent technology, and strategies for treating carotid artery disease. Ideal management of recurrent stenosis has not yet been established. Conservative management with best medical therapy (BMT), repeated percutaneous transluminal angioplasty with or without stenting (rePTA/S), and surgical management—carotid endarterectomy with stent removal—may be the method of choice.

A previous review indicates the most common management of rePTA is combination with regular balloon angioplasty [19]. However, stent placement is limited by the frequent recurrence of ISR, leading to repeated interventions. According to the Carotid and Vertebral Artery Transluminal Angioplasty Study (CAVATAS), a significant 70%–90% restenosis rate was demonstrated in 14% of patients who underwent angioplasty with or without stent placement, compared to 4% of patients who underwent surgery [20]. Newer endovascular methods for the management of ISR include drug-coated balloon angioplasty (DCB), which has lower restenosis rates in most indications. It has the advantage of immediate drug release without prolonged direct drug contact with the artery vessel and maintaining the original anatomy and flexibility of the vessels [21]. However, to evaluate the effect of DCB, its concept needs to be supported by more preclinical data and monitoring of long-term outcome in patients.

The stent embedded in atherosclerotic plaque can also be removed by a surgical method, carotid endarterectomy with stent removal (CEASR), which has been shown in previous studies to be safe and beneficial for the patient after CAS [15, 22–24]. The first case of CEASR after CAS was described by Vale et al. in 1997. Performing CEASR can be technically more challenging due to the length of exposure required to dissect the metal stent and the potential difficulty in opening and cutting the artery without perforating the vessel wall [25]. In most cases, however, exposure of the ICA is possible and the traditional cleavage plane between the tunica intima and tunica media is well recognized. Some authors report perivascular inflammation, but nerve injury has not been reported. However, during stent removal, n.X and n.XII may adhere to the arterial wall, so distal inspection of ICA and their identification is essential [24].

A recent study comparing CAS and CEA for de novo ICA stenosis and post-intervention restenosis suggested that rePTA/S for moderate stenosis and CEA for severe stenosis should have been indicated [26]. However, based on the available data, it is not possible to determine which ISR treatment is optimal; therefore, a large multicenter analysis is necessary to stratify optimal therapeutic options.

5 Surgical Management of In-Stent Restenosis Technique

Surgical removal of the stent from the internal carotid artery can be performed by several possible techniques, which basically correspond to carotid endarterectomy. That is, in addition to the choice of general or local anaesthesia, through the method of monitoring clinical neurological findings after carotid artery clipping during local anaesthesia through electrophysiological monitoring of somatosensitive evoked potentials (SSEP) and ultrasound monitoring by TCD measurement of perioperative flow on the ipsilateral middle cerebral artery. Also, perioperative intravenous heparin administration has the same recommendations as primo-operation.

Perioperative application of a shunt to the operated artery is technically more challenging than primo-operation for carotid stenosis and sufficient exposure of the artery over the cranial and caudal ends of the stent must be calculated for safe insertion of the shunt. However, high stent deposition may be a contraindication to surgical management of stent restenosis (Figs. 3, 4, and 5).

The arteriotomy itself is performed longitudinally; reversal technique is associated with a greater risk of vessel wall damage in cases of stent restenosis. Subsequently, the vascu-

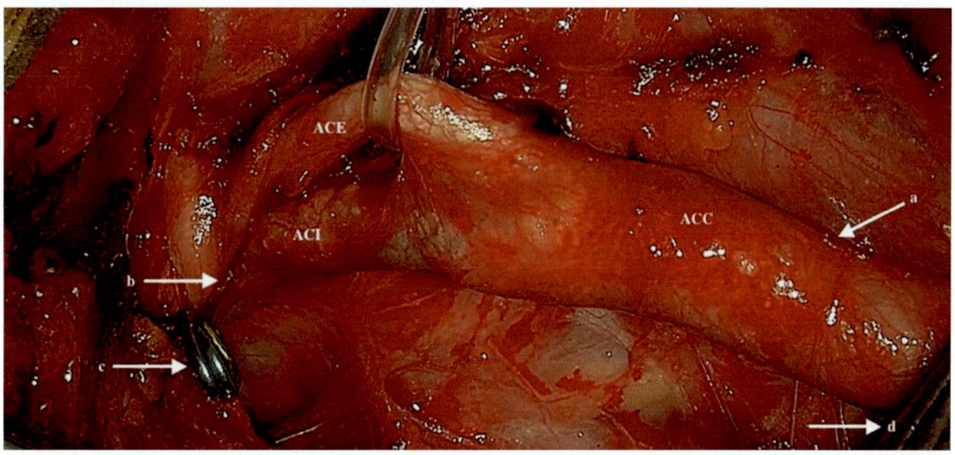

Fig. 3 Intraoperative image of carotid bifurcation with stent in the common and internal carotid arteries before arteriotomy. (**a**) Caudal edge of the stent, (**b**) cranial edge of the stent, (**c**) clipped internal carotid artery, (**d**) clipped common carotid artery

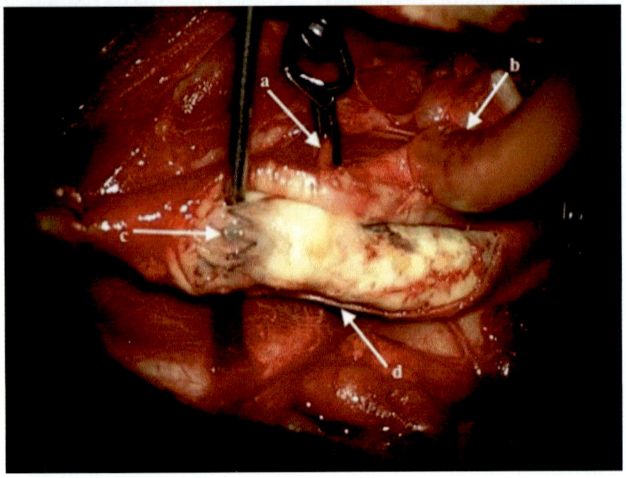

Fig. 4 Intraoperative image of carotid bifurcation with stent extraction from internal carotid artery. (**a**) Clipped superior thyroid artery, (**b**) tourniquet on the external carotid artery, (**c**) stent surrounded by atherosclerotic plaque, (**d**) vascular wall

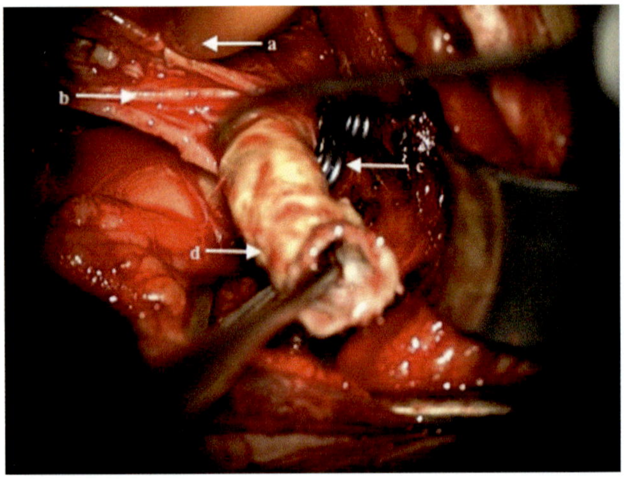

Fig. 5 Intraoperative image of stent removal from the internal carotid artery. (**a**) tourniquet on the external carotid artery, (**b**) internal lumen of the internal carotid artery, (**c**) clipped internal carotid artery, (**d**) atherosclerotic-coated stent removed from the lumen of the internal carotid artery

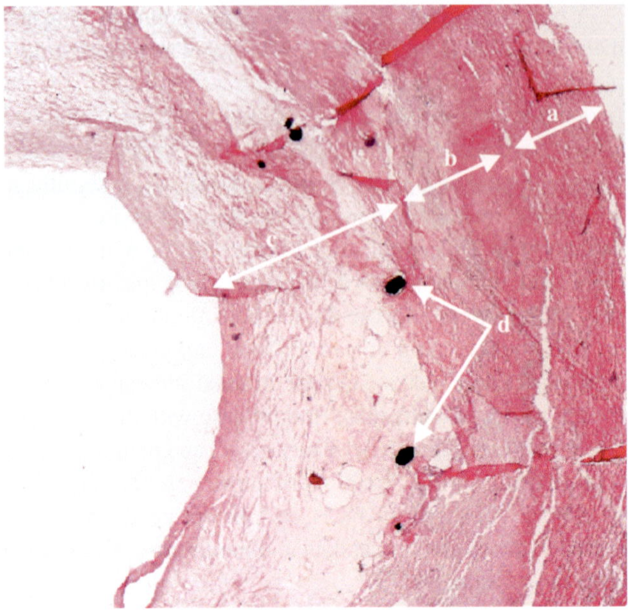

Fig. 6 Histological sample: Microscopic section through the internal carotid artery wall with in-stent restenosis. (**a**) Tunica adventitia of the vascular wall, (**b**) tunica intima and media of the vascular wall, (**c**) atherosclerotic plaque with neointimal hyperplasia, (**d**) stent mesh

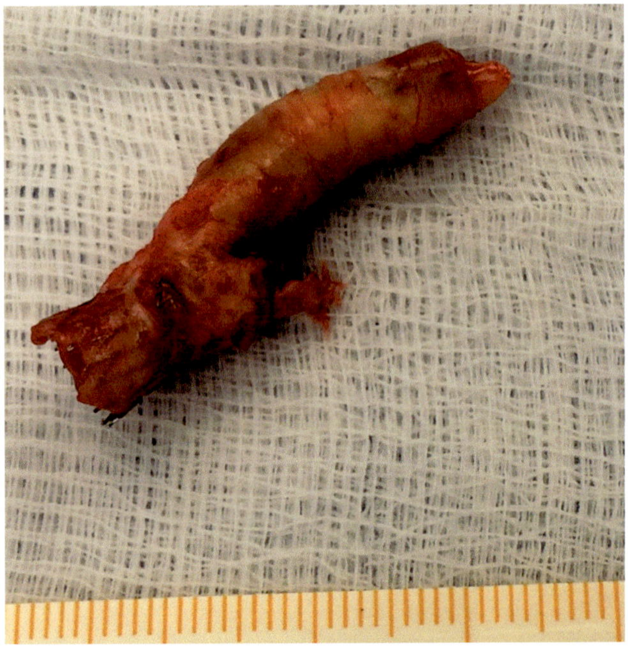

Fig. 7 Extracted stent with in-stent restenosis

lar wall can be detached relatively easily from the stent embedded in the intima, such as atherosclerotic plaque in primary stenosis (Figs. 6 and 7).

Suturing can then be performed as a direct primary suture of a 6/0 monofilament arteriotomy or with a venous or artificial PTFE (Gore-Tex) graft, which is associated with a lower incidence of restenosis.

Some papers report stent dislodgement together with the artery and bridging the missing segment with an autologous or artificial PTFE graft [27, 28].

CAVE: estimating the surgical operability of in-stent restenosis is crucial, in the sense of in-stent exposure of the stent-filled artery mainly cranially. Angiographic stitching provides sufficient orientation, where we assess the relationship of the upper edge of the stent placement to the mandibular angle and the vertebrae of the cervical spine. Stent placement beyond the mandibular angle or above the mid-body of C2 is again surgically unfavourable and it is associated with a high risk of surgical complications.

6 Complications of Surgical Management

As a result of reparative changes in the vessel wall after CAS, stent adherence to the atherosclerotic plaque and arterial wall occurs inside the artery, which increases the technical difficulty of the operation. The degree of adherence to the vessel wall may be influenced by the time interval between CAS and CEASR. Removal of the distal portion of the stent is problematic because it is usually located in the unaffected portion of the ICA, which has a fragmented vessel wall and thus it is predisposed to dissection [23]. An asymptomatic dissecting aneurysm in the distal part of the pars petrosa has also been described in one patient [29].

During surgical management, it is also necessary to identify the nerves, especially the n. vagus and n. hypoglossus, to avoid injury to them, similarly to a conventional carotid endarterectomy [23]. The described lesions of the cranial nerves after CEASR were only transient in nature [30].

Significant stent adhesions to the vessel wall may result in loss of the vessel wall and indication of transposition of the ICA to the ECA. In more complicated cases, a stent is removed together with the damaged artery and replaced with bypass grafting [27, 28].

7 Conclusion: Recommended Course of Action

Recommendations regarding the management of in-stent restenosis after carotid stenting for atherosclerotic involvement as prevention of ischemic stroke are like those for primary carotid artery stenosis according to the latest ESO and AHA guidelines [31–33]. Endovascular or surgical management might be indicated in symptomatic patients with restenosis >50% according to NASCET criteria, and >60% in asymptomatic ones. For restenosis below these values, management is conservative—medical therapy is recommended [31–34].

Regarding the recommendation of different interventional methods, as mentioned above, in most cases the first method of choice for in-stent restenosis is angioplasty or re-stent angioplasty following DSA. In further in-stent restenosis of the carotid artery, a surgical approach is quite legitimate based on the available safety results of surgical management of in-stent restenosis. However, the patient's general condition, comorbidities, and collateral blood flow, may also be impaired by the atherosclerotic process. Finally, the experience of the surgical team with this issue cannot be overlooked.

Declarations

Competing Interests The author(s) has no competing interests to declare that are relevant to the content of this manuscript.

Ethics Approval The author(s) declares that this manuscript does not include primary research with human participants.

References

1. Garg N, Karagiorgos N, White CJ. Carotid in-stent restenosis: from pathophysiology to treatment. J Am Coll Cardiol. 2019;74(11):1245–54.
2. Brott TG, Calvet D, Howard G, Amarenco P. Long-term outcomes of stenting versus endarterectomy for carotid-artery stenosis. N Engl J Med. 2016;374(11):1021–31.
3. Huang H, Wu L, Guo Y, Zhang Y, Zhao J, Yu Z, Luo X. Treatment of the carotid in-stent restenosis: a systematic review. Front Neurol. 2021;12:748304.
4. Fernandes LD, Coelho AB, Peixoto JP, Machado MM, Basílio F, Carvalho P, Silveira D, Canedo A. State of the art on restenosis after carotid artery stenting: incidence, risk factors, mechanisms, diagnosis, and treatment options. Angiol Cir Vasc. 2024;20(1):28–31.
5. Peng ZY, Ji YH, Li Y, Wang F. Meta-analysis of risk factors for restenosis after stent implantation in patients with ischemic cerebrovascular disease. Eur Rev Med Pharmacol Sci. 2024;28(1):402.
6. Zhang K, Li TX, Wang ZL, Gao BL, Gu JJ, Gao HL, Wang YF, Xia JC. Factors affecting in-stent restenosis after angioplasty with the Enterprise stent for intracranial atherosclerotic diseases. Sci Rep. 2021;11:10479.
7. Megaly M, Alani F, Cheng CI, Ragina N. Risk factors for the development of carotid artery in-stent restenosis: multivariable analysis. Cardiovasc Revasc Med. 2021;24:65–9.
8. Gimžauskaitė A, Inčiūra D, Diringytė G, Lukoševičius S, Kaupas R, Pranculis A, Mačiulaitytė A, Basevičius A, Kuprytė M, Stankevičius E, Plisienė J. Assessment of plaque characteristics by contrast-enhanced ultrasound and stent restenosis following carotid artery stenting: a retrospective study. Medicina. 2024;60(5):836.
9. de Borst GJ, Meijer R, Lo RH, Vosmeer HW, Ackerstaff RG, Moll FL. Effect of carotid angioplasty and stenting on duplex velocity measurements in a porcine model. J Endovasc Ther. 2008;15(6):672–9.
10. Bosch FTM, Hendrickse J, Davagnanam I, Bonati L, van der Lugt A, van der Worp HB, et al. Optimal cutoff for duplex ultrasound compared with computed tomography for the diagnosis of restenosis in stented carotid arteries in the International Carotid Stenting Study. Eur Heart J. 2016;2:37–45.
11. Bonati LH, Jongen LM, Haller S, Flach HZ, Dobson J, Nederkoorn PJ, et al. New ischemic brain lesions on MRI after stenting or endarterectomy for symptomatic carotid stenosis: a substudy of the International Carotid Stenting Study (ICSS). Lancet Neurol. 2012;9(4):353–62.
12. Lal BK, Beach KW, Roubin GS, Moore WS, Voeks JH. Restenosis after carotid artery stenting and endarterectomy: a secondary analysis of CREST, a randomized controlled trial. Lancet Neurol. 2013;12(6):530–8.
13. Naylor R, Rantner B, Ancetti S, de Borst GJ, De Carlo M, Halliday A, Kakkos SK, Markus HS, McCabe DJ, Sillesen H, van den Berg JC. Editor's choice—European Society for Vascular Surgery (ESVS) 2023 clinical practice guidelines on the management of atherosclerotic carotid and vertebral artery disease. Eur J Vasc Endovasc Surg. 2023;65(1):7–111.

14. Arko FR, Lim RP, Eskandari MK. Carotid artery in-stent restenosis: current treatments. Ann Vasc Surg. 2020;66:265–75.
15. Hrbáč T, Fiedler J, Procházka V, Jonszta T, Roubec M, Pakizer D, Václavík D, Netuka D, Heryán T, Školoudík D. Comparison of carotid endarterectomy and repeated carotid angioplasty and stenting for in-stent restenosis (CERCAS trial): a randomised study. Stroke Vasc Neurol. 2023;8(5):399.
16. Moulakakis KG, Lazaris AM. Emergent carotid stent removal after carotid stent thrombosis. Ann Vasc Surg. 2018;46:401–6.
17. Coelho AP, Lobo M, Nogueira C, Gouveia R, Campos J, Augusto R, Coelho N, Semião AC, Canedo A. Overview of evidence on risk factors and early management of acute carotid stent thrombosis during the last two decades. J Vasc Surg. 2019;69(3):952–64.
18. Meena D, Patel S, Chandolia P, Tiwari S, Mathur A, Sharma AK. Emergency carotid endarterectomy with stent retrieval in a patient with stent migration following failed carotid artery stenting. Indian J Thorac Cardiovasc Surg. 2024;41(2):1–4.
19. Pourier VE, de Borst GJ. Technical options for treatment of in-stent restenosis after carotid artery stenting. J Vasc Surg. 2016;64:1486–96.
20. Ederle J, Bonati LH, Dobson J, et al. Endovascular treatment with angioplasty or stenting versus endarterectomy in patients with carotid artery stenosis in the Carotid and Vertebral Artery Transluminal Angioplasty Study (CAVATAS): long-term follow-up of a randomised trial. Lancet Neurol. 2009;8:898–907.
21. Marzullo R, Aprile A, Clementi F, Stella P, Modena MG, Sangiorgi GM. Paclitaxel eluting balloon: from bench to bedside. Minerva Cardioangiol. 2009;57:597–609.
22. Xu B, Liu R, Jiao L, Yu J. Carotid endarterectomy for in-stent restenosis: a case report and literature review. Biomed Rep. 2017;7(2):128–32.
23. Reichmann BL, van Laanen JH, de Vries JPP, Hendriks JM, Verhagen HJ, Moll FL, de Borst GJ. Carotid endarterectomy for treatment of in-stent restenosis after carotid angioplasty and stenting. J Vasc Surg. 2011;54(1):87–92.
24. Zheng J, Zhao J. Response to 'Re. Carotid endarterectomy with stent removal in management of in-stent restenosis: a safe, feasible, and effective technique'. Eur J Vasc Endovasc Surg. 2014;48(1):108–9.
25. Vale FL, Fisher WS, Jordan WD, Palmer CA, Vitek J. Carotid endarterectomy performed after progressive carotid stenosis following angioplasty and stent placement: case report. J Neurosurg. 1997;87(6):940–3.
26. Wangqin R, Krafft PR, Piper K, Kumar J, Xu K, Mokin M, et al. Management of de novo carotid stenosis and postintervention restenosis-carotid endarterectomy versus carotid artery stenting—a review of literature. Transl Stroke Res. 2019;10:460–74.
27. Owens EL, Kumins NH, Bergan JJ, Sparks SR. Surgical management of acute complications and critical restenosis following carotid artery stenting. Ann Vasc Surg. 2002;16:168–75.
28. Brown KR, Desai TR, Schwartz LB, Gewertz BL. Operative intervention for recurrent stenosis after carotid stent angioplasty: a report. Ann Vasc Surg. 2002;16(5):575–8.
29. Yu LB, Yan W, Zhang Q, Zhao JZ, Zhang Y, Wang R, Shao JS, Zhang D. Carotid endarterectomy for treatment of carotid in-stent restenosis: long-term follow-up results and surgery experiences from one single centre. Stroke Vasc Neurol. 2017;2(3):140–6.
30. de Marino PM, Lopez IM, Mateo MMH, Artero IC, Fernandez MC, Gutierrez MTR, Hernando FJS. Open versus endovascular treatment for patients with post-carotid endarterectomy restenosis: early and long-term results. Ann Vasc Surg. 2016;36:159–65.
31. Bushnell C, Kernan WN, Sharrief AZ, Chaturvedi S, Cole JW, Cornwell WK 3rd, Cosby-Gaither C, Doyle S, Goldstein LB, Lennon O, Levine DA, Love M, Miller E, Nguyen-Huynh M, Rasmussen-Winkler J, Rexrode KM, Rosendale N, Sarma S, Shimbo D, Simpkins AN, Spatz ES, Sun LR, Tangpricha V, Turnage D, Velazquez G, Whelton PK. 2024 Guideline for the primary prevention of stroke: a guideline from the American Heart Association/American Stroke Association. Stroke. 2024;55(12):e344–424.
32. Kleindorfer DO, Towfighi A, Chaturvedi S, Cockroft KM, Gutierrez J, Lombardi-Hill D, Kamel H, Kernan WN, Kittner SJ, Leira EC, Lennon O, Meschia JF, Nguyen TN, Pollak PM, Santangeli P, Sharrief AZ, Smith SC Jr, Turan TN, Williams LS. 2021 Guideline for the prevention of stroke in patients with stroke and transient ischemic attack: a guideline from the American Heart Association/American Stroke Association. Stroke. 2021;52(7):e364–467.
33. Fonseca AC, Merwick Á, Dennis M, Ferrari J, Ferro JM, Kelly P, Lal A, Ois A, Olivot JM, Purroy F. European Stroke Organisation (ESO) guidelines on management of transient ischaemic attack. Eur Stroke J. 2021;6(2):CLXIII–XXVI.
34. Naylor R, Rantner B, Ancetti S, de Borst GJ, De Carlo M, Halliday A, Kakkos SK, Markus HS, DJH MC, Sillesen H, van den Berg JC, Vega de Ceniga M, Venermo MA, FEG V, Esvs Guidelines Committee, Antoniou GA, Bastos Goncalves F, Bjorck M, Chakfe N, Coscas R, Dias NV, Dick F, Hinchliffe RJ, Kolh P, Koncar IB, Lindholt JS, BME M, Resch TA, Trimarchi S, Tulamo R, Twine CP, Wanhainen A, Document Reviewers, Bellmunt-Montoya S, Bulbulia R, Darling RC 3rd, Eckstein HH, Giannoukas A, MJW K, Lindström D, Schermerhorn M, Stone DH. Editor's choice—European Society for Vascular Surgery (ESVS) 2023 clinical practice guidelines on the management of atherosclerotic carotid and vertebral artery disease. Eur J Vasc Endovasc Surg. 2023;65(1):7–111.

Management of Simultaneous Coronary Bypass and Carotid Surgery

Vladimir Priban, Jiri Dostal, and Jan Mracek

1 Introduction

Carotid endarterectomy has a clearly defined place in the prevention of ischemic stroke. Multicenter studies have repeatedly demonstrated its benefit for symptomatic stenoses and less convincingly for asymptomatic stenoses [1–4]. These are mainly elective procedures. A prerequisite for an effective procedure is low perioperative morbidity/mortality, which should not exceed 3% for asymptomatic and 6% for symptomatic internal carotid stenoses [5, 6]. Patients who have simultaneous carotid and coronary artery involvement represent a high-risk group for whom the treatment strategy is not clearly defined. Between 3% and 16% of patients with coronary artery stenosis have simultaneous significant carotid involvement [7, 8]. Conversely, up to 50% of patients with significant carotid stenosis have substantial coronary artery involvement [9, 10]. The risk of stroke during coronary revascularization in patients with concomitant carotid artery involvement is as high as 14% [11]. Similarly, patients referred for CEA with concomitant coronary artery involvement have a non-negligible risk of myocardial infarction after the procedure [12]. The surgical strategy when carotid and coronary arteries are simultaneously involved is controversial. A possible option is staged surgery prioritizing CEA, however the interval between both procedures is not clearly defined and usually takes several weeks. The procedure is performed in order to reduce the risk of postoperative stroke. Disadvantage of this strategy is a higher rate of coronary complications. Another option is to perform a reverse-staged CEA operation prioritizing CABG. These procedures have a reduced incidence of cardiac complications but an increased risk of ischemic stroke. The interval between procedures is identical to the staged CEA surgery. A combined CEA/CABG procedure during a single anaesthesia can eliminate the disadvantages of previous procedures. However, it also represents a higher surgical burden for high-risk patients [13]. The literature data do not provide strict recommendations; thus, the indication strategy varies from department to department based on individual experience and complication rates. The following section presents an indication strategy by analyzing the results of literature and complications of combined carotid and coronary revascularization.

2 Historical Notes

The first revascularization for ischemic stroke due to carotid artery stenosis was performed in 1951 by Raúl Carrea in Argentina. He resected a portion of the internal carotid artery with a plaque and sewed it end-to-end to the external carotid artery. Eastcott published a resection of the internal carotid artery with a plaque followed by an end-to-end suture to the common carotid artery in 1954. The first classic carotid endarterectomy was performed by DeBakey in 1953. He published a compilation of patients 20 years apart [14].

The first coronary revascularization was performed by Goetz in 1960 and early thereafter by Sabiston [15]. The first series of 16 combined coronary and carotid operations was published by Bernhardt in 1972. He operated with zero mortality in the absence of stroke.[16]. A few years later, Cambria reported perioperative stroke in 4.2% and mortality in 2.8% in his cohort of 71 patients with symptomatic or asymptomatic carotid stenosis ≥70%. He observed no difference versus isolated CABG and recommended simultaneous surgery for combined coronary and carotid lesions [17].

V. Priban (✉) · J. Dostal · J. Mracek
Department of Neurosurgery, University Hospital and Faculty of Medicine in Pilsen, Charles University, Pilsen, Czech Republic
e-mail: pribanv@fnplzen.cz; dostalj@fnplzen.cz; mracek@fnplzen.cz

V. Beneš, D. Netuka (eds.), *Surgical and Interventional Treatment of Cerebral Ischemia*, https://doi.org/10.1007/978-3-032-08934-2_15

Table 1 Prevalence of carotid stenosis in CABG patients

Author	Year	No pts.	% stenosis (DUSG)	% with stenosis (DUSG)
Brener	1987	4047	>50%	3.8 (DUSG, AG)
Faggioli	1990	539	>75%	8.7
Berens	1992	1087	>50% >80%	17 5.9
Riccota	1994	1179	>50%	14.7
Salasidis	1995	387	>80%	8.5
Schwartz	1995	582	>50% >80%	22 12
Abboyans	2009	Review	>60%	9

3 Prevalence of Carotid Stenosis in CABG Patients

In the early 1980s, Brener presented a 3.8% prevalence of hemodynamically significant carotid stenoses (≥50% on DUSG) in his coronary bypass cohort [18]. Faggioli sonographically examined 539 patients before CABG in 1995 and found carotid stenosis ≥50% in 19% of patients and "severe carotid stenosis" ≥80% in 8.7% of patients [7]. Berens described carotid stenosis ≥50% in 17% of 1087 patients over 65 years and carotid stenosis ≥80% in 5.9% of patients [19]. Riccota analyzed 1179 patients and found ≥50% carotid stenosis in 14.7% of patients [20]. Salasidis analyzed 387 patients and found ≥80% carotid stenosis in 8.5% of patients [21]. Schwartz examined 582 patients and found ≥50 carotid stenosis in 22% and ≥80% stenosis in 12% of patients [22]. The role of carotid ultrasound screening is debated and sometimes questioned. In high-risk groups (age ≥65 years, peripheral vascular disease, previous stroke), screening is surely warranted. Aboyans in 2009, published a prevalence of carotid stenosis ≥60% in 9% of patients undergoing CABG. He highlighted risk factors for stroke, such as hypoechogenicity and plaque echolucency on sonography [23] (Table 1).

4 Incidence of Ischemic Stroke in CABG Patients: Risk Factors Associated with Perioperative Stroke

Ischemic stroke is one of the major causes of non-cardiac morbidity in patients after CABG. The incidence of stroke after coronary procedures is generally reported to be up to 2% [19]. However, when the incidence of perioperative stroke after CABG is followed prospectively, the incidence is reported to be around 5% [24]. The variance in the incidence of stroke is considerable and depends on the type of surgery performed (isolated CABG, combined CEA/CABG, staged CEA, reverse-staged CEA). In 2005, Dacey reviewed a database of 35,000 patients undergoing CABG alone and reported strokes in 1.3% of cases [25]. Contrast to this, Udesh reported an incidence of stroke of 6.17% and mortality in 4.96% of combined CEA/CABG procedures [26]. Outcome assessment is complicated, with individual cohorts being heterogeneous regarding elective, acute, and emergent surgeries. These factors significantly affect results and make evaluation extremely difficult. Patient age is a key risk factor for stroke [7]. The incidence of stroke in patients over 60 years of age with carotid stenosis ≥75% was 15%. This is related to the development of atherosclerotic changes in the aortic arch, carotid arteries and intracranial circulation. Other factors increasing the incidence of stroke were atrial fibrillation and prolonged cardiopulmonary bypass time [27]. A history of ischemic stroke increases the risk of perioperative stroke fourfold [28]. Despite the possible multifactorial aetiology of ischemic stroke, carotid stenosis is considered a significant risk factor [29]. The incidence of carotid stenosis ≥50% is reported to be around 20% in coronary revascularization series; the incidence of stenosis ≥70% is approximately 10% [12]. D'Agostino demonstrated that perioperative stroke risk after CABG depends on the degree of stenosis. Carotid stenosis below 50% carries a risk of less than 2%. Carotid stenosis of 50-80% carries a risk of stroke of 10%, and stenosis above 80% carries a risk of 19% [30]. Bilateral ACI stenosis again carries an increased risk of stroke during coronary revascularization. A meta-analysis of 11 studies by Brener showed an incidence of stroke with unilateral carotid stenosis of 6.9%, while bilateral carotid stenosis increased the risk to 12.7%. The risk of stroke with contralateral carotid occlusion was 15.6% and even 33% with bilateral carotid occlusion [18]. Ricotta reported a relatively low combined morbidity for stroke and mortality of 3.1%. He cites carotid stenosis ≥50% as a significant predictor of complications along with the presence of peripheral vascular disease and prolonged extracorporeal circulation time [20]. Salasidis lists severe carotid stenosis ≥80% (SCD) as a risk factor, followed by peripheral vascular disease and previous CEA. In patients with SCD, the incidence of stroke was 18% [21]. In 582 patients with asymptomatic carotid stenosis, Schwartz reported stroke in 2.1% of patients with carotid stenosis ≥50% and in 6.2% of patients with carotid stenosis ≥80%. Stroke was never reported in asymptomatic unilateral stenosis of 50%–80% [22].

5 Indications and Timing of Carotid Stenosis Surgery in CABG Patients

As mentioned, the following treatment options are available for patients undergoing CABG with concomitant carotid stenosis: staged CEA followed by CABG, combined CEA/

CABG, reverse-staged CEA and CABG, staged CAS followed by CABG, and combined CAS/CABG.

Generally speaking, comparing different series is not simple because of group heterogeneity. Different percentages of symptomatic or asymptomatic stroke patients, different anatomical situations, severity of carotid stenosis, presence of bilateral carotid stenosis, presence of contralateral carotid occlusion and clinical course of cardiac disease (stable vs. unstable angina) make simple solutions impossible.

Data Analysis

Hertzer analyzed 275 patients in a prospective randomized trial in 1989. Thirty percent of patients with carotid stenosis had a stroke before surgery. Twenty-four patients with cardiac stable disease underwent staged CEA/CABG (Group I). One hundred twenty-nine patients had cardiac instability and asymptomatic carotid stenosis (Group II). These patients were randomized—71 underwent simultaneous surgery (Group IIa), and 58 underwent reverse-staged CEA (Group IIb). The remainder acted as a non-randomized control group III of 122 patients. Postoperative stroke was noted in 4.7% of patients in groups I and II. Reverse-staged CEA resulted in a stroke in 14%. The vast majority occurred when CEA was performed within 2 weeks of the first operation [11].

Rizzo evaluated 127 patients with simultaneous CEA/CABG surgery. Before surgery, 68% had TIA/stroke, 60% had bilateral carotid stenosis, and 16% had contralateral carotid occlusion. Mortality was 5.5% and the stroke rate was also 5.5% [31]. Trachiotis performed 88 simultaneous procedures in patients with symptomatic carotid stenosis, asymptomatic carotid stenosis+contralateral carotid occlusion, and asymptomatic stenosis ≥80%. The mortality and permanent stroke rate was 6.8% [32]. Evangelopoulos reported a perioperative mortality of 8.9%, stroke rate of 2.2% and myocardial infarction of 4.2% in 313 patients with combined procedures [33]. Kolh demonstrated a mortality of 6% and stroke rate of 3.8% in 311 patients with simultaneous surgery. A history of TIA/stroke was present in 23% of patients, and another 20% had bilateral carotid stenosis [34].

Modugno, reported a mortality of 4.1% and stroke of 3.2% in a cohort of 222 patients with combined surgery. Five of the seven stroke cases were contralateral to the CEA [35].

Of great interest is a paper comparing the results of combined procedures from a single institution in three periods: Group I of 100 patients from 1984 to 1994, group II had 74 patients from 1994 to 1999, and Group III had 91 patients from 2006 to 2018. Patients in Group III were much less symptomatic in terms of stroke due to a more relaxed policy with knowledge of previous low complication rates (55% vs 31% vs 4.4%). Unilateral asymptomatic carotid stenosis was represented in 20% in Group I, 55% in Group II and 78% in Group III). Perioperative mortality was: I—8%, II—3%, III—2.2%. Perioperative stroke was reported in 9% of Group I, 1.4% in Group II and 2.2% in Group III [36].

In 2023, Haywood compared the outcomes of combined operations (n = 643, staged CEA 309 and reverse-staged CEA106). Combined mortality, stroke and MI did not differ between groups. Stroke was logically more frequent in the reverse-staged CEA group, whereas MI was more frequent in the staged CEA group [12].

Several studies have compared combined surgery vs CABG only. Kougias, in 2007 reported a mortality rate of 3.6% and a stroke rate of 2.8% in a cohort of 277 patients with carotid stenosis ≥70%, after combined surgery. The risk factor was contralateral carotid occlusion, where the incidence of stroke was 13.6%. In the CABG-only group, mortality occurred in 1.7%, and stroke in 1.28%. The authors concluded that combined procedures were justified [37]. In contrast, Klarin found no statistically significant reduction in perioperative stroke with carotid stenosis ≥80% in combined procedures compared with CABG only [38]. Tsukagoshi reached the same conclusions in an analysis of 32,473 patients [39].

The criticism of reverse-staged CEA stems from the higher stroke rate than staged CEA or CEA/CABG [11, 40]. Ischemic stroke predominantly occurs when CEA is performed early within 2 weeks after CABG [11].

Some studies oppose combined procedures. Chan reviewed 11 articles in 2019 with 67,953 patients who underwent staged CEA and combined CEA/CABG surgery. The primary outcome was postoperative stroke, and the secondary outcome was myocardial infarction and mortality. Postoperative stroke occurred in 3.64% for combined operations, 2.83% for staged CEA (OR 0.72, P 0.001) mortality was 4.40% vs 3.58% (OR 0.86, P 0.006). Mortality, TIA and myocardial infarction did not differ. Thus the authors preferred staged CEA [41].

Tzoumas processed 11 publications containing 44,895 patients in 2020. Of these, 27,000 underwent simultaneous surgery, and 21,000 underwent staged CEA. Patients undergoing simultaneous surgery had a higher incidence of postoperative stroke and mortality; in contrast, the incidence of MI was lower. The author recommends RCTs to refine the indication for each type of procedure [42].

6 Asymptomatic Carotid Stenosis in CABG Patients

The occurrence of asymptomatic ICA stenosis in patients indicated for CABG presents a dilemma. The indication for each type of surgery is controversial. In one hand, we know that the more severe the carotid stenosis, the higher the incidence of perioperative stroke. Bilateral ICA stenosis, especially asymptotic carotid stenosis + contralateral carotid occlusion, increases this risk. On the other hand, sole CABG surgery of patients with asymptomatic ICA stenosis does not result in a higher incidence of stroke in many series [38, 39].

Ogutu analyzed 20 papers, including two RCTs. As previously mentioned, the partially randomized trial by Hertzer demonstrated that combined CEA/CABG procedures are safer than reverse-staged procedures. Compared to CABG only, combined procedures are burdened with a lower risk of perioperative stroke and a somewhat higher risk of morbidity [43]. Byrne compared the outcomes of combined procedures in patients with symptomatic versus asymptomatic ICA stenosis. Asymptomatic patients had a 30-day stroke-related mortality of 4.3%, while symptomatic patients had a mortality of 6.1% [44]. In a second RCT, Illuminati divided 185 patients with asymptomatic stenosis ≥70% into two groups: group A—CEA/CABG patients,79 combined, 15 staged CEA; group B: 91 reverse-staged CEA. In group A the mortality and stroke rates were 1% and 0% respectively; in group B, the mortality and stroke rates were respectively 1.1% and 7.7%. The outcome of stroke prevention in asymptomatic carotid stenosis was worse in reverse-staged surgery [40]. Kougias evaluated 277 simultaneous operations in patients with ≥70% carotid stenosis unilateral, bilateral and carotid stenosis +contralateral carotid occlusion. The unilateral and bilateral groups did not present a higher risk of stroke and mortality than CABG alone [37]. Kaul reported a mortality rate of 2.45% for simultaneous procedures in patients with asymptomatic carotid stenosis (unilateral, bilateral, contralateral carotid occlusion). He recommended simultaneous procedures as safe for these patients [45]. Naylor did not demonstrate a benefit of prophylactic unilateral CEA in asymptomatic carotid stenosis. Preventive surgery in bilateral stenosis is worth considering [46]. Risk factors for stroke in asymptomatic carotid stenosis are an essential parameter in deciding whether to indicate isolated surgery—CEA. Similarly, they should be considered for all types of combined procedures. A life expectancy of more than 5 years and the presence of at least one of the factors listed subsequently justifies a proactive approach. Risk factors are (1) silent infarcts on MRI or CT, (2) progression of carotid stenosis, (3) juxtaluminal black area, (4) intraplaque haemorrhage on MRI, (5) exhausted cerebrovascular reserve capacity, (6) plaque lucency on DUSG, (7) ≥1 microembolic signal on TCD per hour, (8) contralateral carotid TIA/stroke [6].

Selective series of combined CEA/CABG are listed in Table 2.

Table 2 Combined CEA/CABG selected series

Author	Year	No pts	Death (%)	Stroke (%)	MI (%)	Comments
Rizzo	1992	127	5.5	5.5	4.7	
Trachiotis	1997	88	3.4	3.4	0	
Evangelopoulos	2000	313	8.9	2.2	4.2	
Kohl	2006	311	6.1	3.9	2.2	
Kougias	2007	277	3.6	2.8	0.72	
Illuminati	2011 [a]RCT Asymp. ICA stenosis >70%	185 Group A Combined + staged CEA	1	0	–	Favors combined and staged CEA
		Group B Reverse-staged CEA	1.1	7.7	–	
Modugno	2022	222	4.1	4.1	0.9	
Minisandran	1984–1994 (group I)	100	8	9	–	
	1994–1999 (group II)	74	3	1.4	–	
	2006–2018 (group III)	91	2.2	2.2	–	
Chan	2019 Asymp. ICA stenosis >80%	67,953	4.4. (C) 3.58 (S)	3.6 (C) 2.8 (S)	– –	Favors staged CEA
Haywood	2023	Combined 643	7.0	4.6	5.5	Favors combined CEA
		Staged CEA + reverse-staged CEA 415	5.0	4.1	11.5	

[a]*RCT* randomized control trial, *C* combined CEA/CABG, *S* staged CEA followed by CABG

7 Carotid Artery Stenting and CABG

A hybrid strategy is a potentially advantageous technique that requires shorter surgical time and less extensive surgical trauma. The disadvantage is the need for dual antiplatelet therapy and, thus, a higher risk of perioperative bleeding. The combination of CAS and CABG is a potential alternative to CEA/CABG. In the Sharp study, Versaci demonstrated favourable outcomes in a small cohort of patients who underwent CAS followed by CABG. Stroke was reported in 2%, and mortality was 2% [47]. Van der Heyden reported combined morbidity (stroke, MI) and mortality of 12.3% in a cohort of 57 patients with CAS and delayed CABG [48].

In contrast, Vellisaris had a stroke rate of 1.1% and a mortality rate of 1.1% in his group of 90 CAS/CABG patients [49]. Giannopoulos analyzed combined CEA/CABG vs staged CAS and CABG in 5 studies comprising 16712 patients. Stroke, MI and TIA were comparable in both groups, but perioperative mortality was higher in the CEA/CABG group [50]. In contrast, Tsukagoshi, found a lower incidence of perioperative stroke/TIA in CEA/CABG patients compared with CAS/CABG in a systematic review and meta-analysis of two RCTs and 23 observational studies comprising 32,473 patients. No strategy showed a significant advantage over CABG-only surgery for perioperative TIA/stroke [39].

Nardi published a study of 31 patients with early-stage CAS prior to CABG. The interval between interventions was 1–2 days. Combined morbidity/mortality was very low—3.2%. The CABG-only group had a morbidity/mortality of 5.9% [51].

A new promising technique of CAS is transcarotid artery revascularization (TCAR), which is performed through direct transcervical carotid access under local anaesthesia. This technique minimizes the chance of arch manipulation and consequent antegrade embolic stroke rate. CABG is then immediately performed in the operating room [52].

8 Author's Personal Experience

1. *Staged CEA followed by CABG*
   In our institution cardiologically stable patients with elective coronary revascularization and presenting with a coincidental symptomatic ICA stenosis, staged CEA followed by coronary bypass is preferred. The same procedure is indicated for bilateral asymptomatic ICA stenosis, with initial surgery performed at the more severely stenosed site. Similar timing applies to asymptomatic significant ICA stenosis and contralateral carotid occlusion. Sequential operations prioritizing CEA reduce the risk of stroke but increase the risk of cardiac complications. These procedures are indicated in a situation of acceptable cardiac risk. When these conditions are met, the combined morbidity/mortality is acceptably low.
2. *Combined CEA/CABG*
   Simultaneous surgery is indicated in patients with unstable angina pectoris and
   1. symptomatic significant ICA stenosis ≥50%,
   2. bilateral asymptomatic ICA stenosis ≥70%,
   3. asymptomatic ICA stenosis ≥ 70% and contralateral carotid occlusion; see Table 3.
3. *Reverse-staged CABG followed by CEA*
   Patients after cardiac surgery are sent for CEA on an individual basis depending on stroke risk factors in asymptomatic carotid stenosis. Communication between cardiologists, neurologists, cardiac surgeons and neurosurgeons is essential.

Surgical Technique

CEA is performed initially, followed immediately by CABG in the same operating room. The cardiac surgeon harvests the venous donor at the same time as CEA starts. From vessel dissection to arteriotomy closure, a microscope and microsurgical technique were used; see Fig. 1.

The primary arteriotomy closure was performed with a running suture in all cases.

Table 3 The authors' strategy in carotid and coronary revascularization procedures

Staged CEA surgery: CEA prior CABG	Cardiac stability	1.	ICA stenosis ≥50% sympt.
		2.	ICA stenosis ≥70% asympt. bilat.
		3.	ICA stenosis ≥70% asympt. + CCO
Reverse staged CEA surgery: CABG first	Cardiac instability	ICA stenosis ≥70% asympt.	
Simultaneous CEA/CABG surgery	Cardiac instability	1.	ICA stenosis ≥50% sympt.
		2.	ICA stenosis ≥70% asympt bilat.
		3.	ICA stenosis ≥70% asympt. + CCO

CCO contralateral ICA occlusion

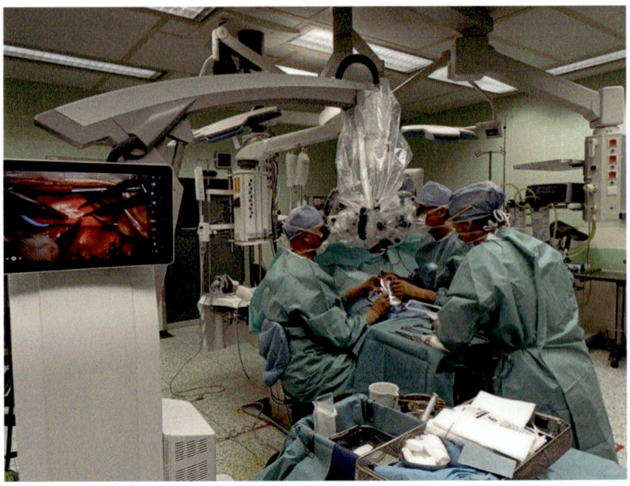

Fig. 1 CEA with the use of microscope

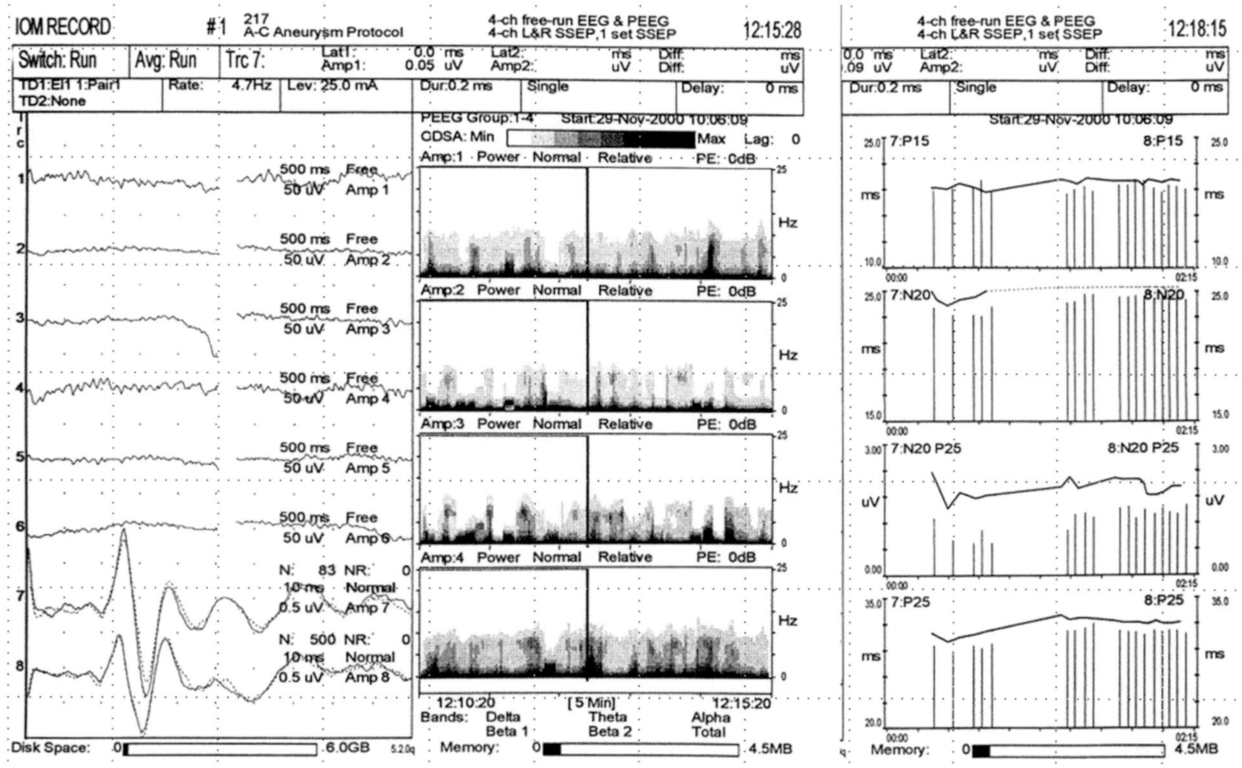

Fig. 2 Monitoring of somatosensory evoked potentials

The shunt is used selectively. Its need was determined in the initial group by combining carotid stump back pressure measurement and near-infrared spectroscopy (NIRS) [53].

Subsequently, somatosensory evoked potentials were used and monitored throughout the combined operation, see Fig. 2. The neck wound is closed at the end of the combined procedure [54].

9 Conclusions and Recommendations

SVS guidelines summarized the recommendations as follows

- Patients requiring CABG with symptomatic carotid stenosis ≥50% are indicated for staged CEA or simultaneous CEA/CABG (*Class II, Level C*).
- Patients with asymptomatic bilateral carotid stenosis 70%–99% or asymptomatic ICA stenosis and contralateral carotid occlusion are indicated for staged CEA or simultaneous CEA/CABG (*Class II, Level C*) [55].

ESVS guidelines have similar conclusions. In addition:

- Asymptomatic carotid stenosis is 70%–99%; they do not recommend staged CEA or CEA/CABG to prevent postoperative stroke (*Class III, Level B*) [6, 56].

In cases where risk factors are present for asymptomatic carotid stenosis ≥70%, the patient's life expectancy is above 5 years, and one of the risk factors for stroke is present; the author believes that an active approach of staged CEA or CEA/CABG can also be beneficial.

Acknowledgments Authors thank to cardiac surgeons V. Kuntscher and V. Zlocha for critical review of the manuscript.

Declarations

Competing Interests The author(s) has no competing interests to declare that are relevant to the content of this manuscript.

Ethics Approval The author(s) declares that this manuscript does not include primary research with human participants.

References

1. Barnett HJ, et al. Benefit of carotid endarterectomy in patients with symptomatic moderate or severe stenosis. North American Symptomatic Carotid Endarterectomy Trial Collaborators. N Engl J Med. 1998;339(20):1415–25.
2. Jensen TS. MRC European Carotid Surgery Trial: interim results for symptomatic patients with severe (70-99%) or with mild (0-29%) carotid stenosis. European Carotid Surgery Trialists' Collaborative Group. Lancet. 1991;337(8752):1235–43.
3. Walker MD, et al. Endarterectomy for asymptomatic carotid artery stenosis. Executive Committee for the Asymptomatic Carotid Atherosclerosis Study. JAMA. 1995;273(18):1421–8.
4. Brott TG, et al. 2011 ASA/ACCF/AHA/AANN/AANS/ACR/ASNR/CNS/SAIP/SCAI/SIR/SNIS/SVM/SVS guideline on the management of patients with extracranial carotid and vertebral artery disease: executive summary: a report of the American College of Cardiology Foundation/American Heart Association Task Force on practice guidelines, and the American Stroke Association, American Association of Neuroscience Nurses, American Association of Neurological Surgeons, American College of Radiology, American Society of Neuroradiology, Congress of Neurological Surgeons, Society of Atherosclerosis Imaging and Prevention, Society for Cardiovascular Angiography and Interventions, Society of Interventional Radiology, Society of NeuroInterventional Surgery, Society for Vascular Medicine, and Society for Vascular Surgery. J Am Coll Cardiol. 2011;57(8):1002–44.
5. Kleindorfer. Correction to: 2021 guideline for the prevention of stroke in patients with stroke and transient ischemic attack: a guideline from the American Heart Association/American Stroke Association. Stroke. 2021;52(7):e483–4.
6. Naylor R, et al. Editor's choice—European Society for Vascular Surgery (ESVS) 2023 clinical practice guidelines on the management of atherosclerotic carotid and vertebral artery disease. Eur J Vasc Endovasc Surg. 2023;65(1):7–111.
7. Faggioli GL, Curl GR, Ricotta JJ. The role of carotid screening before coronary artery bypass. J Vasc Surg. 1990;12(6):724–9; discussion 729–31.
8. Reul GJ Jr, et al. The effect of coronary bypass on the outcome of peripheral vascular operations in 1093 patients. J Vasc Surg. 1986;3(5):788–98.
9. Brener BJ, et al. A four-year experience with preoperative noninvasive carotid evaluation of two thousand twenty-six patients undergoing cardiac surgery. J Vasc Surg. 1984;1(2):326–38.
10. Hertzer NR, et al. Coronary angiography in 506 patients with extracranial cerebrovascular disease. Arch Intern Med. 1985;145(5):849–52.
11. Hertzer NR, et al. Surgical staging for simultaneous coronary and carotid disease: a study including prospective randomization. J Vasc Surg. 1989;9(3):455–63.
12. Haywood NS, et al. Operative and long-term outcomes of combined and staged carotid endarterectomy and coronary bypass. J Vasc Surg. 2023;77(5):1424.e1–33.e1.
13. Vassilidze TV, et al. Simultaneous coronary artery bypass and carotid endarterectomy. Determinants of outcome. Tex Heart Inst J. 1994;21(2):119–24.
14. Friedman SG. The first carotid endarterectomy. J Vasc Surg. 2014;60(6):1703–8.e1-4.
15. Doenst T, et al. The treatment of coronary artery disease. Dtsch Arztebl Int. 2022;119(42):716–23.
16. Bernhard VM, Johnson WD, Peterson JJ. Carotid artery stenosis. Association with surgery for coronary artery disease. Arch Surg. 1972;105(6):837–40.
17. Cambria RP, et al. Simultaneous carotid and coronary disease: safety of the combined approach. J Vasc Surg. 1989;9(1):56–64.
18. Brener BJ, et al. The risk of stroke in patients with asymptomatic carotid stenosis undergoing cardiac surgery: a follow-up study. J Vasc Surg. 1987;5(2):269–79.
19. Berens ES, et al. Preoperative carotid artery screening in elderly patients undergoing cardiac surgery. J Vasc Surg. 1992;15(2):313–21; discussion 322–3.
20. Ricotta JJ, et al. Risk factors for stroke after cardiac surgery: Buffalo Cardiac-Cerebral Study Group. J Vasc Surg. 1995;21(2):359–63; discussion 364.
21. Salasidis GC, et al. Carotid artery duplex scanning in preoperative assessment for coronary artery revascularization: the association between peripheral vascular disease, carotid artery stenosis, and stroke. J Vasc Surg. 1995;21(1):154–60; discussion 161–2.
22. Schwartz LB, et al. Asymptomatic carotid artery stenosis and stroke in patients undergoing cardiopulmonary bypass. J Vasc Surg. 1995;21(1):146–53.
23. Aboyans V, Lacroix P. Indications for carotid screening in patients with coronary artery disease. Presse Med. 2009;38(6):977–86.
24. Shaw PJ, et al. Early neurological complications of coronary artery bypass surgery. Br Med J (Clin Res Ed). 1985;291(6506):1384–7.
25. Dacey LJ, et al. Perioperative stroke and long-term survival after coronary bypass graft surgery. Ann Thorac Surg. 2005;79(2):532–6; discussion 537.
26. Udesh R, et al. Perioperative strokes following combined coronary artery bypass grafting and carotid endarterectomy: a nationwide perspective. Neurol India. 2018;66(1):57–64.
27. Likosky DS, et al. Intraoperative and postoperative variables associated with strokes following cardiac surgery. Heart Surg Forum. 2004;7(4):E271–6.
28. Hertzer NR. Basic data concerning associated coronary disease in peripheral vascular patients. Ann Vasc Surg. 1987;1(5):616–20.
29. Borger MA, Fremes SE. Management of patients with concomitant coronary and carotid vascular disease. Semin Thorac Cardiovasc Surg. 2001;13(2):192–8.
30. D'Agostino RS, et al. Screening carotid ultrasonography and risk factors for stroke in coronary artery surgery patients. Ann Thorac Surg. 1996;62(6):1714–23.
31. Rizzo RJ, et al. Combined carotid and coronary revascularization: the preferred approach to the severe vasculopath. Ann Thorac Surg. 1992;54(6):1099–108; discussion 1108–9.
32. Trachiotis GD, Pfister AJ. Management strategy for simultaneous carotid endarterectomy and coronary revascularization. Ann Thorac Surg. 1997;64(4):1013–8.
33. Evagelopoulos N, et al. Simultaneous carotid endarterectomy and coronary artery bypass grafting in 313 patients. Cardiovasc Surg. 2000;8(1):31–40.
34. Kolh PH, et al. Concurrent coronary and carotid artery surgery: factors influencing perioperative outcome and long-term results. Eur Heart J. 2006;27(1):49–56.
35. Modugno P, et al. Combined treatment with carotid Endoarterectomy and coronary artery bypass grafting: a single-institutional experience in 222 patients. Vasc Endovasc Surg. 2022;56(6):566–70.
36. Minisandram A, et al. Lessons learned during a 30-year experience with simultaneous carotid endarterectomy and coronary artery bypass grafting. J Vasc Surg. 2021;73(2):542–7.
37. Kougias P, et al. Simultaneous carotid endarterectomy and coronary artery bypass grafting: results in specific patient groups. Ann Vasc Surg. 2007;21(4):408–14.
38. Klarin D, et al. Concomitant carotid endarterectomy and cardiac surgery does not decrease postoperative stroke rates. J Vasc Surg. 2020;72(2):589–596.e3.
39. Tsukagoshi J, et al. Systematic review and meta-analysis of the treatment strategies for coronary artery bypass graft patients with concomitant carotid artery atherosclerotic disease. J Vasc Surg. 2023;78(4):1083–1094.e8.

40. Illuminati G, et al. Short-term results of a randomized trial examining timing of carotid endarterectomy in patients with severe asymptomatic unilateral carotid stenosis undergoing coronary artery bypass grafting. J Vasc Surg. 2011;54(4):993–9; discussion 998–9.
41. Chan JSK, et al. Concomitant severe carotid and coronary artery diseases: a separate management or concomitant approach. J Card Surg. 2019;34(9):803–13.
42. Tzoumas A, et al. Synchronous versus staged carotid endarterectomy and coronary artery bypass graft for patients with concomitant severe coronary and carotid artery stenosis: a systematic review and meta-analysis. Ann Vasc Surg. 2020;63:427.e1–38.e1.
43. Ogutu P, et al. Should patients with asymptomatic significant carotid stenosis undergo simultaneous carotid and cardiac surgery? Interact Cardiovasc Thorac Surg. 2014;18(4):511–8.
44. Byrne J, et al. Combined carotid endarterectomy and coronary artery bypass grafting in patients with asymptomatic high-grade stenoses: an analysis of 758 procedures. J Vasc Surg. 2006;44(1):67–72.
45. Kaul TK, et al. Coexistent coronary and cerebrovascular disease: results of simultaneous surgical management in specific patient groups. Cardiovasc Surg. 2000;8(5):355–65.
46. Naylor AR, Bown MJ. Stroke after cardiac surgery and its association with asymptomatic carotid disease: an updated systematic review and meta-analysis. Eur J Vasc Endovasc Surg. 2011;41(5):607–24.
47. Versaci F, et al. Simultaneous hybrid revascularization by carotid stenting and coronary artery bypass grafting: the SHARP study. JACC Cardiovasc Interv. 2009;2(5):393–401.
48. Van der Heyden J, et al. Carotid artery stenting and cardiac surgery in symptomatic patients. JACC Cardiovasc Interv. 2011;4(11):1190–6.
49. Velissaris I, Kiskinis D, Anastasiadis K. Synchronous carotid artery stenting and open heart surgery. J Vasc Surg. 2011;53(5):1237–41.
50. Giannopoulos S, et al. Synchronous carotid endarterectomy and coronary artery bypass graft versus staged carotid artery stenting and coronary artery bypass graft for patients with concomitant severe coronary and carotid stenosis: a systematic review and meta-analysis. Ann Vasc Surg. 2020;62:463–473.e4.
51. Nardi P, et al. Early-staged carotid artery stenting prior to coronary artery bypass grafting: analysis of the early and mid-term results in comparison with a consecutive cohort of isolated coronary artery surgery patients. J Clin Med. 2024;13(2):480.
52. Vyas Y, et al. Evaluating the safety of transcarotid artery revascularization under local anesthesia prior to coronary artery bypass grafting surgery. Ann Vasc Surg. 2023;91:176–81.
53. Hejčl A, et al. Selective internal carotid artery cross-clamping increases the specificity of cerebral oximetry for indication of shunting during carotid endarterectomy. Acta Neurochir. 2021;163(6):1807–17.
54. Pribán V, et al. Simultaneous carotid endarterectomy and coronary revascularization: indications and results. Rozhl Chir. 2011;90(1):67–72.
55. AbuRahma AF, et al. Society for Vascular Surgery clinical practice guidelines for management of extracranial cerebrovascular disease. J Vasc Surg. 2022;75(1s):4s–22s.
56. Ashrafi M, et al. Carotid endarterectomy for critical stenosis prior to cardiac surgery: should it be done? A retrospective cohort study. Int J Surg. 2016;26:53–7.

Management of Carotid Restenosis

Aleš Hejčl, Filip Cihlář, and Martin Sameš

1 Introduction

Carotid artery restenosis may occur after ipsilateral carotid endarterectomy (CEA) or carotid stenting (CAS). While many studies established the role of both CEA and CAS for carotid stenosis, less is known about restenosis and its management after either of these methods [1, 2]. Restenosis after CAS and CEA has been reported in a range of 5%–36% [3–6] and is dependent on the definition of restenosis and duration of follow-up. There is no clear consensual definition of carotid restenosis and various studies propose values ranging from 50% to 70% of carotid lumen stenosis [3, 7]. Most studies define moderate restenosis as a lumen reduction of at least 50% and severe restenosis a lumen reduction by 70% [8]. Optimal management of carotid restenosis still needs to be established as literature concerning these cases is much scarcer, compared to the treatment of primary carotid stenosis. It is unclear whether conservative therapy, CAS or a repeat CEA (redoCEA) is the best treatment strategy for carotid artery restenosis given the absence of randomized controlled trials (RCTs) or guidelines on this topic.

A. Hejčl (✉)
Department of Neurosurgery, Masaryk Hospital, J. E. Purkyně University, Ústí nad Labem, Czech Republic

International Clinical Research Center, St. Anne's Hospital, Brno, Czech Republic

F. Cihlář
Department of Radiology, Masaryk Hospital, J. E. Purkyně University, Ústí nad Labem, Czech Republic
e-mail: filip.cihlar@kzcr.eu

M. Sameš
Department of Neurosurgery, Masaryk Hospital, J. E. Purkyně University, Ústí nad Labem, Czech Republic
e-mail: martin.sames@kzcr.eu

2 Pathophysiological Background

The incidence of carotid restenosis after CEA ranges from 6% to 16% [6, 7, 9, 10]. Restenosis after CEA was reported in up to 20% of patients in early papers [11], but subsequent studies reported lower values (2.6%–10% at 5 years) [12–14].

Carotid restenosis has several etiologies, which differ in pathophysiology and the time frame within which restenosis develops. Early restenosis (within the first 24 months) is mostly attributed to neo-intimal hyperplasia, while late restenosis (occurring more than 2 years after carotid intervention) is thought to originate from recurrent or ongoing carotid atherosclerosis [15]. If restenosis is diagnosed within the first month of carotid intervention, it is attributed to residual atherosclerosis.

The pathophysiology of carotid restenosis is still not fully understood [16]. Neo-intimal hyperplasia most likely results from vessel trauma causing endothelial dysfunction and chronic inflammation. The clinical impact of neointimal hyperplasia is uncertain, but it is thought to have reduced potential for embolization compared to native lesions. On the other hand, late carotid restenosis is mainly attributed to recurrence or progression of carotid atherosclerotic disease and the pathophysiology does not significantly differ from primary atherosclerotic lesions.

Several risk factors have been associated with the development of carotid restenosis [5, 6, 17–19]. These may be classified into different subtypes. Age over 65 years, female sex and family history of stroke are three non-modifiable risk factors [8, 17]. Medical conditions associated with carotid restenosis are non-insulin dependent diabetes, high cholesterol, hypertension and history of angina [8]. Smoking predicts an increased rate of restenosis after carotid endarterectomy but not after CAS [7]. Vascular risk factors include contralateral stenosis and the presence of a calcified plaque [8, 18]. Also, patients operated for asymptomatic carotid plaque (stable plaque) have an increased risk of carotid restenosis [19]. Further studies showed that possibly high pre-operative values of inflammatory biomarkers within

V. Beneš, D. Netuka (eds.), *Surgical and Interventional Treatment of Cerebral Ischemia*,
https://doi.org/10.1007/978-3-032-08934-2_16

the carotid plaque are strong independent factors predicting the risk of 12-month restenosis [20]. It is generally accepted that asymptomatic lesions have a more stable plaque composition, characterized by less inflammation and lower lipid content.

2.1 Pathophysiology of In-Stent Restenosis

Stents implanted within a carotid plaque will induce permanent alterations of flow physiology [21]. The enhanced stiffness of the stented segment, positive arterial remodeling caused by stent expansion, changes in the wall shear stress or mismatch between the native and stented segment leads to endothelial dysfunction resulting in intimal hyperplasia and development of restenosis [22–26]. Another mechanism leading to the development of restenosis results from underexpansion of the implanted stent due to external compression [27]. This is typical in cases of significant plaque calcifications.

3 Diagnostic Imaging and Criteria

The primary and probably the most commonly used diagnostic technique to follow patients after CEA or CAS is duplex ultrasound, DUS. The advantages of DUS for patient follow-up is its non-invasive nature, no risk of complications, availability in vascular laboratories with fast examination of the lesion. Because of its extended and long-time use in primary carotid stenosis evaluation, specific velocity criteria used to determine the level of stenosis have been established long time ago [28].

On the other hand, precise evaluation of carotid in-stent restenosis is more complicated. Stent implantation alters the biomechanical properties of the carotid wall by reducing its compliance [29]. The stent-arterial wall complex is more stiff compared to the natural arterial wall, which results in increased velocities. Furthermore, more emphasis is placed on B-mode imaging for both situations, post CAS and post CEA.

According to the Society for Vascular Surgery recommendations, an assessment should be made of stent apposition to the surrounding plaque, expansion of the lumen, and luminal encroachment due to neointimal hyperplasia [30]. The morphology of any hyperplastic lesion can be mapped based on this classification. Velocity waveforms and luminal diameter measurements should be obtained at multiple locations.

CT angiography and MR angiography are alternative methods usually used to confirm restenosis mostly when considering a possible re-intervention [30]. They are not used for regular follow-up due to the risks associated with radiation during CT angiography, nephrotoxic contrast agents, and expensive nature. However, they are useful for assessing the anatomy of the carotid plaque, the proximal common carotid artery as well as the aortic arch. Further they allow assessment of distances between the plaque related to the CCA bifurcation and the skull base when considering a surgical approach.

Cervical contrast angiography is in general only used in the event of a therapeutic intervention and less commonly for diagnostic purposes.

3.1 Diagnosis of In-Stent Restenosis

Multiple imaging methods can be performed to diagnose carotid ISR, including carotid duplex ultrasound, CTA, MRA, and digital subtraction angiography. Most institutions initially perform duplex ultrasound as it is noninvasive, does not require contrast agents or radiation exposure, and has relatively high sensitivity and specificity compared to digital subtraction angiography or CTA [1]. The accuracy of carotid ultrasound has not been well established in predicting in-stent restenosis (ISR) after carotid artery stenting (CAS) [31].

Setacci et al. [26] performed a 6 year prospective study, which aimed to determine the accuracy of predicting in-stent restenosis after carotid artery stenting using ultrasound. They compared ultrasound velocity criteria to the percentage of stenosis at angiography. The study found strong correlations between angiographic measurements and ultrasound velocity criteria, with high sensitivity and specificity for the identified thresholds. The peak systolic velocity (PSV) for carotid restenosis of 50%–70% was set at 175–299 cm/s, while severe restenosis >70%, correlated with the PSV higher than 300 cm/s.

4 Risk of Stroke Associated with Carotid Restenosis

There is only scarce data on the occurrence of stroke in patients with carotid restenosis. The most robust study is most likely derived from secondary analysis of the ISASS (International Carotid Stenting Study) [8]. The level or restenosis was defined as either moderate (≥50%) or severe (≥70%). It this study, authors found that patients with at least moderate restenosis after either CEA or CAS had a higher risk of ipsilateral stroke, with a cumulative risk at 6 years of 6.9% versus 2.5% for patients without restenosis. The 6-year cumulative risk of stroke in any territory was also increased to 9.6% in patients with moderate or higher restenosis after either CEA or CAS versus 5.6% in patients without restenosis.

Furthermore, in this study the risk of stroke was analyzed based on treatment modality. Patients in the post-endarterectomy group with moderate or higher (≥50%) restenosis had a 6-year cumulative risk of ipsilateral stroke of 5.8% compared to 1.3% in patients without restenosis. Furthermore, patients with at least moderate (≥50%) restenosis had a 6.5% 6-year risk of any stroke compared to a 3.4% in patients without restenosis. Both complications reached statistical significance. No significant increase in risk of ipsilateral stroke was noted in the stenting group, with 6-year cumulative risk of 7.8% in patients with at least moderate (≥50%) restenosis versus 3.8% in those without restenosis. Furthermore, the risk of any stroke was 12.0% in patients with moderate or higher (≥50%) restenosis versus 8.1% in patients after CAS without restenosis.

5 Treatment of Patients with Carotid Restenosis After Previous CEA

As stated above, patients with carotid restenosis have an increased risk of stroke compared to patients without restenosis [8]. This necessitates specific management of individuals with restenosis after CEA. On the other hand, we need to balance the relatively low overall risk of stroke in these patients (approximately 6% in 6 years) with the risk of interventions. Therefore, regular follow up with management of risk factors is a common strategy. This includes antiplatelet therapy and management of risk factors (treatment of hypertension, hypercholesterolemia, diabetes management, quitting smoking, etc.).

The ambiguity surrounding indications for intervention in the real world was demonstrated in a systematic review on 50 studies reporting post-CEA or CAS restenosis [32]. The recent guidelines of the European Society for Vascular Surgery state that in patients experiencing ipsilateral stroke or transient ischemic attack in the presence of an ipsilateral 50%–99% re-stenosis, re-do carotid endarterectomy or carotid artery stenting is recommended [2] (Fig. 1a, b).

In 2018 a meta-analysis was published which combined information from 13 observational studies comparing patients either treated with redoCEA or CAS [33]. When comparing the risk of stroke between both modalities, 2.3% of patients after redoCEA and 1.7% after CAS suffered strokes. In terms of TIA, 2.1% of patients after redoCEA group and 3.8% in the CAS group suffered TIA. There was no statistically significant difference between these two groups for TIA or stroke. Also, 1.2% of patients in the redoCEA group and 0.9% in the CAS group suffered MI. When considering mortality, 1% of patients in the redoCEA group and 0.5% in the CAS group died. There were no statistically significant differences between any of these indicators. The difference between redoCEA and CAS was in the risk of postoperative cranial nerve (CN) injuries. Patients after redoCEA had a significantly higher risk of CN injuries (6%). However, most of the injures were reversible within 6 months leaving only 1.3% of patients with permanent CN injuries, which was not a statistically significant compared to CAS. Nonetheless, despite reports on similar outcomes after both redoCEA and CAS in patient with carotid restenosis, the advancement of endovascular techniques resulted in an increased number of patients with carotid restenosis treated via carotid stenting.

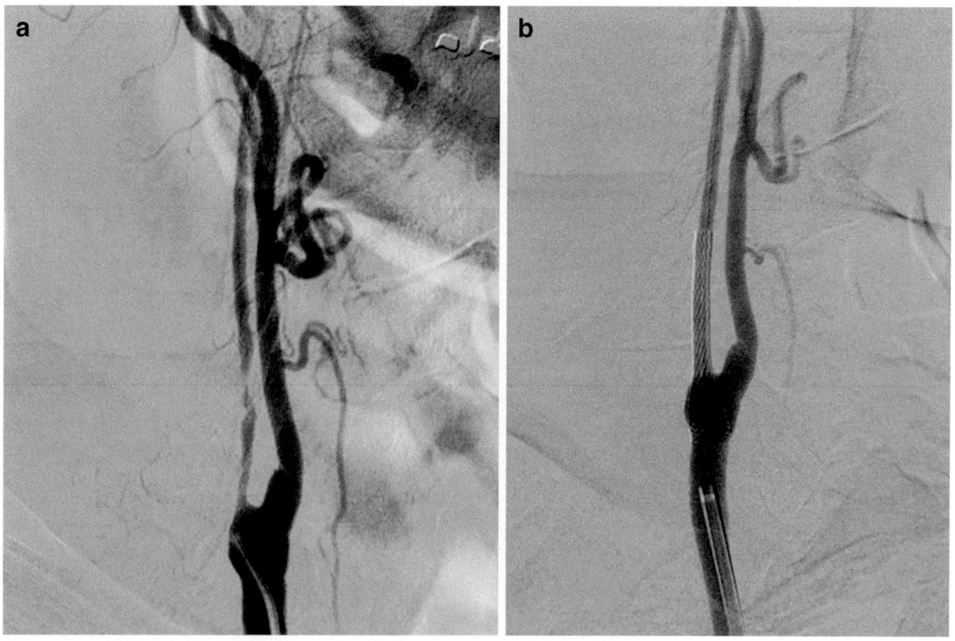

Fig. 1 (**a**) Symptomatic restenosis after primary CEA. Treated with intravenous thrombolysis after at the acute stage. (**b**) Later the carotid restenosis was treated with a stent (Carotid Wallstent) after saturating the patient with double antiplatelet therapy

5.1 Patients with Asymptomatic Re-stenosis

The management of patients with asymptomatic re-stenosis is even more controversial. There are currently no RCTs to guide the clinical practice. Despite the fact that carotid restenosis is generally considered to be a benign lesion a large study showed that over 40% of patients treated for carotid restenosis are asymptomatic [32]. The same study also demonstrated that patients were generally treated when the degree of restenosis exceeded 80%, However, the latest ESVS guidelines recommend that in cases of asymptomatic re-stenosis >70%, re-intervention should be considered following a multidisciplinary team review. The decision-making process should include factors such as age, medical conditions, morphology of the plaque, possibilities for further intensification of medical therapy, etc.

6 Treatment of Patients with In-Stent Restenosis

Since its development, endovascular treatment of carotid atherosclerotic plaques has been associated with in-stent restenosis. There remains a large debate on the optimal treatment algorithm, which stems from the lack of data from large, randomized trials, that would help create generally accepted treatment protocols [1].

The indication for re-interventional therapy is still a matter of debate. In symptomatic patients despite best medical therapy, ISR > 50% has been considered a reasonable cut off value for re-intervention [2]. For asymptomatic patients, the decision is more complicated. Most studies consider re-intervention in patients with restenosis of at least 80% despite best medical treatment [32].

Nonetheless, we need to bear in mind the low rate of late ipsilateral stroke of 0.8% over 50 months in patients with untreated asymptomatic >70% CAS ISR, as demonstrated in a systematic review and meta-analysis [7]. In addition, the use of a percutaneous intervention for CAS ISR does not appear to improve outcomes compared with nonoperative management [34]. Also, patients with CAS ISR have more comorbidities compared to a patients indicated for primary stenting of de novo carotid atherosclerotic lesions [35]. On the other hand, the re-stent procedure seems to be associated with lower event rates compared to CAS for primary atherosclerotic lesions.

Certainly, identifying and treating the modifiable risk factors is the first step in patients with carotid restenosis [16]. Medical management with antiplatelet agents, high-intensity statin therapy, blood pressure control and tobacco cessation represent the first line of treatment.

The technical possibilities for treating patients with ISR include PTA using different types of balloons (cutting balloons, drug-eluting balloons) (Fig. 2a, b), repeated CAS (rCAS) or CEA with stent removal. Twenty years ago, CEA was the second most common procedure, but its use declined due to increased use of endovascular techniques. Other alternative methods to endovascular techniques include carotid artery bypass or external beam radiotherapy. A systematic review showed that the rates of TIA and stroke are similar for all 3 major treatment modalitites (rCAS, PTA and CEA) during the periprocedural period [1]. CEA was associated with a slightly higher risk of mortality compared to rCAS. Importantly, PTA was associated with a significantly higher risk of recurrent restenosis and long-term risk of TIA and stroke compared to rCAS and significantly higher risk of restenosis compared to both alternative methods, rCAS and CEA. In view of the results above, rCAS is today the most common treatment modality for patients with in-stent restenosis.

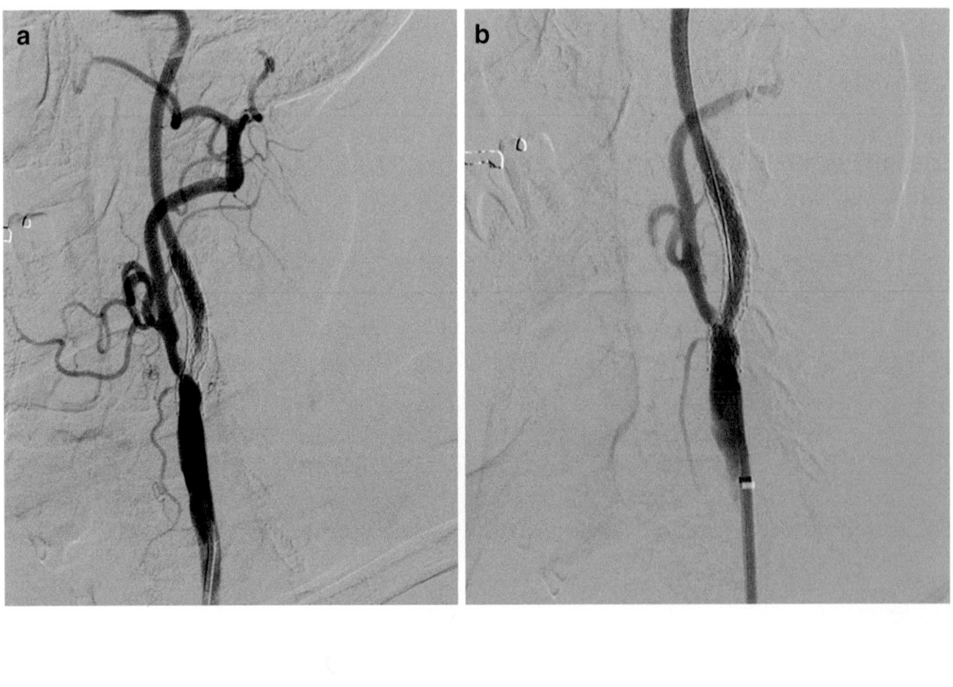

Fig. 2 (a) In-stent restenosis. (b) The in-stent restenosis was treated with a drug-eluting balloon

7 Future Research and Development

Carotid restenosis is not uncommon after previous CEA or CAS, however RCTs on this topic are scarce. Well-designed RCTs that would provide information on the risk of stroke associated with carotid restenosis as well as morbidity and mortality associated with treating carotid restenosis are needed. Balancing the risks of natural progression and various kinds of treatments, which would stem from these RCTs may then guide the development of clinical protocols for patients with carotid restenosis. This would also influence recommendations regarding the follow up protocols after CEA or CAS.

Declarations

Competing Interests The author(s) has no competing interests to declare that are relevant to the content of this manuscript.

Ethics Approval The author(s) declares that this manuscript does not include primary research with human participants.

References

1. Huang H, Wu L, Guo Y, Zhang Y, Zhao J, Yu Z, et al. Treatment of the carotid in-stent restenosis: a systematic review. Front Neurol. 2021;12:748304.
2. Naylor R, Rantner B, Ancetti S, de Borst GJ, De Carlo M, Halliday A, et al. Editor's choice—European Society for Vascular Surgery (ESVS) 2023 clinical practice guidelines on the management of atherosclerotic carotid and vertebral artery disease. Eur J Vasc Endovasc Surg. 2023;65(1):7–111.
3. Vos JA, de Borst GJ, Overtoom TT, de Vries JP, van de Pavoordt ED, Zanen P, et al. Carotid angioplasty and stenting: treatment of postcarotid endarterectomy restenosis is at least as safe as primary stenosis treatment. J Vasc Surg. 2009;50(4):755–61 e1.
4. Lal BK, Hobson RW 2nd, Goldstein J, Geohagan M, Chakhtoura E, Pappas PJ, et al. In-stent recurrent stenosis after carotid artery stenting: life table analysis and clinical relevance. J Vasc Surg. 2003;38(6):1162–8; discussion 9.
5. Bonati LH, Ederle J, McCabe DJ, Dobson J, Featherstone RL, Gaines PA, et al. Long-term risk of carotid restenosis in patients randomly assigned to endovascular treatment or endarterectomy in the Carotid and Vertebral Artery Transluminal Angioplasty Study (CAVATAS): long-term follow-up of a randomised trial. Lancet Neurol. 2009;8(10):908–17.
6. Lattimer CR, Burnand KG. Recurrent carotid stenosis after carotid endarterectomy. Br J Surg. 1997;84(9):1206–19.
7. Lal BK, Beach KW, Roubin GS, Lutsep HL, Moore WS, Malas MB, et al. Restenosis after carotid artery stenting and endarterectomy: a secondary analysis of CREST, a randomised controlled trial. Lancet Neurol. 2012;11(9):755–63.
8. Bonati LH, Gregson J, Dobson J, McCabe DJH, Nederkoorn PJ, van der Worp HB, et al. Restenosis and risk of stroke after stenting or endarterectomy for symptomatic carotid stenosis in the International Carotid Stenting Study (ICSS): secondary analysis of a randomised trial. Lancet Neurol. 2018;17(7):587–96.
9. Mantese VA, Timaran CH, Chiu D, Begg RJ, Brott TG, Investigators C. The carotid revascularization endarterectomy versus stenting trial (CREST): stenting versus carotid endarterectomy for carotid disease. Stroke. 2010;41(10 Suppl):S31–4.
10. Keagy BA, Edrington RD, Poole MA, Johnson G. Incidence of recurrent or residual stenosis after carotid endarterectomy. Am J Surg. 1985;149(6):722–5.
11. Zierler RE, Bandyk DF, Thiele BL, Strandness DE Jr. Carotid artery stenosis following endarterectomy. Arch Surg. 1982;117(11):1408–15.
12. LaMuraglia GM, Stoner MC, Brewster DC, Watkins MT, Juhola KL, Kwolek C, et al. Determinants of carotid endarterectomy anatomic durability: effects of serum lipids and lipid-lowering drugs. J Vasc Surg. 2005;41(5):762–8.
13. Goodney PP, Nolan BW, Eldrup-Jorgensen J, Likosky DS, Cronenwett JL, Vascular Study Group of Northern New England. Restenosis after carotid endarterectomy in a multicenter regional registry. J Vasc Surg. 2010;52(4):897–904, 5 e1–2; discussion 5.
14. Dorigo W, Pulli R, Fargion A, Pratesi G, Angiletta D, Aletto I, et al. Comparison of open and endovascular treatments of post-carotid endarterectomy restenosis. Eur J Vasc Endovasc Surg. 2013;45(5):437–42.
15. Fericks H, Kievit J, van Baalen JM, van Bockel JH. Carotid recurrent stenosis and risk of ipsilateral stroke: a systematic review of the literature. Stroke. 1998;29(1):244–50.
16. Stilo F, Montelione N, Calandrelli R, Distefano M, Spinelli F, Di Lazzaro V, et al. The management of carotid restenosis: a comprehensive review. Ann Transl Med. 2020;8(19):1272.
17. Ladowski JS, Shinabery LM, Peterson D, Peterson AC, Deschner WP. Factors contributing to recurrent carotid disease following carotid endarterectomy. Am J Surg. 1997;174(2):118–20.
18. Moon K, Albuquerque FC, Levitt MR, Ahmed AS, Kalani MY, McDougall CG. The myth of restenosis after carotid angioplasty and stenting. J Neurointerv Surg. 2016;8(10):1006–10.
19. van Lammeren GW, Peeters W, de Vries JP, de Kleijn DP, De Borst GJ, Pasterkamp G, et al. Restenosis after carotid surgery: the importance of clinical presentation and preoperative timing. Stroke. 2011;42(4):965–71.
20. Niculescu R, Russu E, Arbanasi EM, Kaller R, Arbanasi EM, Melinte RM, et al. Carotid plaque features and inflammatory biomarkers as predictors of restenosis and mortality following carotid endarterectomy. Int J Environ Res Public Health. 2022;19(21):13934.
21. Kokkalis E, Aristokleous N, Houston JG. Haemodynamics and flow modification stents for peripheral arterial disease: a review. Ann Biomed Eng. 2016;44(2):466–76.
22. Lal BK, Hobson RW 2nd, Goldstein J, Chakhtoura EY, Duran WN. Carotid artery stenting: is there a need to revise ultrasound velocity criteria? J Vasc Surg. 2004;39(1):58–66.
23. Vernhet H, Jean B, Lust S, Laroche JP, Bonafe A, Senac JP, et al. Wall mechanics of the stented extracranial carotid artery. Stroke. 2003;34(11):e222–4.
24. Willfort-Ehringer A, Ahmadi R, Gruber D, Gschwandtner ME, Haumer A, Haumer M, et al. Arterial remodeling and hemodynamics in carotid stents: a prospective duplex ultrasound study over 2 years. J Vasc Surg. 2004;39(4):728–34.
25. Willfort-Ehringer A, Ahmadi R, Gschwandtner ME, Haumer A, Heinz G, Lang W, et al. Healing of carotid stents: a prospective duplex ultrasound study. J Endovasc Ther. 2003;10(3):636–42.
26. Setacci C, Chisci E, Setacci F, Iacoponi F, de Donato G. Grading carotid intrastent restenosis: a 6-year follow-up study. Stroke. 2008;39(4):1189–96.

27. Nicoud F, Vernhet H, Dauzat M. A numerical assessment of wall shear stress changes after endovascular stenting. J Biomech. 2005;38(10):2019–27.
28. Faught WE, Mattos MA, van Bemmelen PS, Hodgson KJ, Barkmeier LD, Ramsey DE, et al. Color-flow duplex scanning of carotid arteries: new velocity criteria based on receiver operator characteristic analysis for threshold stenoses used in the symptomatic and asymptomatic carotid trials. J Vasc Surg. 1994;19(5):818–27; discussion 27–8.
29. Timmins LH, Meyer CA, Moreno MR, Moore JE. Effects of stent design and atherosclerotic plaque composition on arterial wall biomechanics. J Endovasc Ther. 2008;15(6):643–54.
30. Zierler RE, Jordan WD, Lal BK, Mussa F, Leers S, Fulton J, et al. The Society for Vascular Surgery practice guidelines on follow-up after vascular surgery arterial procedures. J Vasc Surg. 2018;68(1):256–84.
31. Zhou W, Felkai DD, Evans M, McCoy SA, Lin PH, Kougias P, et al. Ultrasound criteria for severe in-stent restenosis following carotid artery stenting. J Vasc Surg. 2008;47(1):74–80.
32. Bekelis K, Moses Z, Missios S, Desai A, Labropoulos N. Indications for treatment of recurrent carotid stenosis. Br J Surg. 2013;100(4):440–7.
33. Texakalidis P, Giannopoulos S, Jonnalagadda AK, Kokkinidis DG, Machinis T, Reavey-Cantwell J, et al. Carotid artery endarterectomy versus carotid artery stenting for restenosis after carotid artery endarterectomy: a systematic review and meta-analysis. World Neurosurg. 2018;115:421–9 e1.
34. Chung J, Valentine W, Sharath SE, Pathak A, Barshes NR, Pisimisis G, et al. Percutaneous intervention for carotid in-stent restenosis does not improve outcomes compared with nonoperative management. J Vasc Surg. 2016;64(5):1286–94 e1.
35. Zahn R, Ischinger T, Zeymer U, Brachmann J, Jung J, Haase H, et al. Carotid artery interventions for restenosis after prior stenting: is it different from interventions of de novo lesions? Results from the carotid artery stent (CAS)—registry of the Arbeitsgemeinschaft Leitende Kardiologische Krankenhausarzte (ALKK). Clin Res Cardiol. 2010;99(12):809–15.

Other Surgeries at the Carotid Bifurcation Region

Vladimír Beneš, Adéla Bubeníková, David Netuka, and Tomáš Hrbáč

1 Introduction

Carotid endarterectomy (CEA) is widely regarded as the cornerstone of surgical management for carotid artery disease at the bifurcation [1]. However, other surgical interventions, though infrequent and highly specific, remain within the surgeon's repertoire for treating various carotid pathologies. Although these surgeries are less commonly performed, they remain essential components of a vascular surgeon's repertoire when managing complex cases of carotid disease. This chapter aims to provide a concise overview of these alternative surgical techniques, their indications, and their role in contemporary vascular surgery.

2 Carotid Sympathectomy

Carotid sympathectomy was historically performed with the aim of improving cerebral blood flow by severing the sympathetic nerve fibers running along the carotid bifurcation [2]. This procedure involved surgical exposure of the carotid bifurcation, followed by removal of the carotid sheath. At the time, it was hypothesized that interruption of sympathetic innervation could enhance cerebral perfusion.

However, advances in vascular physiology and a deeper understanding of cerebrovascular circulation have rendered carotid sympathectomy obsolete. Subsequent studies demonstrated that the procedure did not confer significant benefits, and safer, more effective alternatives have supplanted it [3, 4]. As such, carotid sympathectomy is no longer performed in modern surgical practice.

3 Carotid Resection

Carotid resection was another procedure employed in the past, primarily for patients with carotid occlusion. This surgery involved the excision of the internal carotid artery (ICA) at the bifurcation, often between ligatures, in the belief that it could improve collateral circulation or prevent thromboembolic events [5].

However, like sympathectomy, carotid resection has been discontinued due to a lack of evidence supporting its efficacy and its associated risks. Modern approaches to carotid occlusion have focused on more targeted and physiologically beneficial interventions, relegating carotid resection to historical relevance [5].

4 Carotid Stumpectomy

Carotid stumpectomy is an uncommon procedure indicated for patients with carotid occlusion who have a residual stump that serves as a source of emboli [6]. Emboli originating from this stump can travel via the external carotid artery (ECA), leading to transient ischemic attacks (TIAs) or retinal ischemia.

This procedure is considered when conservative medical management fails to prevent repeated ocular TIAs. During the surgery, the carotid bifurcation is exposed using standard surgical techniques. An arteriotomy is created, extending from the common carotid artery (CCA) to the ECA. Endarterectomy is then performed on both the CCA and ECA. The residual ICA stump is securely closed using a

V. Beneš (✉) · D. Netuka
Department of Neurosurgery and Neurooncology, First Medical Faculty, Charles University, Prague, Czech Republic
e-mail: beneseva@volny.cz

A. Bubeníková
Department of Neurosurgery, Second Faculty of Medicine, Charles University and Motol University Hospital, Prague, Czech Republic

T. Hrbáč
Department of Neurosurgery, University Hospital Ostrava, Ostrava, Czech Republic

Department of Anatomy, Faculty of Medicine, University of Ostrava, Ostrava, Czech Republic

V. Beneš, D. Netuka (eds.), *Surgical and Interventional Treatment of Cerebral Ischemia*,
https://doi.org/10.1007/978-3-032-08934-2_17

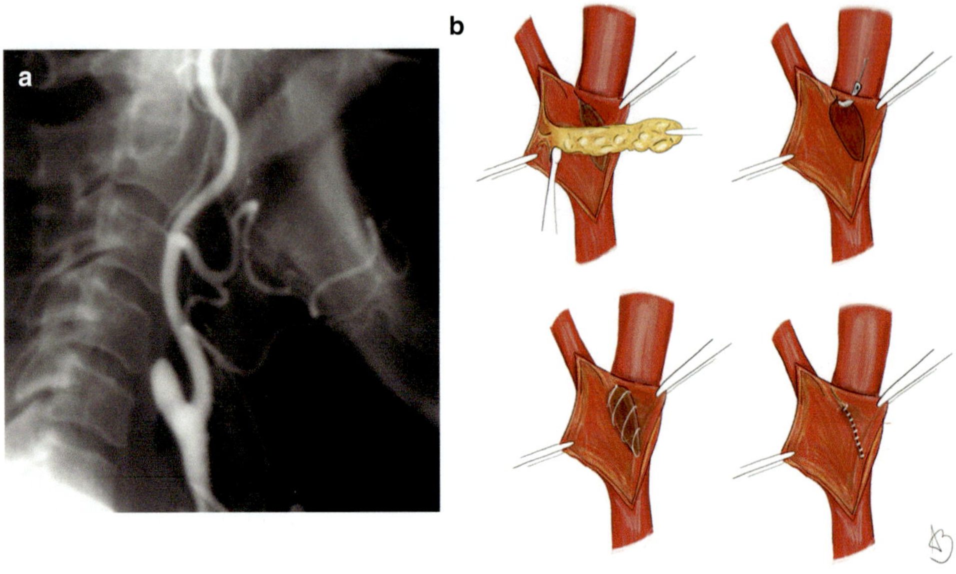

Fig. 1 (**a**) Illustrative example of the carotid stump. (**b**) Procedure description highlighting the application of the suture from the external surface inward

running suture applied from the external surface inward. Finally, the arteriotomy is closed in the usual manner (Fig. 1).

In certain rare cases, an ECA endarterectomy performed during a stumpectomy may serve as a preparatory step for an extracranial-to-intracranial (EC-IC) bypass procedure, which is indicated in patients with advanced cerebrovascular disease and insufficient collateral circulation [6].

5 Carotid Kinks and Coils

Carotid coils, which represent looped deviations in the ICA, are typically asymptomatic and do not generally require surgical intervention [7] (Fig. 2). When surgery is necessary, the coil is excised, and the ICA is reimplanted into the CCA to restore normal blood flow.

In contrast, carotid kinks are more likely to be symptomatic and can cause both hemodynamic compromise and embolic events [8] (Fig. 3). Hemodynamic symptoms occur because the kinked artery may temporarily occlude during neck movements, leading to transient ischemic attacks (TIAs). Furthermore, turbulent blood flow at the apex of the kink can promote the formation of emboli, potentially resulting in cerebrovascular events [8].

Surgical management of carotid kinks depends on the underlying pathology [9]. If the kink is associated with atherosclerotic stenosis, the procedure may involve endarterectomy combined with resection of the kinked segment (Fig. 4). The ICA is then reimplanted into the CCA. Alternatively, in cases without significant atherosclerotic involvement, straightening of the artery can be achieved by anchoring the carotid adventitia to surrounding muscles such as the omohyoid or sternocleidomastoid. This technique effectively relieves the kink and restores normal arterial flow dynamics.

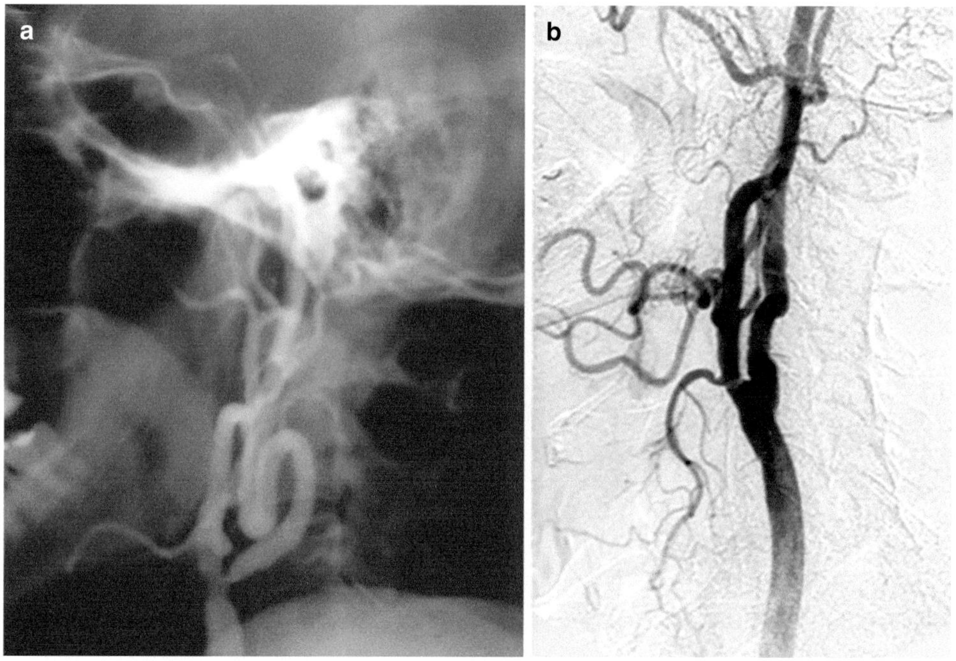

Fig. 2 (**a**) Carotid coil distal to the carotid stenosis. TIAs. (**b**) After the CEA coil resection and ICA reimplantation into the CCA

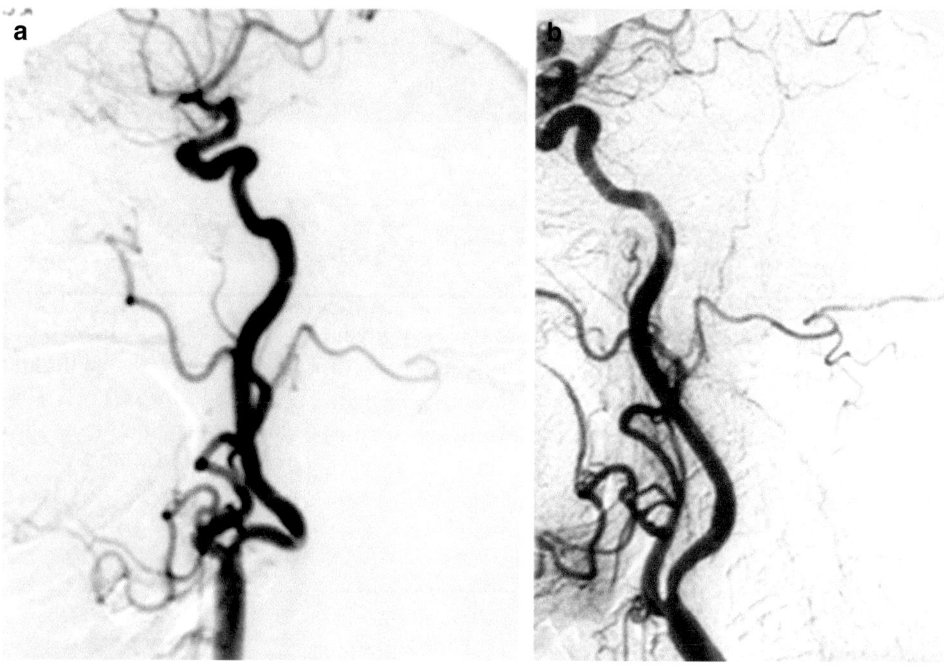

Fig. 3 Carotid kink before (**a**) and after surgery (**b**). The kink has only been straightened, no cross-clamping, no vessel opening

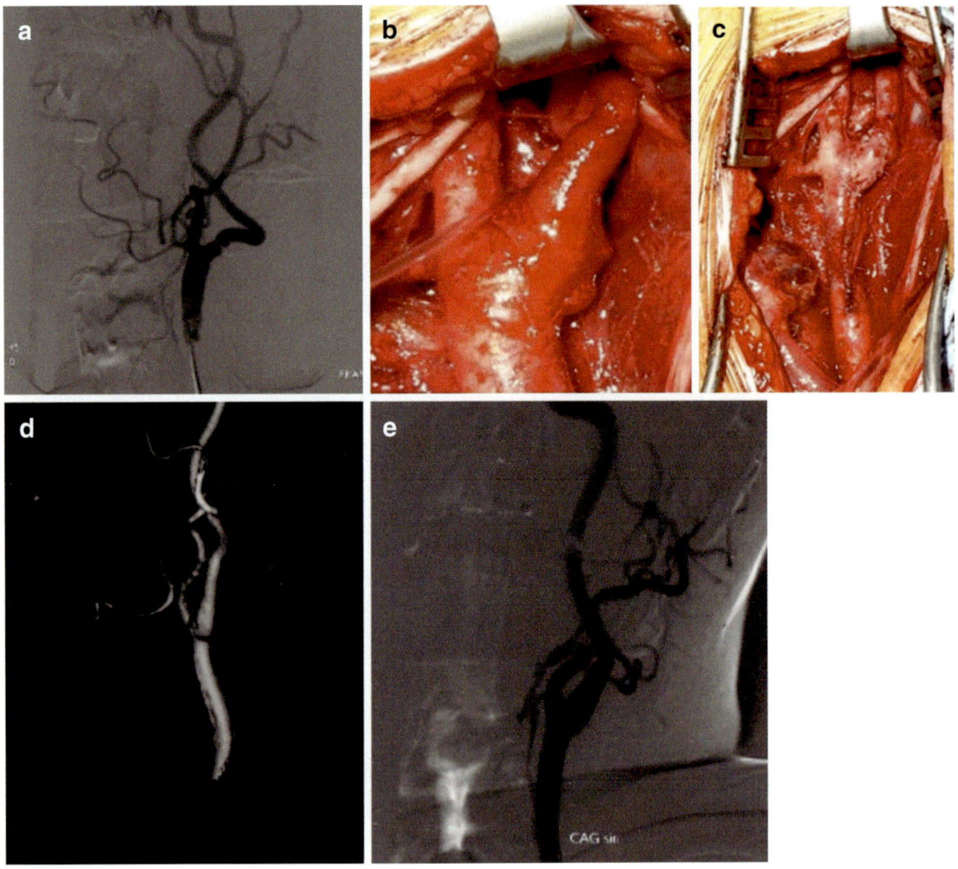

Fig. 4 Carotid kink and carotid stenosis. (**a**) Before surgery. (**b**) Exposed carotid bifurcation, the kink is apparent. (**c**) After the CEA, reimplantation of ICA and arterial closure using patch. (**d**) Postoperative MRA. (**e**) Postoperative angiography

6 Carotid Occlusion and Pseudoocclusion

Carotid occlusion and pseudoocclusion are typically urgent conditions that require immediate intervention [10]. However, in rare instances, elective surgery may be indicated. Elective interventions are considered only when retrograde blood flow in the ICA is detectable up to the level of the foramen lacerum, suggesting a possibility for recanalization.

Pseudoocclusion is best diagnosed using digital subtraction angiography (DSA), which provides superior clarity compared to CT angiography (CTA) or MR angiography (MRA) (Figs. 5, 6, and 7). During surgical intervention, the ICA is exposed, and thrombus removal is performed using a Fogarty catheter [11]. The procedure requires precise and gentle manipulation of the catheter to avoid damage to the fragile vessel walls.

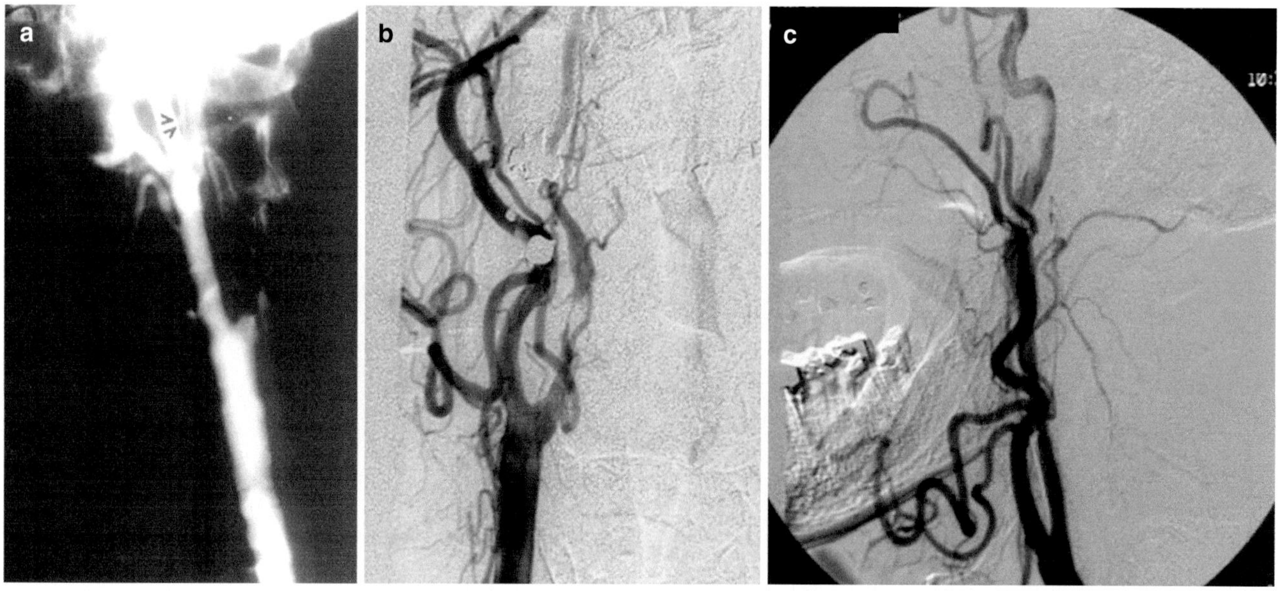

Fig. 5 Carotid pseudoocclusion before and after the stenting

Fig. 6 Carotid pseudoocclusion at the level of carotid bifurcation. After the CEA the thrombus filling the ICA was found and removed using Fogarty catheter. Unfortunatelly, the A-V fistula was caused by catheter manipulation and the vessel had to be occluded

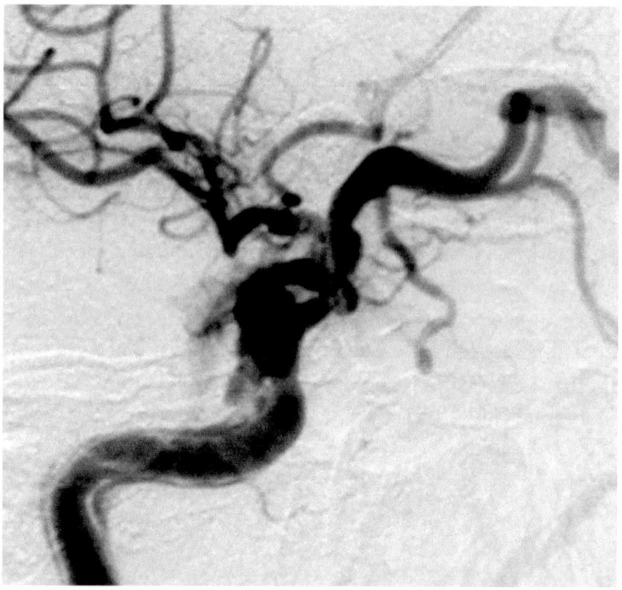

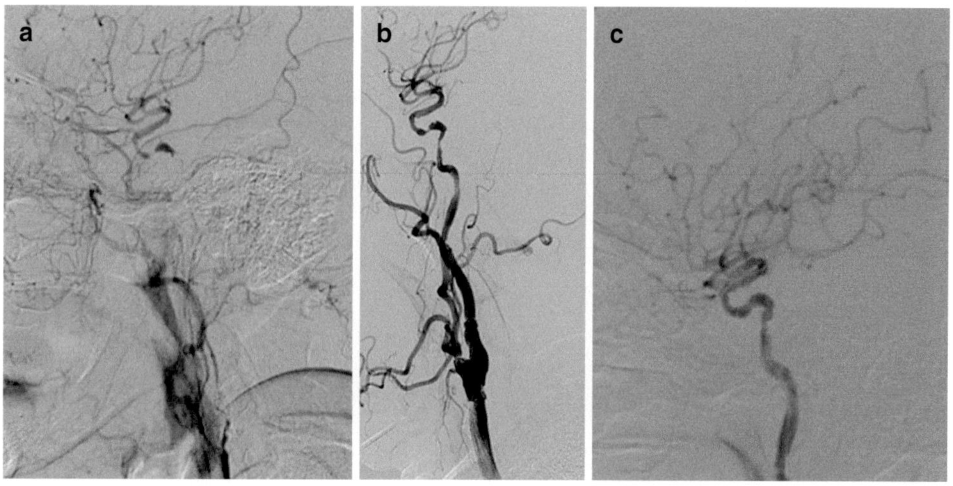

Fig. 7 (**a**) Carotid pseudoocclusion and tandem lesion. Some traces of contrast media are apparent. The tandem lesion has not been properly evaluated and CEA was performed. (**b**) After the CEA the tandem lesion is apparent. (**c**) Distal stenosis after the endovascular treatment. It is obvious the patient should have been treated primarily by endovascular means

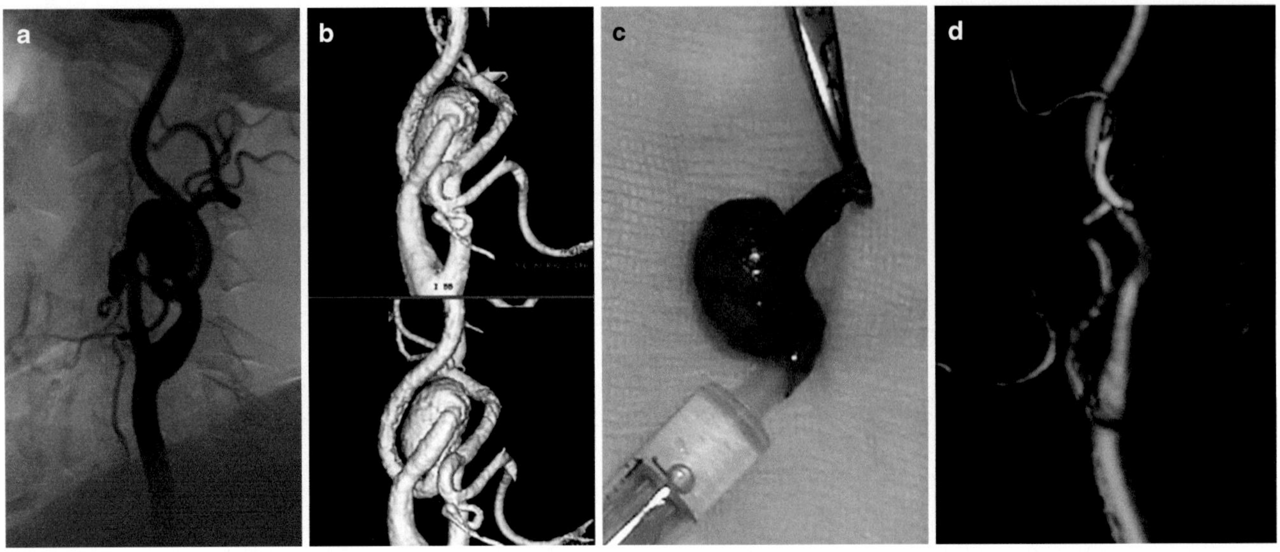

Fig. 8 Carotid aneurysm. (**a**) Angiography. (**b**) CT AG. (**c**) Surgical specimen. (**d**) Postoperative MR AG

7 Carotid Aneurysms

True aneurysms of the carotid artery are exceedingly rare and more commonly pose a risk of ischemic events than rupture [12]. Surgical treatment is preferred in these cases due to its ability to provide definitive resolution (Fig. 8).

The procedure involves exposing the aneurysm and the affected segment of the ICA. The aneurysmal section is excised, and the artery is reconstructed using an end-to-end anastomosis. This approach ensures long-term durability and reduces the risk of recurrence compared to endovascular techniques [13].

8 Carotid Dissections and Pseudoaneurysms

Carotid dissections and pseudoaneurysms are most often managed with endovascular techniques such as stenting or coil embolization (Figs. 9 and 10). Surgical options are limited, as the affected vessels are typically friable and difficult to repair [14].

Observation is appropriate in asymptomatic dissections, as the majority heal spontaneously with conservative management. Surgical resection of pseudoaneurysms is rarely successful due to the degenerative nature of the surrounding arterial tissue, making primary repair challenging [15].

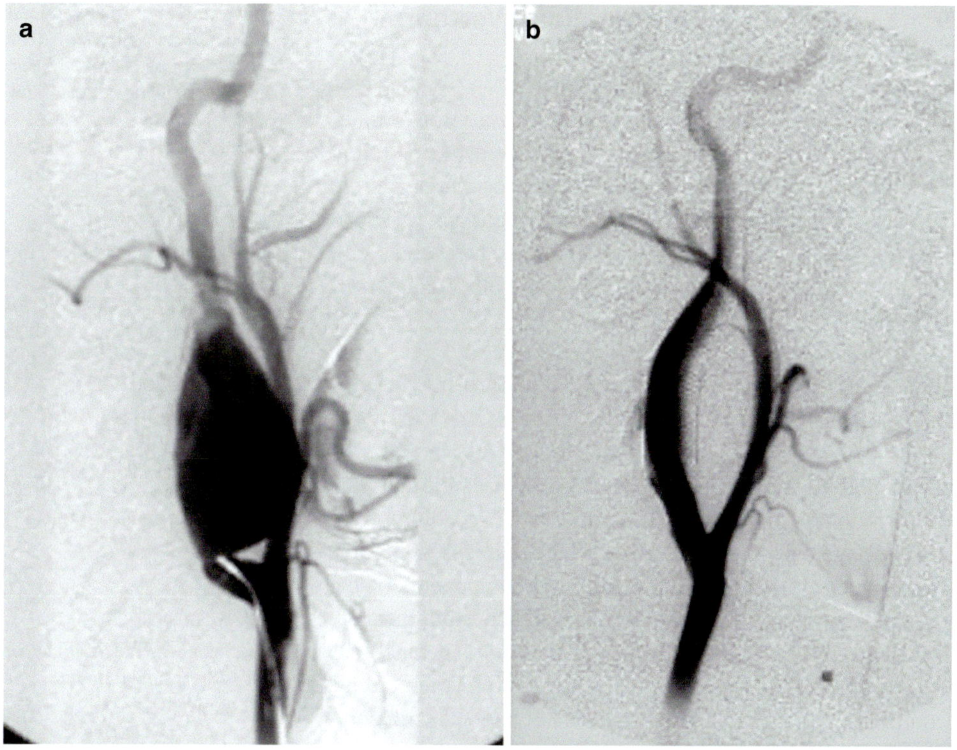

Fig. 9 Carotid pseudoaneurysm treated by stent

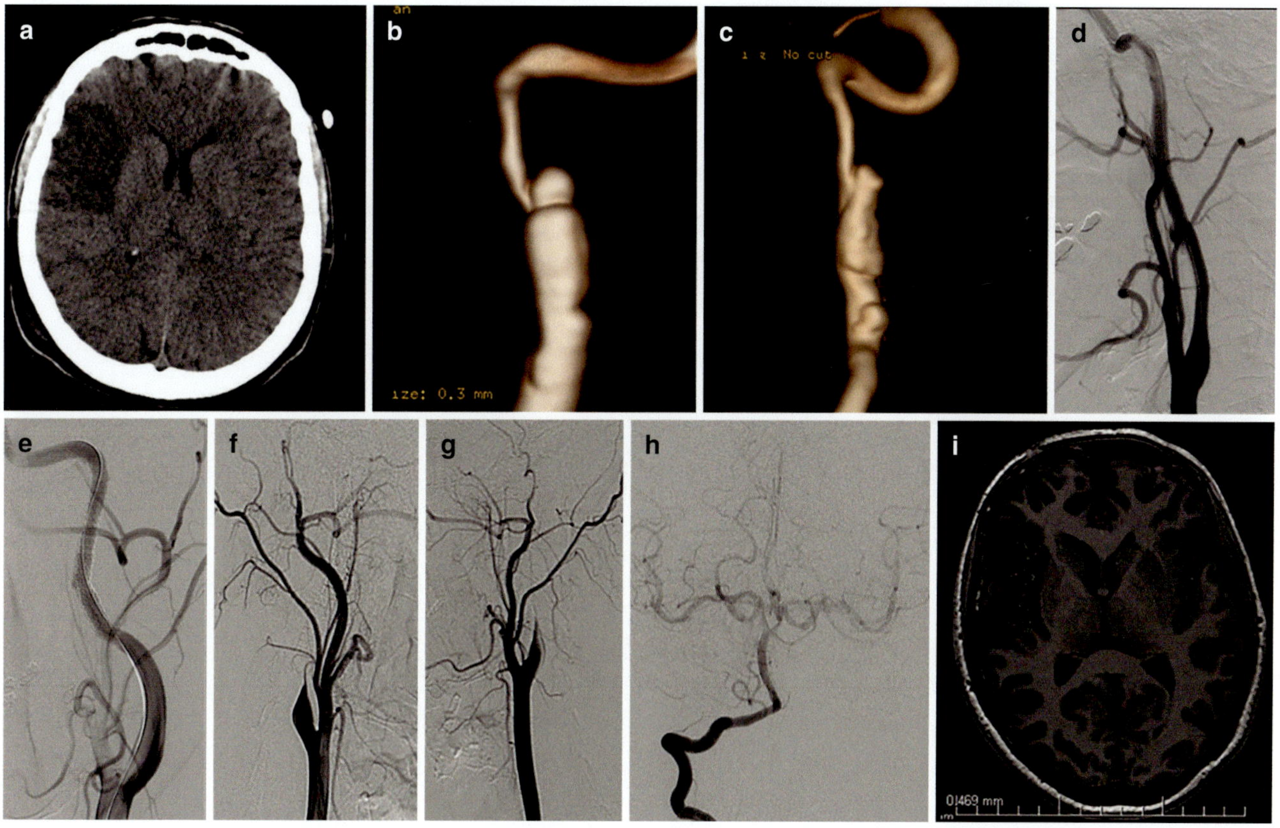

Fig. 10 Bilateral carotiod dissection after the neck trauma. 47-year-old female was admitted at the Neurology Department neurologically intact. Bilateral carotid dissection was treated endovascularly. Within a year, both carotid arteries got occluded. Collateral flow through vertebral arteries, while the patient remains asymptomatic. (**a**) Initial CT. (**b**) Right ICA dissection. (**c**) Left ICA dissection. (**d**) After the stenting on the right. (**e**) After the stenting on the left. (**f**) One year later, right side. (**g**) One year later, left side. (**h**) Collateral flow through the right vertebral artery. (**i**) Infarction in the right frontotemporal region

9 Additional Considerations: Vertebral Artery Pathologies

Vertebral artery kinks and conditions such as Bow-Hunter Syndrome may necessitate surgical management, including vertebral artery transposition [16]. These procedures are rare but essential for treating patients with rotational vertebrobasilar insufficiency when conservative measures fail. Details of these procedures are described in other chapters of this book.

10 Conclusion

Compared to the frequency of CAE, alternative surgical interventions at the carotid bifurcation are exceedingly rare and are typically reserved for specific clinical scenarios. Nevertheless, these procedures are vital components of the vascular surgeon's armamentarium. When appropriately indicated, they can be performed with risks and outcomes comparable to those of standard carotid endarterectomy, contributing to the comprehensive care of patients with complex carotid artery pathologies.

References

1. Sehgal VS, Ting W. The evolution of carotid surgery. Ann Vasc Surg. 2024;113:287–93.
2. Jennings DB, Szlyk PC. Carotid bifurcation sympathectomy and deafferentation: respiration during hypercapnia. Am J Phys. 1988;255(2 Pt 2):R252–8.
3. Eseoglu M, et al. The role of sympathectomy on the regulation of basilar artery volume changes in stenoocclusive carotid artery modeling after bilateral common carotid artery ligation: an animal model. Acta Neurochir. 2014;156(5):963–9.
4. Briasoulis A, Bakris G. The future of interventional management of hypertension: threats and opportunities. Curr Vasc Pharmacol. 2014;12(1):69–76.
5. Tallarita T, et al. History of carotid surgery: from ancient greeks to the modern era. Perspect Vasc Surg Endovasc Ther. 2013;25(3–4):57–64.
6. McCormick PW, et al. Thromboendarterectomy of the symptomatic occluded internal carotid artery. J Neurosurg. 1992;76(5):752–8.
7. Ovchinnikov NA, Rao RT, Rao SR. Unilateral congenital elongation of the cervical part of the internal carotid artery with kinking and looping: two case reports and review of the literature. Head Face Med. 2007;3:29.
8. Liu Y, et al. Association between internal carotid artery kinking and ischemic stroke: a population-based cross-sectional study. J Stroke Cerebrovasc Dis. 2023;32(12):107417.
9. van Alphen HA. Kinking of the carotid artery: indications for surgery and surgical procedure. Clin Neurol Neurosurg. 1977;80(2):92–9.
10. Kim HJ, et al. Stent implantation of multichanneled pseudo-occlusion of the internal carotid artery. J Vasc Interv Radiol. 2009;20(3):391–5.
11. Berman SS, et al. Critical carotid artery stenosis: diagnosis, timing of surgery, and outcome. J Vasc Surg. 1994;20(4):499–508. discussion 508–10
12. Pourier VE, De Borst GJ. Which carotid artery aneurysms need to be treated (and how)? J Cardiovasc Surg. 2016;57(2):152–7.
13. Davidovic L, et al. Carotid artery aneurysms. Vascular. 2004;12(3):166–70.
14. Wang GH, et al. Traumatic pseudoaneurysms of external carotid artery branch: case series and treatment considerations. Chin J Traumatol. 2021;24(6):368–73.
15. Deng D, et al. Clinical characteristics of internal carotid artery pseudoaneurysms in the sphenoid sinus. Am J Otolaryngol. 2019;40(1):106–9.
16. Xue S, et al. Bow Hunter's syndrome combined with ipsilateral vertebral artery dissection/pseudoaneurysm: case study and literature review. Br J Neurosurg. 2023;37(4):911–5.

Elective Endovascular Intracranial Procedures in Occlusive Diseases

Kota Kurisu, Toshiya Osanai, Yusuke Shimoda, and Miki Fujimura

1 Introduction

Intracranial artery stenosis (ICAS), characterized by atherosclerotic narrowing of major intracranial arteries, is a one of the significant pathological conditions that can cause ischemic stroke [1, 2]. Intracranial artery stenosis commonly affects the basilar artery (BA), internal carotid arteries (ICA), middle cerebral arteries (MCA), intracranial vertebral arteries (VA), and other intracranial arteries, in decreasing order of frequency [1]. This pathology is particularly prevalent among Asian populations [3, 4]. While many cases are diagnosed following transient ischemic attacks (TIA) or ischemic stroke, there is also an increasing number of asymptomatic cases identified through screening with magnetic resonance (MR) angiography. Better understanding of the etiology of ICAS would be essential to provide appropriate treatment for prevention of future severe cerebrovascular events.

Despite its clinical significance, ICAS remains less understood compared to cervical internal carotid artery stenosis, which is similar atherosclerotic lesion contributing to stroke. The mechanisms, treatment options, including medical and surgical management—in particular the role of elective endovascular treatment (EVT)—remain controversial [2, 5]. The efficacy and safety of EVT for ICAS are not still under investigation.

In this chapter, we will provide an overview of the clinical characteristics of ICAS, including its presentation, etiology, and diagnostic trends. Additionally, we will introduce some important clinical trials that investigated the role of EVT in treatment of ICA. Moreover, techniques and devices for EVT will also be presented with some illustrative cases.

K. Kurisu · T. Osanai · M. Fujimura (✉)
Department of Neurosurgery, Hokkaido University Graduate School of Medicine, Sapporo, Hokkaido, Japan
e-mail: osanait@med.hokudai.ac.jp; fujimur@med.hokudai.ac.jp

Y. Shimoda
Department of Neurosurgery, Sapporo Asabu Neurosurgical Hospital, Sapporo, Hokkaido, Japan

2 Epidemiology

ICAS is one of the most common cause of ischemic stroke worldwide, primarily due to its high prevalence among Asian patients [3]. Reports from China [4, 6] indicate that 20%–46% of ischemic stroke patients have ICAS, whereas reports from the United States [7] indicate a prevalence of ICAS among all stroke patients was 8%–10%. This difference of prevalence based on racial differences in prevalence could be explained by genetic predispositions, and also higher rates of risk factors including smoking, diabetes, hypertension, dyslipidemia, and obesity [8–10].

3 Pathophysiology

The pathophysiological progression of ICAS is thought to be similar to extracranial vascular lesions, particularly cervical internal carotid artery lesions, as proposed by Russell Ross's theory [11]. The progression occurs in the following stages: endothelial dysfunction, fatty streak formation, formation of advanced, complicated lesions, and development of unstable fibrous plaques [11]. Autopsy studies have provided early evidence of atherosclerosis in cerebral arteries, examining 200 patients ranging in age from newborn to 80 years [12]. Initial signs of atherosclerosis, such as lipid streaks or spots, were observed in intracranial arteries starting from the fourth decade of life, which is roughly two decades later than in coronary arteries. A separate postmortem study involving 334 patients indicated that intimal necrosis might occur early in the development of cerebral artery atherosclerosis, preceding the appearance of fatty streaks and fibromuscular plaques, which are thought to be secondary phenomena [13]. In cerebral arteries, intimal thickening and proliferative changes in the basement membrane and adventitia were more frequently identified compared to fatty infiltrations [2, 14]. With advancing age (after the fifth decade), more pronounced fibrous plaques and complex lesions, such as calcifications and plaque rupture, were seen primarily in the

V. Beneš, D. Netuka (eds.), *Surgical and Interventional Treatment of Cerebral Ischemia*,
https://doi.org/10.1007/978-3-032-08934-2_18

proximal segments of the basilar, vertebral, and internal carotid arteries, whereas necrotic and hemorrhagic changes were comparatively uncommon in cerebral arteries [15].

In addition, ICAS contributes to the occurrence of ischemic stroke through several mechanisms. The etiology of stroke related to ICAS can be classified into the following five types: hemodynamic ischemia, in situ thrombosis, artery-to-artery embolism, perforator vessel occlusion, and complex of these mechanisms [2, 5, 16]. Understanding these underlying processes is crucial for effective management and treatment of ICAS, since these provide insight into both preventive strategies and therapeutic interventions.

Structural and functional features that differ to extracranial artery stenosis include: a reduced number of elastic fibers in the media for muscular arteries, a thinner media, lack of an external elastic lamina, the presence of vasa vasorum only in large vessels such as the ICA and VA, surrounding by cerebrospinal fluid, tight junctions, decreased endothelial permeability, and well-developed defense mechanisms against oxidative stress [15]. When treating ICAS, especially by endovascular approach, it is important to fully understand these differences, compared to extracranial arteries.

4 Diagnosis and Imaging

The diagnosis of ICAS involves multiple imaging modalities and assessments to accurately determine the presence, severity, and location of the stenosis. Accurate diagnosis is crucial for selecting the appropriate treatment to prevent the future ischemic events.

4.1 Non-invasive Imaging

Intracranial arterial stenosis could be often detected by non-invasive imaging examinations, in patients who developed stroke or transient ischemic attacks. However, recently, opportunity to treat asymptomatic ICAS are increasing, which are detected by other symptoms or by screening intracranial vascular imaging examinations [2]. In addition to the diagnosis by magnetic resonance (MR) Angiography and computed tomography (CT) Angiography, it has been reported that intracranial arterial stenosis can also be detected by ultrasound (US) examination by the presence of reduced end-diastolic velocity (EVD) and its left-right difference (ED ratio) which are able to be measured in the common carotid artery [17, 18].

4.2 Cerebral Angiography

Although an invasive imaging modality, cerebral angiography is often required for a detailed assessment of the degree of stenosis, plaque characteristics, and cerebral hemodynamics. These findings would be useful in diagnosing stroke etiology, and determining the optimal management strategy.

To evaluate the degree of stenosis, the method used in WASID (Warfarin-Aspirin Symptomatic Intracranial Disease) trial is commonly applied (Fig. 1) [19, 20]. Briefly, degree of stenosis would be calculated as below; Degree of stenosis (percentage) = [(1 − (D (diameter) stenosis/D normal)) × 100. The settings of D stenosis and D normal differ according to the location of the lesions, thus some examples of measurement of stenotic degree using WASID method is shown in Fig. 1.

And for the assessment of plaque characteristics of ICAS, Mori classification [21], which were modified classification for coronary artery stenosis are commonly adapted (Table 1). Report that argued this classification [21] which was a retrospective observational cohort study of 42 symptomatic ICAS patients treated with elective EVT demonstrated that successful treatment was achieved in 92%, 86%, and 33% of patients with type A, type B and type C lesions, respectively. The cumulative risk of ipsilateral stroke occurrence and bypass surgery requirement was 8%, 26%, and 87% for type A, type B and type C lesions, respectively. The restenosis rate after 1 year of EVT was also 0%, 33%, and 100% in type A, type B and type C lesions, respectively. These results suggest that type A lesions would be a better indication for EVT to achieve a favorable clinical outcome, although this is still controversial.

4.3 Differential Diagnosis

In addition to atherosclerotic lesions, other conditions that can cause ICAS include vasculitis, arterial dissection, and moyamoya disease. Moyamoya disease, in particular, has been linked to RNF213 gene mutations, which have also been associated with atherosclerotic ICAS [22–25]. To differentiate atherosclerotic ICAS from other pathological ICAS lesions, the feasibility of vessel wall imaging (VWI) has recently gained attention. The VWI is an imaging technique that suppresses blood signals within the vessel and cerebrospinal fluid signals outside the vessel, allowing assessment of vessel walls that cannot be assessed by cerebral angiography or conventional MR imaging [26, 27].

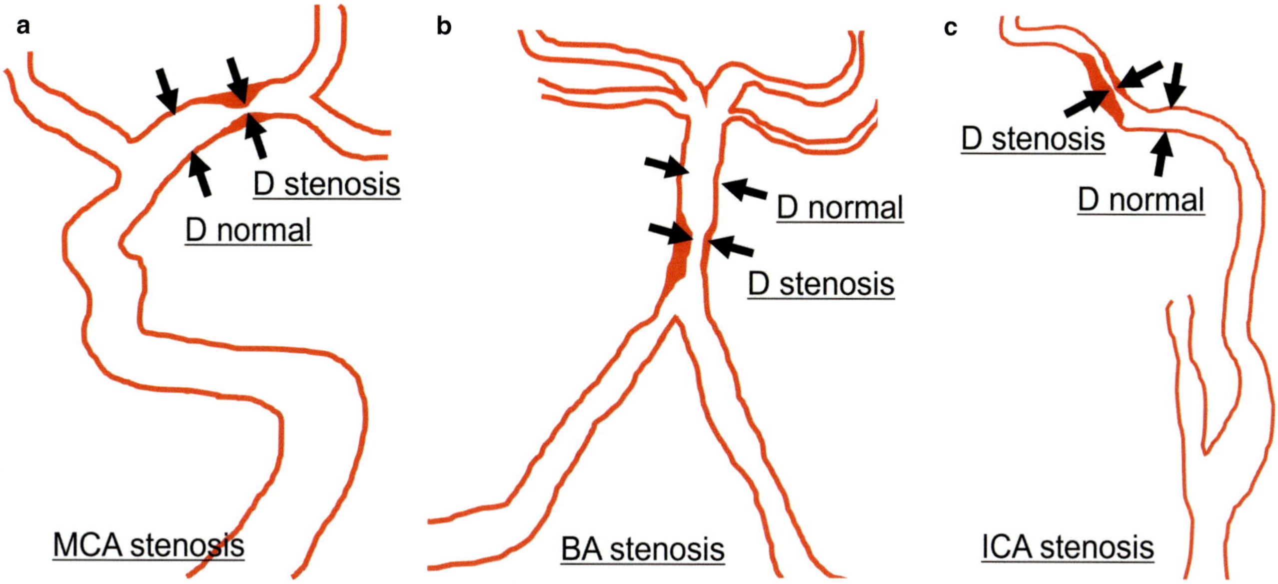

Fig. 1 Measurement method to evaluate the percentage of stenosis using WASID (Warfarin-Aspirin Symptomatic Intracranial Disease) study method. The degree of stenosis would be calculated as; degree of stenosis (percentage) = [(1 − (D (diameter) stenosis/D normal)) × 100. (**a**) In case when stenosis is located in the MCA (middle cerebral artery). (**b**) In case when stenosis is located in BA (basilar artery). (**c**) In case when stenosis is locating in ICA (internal carotid artery)

Table 1 Summary of intracranial artery stenosis classification (Mori classification)

Type	Stenosis length (mm)	Angiographical characteristics
A	<5	Concentric stenosis
B	5–10	A tubular lesion Extreme eccentric lesion
C	>10	Diffuse lesion

In atherosclerotic ICAS lesions, VWI shows the presence of locally ubiquitous plaques, with variable contrast enhancement. Generally, symptomatic lesions appear to have more contrast enhancement, and outward remodeling, irregularity and intraplaque hemorrhage have also been documented as indicators of plaque vulnerability [26, 27]. Vasculitis is characterized by multiple, segmental, smooth, circumferential contrast enhancing lesions and vessel wall thickening. Contrast enhancement is characteristically seen not only at the site of stenosis, but also in areas without stenosis. In arterial dissection, VWI may also show a 'pearl and string sign' with an intimal flap, double lumen and intramural hematoma [26, 27]. In general, the contrast enhancement in the dissection lesion is obvious and homogenous.

5 Clinical Evidences

This section outlines the content and results of several important clinical trials. Among these trials, large representative RCTs that compared efficacy of EVT for ICAS are also summarized in Table 2.

5.1 WASID Trial [19]

The WASID trial [19], published in 2005, compared the efficacy of warfarin and aspirin in ICAS patients with 50%–99% stenosis. Death, major hemorrhage, sudden death and myocardial infarction were all significantly lower in the aspirin group. The primary endpoint of occurrence of ischemic stroke did not differ between the two groups. This study demonstrated that antiplatelet therapy would be the first-line medical treatment for ICAS patients. Furthermore, the results of this study suggest that ICAS is associated with a high risk of stroke recurrence and a poor clinical outcome. The results of this clinical trial also suggest that the development of feasible surgical or endovascular treatment for ICAS is warranted.

Table 2 Summary of representative randomised clinical trials regarding the efficacy of endovascular treatment for intracranial artery stenosis (ICAS)

Study name	SAMPRIS, 2011	VISSIT, 2015	CASSISS, 2022
No of patients	541	111	380
Primary endpoint	Stroke or death within 30 days Stroke beyond 30 days	Stroke or TIA within 1 year	Stroke or death within 30 days Stroke beyond 30 days through 1 year
Used device	Self expandable stent	Balloon expandable stent	Self-expandable stent
Results Patients with events	15% in medical group 23% in stent group	15% in medical group 36% in stent group	7% in medical group 8% in stent group

5.2 SAMPRIS Trial [28, 29]

The trial included patients with TIA or stroke within 30 days of onset with 70%–99% stenosis of the major intracranial arteries (ICA, MCA, M1, VA, BA) who were randomized to receive an aggressive medical treatment (antiplatelet therapy, intensive management of vascular risk factors, and a lifestyle-modification program) or aggressive medical management plus endovascular treatment (PTA/stenting (self-expandable Wingspan stent (Stryker, Kalamazoo, MI)) (PTAS) group. 451 patients were enrolled, and the primary endpoint of stroke or death at 30 days was significantly higher in the PTAS group (14.7%) compared to the medical group (5.8%). This result was thought to be due to the higher rate of peri-operative stroke in the PTAS group. In the final report [28] with a median follow-up of 32.4 months, the primary endpoint (stroke or death within 30 days after enrolment, ischemic stroke in the territory of the qualifying artery beyond 30 days of enrolment, or stroke or death within 30 days after a revascularization procedure of the qualifying lesion during follow-up) was predominantly lower in the medical group (15%) and in the PTAS group (23%) ($p = 0.0252$). The absolute difference in the incidence of the primary endpoints between the two groups was 7.1% at 1 year ($p = 0.0428$), 6.5% at 2 years ($p = 0.07$%) and 9.0% at 3 years ($p = 0.0193$). The incidence of all strokes (26% in the PTAS group vs 19% in the medical group, $p = 0.0468$) and major bleeding (13% in the PTAS group vs 4% in the medical group, $p = 0.00009$) was markedly lower in the medical treatment group. These results indicates the superiority of aggressive medical treatment also in terms of long-term prognosis.

5.3 VISSIT Trial [30]

This trial is also a large RCT comparing the effectiveness of endovascular treatment (stenting with balloon-expandable stents) and aggressive medical treatment for ICAS. In this study, symptomatic ICAS of ≥70% was enrolled, with 59 patients receiving stenting in addition to medical therapy (stent group) and 53 patients receiving medical therapy alone (medical group). The primary outcome was a composite of stroke in the same region within 12 months after randomization or transient ischemic attack (TIA) in the same region from day 2 to 12 months after randomization, which was significantly higher in the stent group compared with the medical group (36.2% in the stent group and 15.1% in the medical group, $p = 0.02$). The primary safety endpoint, defined as a composite of any stroke, death or intracranial hemorrhage within 30 days of randomization and any major TIA between days 2 and 30 of randomization, was significantly lower in the medical group compared to the stent group (34.5% in stent group vs. 9.4% in medical group, $p = 0.05$). In line with the SAMPRIS trial [28, 29], this study also failed to demonstrate the efficacy of endovascular treatment in the treatment of ICAS.

5.4 CASSIS Trial [31, 32]

This RCT, conducted in China, compared the efficacy of endovascular treatment (PTAS group) with medical treatment (medical group) in patients with TIA or ICAD (>70% stenosis) within 1 year of stroke onset. The trial allowed 1 year from ischemic event to allocation (longer than previous trials), with strict inclusion criteria (excluding cases of perforating branch infarction) and operator selection, and compared the incidence of primary outcomes (composite of stroke or death within 30 days or stroke in the qualifying artery territory beyond 30 days to 1 year) in the PTAS group and the medical group. However, the results showed that there was no significant difference in the primary outcome (8.0% in the PTAS group vs 7.2% in the medical group; $p = 0.82$). And also, there were no significant differences between the two groups in other secondary endpoints. Based on these results, the authors concluded that their findings do not support the addition of PTAS to medical therapy for the treatment of patients with symptomatic severe intracranial atherosclerotic stenosis.

5.5 VISIT Trial [33]

In this study, patients with posterior circulation TIA or stroke within 180 days (later changed to 90 days) of onset with >50% stenosis in the extracranial and intracranial VA were allocated to the medical treatment group (n = 88) and PTAS group (Aggressive medical treatment plus PTA/stenting, n = 91 (intracranial n = 17, extracranial n = 74)). With a median follow-up of 3.5 years, the primary endpoint of fatal or non-fatal stroke occurred in 5 patients in the stent group vs 12 in the medical group (hazard ratio 0.40, p = 0. 08), with an absolute risk reduction of 25 strokes per 1000 person-years. The results of this study suggest that PTAS has a low complication rate in symptomatic VA stenosis, especially in extracranial lesions, and would be one of the considerable treatment options.

5.6 WEAVE [34], WOVEN [35] Trial

These studies are prospective, single-arm, consecutive registry post-market surveillance studies of the Wingspan stent, a self-expanding stent for ICAS. Patients with symptomatic and severe (70%–99%) intracranial artery stenosis (intracranial ICA, MCA M1, intracranial VA, BA) with at least two previous stroke events (at least one during antiplatelet therapy) and who had undergone endovascular revascularization with Wingspan stenting after day 8 of the last ischemic event were enrolled in this study. The degree of stenosis was improving from an average of 83–28% with endovascular treatment in an analysis of 152 patients. Perioperative (within 72 h postoperatively) stroke/hemorrhage/death was 2.6%, which was lower than expectations, allowing the study to be terminated earlier than expected. Furthermore, this complication was not observed in high-volume institutes (more than 50 cases), while it was observed in 4.8% in other institutes. The results suggest that this endovascular revascularization may be safer and more effective when performed by an experienced surgeon in a high-volume center.

WOVEN is a post-hoc study using the WEAVE cohort for follow-up and imaging analysis for up to 1 year. The patients included 50% of the WEAVE study enrolment institutes, 12 sites and 129 patients. During the 1-year follow-up period, stroke occurred in seven patients (six mild and one severe). Including the four perioperative events observed in WEAVE trial, 8.5% (11 of 129 patients) had a stroke or death at 1 year.

5.7 Current Standpoint of EVT for ICAS and Future Prospect

According to previous large clinical trials described in the sections above, the position of EVT in ICAS remains controversial. One of the reasons for this is the unexpectedly high efficacy of aggressive medical treatment observed in previous trials. Current national and international guidelines [36–38] recommend best medical treatment even for symptomatic severe (70%–99%) stenotic lesions, whereas EVT (stenting or PTA) is not currently recommended.

Based on these recommendations, the possible conditions that would constitute a clinical indication for EVT of the ICAS are as follows; (1) performed by an experienced operator in an experienced institution, (2) refractory to aggressive medical treatment, including DAPT, (3) severe (70%–99%) symptomatic lesion classified as Mori type A, (4) performing at least 8 days after stroke onset.

However, to establish the role of EVT in severe and symptomatic ICAS patients, future well-designed large clinical trials are warranted.

6 Treatment Strategy

6.1 Antiplatelet Therapy

For elective endovascular revascularization treatment, dual antiplatelet treatment (DAPT) using aspirin, clopidogrel, prasugrel or cilostazol should be initiated at least 1 week before, and preferably 2 weeks before the procedure to ensure adequate antiplatelet effect. Problems that we should be aware of with antiplatelet therapy include the existence of 'hypo-responders' and the occurrence of 'hemorrhagic complications'.

Clopidogrel is metabolized in the liver by CYP2C19, a drug-metabolizing enzyme, to exert its effects. And it is known that genetic polymorphisms in CYP2C19 may result in low metabolic activity and in effectiveness. This clopidogrel poor metabolizer and is more common in Asians, 3–5% in Western populations and 12%–23% in Eastern populations [39]. Currently, VerifyNow (Accumetries, San Diego, CA) is commonly used to test the drug efficacy for clopidogrel and aspirin. A PRU (P2Y12 Reaction Unit) of less than 230 for clopidogrel, and an ARU (Aspirin Reaction Unit) of less than 550 for aspirin, are considered to be indicating sufficient antiplatelet effect provided by the drugs.

On the other hand, the 'hyper-responder' to clopidogrel has also recently been highlighted, where it has been considered that there is a risk of 'hemorrhagic complications'. Previous reports [40] have shown the relationship between the effect of antiplatelet therapy and hemorrhagic complications in patients undergoing endovascular treatment. The results demonstrated a significantly higher antiplatelet effect (63.5%) in patients who had a hemorrhagic event, compared with 19% in those who did not have a hemorrhagic complication. To address this issue, prasugrel, a prodrug of the thienopyridine family that is less affected by genetic polymorphisms in CYP2C19, has also been the focus of interest in the field of stroke and neurointerventional therapy. As this prodrug has less individual variability in antiplatelet efficacy, its use has spread widely and rapidly.

6.2 Percutaneous Transluminal Angioplasty (PTA)

Balloons for PTA that can be used for ICAS are the Gateway balloon (over the wire type (OTW), monorail type) (Stryker, Kalamazoo, MI) and the Unryu balloon (Kaneka medics, Osaka, JPN). Both are classified as semi-compliant balloons. The characteristics of these PTA balloons are summarized in Table 3.

When performing a PTA, it is recommended to select a balloon smaller than 80% of the target vessel diameter and to inflate the balloon at less than nominal pressure. Particularly when treating the M1 segment of the MCA, where the vessel diameter tends to be small, the use of a 1.5 or 2.0 mm PTA balloon should be appropriate. During balloon inflation, the balloon should be inflated at a rate of approximately 1 atm/10 s and maintained at nominal pressure for approximately 30 s. After deflation of the PTA balloon, the balloon should be positioned proximally while maintaining the position of the micro guidewire distal to the stenosis. The vasodilating effect of PTA is then assessed. Although favorable vasodilatation is confirmed immediately after PTA, it is also important to wait (approximately 15 min) and reassess the status of the treated lesion, as delayed vessel dissection or restenosis due to elastic recoil may occur.

Table 3 Summary of representative Percutaneous Transluminal Angioplasty (PTA) balloon

	Stryker		Kaneka medics
Device	Gateway over the wire	Gateway monorail	Unryu monorail
Baloon size variations			
Diameter (mm)	1.5, 2.0. 2.5, 3.0, 3.5, 4.0	2.0. 2.5, 3.0, 3.5, 4.0	1.5, 2.0, 2.5
Length (mm)	9, 12	9, 12, 15, 20	10
System length	135 cm	140 cm	150 cm
Compatible guidewire	0.014 inch	0.014 inch	0.014 inch
Compatible guiding	0.064 inch	0.058 inch	0.067 inch
Nominal pressure	6 atm	6 atm	6 atm

6.3 Intracranial Artery Stenting

The Wingspan Stent System is currently the only approved stent for ICAS. However, its use in Japan is strictly limited and is currently only approved for: (1) rescue stenting for dissection, acute occlusion or high risk of occlusion followed by balloon PTA, (2) refractory intracranial arterial stenosis after PTA when no other effective treatment is available. Wingspan is a self-expandable stent with an open cell structure and made of Nitinol (nickel-titanium alloy). The range of stent diameters and lengths is shown in Table 4.

Platinum-iridium alloy impermeable markers are attached to the distal and proximal ends of the stent, and housed in a delivery system that can be navigated using with a 0.014″ micro guidewire. Stent size selection should be based on the larger normal vessel diameter either distal or proximal to the stenotic lesion. The stent should be carefully navigated to the stenotic lesion using the micro guidewire used for the just performed PTA. When navigating the stent toward intracranial stenotic lesion, the operator should be aware that there may be some resistance at the point where the stent passes the siphon of ICA. Once in the appropriate position, the stent should be deployed using the un-sheathing technique. As the Wingspan Stent is an open cell stent, it is important to note that it cannot be re-sheathed.

Table 4 Wingspan stent system profile

Stent profile					Compatible devices	
Diameter (mm)	Length (mm)	Recommended vessel size (mm)	Maximum diameter after deployment (mm)	System length	Microguidewire	Guiding system
2.5	9	2.0–2.5	2.8	135 cm	0.36 mm (0.014 inch)	1.63 mm (0.064 inch)
	15					
3.0	9	2.5–3.0	3.4			
	15					
	20					
3.5	15	3.0–3.5	3.9			
	20					
4.0	15	3.5–4.0	4.4			
	20					
4.5	15	4.0–4.5	4.9			
	20					

7 Illustrative Cases

7.1 Case 1: PTA for MCA Stenosis

The patient is an 80-year-old man with a history of hypertension, hyperlipidemia, and coronary artery disease. The patient had been treated with statins, antihypertensives, and dual antiplatelet agents. He developed progressive right upper and lower limb weakness over several days and was transferred to our department by ambulance. Severe MCA stenosis (Fig. 2a) was observed on admission, and the patient was treated with additional antithrombotic agents. However, he experienced worsening left hemiparesis, and MR imaging revealed enlargement of the ischemic lesion (Fig. 2b). Cerebral blood flow (CBF) assessed by IMP-SPECT (Fig. 2c) showed a severe decrease in CBF in the left MCA territory. Given these findings, we decided to perform elective EVT for the left M1 stenosis 8 days after his admission.

Images obtained during EVT are shown in Fig. 3. The procedure was performed under sedation with local anesthesia. Dual antiplatelet therapy (DAPT) was maintained throughout the peri-procedural period, and additional heparinization was administered during EVT. A 6Fr distal access catheter was navigated to the cavernous segment of the ICA. The pre-procedural angiogram (Fig. 3a) showed a severe but localized M1 stenosis (Mori type A, WASID 82.7% stenosis). A PTA balloon, UNRYU 1.5 mm, was navigated to the stenotic lesion with a 0.014-inch micro guidewire, and the balloon was inflated to 6 atm (Fig. 3b). Additionally, another PTA balloon, UNRYU 2.0 mm, was re-navigated to the lesion and inflated to 6 atm (Fig. 3c). The final angiogram after PTA showed favorable vessel dilation (Fig. 3d).

The patient's post-operative course was uneventful with continuation of DAPT. The patient was transferred to another hospital 2 weeks after the procedure for further rehabilitation. He is currently being followed up in our outpatient clinic without any recurrence of stroke.

7.2 Case 2: Stenting for ICA Petrous Portion Stenosis

The patient is a 76-year-old man with a history of hypertension, hyperlipidemia, and a previous ischemic stroke. Thirteen years previously, he had undergone superficial temporal artery—MCA bypass surgery for right ICA occlusion. The patient developed right-sided hemiparesis, and was transferred to our hospital by ambulance. MR imaging showed acute ischemic lesions in both frontal lobes (Fig. 4a, arrows). MR angiography showed progression of the left ICA stenosis, as evidenced by decreased signal intensity of the ICA, MCA, and ACA compared with the image obtained at follow-up (Fig. 4b, circled dashed line). Despite initiation of DAPT, the patient experienced recurrent TIAs during hospitalization. Given this clinical course, we decided to perform elective EVT for the ICA stenosis 14 days after his admission.

The images obtained during the procedure are shown in Fig. 5. The procedure was performed under sedation with local anesthesia. Dual antiplatelet therapy (DAPT) was maintained throughout the peri-procedural period, and additional heparinization was administered during EVT. A 6Fr distal access catheter was placed proximal to the ICA stenosis. The preprocedural angiogram showed a severe but localized ICA stenosis in the petrous portion (Mori type A, WASID 93.0% stenosis) (Fig. 5a). The PTA was first performed with a Gateway monorail balloon (2.5 mm × 15 mm), inflated at 4 atm (Fig. 5b). A Wingspan stent (4.0 mm × 20 mm) was then navigated to the stenotic lesion, and deployed to the lesion (Fig. 5c). The final angiogram showed a favorable vessel dilatation (Fig. 5d).

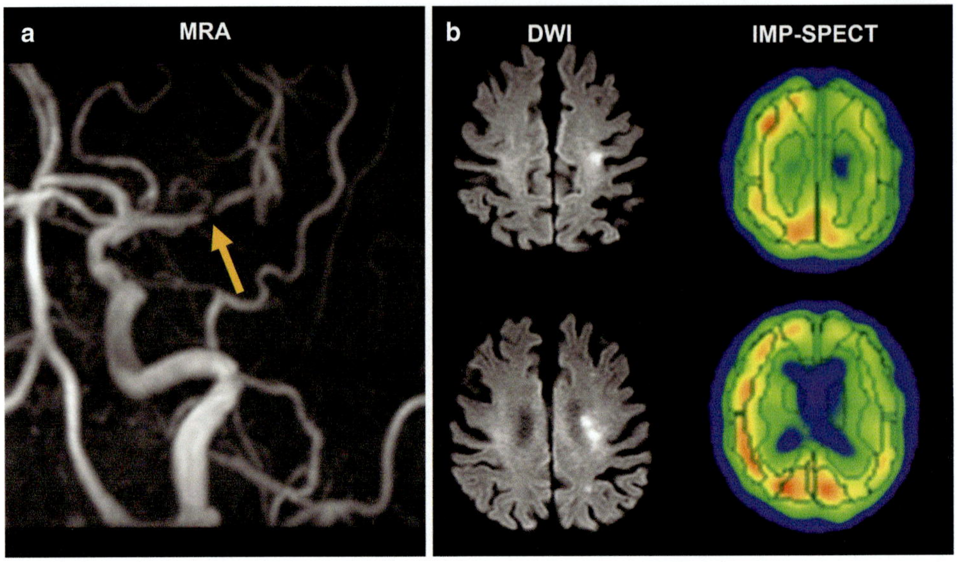

Fig. 2 Pre-operative images of 80-year-old man with middle cerebral artery (MCA) stenosis. (**a**) Severe MCA stenosis was observed on magnetic resonance angiography. (**b**) MR imaging revealed enlargement of the ischemic lesion. (**c**) The SPECT study revealed severe decrease in CBF in the left MCA territory

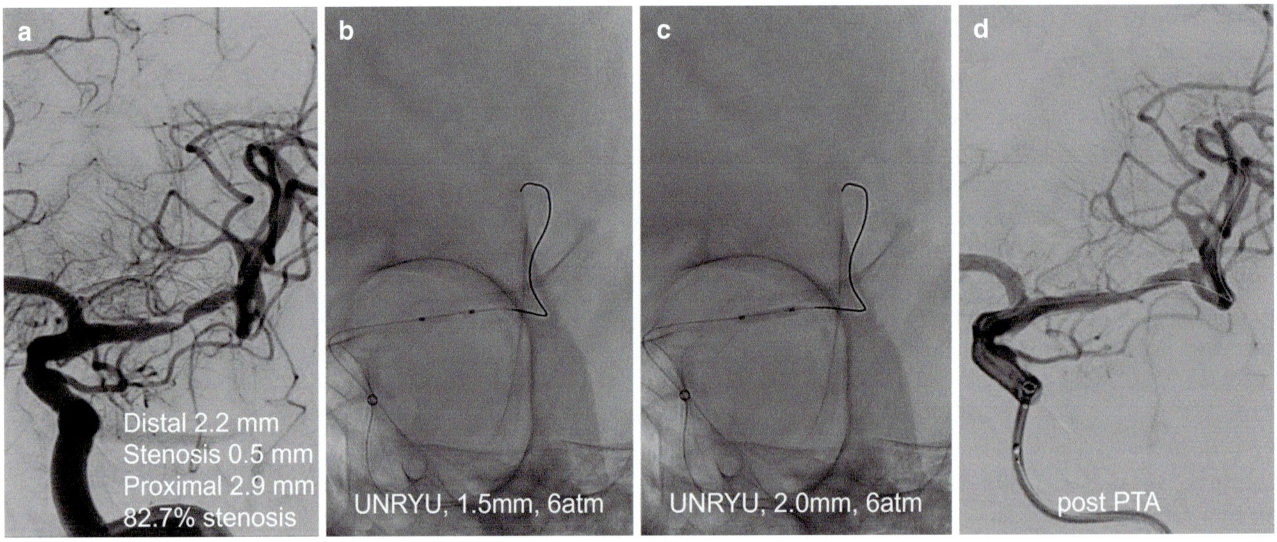

Fig. 3 Operative images percutaneous transluminal angioplasty (PTA) for middle cerebral artery (MCA) stenosis. (**a**) The angiogram showed a severe but localized MCA stenosis (Mori type A, WASID 82.7% stenosis). (**b**) PTA balloon, UNRYU 1.5 mm, was navigated to the stenotic lesion, and the balloon was inflated to 6 atm. (**c**) Additionally, UNRYU 2.0 mm, was re-navigated to the lesion and inflated to 6 atm. (**d**) The angiogram after PTA showed favorable vessel dilation

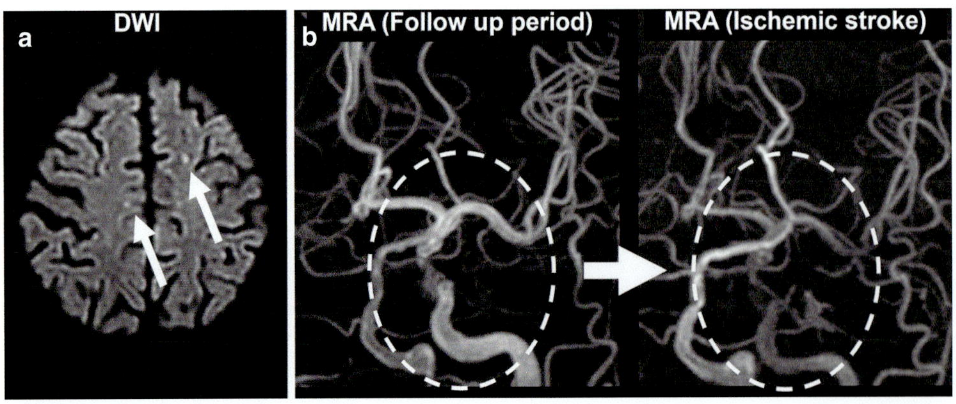

Fig. 4 Pre-operative images of 76-year-old man with internal carotid artery (ICA) stenosis. (**a**) Magnetic resonance (MR) imaging showed acute ischemic lesions in both frontal lobes (arrows). (**b**) MR angiography showed progression of the left ICA stenosis (circled dashed line), as evidenced by decreased signal intensity of intracranial arteries compared with the image obtained at follow-up

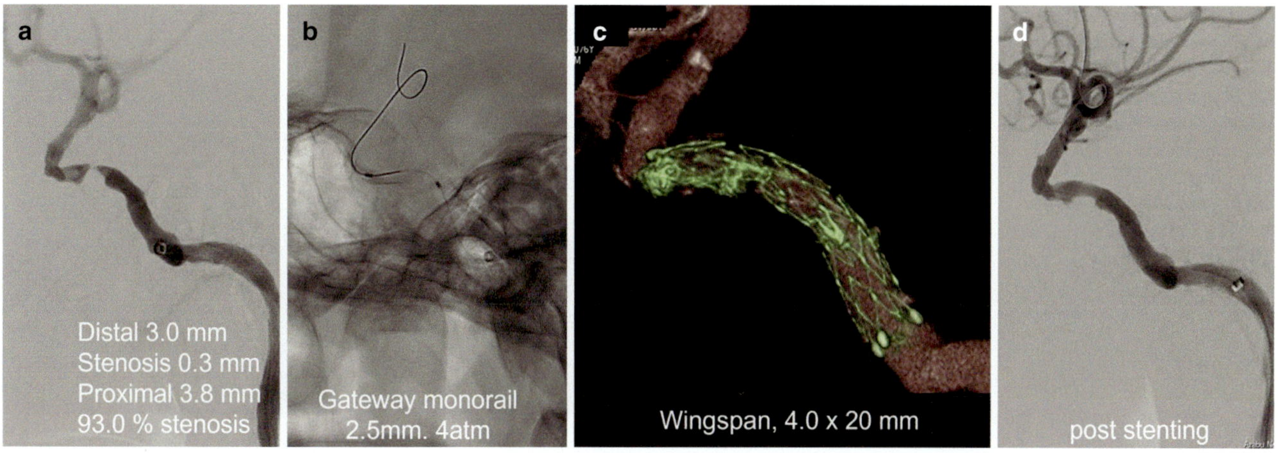

Fig. 5 Operative images percutaneous stenting for internal carotid artery (ICA) stenosis. (**a**) The angiogram showed a severe but localized ICA stenosis (Mori type A, WASID 93.0% stenosis). (**b**) The percutaneous transluminal angioplasty was first performed with a Gateway monorail balloon (2.5 mm × 15 mm), inflated at 4 atm. (**c**) A Wingspan stent (4.0 mm × 20 mm) was then navigated to the stenotic lesion, and deployed at the stenotic lesion. (**d**) The final angiogram showed a favorable vessel dilatation

Post-operatively, the patient's clinical course was uneventful with complete resolution of TIA. He was discharged 2 weeks after the procedure, and continued to be followed in our outpatient clinic without any stroke events.

7.3 Case 3: Stenting for VA Stenosis

The patient is a 73-year-old man with a history of hypertension, hyperlipidemia, and diabetes mellitus. The patient developed sudden vertigo and vomiting, and was transferred to our hospital by ambulance. MR imaging showed acute ischemic lesions in left cerebellar (Fig. 6a). MR angiography showed severe stenosis of the left VA, which was the dominant side (Fig. 6b). In addition, the right VA, the non-dominant side, was hypoplastic. After the admission, antiplatelet therapy was initiated and maintained. However, the patient experienced several episodes of dizziness and fainting, which were considered to be transient ischemic symptoms due to insufficient posterioe circulation blood flow. Therefore, we decided to perform EVT for the VA stenosis 17 days after his admission.

The images obtained during the procedure are shown in Fig. 7. The procedure was performed under sedation with local anesthesia. A 6Fr distal access catheter was placed proximal to the VA stenosis. The preprocedural angiogram showed a severe but localized VA stenosis in the V3 segment (Mori type A, WASID 91.0% stenosis) (Fig. 7a). The PTA was initially performed with a Gateway monorail balloon (2.5 mm × 15 mm), inflated at 6 atm (Fig. 7b). A coronary stent (3.0 mm × 18 mm) was then navigated to the stenotic lesion, and deployed at the stenotic lesion (Fig. 7c). The final angiogram showed a favorable vessel dilatation (Fig. 7d).

Post-operatively, the patient's clinical course was uneventful with no neurological deficits. He was discharged 2 weeks after the procedure, and has been followed in our outpatient clinic without any stroke events.

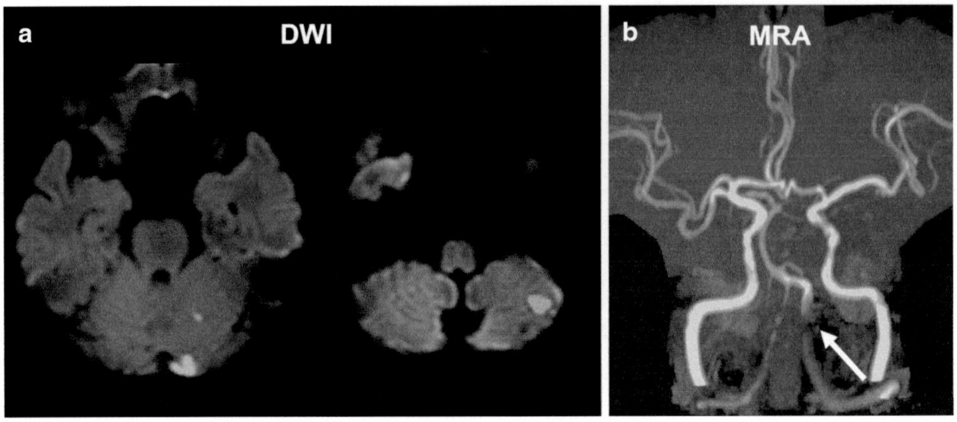

Fig. 6 Pre-operative images of 73-year-old man with vertebral artery (VA) stenosis. (**a**) Magnetic resonance (MR) imaging showed acute ischemic lesions in left cerebellar. (**b**) MR angiography showed severe stenosis of the left VA (arrow), which was the dominant side

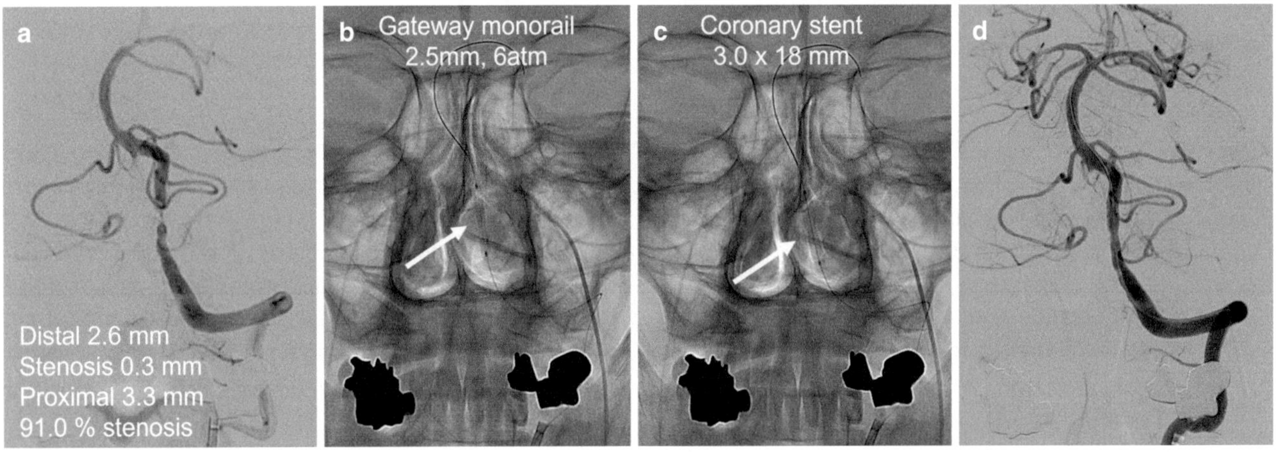

Fig. 7 Operative images percutaneous stenting for internal carotid artery (ICA) stenosis. (**a**) The angiogram showed a severe but localized VA stenosis in the V3 segment (Mori type A, WASID 91.0% stenosis). (**b**) The percutaneous transluminal angioplasty (PTA) was performed with a Gateway monorail balloon (2.5 mm × 15 mm), inflated at 6 atm. (**c**) A coronary stent (3.0 mm × 18 mm) was then navigated to the stenotic lesion, and deployed at the stenotic lesion. (**d**) The final angiogram showed a favorable vessel dilatation

Declarations

Competing Interests The author(s) has no competing interests to declare that are relevant to the content of this manuscript.

Ethics Approval The author(s) declares that this manuscript does not include primary research with human participants.

References

1. Gutierrez J, Turan TN, Hoh BL, Chimowitz MI. Intracranial atherosclerotic stenosis: risk factors, diagnosis, and treatment. Lancet Neurol. 2022;21(4):355–68. https://doi.org/10.1016/S1474-4422(21)00376-8.
2. Tekle WG, Hassan AE. Intracranial atherosclerotic disease: current concepts in medical and surgical management. Neurology. 2021;97(20 Suppl 2):S145–S57. https://doi.org/10.1212/WNL.0000000000012805.
3. Wong LK. Global burden of intracranial atherosclerosis. Int J Stroke. 2006;1(3):158–9. https://doi.org/10.1111/j.1747-4949.2006.00045.x.
4. Wang Y, Zhao X, Liu L, Soo YO, Pu Y, Pan Y, et al. Prevalence and outcomes of symptomatic intracranial large artery stenoses and occlusions in China: the Chinese Intracranial Atherosclerosis (CICAS) Study. Stroke. 2014;45(3):663–9. https://doi.org/10.1161/STROKEAHA.113.003508.
5. Kurisu K, Uchida K, Okuyama T, Miyata K, Yamaguchi Y, Ajiki M, et al. Clinical characteristics of endovascular treatment for acute ischemic stroke with atherosclerotic etiology: factors associating its clinical outcome. Clin Neurol Neurosurg. 2023;228:107680. https://doi.org/10.1016/j.clineuro.2023.107680.
6. Wang ZL, Gao BL, Li TX, Cai DY, Zhu LF, Xue JY, et al. Outcomes of middle cerebral artery angioplasty and stenting with Wingspan at a high-volume center. Neuroradiology. 2016;58(2):161–9. https://doi.org/10.1007/s00234-015-1611-8.

7. Sacco RL, Kargman DE, Gu Q, Zamanillo MC. Race-ethnicity and determinants of intracranial atherosclerotic cerebral infarction. The Northern Manhattan Stroke Study. Stroke. 1995;26(1):14–20. https://doi.org/10.1161/01.str.26.1.14.
8. White H, Boden-Albala B, Wang C, Elkind MS, Rundek T, Wright CB, et al. Ischemic stroke subtype incidence among whites, blacks, and Hispanics: the Northern Manhattan Study. Circulation. 2005;111(10):1327–31. https://doi.org/10.1161/01.CIR.0000157736.19739.D0.
9. Qureshi AI, Caplan LR. Intracranial atherosclerosis. Lancet. 2014;383(9921):984–98. https://doi.org/10.1016/S0140-6736(13)61088-0.
10. Flusty B, de Havenon A, Prabhakaran S, Liebeskind DS, Yaghi S. Intracranial atherosclerosis treatment: past, present, and future. Stroke. 2020;51(3):e49–53. https://doi.org/10.1161/STROKEAHA.119.028528.
11. Ross R. The pathogenesis of atherosclerosis—an update. N Engl J Med. 1986;314(8):488–500. https://doi.org/10.1056/NEJM198602203140806.
12. Mathur KS, Kashyap SK, Kumar V. Correlation of the extent and severity of atherosclerosis in the coronary and cerebral arteries. Circulation. 1963;27:929–34. https://doi.org/10.1161/01.cir.27.5.929.
13. Velican C, Velican D. Atherosclerotic involvement of human intracranial arteries with special reference to intimal necrosis. Atherosclerosis. 1982;43(1):59–69. https://doi.org/10.1016/0021-9150(82)90099-5.
14. Stehbens WE. Cerebral atherosclerosis. Intimal proliferation and atherosclerosis in the cerebral arteries. Arch Pathol. 1975;99(11):582–91.
15. Ritz K, Denswil NP, Stam OC, van Lieshout JJ, Daemen MJ. Cause and mechanisms of intracranial atherosclerosis. Circulation. 2014;130(16):1407–14. https://doi.org/10.1161/CIRCULATIONAHA.114.011147.
16. Barnard ZR, Alexander MJ. Update in the treatment of intracranial atherosclerotic disease. Stroke Vasc Neurol. 2020;5(1):59–64. https://doi.org/10.1136/svn-2019-000279.
17. Zhang X, Wu D, Li H, Fang Y, Xiong H, Li Y. Early diagnosis of intracranial internal carotid artery stenosis using extracranial hemodynamic indices from carotid Doppler ultrasound. Bioengineering (Basel). 2022;9(9):422. https://doi.org/10.3390/bioengineering9090422.
18. Sharma VK, Tsivgoulis G, Lao AY, Malkoff MD, Alexandrov AV. Noninvasive detection of diffuse intracranial disease. Stroke. 2007;38(12):3175–81. https://doi.org/10.1161/STROKEAHA.107.490755.
19. Chimowitz MI, Lynn MJ, Howlett-Smith H, Stern BJ, Hertzberg VS, Frankel MR, et al. Comparison of warfarin and aspirin for symptomatic intracranial arterial stenosis. N Engl J Med. 2005;352(13):1305–16. https://doi.org/10.1056/NEJMoa043033.
20. Samuels OB, Joseph GJ, Lynn MJ, Smith HA, Chimowitz MI. A standardized method for measuring intracranial arterial stenosis. AJNR Am J Neuroradiol. 2000;21(4):643–6.
21. Mori T, Fukuoka M, Kazita K. Follow-up study after intracranial percutaneous transluminal cerebral balloon angioplasty. Interv Neuroradiol. 2000;6(Suppl 1):243–9. https://doi.org/10.1177/15910199000060S141.
22. Matsuda Y, Mineharu Y, Kimura M, Takagi Y, Kobayashi H, Hitomi T, et al. RNF213 p.R4810K variant and intracranial arterial stenosis or occlusion in relatives of patients with Moyamoya disease. J Stroke Cerebrovasc Dis. 2017;26(8):1841–7. https://doi.org/10.1016/j.jstrokecerebrovasdis.2017.04.019.
23. Uchiyama S, Fujimura M. Adult Moyamoya disease and Moyamoya syndrome: what is new? Cerebrovasc Dis Extra. 2024;14(1):86–94. https://doi.org/10.1159/000540254.
24. Tashiro R, Fujimura M, Sakata H, Endo H, Tomata Y, Sato-Maeda M, et al. Genetic analysis of ring finger protein 213 (RNF213) c.14576G>A polymorphism in patients with vertebral artery dissection: a comparative study with Moyamoya disease. Neurol Res. 2019;41(9):811–6. https://doi.org/10.1080/01616412.2019.1615726.
25. Fujimura M, Bang OY, Kim JS. Moyamoya disease. Front Neurol Neurosci. 2016;40:204–20. https://doi.org/10.1159/000448314.
26. Kern KC, Liebeskind DS. Vessel wall imaging of cerebrovascular disorders. Curr Treat Options Cardiovasc Med. 2019;21(11):65. https://doi.org/10.1007/s11936-019-0782-8.
27. van der Kolk AG, Zwanenburg JJ, Denswil NP, Vink A, Spliet WG, Daemen MJ, et al. Imaging the intracranial atherosclerotic vessel wall using 7T MRI: initial comparison with histopathology. AJNR Am J Neuroradiol. 2015;36(4):694–701. https://doi.org/10.3174/ajnr.A4178.
28. Derdeyn CP, Chimowitz MI, Lynn MJ, Fiorella D, Turan TN, Janis LS, et al. Aggressive medical treatment with or without stenting in high-risk patients with intracranial artery stenosis (SAMMPRIS): the final results of a randomised trial. Lancet. 2014;383(9914):333–41. https://doi.org/10.1016/S0140-6736(13)62038-3.
29. Chimowitz MI, Lynn MJ, Derdeyn CP, Turan TN, Fiorella D, Lane BF, et al. Stenting versus aggressive medical therapy for intracranial arterial stenosis. N Engl J Med. 2011;365(11):993–1003. https://doi.org/10.1056/NEJMoa1105335.
30. Zaidat OO, Fitzsimmons BF, Woodward BK, Wang Z, Killer-Oberpfalzer M, Wakhloo A, et al. Effect of a balloon-expandable intracranial stent vs medical therapy on risk of stroke in patients with symptomatic intracranial stenosis: the VISSIT randomized clinical trial. JAMA. 2015;313(12):1240–8. https://doi.org/10.1001/jama.2015.1693.
31. Gao P, Wang T, Wang D, Liebeskind DS, Shi H, Li T, et al. Effect of stenting plus medical therapy vs medical therapy alone on risk of stroke and death in patients with symptomatic intracranial stenosis: the CASSISS randomized clinical trial. JAMA. 2022;328(6):534–42. https://doi.org/10.1001/jama.2022.12000.
32. Gao P, Zhao Z, Wang D, Wu J, Cai Y, Li T, et al. China Angioplasty and Stenting for Symptomatic Intracranial Severe Stenosis (CASSISS): a new, prospective, multicenter, randomized controlled trial in China. Interv Neuroradiol. 2015;21(2):196–204. https://doi.org/10.1177/1591019915581778.
33. Markus HS, Larsson SC, Kuker W, Schulz UG, Ford I, Rothwell PM, et al. Stenting for symptomatic vertebral artery stenosis: the Vertebral Artery Ischaemia Stenting Trial. Neurology. 2017;89(12):1229–36. https://doi.org/10.1212/WNL.0000000000004385.
34. Alexander MJ, Zauner A, Chaloupka JC, Baxter B, Callison RC, Gupta R, et al. WEAVE trial: final results in 152 on-label patients. Stroke. 2019;50(4):889–94. https://doi.org/10.1161/STROKEAHA.118.023996.
35. Alexander MJ, Zauner A, Gupta R, Alshekhlee A, Fraser JF, Toth G, et al. The WOVEN trial: Wingspan one-year vascular events and neurologic outcomes. J Neurointerv Surg. 2021;13(4):307–10. https://doi.org/10.1136/neurintsurg-2020-016208.
36. Eskey CJ, Meyers PM, Nguyen TN, Ansari SA, Jayaraman M, McDougall CG, et al. Indications for the performance of intracranial endovascular neurointerventional procedures: a scientific statement from the American Heart Association. Circulation. 2018;137(21):e661–e89. https://doi.org/10.1161/CIR.0000000000000567.

37. Psychogios M, Brehm A, Lopez-Cancio E, Marco De Marchis G, Meseguer E, Katsanos AH, et al. European Stroke Organisation guidelines on treatment of patients with intracranial atherosclerotic disease. Eur Stroke J. 2022;7(3):III–IV. https://doi.org/10.1177/23969873221099715.
38. Miyamoto S, Ogasawara K, Kuroda S, Itabashi R, Toyoda K, Itoh Y, et al. Japan Stroke Society guideline 2021 for the treatment of stroke. Int J Stroke. 2022;17(9):1039–49. https://doi.org/10.1177/17474930221090347.
39. Musallam KM, Charafeddine K, Bitar A, Khoury M, Assaad S, Beresian J, et al. Resistance to aspirin and clopidogrel therapy. Int J Lab Hematol. 2011;33(1):1–18. https://doi.org/10.1111/j.1751-553X.2010.01268.x.
40. Goh C, Churilov L, Mitchell P, Dowling R, Yan B. Clopidogrel hyper-response and bleeding risk in neurointerventional procedures. AJNR Am J Neuroradiol. 2013;34(4):721–6. https://doi.org/10.3174/ajnr.A3418.

The Vertebral Arteries: Anatomy, Pathophysiology, and Ischemic Disorders

Laura Stone McGuire, Tatiana Abou-Mrad, Richard Bram, Gursant S. Atwal, Ali Alaraj, and Fady T. Charbel

1 Introduction

The vertebral arteries (VAs) play a critical role in supplying blood to the brain's posterior circulation, which includes essential structures such as the brainstem, cerebellum, and occipital lobes. Disorders affecting these arteries can lead to ischemia, resulting in transient or permanent neurological deficits. Understanding the anatomy, physiology, and pathophysiology of the VAs is vital for recognizing and managing conditions that may compromise their function.

2 Anatomy of the Vertebral Arteries

2.1 Gross Anatomy

The vertebral artery is commonly divided into four segments:

1. V1 segment (extraosseous): from its origin, typically at the subclavian artery, to its entry into the cervical transverse foramen
2. V2 segment (foraminal): from its entry into the transverse foramen, typically at C6, to its exit at C1 transverse foramen
3. V3 segment (extraspinal): from its exit at the transverse foramen at C1, as it courses posteromedially at the sulcus arteriosus, before its dural entry
   (a) *Note that different texts define the start of V3 segment at the artery's exit from the C2 transverse foramen, while the definition used in this chapter has been adopted from Osburn, such that the V3 segment begins at the artery's exit from the C1 transverse foramen.* [33, 35]
4. V4 segment (intradural): from its entry into the dura at the foramen magnum to its merger with the contralateral VA to become the basilar artery

The vertebral arteries originate as the first branches of the subclavian arteries. The VAs arise from the superior aspect of the subclavian arteries in nearly half of cases (47%) and otherwise come from the ventral, caudal, or dorsal surfaces. Variant origins also exist. The VA can arise from the brachiocephalic artery rather than the subclavian on the right, and it can arise directly from the aortic arch in 6% of cases, usually on the left. [46].

They ascend vertically through the transverse foramina of the cervical vertebrae, typically entering the transverse foramen at C6. Upon reaching the atlas (C1), the arteries curve posteromedially, travelling in the sulcus arteriosus of the posterior ring, and pass through the suboccipital triangle before penetrating the dura mater and entering the cranial cavity via the foramen magnum. Once inside the skull, the VAs course anteromedially and then converge at the pontomedullary junction to form the basilar artery, behind the clivus.

Ultimately, the course of the vertebral arteries, alternating through fixed boney foramina, makes them vulnerable to mechanical forces and injury, which will be discussed later. Further, the unique path of two large arteries merging to become the basilar artery creates hemodynamic forces that may make them prone to pathological changes [19].

L. S. McGuire (✉)
Department of Neurosurgery, University of Illinois at Chicago, Chicago, IL, USA

Department of Neurological Surgery, University of Wisconsin-Madison, Madison, WI, USA
e-mail: mcguire@neurosurgery.wisc.edu

T. Abou-Mrad · R. Bram · G. S. Atwal · A. Alaraj · F. T. Charbel
Department of Neurosurgery, University of Illinois at Chicago, Chicago, IL, USA
e-mail: tamrad@uic.edu; rbram3@uic.edu; gatwal@uic.edu; alaraj@uic.edu; fcharbel@uic.edu

V. Beneš, D. Netuka (eds.), *Surgical and Interventional Treatment of Cerebral Ischemia*,
https://doi.org/10.1007/978-3-032-08934-2_19

2.2 Surrounding Structures and Other Anatomic Relationships

The vertebral arteries are intimately associated with several critical anatomical structures, including the cervical vertebrae, the longus colli and capitis muscles, and the sympathetic nerve plexus. The vertebral arteries pass behind the anterior scalene muscles and common carotid arteries.

As they ascend through the cervical transverse foramina, they are found adjacent to the uncinate process and pass anterior to the ventral rami of each of the cervical spinal nerves. Within the transverse foramen, the vertebral arteries are surrounded by a venous plexus. Once the vertebral arteries leave the V2 segment, passing from the transverse foramina of C1, they travel posteromedially within the sulcus arteriosus of the posterior arch of C1. A complete bony ring may form around the sulcus arteriosus, named a "ponticulus posticus," in 16.7% of individuals [15].

After passing posteriorly at C1, the vertebral arteries then turn course anteromedially to then cross the atlanto-occipital membrane and enter the dura of the foramen magnum. Once intradural, the vertebral arteries pass anterior to the hypoglossal nerve roots. The bilateral vertebral arteries then converge to form the basilar artery at approximately the pontomedullary junction, which is usually at or near the inferior margin of the clival portion of the occipital bone.

2.3 Branching Patterns

The branches of the vertebral arteries can be grouped as cervical, meningeal, and intracranial.

2.3.1 Cervical Branches

The cervical spine receives blood supply from branches of the vertebral arteries and the external carotid arteries, which commonly anastomose with one another. From the vertebral arteries, there are spinal segmental branches and muscular branches.

- Spinal segmental branches: Supply the cervical spinal cord and often anastomose with the segmental branches of neighboring levels
- Muscular branches: Support the muscles in the suboccipital region

2.3.2 Meningeal Branches

The meningeal branches provide blood supply to the dura mater of the posterior cranial fossa and upper spinal cord. There are both anterior and posterior meningeal branches that may arise from the distal V2 segment or V3 segments, respectively. These meningeal branches may anastomose with one another and other meningeal branches from the anterior circulation, such as the middle meningeal artery.

- Anterior meningeal branch: Smaller branch and supplies the dura of the foramen magnum
- Posterior meningeal branch: Larger branch and often easily seen on angiography taking a superomedial course to the dura of the posterior fossa and falx cerebelli

2.3.3 Intracranial Branches

The major intracranial branches include the anterior and posterior spinal arteries, the posterior inferior cerebellar artery (PICA), and several small perforating arteries to the brainstem.

- Anterior spinal artery: Branch from the distal VA that merges medially with its contralateral counterpart to run in the anteromedian fissure of the spinal cord, supplying the anterior upper spinal cord and inferior medulla
- Posterior spinal artery: Branch from the distal VA or PICA that travel on the dorsal surface of the medulla and spinal cord, supplying the posterior surface of the spinal cord
- Posterior inferior cerebellar artery (PICA): The largest branch, which supplies the cerebellum, medulla, and choroid plexus of the fourth ventricle
- Perforating or penetrating branches: Multiple small branches that supply a portion of the medulla, olives, and inferior cerebellar peduncle

2.3.4 Posterior Inferior Cerebellar Artery

The posterior inferior cerebellar artery (PICA) has a highly variable origin and course, relative to the other cerebellar arteries, and it is generally the largest branch from the VA. The PICA branches from the distal VA, and 5–20% may have an extradural origin, which should be noted preoperatively prior to surgeries of the upper cervical spine and posterior fossa [16].

There are several perforators from PICA throughout its course, including supply to the lateral medulla proximally and choroid plexus distally.

There are 4 segments and 2 loops associated with the PICA:

- Anterior medullary segment: From the PICA origin, coursing posterolaterally in the medullary cistern
- Lateral medullary segment (caudal or tonsillar loop): Caudal loop within the cerebellomedullary fissure that then continues posteriorly
- Posterior medullary segment: Once PICA reaches the posterior border of the medulla and continues to the posterior medullary velum

- Supratonsillar segment (cranial loop): Cranially directed loop whereby the PICA courses above and around the tonsil and then divides after the cranial loop with lateral (tonsillohemispheric) and medial (vermian) branches

2.4 Blood Supply

The vertebral arteries contribute approximately 26–27% of the brain's total blood flow [2, 3]. They play a critical role in supplying oxygenated blood to the posterior circulation, which includes the brainstem, cerebellum, occipital lobes, thalamus, and parts of the spinal cord. This distinct vascular territory makes the vertebral arteries indispensable for maintaining vital functions such as respiration, coordination, and vision.

2.5 Developmental Variations

Anatomical variations in the vertebral arteries and their branches are common and can sometimes be clinically significant. These include:

- Unilateral dominance: One vertebral artery is significantly larger or provides the majority of posterior circulation flow. The left vertebral artery is usually dominant.
- Hypoplasia: One vertebral artery may be underdeveloped, and 5% of vertebral arteries will terminate in PICA (Fig. 1).
- Aberrant origins: The vertebral artery may arise directly from the aortic arch or other unusual locations. The left vertebral artery may originate directly from the aorta in 6% of cases [46]
- Duplicated origin of the vertebral artery: The origin of the vertebral artery may be duplicated or fenestrated (Fig. 2).

The PICA also has several variations [35], some of which include:

- Extradural PICA: The origin of the PICA originates on the V3 segment, rather than the V4 segment, and may occur in 5–18% of cases. Of note, the PICA may also have a normal intradural origin with a caudal loop that travels below the foramen magnum (Figs. 3 and 4).
- AICA-PICA: The AICA and PICA share a common origin, usually on the basilar trunk (Fig. 5).
- Singular PICA: One PICA supplies both right and left cerebellar hemispheres.
- Duplicated PICA: The PICA may be duplicated.

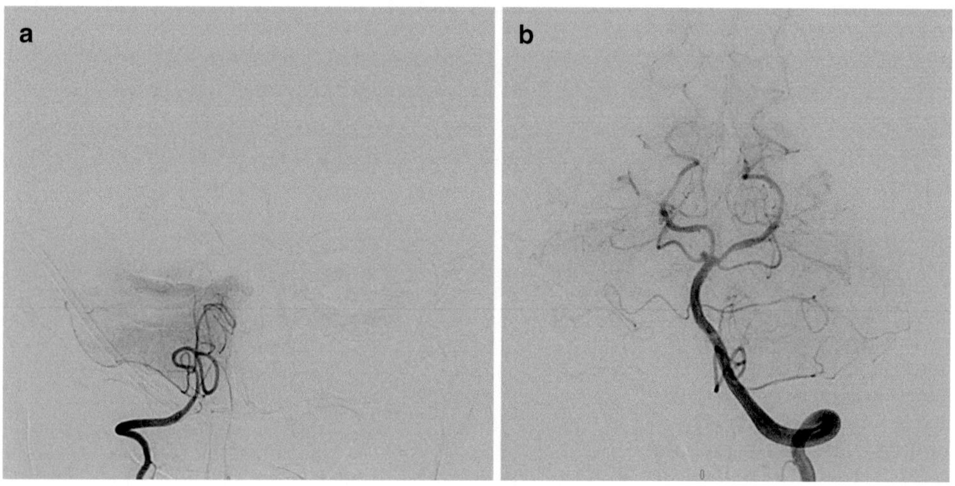

Fig. 1 DSA of right vertebral artery in AP view (**a**), demonstrating its termination in the PICA. DSA of the left vertebral artery in the same patient in AP view (**b**), showing no filling of the right PICA or right vertebrobasilar junction. Incidentally, DSA of the left vertebral artery shows an aneurysm of the right superior cerebellar artery

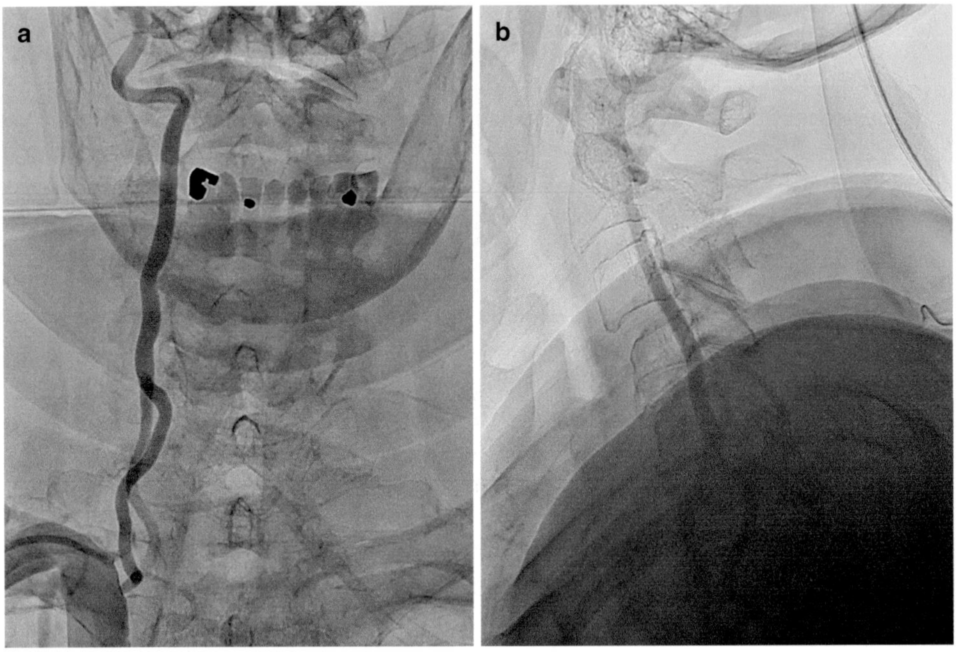

Fig. 2 DSA of the right subclavian artery in AP and lateral views (**a**, **b**), showing a duplicated origin of the right vertebral artery (black arrows) and its convergence at the inferior border of cervical level 5

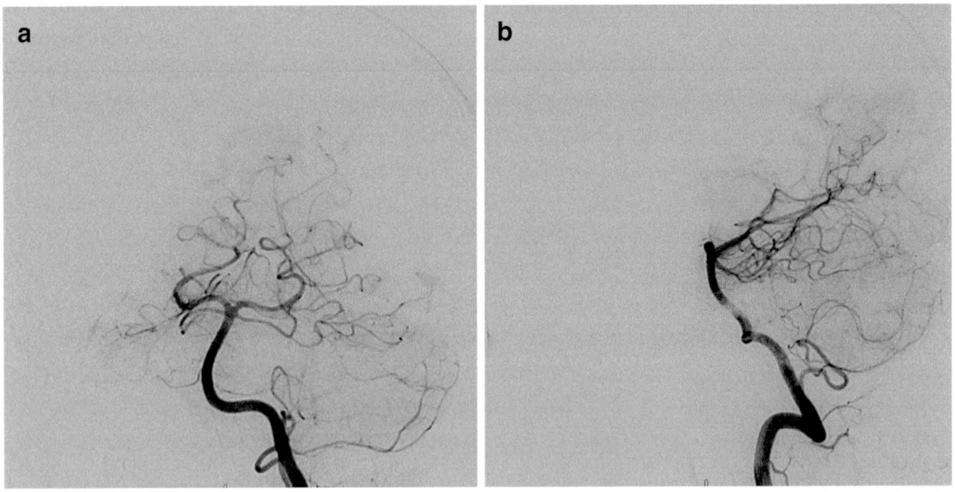

Fig. 3 DSA of the left vertebral artery in AP and lateral views (**a**, **b**), showing an extradural origin of the left PICA (black arrow)

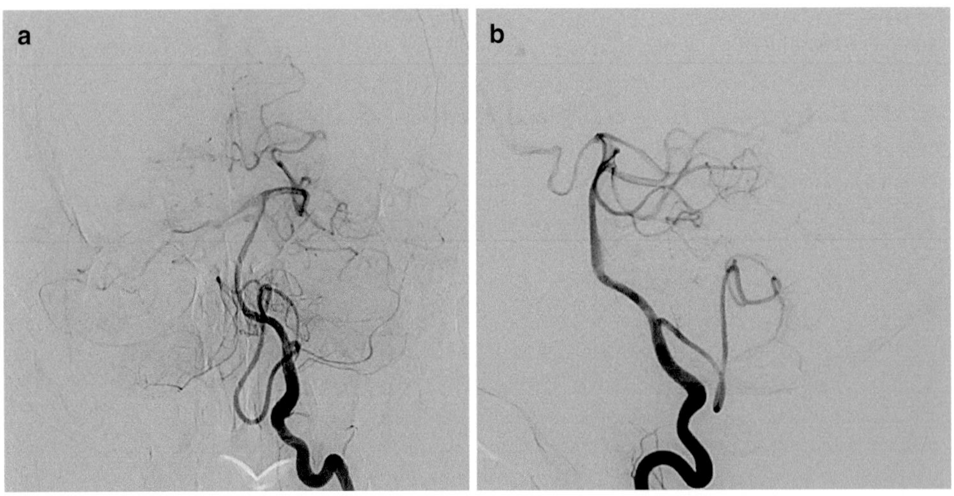

Fig. 4 DSA of the left vertebral artery in AP and lateral views (**a**, **b**), showing an intradural origin of the left PICA but descent of the caudal loop extending below the foramen magnum (black arrow)

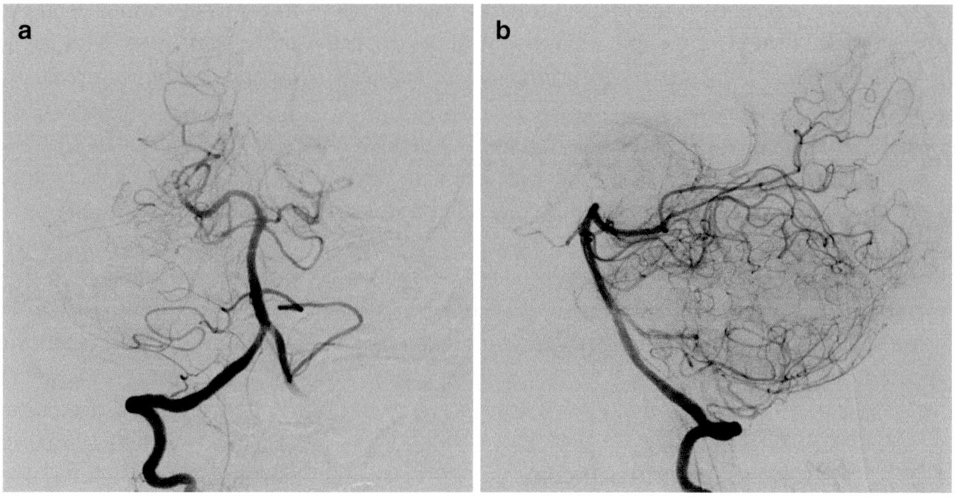

Fig. 5 DSA of the right vertebral artery in AP and lateral views (**a**, **b**), demonstrating bilateral AICA-PICA variants (black stars). The AP view also demonstrates a duplicated right superior cerebellar artery

3 Physiology of the Vertebrobasilar System

The vertebral arteries ensure adequate blood flow to the posterior brain under varying physiological demands. Autoregulatory mechanisms maintain constant perfusion despite fluctuations in systemic blood pressure. The collateral circulation provided by the Circle of Willis allows compensation in cases of partial occlusion or reduced flow.

3.1 Hemodynamics

The basilar artery represents the only large artery formed at the merger of two other large arteries. The vertebral arteries have equal diameters in 6–26% of cases, but the dominant VA is found more frequently on the left [20]. Accordingly, blood flow tends to be greater on the left compared to the right [2, 3, 20]. According to Amin-Hanjani et al. [2, 3], blood flow as measured on quantitative MRA is approximately 138 mL/min in the basilar artery, 100 mL/min in the left VA, and 88 mL/min in the right VA. Similar reference values have been shown using duplex ultrasonography with 105 mL/min flow volume in the left VA and 77 mL/min in the right VA [41]. The difference in diameters of each VA may contribute to the directionality and degree of curvature of the basilar artery [19].

3.2 Impact of Sex and Aging

In a study using duplex ultrasonography on healthy subjects, women were noted to have significantly smaller VA diameters, higher flow velocities, and lower resistance indices, compared to men [20].

The literature has shown conflicting results on the impact of age in VA flow volume on ultrasonography. Some have shown an age-dependent decrease in VA flow volume [14, 47], while others have not identified a correlation between VA flow volume and aging [20, 27, 39, 41]. In a study of 325 healthy subjects using quantitative MRA, total VA blood flow, in addition to total cerebral blood flow, declined with increasing age [2, 3]; this effect was seen in blood flow measurements of individual vessels also, including the basilar artery and left VA.

3.3 Impact of Movement

The impact on blood flow within the vertebral arteries during movement in the cervical spine has been debated, especially in healthy individuals. A meta-analysis of Doppler studies of VA blood flow velocity during cervical movement found that VA blood flow velocity could become compromised during contralateral rotation, in particular sustained full rotation of the cervical spine [31]. Mitchell reported that this effect was more prominent in patients, rather than in healthy participants. A more recent systematic review with broader inclusion criteria cast doubt on this, however Kranenburg et al. [25]. [25], notes that majority of the published studies on this topic ($n = 16$) did not find hemodynamic alterations with maximal rotation of the neck, while 8 of the studies did observe a decrease in flow during maximal rotation and 4 during maximal extension plus rotation.

4 Pathophysiology of Vertebral Artery Ischemia

4.1 Mechanisms of Ischemia

Ischemia in the vertebral arteries can result from multiple interconnected mechanisms:

- Embolism: Thrombi or atheromatous debris from proximal sites, such as the subclavian artery or heart, can occlude the vertebral arteries or their branches, leading to abrupt ischemic events.
- Thrombosis: Local clot formation occurs due to endothelial injury, hypercoagulability, or turbulence in blood flow, often exacerbated by underlying atherosclerotic disease.
- Hemodynamic Compromise: Severe stenosis, systemic hypotension, or steal phenomena may reduce perfusion, especially in the presence of hypoplastic or anomalous arteries.

4.2 Vertebrobasilar Insufficiency

Vertebrobasilar insufficiency (VBI) is characterized by transient ischemia affecting the posterior circulation. This condition arises from reduced VA flow due to atherosclerosis, dissection, or dynamic compression (e.g., during head rotation). Symptoms include episodic dizziness, vertigo, and ataxia, often precipitated by positional changes.

5 Diseases Affecting the Vertebral Arteries

5.1 Atherosclerosis

Approximately one-third of ischemic strokes arise from the posterior circulation, and a leading cause is vertebrobasilar atherosclerotic disease [1, 10, 37, 44]. Plaque deposition within the arterial wall leads to stenosis, and plaque rupture may trigger acute occlusion or embolization. Up to 30% of patients presenting with ischemic stroke or TIA may be found to have mild, moderate, or severe vertebrobasilar stenosis, and those with higher degree of stenosis carried a higher risk of recurrent stroke [37]. The risk of recurrent stroke due to vertebrobasilar stenosis over 50% has been previously estimated at 10–15% [34, 36, 44].

The VERiTAS study examined patients with symptomatic vertebrobasilar stenosis (≥50%) or occlusion and performed hemodynamic assessments with quantitative MRA [1]. Basilar artery flow was shown to decrease with worsening stenosis, with a threshold of ≥80% narrowing leading to a significant drop in blood flow; furthermore, tandem disease in one or both VA caused the basilar artery flow to significantly worsen [2, 3]. Additionally, in their study, a subgroup of patients vertebrobasilar disease and low blood flow, strict blood pressure control (BP goal <140/90) could increase the risk of stroke [4] (Fig. 6).

5.2 Dissection

Arterial dissections—a tear in the intimal layer of the artery—can occur within the vertebral arteries at a rate of 1–1.5 per 100,000. While cervical arterial dissections of the carotid and vertebral arteries are a rare cause of stroke overall, it is estimated to cause at least 20% of strokes in young adults [38]. Ischemia may be secondary to thromboembolism or stenosis, which might result from intramural hematoma formation [49]. Vessel narrowing may further contribute to ischemia via a disruption of normal blood flow, although blood flow does tend to improve over time [28, 29].

Precipitating events to the VA dissection are commonly described, such as cervical spine trauma (blunt or penetrating), chiropractic manipulation, coughing, or vomiting, and individuals with connective tissue diseases carry an elevated risk. Spontaneous cases tend to occur more frequently in

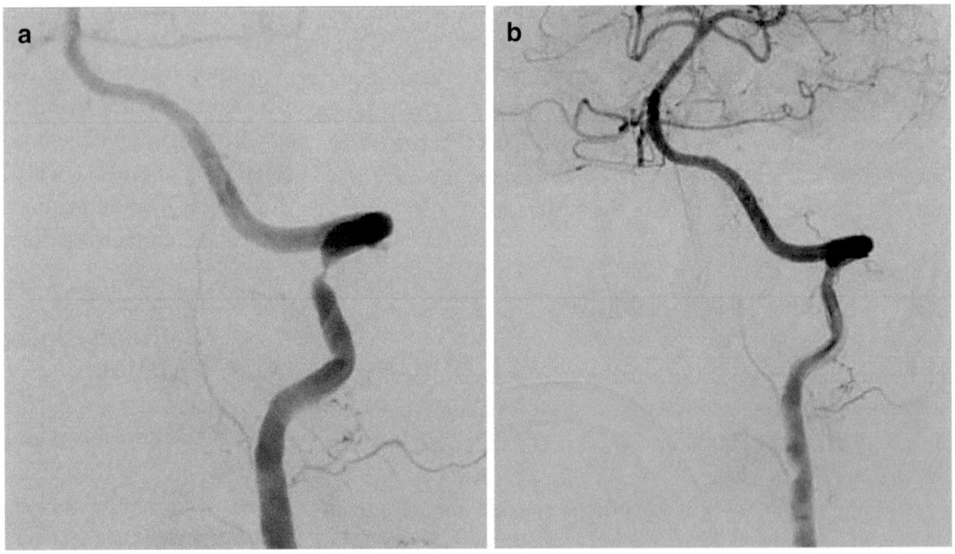

Fig. 6 DSA of the left vertebral artery in AP view, showing severe left V3 stenosis, pre- (**a**) and post-balloon angioplasty (**b**) (black arrows)

middle-aged females and have been associated with fibromuscular dysplasia or hypertension [11]. Following cervical non-penetrating trauma, the incidence of VA dissection reported in the literature varies from 24–46% [17, 48]. Most remain asymptomatic or present with vague musculoskeletal symptoms, such as neck pain or headache. However, when symptomatic, VA dissections can present with neurologic deficit, including lateral medullary syndrome (Wallenberg syndrome), or even be fatal.

5.3 Compression Syndromes

Positional compression of the vertebral arteries, often due to cervical spondylosis or dynamic stenosis during head movements, can transiently reduce blood flow and cause symptoms of VBI. This syndrome is often referred to as "bowhunter syndrome" or "rotary occlusion of the vertebral artery" and was first described in 1978 [43]. Head movements that have been associated with the reproduction of symptoms include contralateral rotation from the affected VA, rotation leading to bilateral VA compression, and neck flexion and extension [12]. Both the upper and subaxial cervical spine have been implicated, although C1–2 is the most frequently encountered single level: a literature review noted 54% of published cases were described at C3–7 with the remaining at C2 and above [40]. Diagnosis typically involves dynamic imaging techniques, such as catheter angiography both with and without the triggering head and neck position [12]. Treatment ranges from conservative management to cervical decompression or instrumentation [40] (Fig. 7).

5.4 Fibromuscular Dysplasia

Fibromuscular dysplasia (FMD) is a non-inflammatory, non-atherosclerotic arteriopathy that involves medium-sized vessels and can affect the vertebral arteries, particularly in younger women [22, 45]. It manifests as focal or multifocal stenosis with a classic "string of beads" appearance on angiography, although there is a spectrum in the degree to which the vessel may be impacted. FMD generally presents in multiple vessels, although a single vessel may be affected, and it can be found in multiple vascular beds. Although commonly asymptomatic and found incidentally, FMD places an individual at a higher risk of dissection, transient ischemic attack, ischemic stroke, and intracranial aneurysms [26, 45]. In a retrospective study, recurrent cerebrovascular events were observed in 23% of patients [26].

5.5 Arteritis

Inflammatory conditions affecting the vertebral arteries include giant cell arteritis (GCA) and Takayasu arteritis. Corticosteroids and immunosuppressive therapies are the mainstays of management, although in severe progressive cases, endovascular and surgical treatments have been described [21, 23, 32, 42].

Giant cell arteritis is an autoimmune vasculitis of the medium- and large vessels surrounding the head and can involve the extracranial vertebral arteries. GCA is primarily observed in older adults and may present with headache, vision loss, or ischemic stroke. Ischemic stroke occurs in

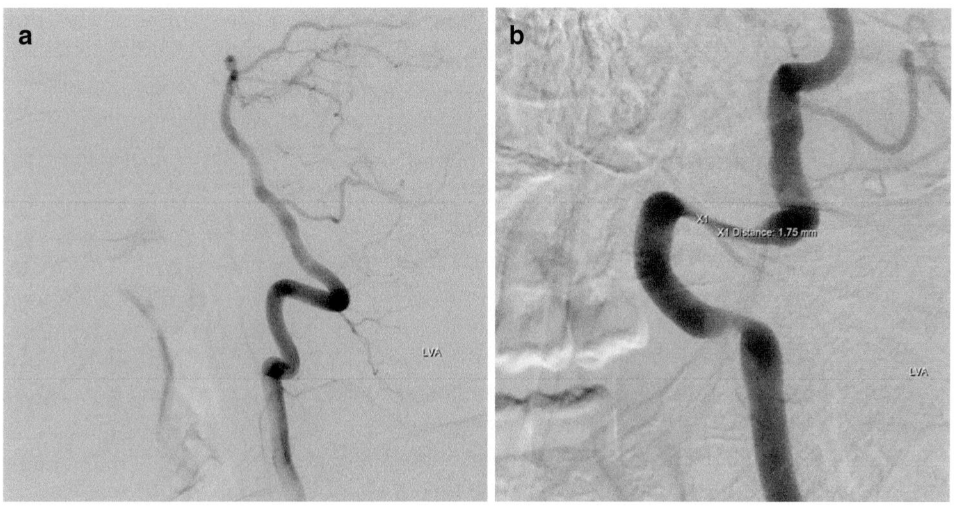

Fig. 7 Dynamic DSA of the left vertebral artery in lateral view with the head in neutral position (**a**) and then turned contralaterally (**b**)

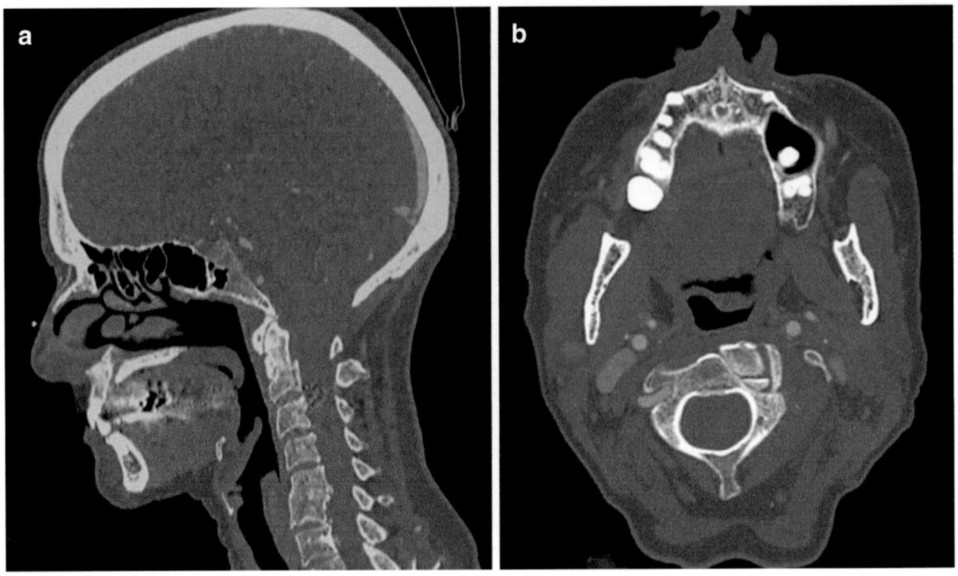

Fig. 8 CT angiography of the head and neck showing a C2 dens fracture (**a**) (black circle) with bony fragment in the transverse foramen and occlusion of the left vertebral artery (**b**) (black circle)

only 3–7% of GCA cases, with the majority in the vertebrobasilar territory [5, 13]. GCA can cause progressive, symptomatic vertebrobasilar stenosis with recurrent ischemic events [5, 32].

Takayasu arteritis is a rare, chronic large-vessel vasculitis predominantly affecting young women of Asian descent, leading to progressive stenosis or occlusion [21, 23, 42]. Takayasu arteritis characteristically affects the aorta but can also impact the coronary, pulmonary, carotid, and vertebral arteries. Approximately 20% of patients with Takayasu arteritis may develop ischemic stroke or transient ischemic attacks, mostly in the carotid territory but can occur in the vertebrobasilar distribution [30].

5.6 Trauma

Blunt or penetrating cervical trauma can damage the vertebral arteries, resulting in dissection (described above), thrombosis, or pseudoaneurysm formation (Fig. 8). The mechanism of extracranial cerebrovascular injury is typically blunt (89.5%) versus penetrating (10.5%), according to a study at a trauma center, and it more frequently involves the VA (66%) [9]. The Biffl scale for blunt injuries classifies the spectrum of disease as the following [6–8]:

- Grade I: minimal luminal irregularity or intramural hematoma/dissection with <25% narrowing
- Grade II: intramural hematoma/dissection with ≥25% narrowing, intraluminal thrombus, or raised intimal flap
- Grade III: pseudoaneurysm
- Grade IV: occlusion
- Grade V: transection with extravasation

Table 1 Expanded Denver criteria for screening trauma patients for vascular injury with CT angiography of the neck

Signs and symptoms	Risk factors
Potential arterial hemorrhage from the neck, nose, or mouth Cervical bruit in <50 years of age Expanding cervical hematoma Focal neurologic deficit Neurologic deficit incongruous with CT head findings Stroke on CT or MRI	High-energy transfer mechanism plus any of the following: Displaced midface fracture (Le fort II or III) Mandible fracture Complex skull, skull base, or occipital condyle fracture Severe traumatic brain injury with Glascow coma scale <6 Cervical spine fracture, subluxation, or ligamentous injury Near hanging with hypoxic-ischemic (anoxic) brain injury Clothesline type injury or seatbelt abrasion with significant swelling, pain, or altered mental status Traumatic brain injury with thoracic injuries Scalp degloving Thoracic vascular injuries Blunt cardiac rupture Upper rib fractures

While this grading system portends a higher stroke risk with increasing grade severity in carotid injury, the risk of stroke does not correlate with increasing VA injury [6–8]. According to Biffl et al., the incidence of posterior circulation stroke was 24%, and the BVI-attributable death rate was 8% [8]. Prompt imaging and possible intervention are critical to prevent ischemic complications.

The Denver criteria represent a set of conditions to screen individuals with trauma via CT angiography of the neck for vascular injury. It was initially published in 1999 and has been revised and expanded multiple times [6, 7, 18, 24]. Presently, the screening criteria include (Table 1):

6 Clinical Manifestations

Symptoms of VA ischemia often reflect dysfunction in the brainstem, cerebellum, occipital lobes, and/or thalamus. These may include:

- Dizziness or vertigo
- Ataxia
- Diplopia or vision loss
- Dysarthria and dysphagia
- Weakness or numbness

Posterior circulation strokes can thus result in complex presentations, an example of which is the lateral medullary syndrome (Wallenberg syndrome). Symptoms of lateral medullary syndrome include:

- Contralateral loss of pain and temperature sensation (spinothalamic tract)
- Ipsilateral loss of pain and temperature sensation (spinal trigeminal nucleus)
- Ipsilateral Horner syndrome, hiccups (sympathetic fibers)
- Palatal clonus (central trigeminal tract)
- Dysphagia, dysphonia, dysarthria, diminished gag reflex (nucleus ambiguus)
- Vertigo, mutlidirectional nystagmus, vomiting (inferior vestibular nucleus)
- Ipsilateral hemiataxia (inferior cerebellar peduncle)

Diagnostic imaging and management strategies will be described in other chapters.

7 Conclusion

The vertebral arteries are vital to the posterior cerebral circulation, and their compromise can result in significant morbidity. Early recognition and management of ischemic disorders affecting these arteries are essential to improving patient outcomes.

Declarations

Competing Interests The author(s) has no competing interests to declare that are relevant to the content of this manuscript.

Ethics Approval The author(s) declares that this manuscript does not include primary research with human participants.

References

1. Amin-Hanjani S, Rose-Finnell L, Richardson D, Ruland S, Pandey D, Thulborn KR, Liebeskind DS, Zipfel GJ, Elkind MS, Kramer J, Silver FL, Kasner SE, Caplan LR, Derdeyn CP, Gorelick PB, Charbel FT, VERiTAS Study Group. Vertebrobasilar flow evaluation and risk of transient Ischaemic attack and stroke study (VERiTAS): rationale and design. Int J Stroke. 2010 Dec;5(6):499–505.
2. Amin-Hanjani S, Du X, Pandey DK, Thulborn KR, Charbel FT. Effect of age and vascular anatomy on blood flow in major cerebral vessels. J Cereb Blood Flow Metab. 2015a Feb;35(2):312–8.
3. Amin-Hanjani S, Du X, Rose-Finnell L, Pandey DK, Richardson D, Thulborn KR, Elkind MS, Zipfel GJ, Liebeskind DS, Silver FL, Kasner SE, Aletich VA, Caplan LR, Derdeyn CP, Gorelick PB, Charbel FT, VERiTAS Study Group. Hemodynamic features of symptomatic Vertebrobasilar disease. Stroke. 2015b Jul;46(7):1850–6.
4. Amin-Hanjani S, Turan TN, Du X, Pandey DK, Rose-Finnell L, Richardson D, Elkind MS, Zipfel GJ, Liebeskind DS, Silver FL, Kasner SE, Gorelick PB, Charbel FT, Derdeyn CP, VERiTAS Study Group. Higher stroke risk with lower blood pressure in hemodynamic Vertebrobasilar disease: analysis from the VERiTAS study. J Stroke Cerebrovasc Dis. 2017 Feb;26(2):403–10.
5. Beuker C, Wankner MC, Thomas C, Strecker JK, Schmidt-Pogoda A, Schwindt W, Schulte-Mecklenbeck A, Gross C, Wiendl H, Barth PJ, Eckert B, Meinel TR, Arnold M, Schaumberg J, Krüger S, Deb-Chatterji M, Magnus T, Röther J, Minnerup J. Characterization of Extracranial Giant cell arteritis with intracranial involvement and its rapidly progressive subtype. Ann Neurol. 2021 Jul;90(1):118–29.
6. Biffl WL, Moore EE, Offner PJ, Brega KE, Franciose RJ, Elliott JP, Burch JM. Optimizing screening for blunt cerebrovascular injuries. Am J Surg. 1999a Dec;178(6):517–22.
7. Biffl WL, Moore EE, Offner PJ, Brega KE, Franciose RJ, Burch JM. Blunt carotid arterial injuries: implications of a new grading scale. J Trauma. 1999b Nov;47(5):845–53.
8. Biffl WL, Moore EE, Elliott JP, Ray C, Offner PJ, Franciose RJ, Brega KE, Burch JM. The devastating potential of blunt vertebral arterial injuries. Ann Surg. 2000 May;231(5):672–81.
9. Boggs HK, Kiang SC, Tran Z, Mukherjee K, Tomihama RT. Analysis of Extracranial cerebrovascular injuries: clinical predictors of management and outcomes. Ann Vasc Surg. 2024 Mar;100:53–9.
10. Caplan LR, Wityk RJ, Glass TA, Tapia J, Pazdera L, Chang HM, Teal P, Dashe JF, Chaves CJ, Breen JC, Vemmos K, Amarenco P, Tettenborn B, Leary M, Estol C, Dewitt LD, Pessin MS. New England Medical Center posterior circulation registry. Ann Neurol. 2004 Sep;56(3):389–98.
11. Chiras J, Marciano S, Vega Molina J, Touboul J, Poirier B, Bories J. Spontaneous dissecting aneurysm of the extracranial vertebral artery (20 cases). Neuroradiology. 1985;27(4):327–33.
12. Choi JW, Qiao Y, Mehta TI, Wilson JN, Torigoe TH, Tsappidi S, Jonathan Zhang Y, Brown SC, Hui FK, Abruzzo T. Safety and efficacy of dynamic catheter-directed cerebral digital subtraction angiography for diagnosis of bowhunter syndrome spectrum disorders: a systematic review of the literature. Interv Neuroradiol. 2024:15910199241236820.
13. de Boysson H, Liozon E, Larivière D, Samson M, Parienti JJ, Boutemy J, Maigné G, Martin Silva N, Ly K, Touzé E, Bonnotte B, Aouba A, Sacré K, Bienvenu B. Giant cell arteritis-related stroke: a retrospective multicenter case-control study. J Rheumatol. 2017 Mar;44(3):297–303.
14. Eicke BM, Tegeler CH. Ultrasonic quantitative flow volumetry of the carotid arteries: initial experience with a color flow M-mode system. Cerebrovasc Dis. 1995;5:145–9.
15. Elliott RE, Tanweer O. The prevalence of the ponticulus posticus (arcuate foramen) and its importance in the Goel-harms procedure: meta-analysis and review of the literature. World Neurosurg. 2014;82(1–2):e335–43.
16. Fine AD, Cardoso A, Rhoton AL Jr. Microsurgical anatomy of the extracranial-extradural origin of the posterior inferior cerebellar artery. J Neurosurg. 1999 Oct;91(4):645–52.
17. Friedman D, Flanders A, Thomas C, Millar W. Vertebral artery injury after acute cervical spine trauma: rate of occurrence as

detected by MR angiography and assessment of clinical consequences. AJR Am J Roentgenol. 1995;164(2):443–7. discussion 448–9
18. Geddes AE, Burlew CC, Wagenaar AE, Biffl WL, Johnson JL, Pieracci FM, et al. Expanded screening criteria for blunt cerebrovascular injury: a bigger impact than anticipated. Am J Surg. 2016;212(6):1167–74. https://doi.org/10.1016/j.amjsurg.2016.09.016. Epub 2016 Sep 29. PMID: 27751528.
19. Hong JM, Chung CS, Bang OY, Yong SW, Joo IS, Huh K. Vertebral artery dominance contributes to basilar artery curvature and peri-vertebrobasilar junctional infarcts. J Neurol Neurosurg Psychiatry. 2009;80(10):1087–92.
20. Jeng JS, Yip PK. Evaluation of vertebral artery hypoplasia and asymmetry by color-coded duplex ultrasonography. Ultrasound Med Biol. 2004 May;30(5):605–9.
21. Jung JH, Lee YH, Song GG, Jeong HS, Kim JH, Choi SJ. Endovascular versus open surgical intervention in patients with Takayasu's arteritis: a meta-analysis. Eur J Vasc Endovasc Surg. 2018;55(6):888–99.
22. Kesav P, Manesh Raj D, John S. Cerebrovascular fibromuscular dysplasia – a practical review. Vasc Health Risk Manag. 2023;19:543–56.
23. Kim YW, Kim DI, Park YJ, Yang SS, Lee GY, Kim DK, Kim K, Sung K. Surgical bypass vs endovascular treatment for patients with supra-aortic arterial occlusive disease due to Takayasu arteritis. J Vasc Surg. 2012 Mar;55(3):693–700.
24. Kim DY, Biffl W, Bokhari F, Brakenridge S, Chao E, Claridge JA, Fraser D, Jawa R, Kasotakis G, Kerwin A, Khan U, Kurek S, Plurad D, Robinson BRH, Stassen N, Tesoriero R, Yorkgitis B, Como JJ. Evaluation and management of blunt cerebrovascular injury: a practice management guideline from the eastern Association for the Surgery of trauma. J Trauma Acute Care Surg. 2020 Jun;88(6):875–87.
25. Kranenburg HAR, Tyer R, Schmitt M, Luijckx GJ, van der Schans C, Hutting N, Kerry R. Effects of head and neck positions on blood flow in the vertebral, internal carotid, and intracranial arteries: a systematic review. J Orthop Sports Phys Ther. 2019 Oct;49(10):688–97.
26. Kythreotou A, Weerakkody RA, Koysombat K, Marzouqa N, Baker DM. A retrospective cohort study of cerebrovascular fibromuscular dysplasia. Ann Vasc Surg. 2023 May;92:104–10.
27. Lovrencic-Huzjan A, Demarin V, Bosnar M, Vukovic V, PodobnikSarkanji S. Color Doppler flow imaging (CDFI) of the vertebral arteries—the normal appearance, normal values and the proposal for the standards. Coll Antropol. 1999;23:175–81.
28. McGuire LS, Ryoo J, Amin-Hanjani S, Atwal G, Charbel FT, Alaraj A. Impact of vessel narrowing and changes in blood flow on the development of ischemia in cervical arterial dissection using quantitative magnetic resonance angiography. Stroke Vasc Interv Neurol. https://doi.org/10.1161/SVIN.122.000372. Epub 23 Jul 2022.
29. McGuire LS, Ryoo J, Amin-Hanjani S, Atwal G, Charbel FT, Alaraj A. Natural history of cerebrovascular flow in cervical arterial dissection using quantitative magnetic resonance angiography. World Neurosurg. 2023 Jan;169:e114–20.
30. Mirouse A, Deltour S, Leclercq D, Squara PA, Pouchelon C, Comarmond C, Kahn JE, Benhamou Y, Mirault T, Mekinian A, Lambert M, Chiche L, Koskas F, Cluzel P, Redheuil A, Cacoub P, Biard L, Saadoun D, French Takayasu network. Cerebrovascular ischemic events in patients with Takayasu arteritis. Stroke. 2022 May;53(5):1550–7.
31. Mitchell J. Vertebral artery blood flow velocity changes associated with cervical spine rotation: a meta-analysis of the evidence with implications for professional practice. J Man Manip Ther. 2009;17(1):46–57.
32. Mizuta R, Saito S, Kawabe K, Seto H, Suzuki T, Sano M, Hasegawa H, Oishi M. Endovascular treatment for aggressive vertebrobasilar stenosis due to giant cell arteritis: illustrative cases. J Neurosurg Case Lessons. 2024;8(17):CASE24404.
33. Morris P. Chapter 14: The extradural vertebral arteries. In: Morris P, editor. Practical neuroangiography. 3rd ed. Philadelphia: Lippincott Williams and Wilkins; 2013. p. 195–205.
34. Moufarrij NA, Little JR, Furlan AJ, Leatherman JR, Williams GW. Basilar and distal vertebral artery stenosis: long-term follow-up. Stroke. 1986;17(5):938–42.
35. Osburn A. Chapter 9: The vertebrobasilar system. In: Osburn a, editor. Diagnostic cerebral angiography. 2nd ed. Philadelphia: Lippincott Williams and Wilkins; 1999. p. 173–94.
36. Qureshi AI, Ziai WC, Yahia AM, Mohammad Y, Sen S, Agarwal P, Zaidat OO, Suarez JI, Wityk RJ. Stroke-free survival and its determinants in patients with symptomatic vertebrobasilar stenosis: a multicenter study. Neurosurgery. 2003;52(5):1033–9. discussion 1039-40
37. Qureshi AI, Qureshi MH, Lien LM, Lee JT, Jeng JS, Hu CJ, Lai TC, Liu CH, Chen CH, Chen PL, Chen TS, Li JY, Lin CL, Hsu CY, Taiwan stroke registry investigators. One-year risk of recurrent stroke and death associated with Vertebrobasilar artery stenosis and occlusion in a cohort of 10,515 patients. Cerebrovasc Dis. 2019;47(1–2):40–7.
38. Schievink WI. Spontaneous dissection of the carotid and vertebral arteries. N Engl J Med. 2001;344(12):898–906.
39. Scho¨ning M, Walter J, Scheel P. Estimation of cerebral blood flow through color duplex sonography of the carotid and vertebral arteries in healthy adults. Stroke. 1994;25:17–22.
40. Schulz R, Donoso R, Weissman K. Rotational vertebral artery occlusion ("bow hunter syndrome"). Eur Spine J. 2021 Jun;30(6):1440–50.
41. Seidel E, Eicke BM, Tettenborn B, Krummenauer F. Reference values for vertebral artery flow volume by duplex sonography in young and elderly adults. Stroke. 1999 Dec;30(12):2692–6.
42. Shin J, Cho A, Han A, Ahn S, Min S, Min SK. Long-term patency and complications of endovascular and surgical revascularization for Takayasu arteritis. Vasc Specialist Int. 2024;40:46.
43. Sorensen BF. Bow hunter's stroke. Neurosurgery. 1978;2(3):259–61.
44. Prognosis of patients with symptomatic vertebral or basilar artery stenosis. The warfarin-aspirin symptomatic intracranial disease (WASID) Study Group. Stroke. 1998 Jul;29(7):1389–92.
45. Touzé E, Southerland AM, Boulanger M, Labeyrie PE, Azizi M, Bouatia-Naji N, Debette S, Gornik HL, Hussain SM, Jeunemaitre X, Joux J, Kirton A, Le Hello C, Majersik JJ, Mocco J, Persu A, Sharma A, Worrall BB, Olin JW, Plouin PF. Fibromuscular dysplasia and its neurologic manifestations: a systematic review. JAMA Neurol. 2019;76(2):217–26.
46. Trattnig S, Matula C, Karnel F, Daha K, Tschabitscher M, Schwaighofer B. Difficulties in examination of the origin of the vertebral artery by duplex and colour-coded Doppler sonography: anatomical considerations. Neuroradiology. 1993;35(4):296–9.
47. Westkott HP, Holsing K. US-based evaluation of hemodynamic parameters in the common carotid artery: a normogram trial. Radiology. 1997;205:353–9.
48. Willis BK, Greiner F, Orrison WW, Benzel EC. The incidence of vertebral artery injury after midcervical spine fracture or subluxation. Neurosurgery. 1994;34(3):435–41; discussion 441-2. https://doi.org/10.1227/00006123-199403000-00008. PMID: 8190218.
49. Yun SY, Heo YJ, Jeong HW, Baek JW, Choo HJ, Seo JH, Kim ST, Lee JY, Jin SC. Spontaneous intracranial vertebral artery dissection with acute ischemic stroke: high-resolution magnetic resonance imaging findings. Neuroradiol J. 2018 Jun;31(3):262–9.

EC-IC Bypass

Bin Xu and Yujun Liao

In modern neurosurgery, extracranial-intracranial (EC-IC) bypass plays a critically important role in the treatment of cerebral ischemia, despite ongoing advancements in medical therapies [1, 2]. Traditional medical management remains a double-edged sword, as it carries a potential risk of hemorrhage, particularly when surgical intervention is required in other organs. Additionally, it is worth noting that some patients exhibit tolerance or resistance to conventional antiplatelet drugs.

The history and technical details of EC-IC bypass have been thoroughly described in numerous manuscripts and textbooks [3–8]. EC-IC bypass can be categorized into high-flow, medium-flow, and low-flow bypass. Based on procedural purpose, it can also be classified into blood flow augmentation bypass and blood flow replacement bypass. Blood flow augmentation bypass is more common in clinical practice, particularly for conditions such as moyamoya vasculopathy (MMV) and chronic cerebral ischemia caused by atherosclerotic cerebrovascular disease (ACVD). Due to the chronic progression of cerebral ischemia, spontaneous collateral develops in the brain, involving both intracranial-intracranial (IC-IC) and EC-IC networks. As a result, the demand for blood flow is relatively lower, and a low-flow bypass is usually sufficient. Conversely, blood flow replacement bypass is utilized in cases involving complex aneurysms or skull base tumors that affect large arteries such as the internal carotid artery (ICA) or middle cerebral artery (MCA). This classification system, based on flow type and procedural purpose, is widely preferred by clinicians in daily practice.

In chronic cerebral ischemia, progressive stenosis or occlusion of a proximal artery leads to a gradual decrease in perfusion pressure within the distal territory. This results in a sequential reduction in blood flow velocity, and a decrease in cerebral blood flow (CBF), [9, 10]. Neurons become dysfunctional when CBF declines beyond a critical threshold, manifesting clinical ischemic symptoms. The mechanism of EC-IC bypass in treating chronic cerebral ischemia lies in restoring perfusion pressure through blood flow supplementation, thereby reversing prior hemodynamic impairment [11]. Consequently, precise evaluation of the hemodynamic status of each candidate for surgical intervention is crucial [12, 13]. The EC-IC bypass trial in 1985 demonstrated the failure of EC-IC bypass for ICA occlusion, primarily due to the lack of advanced radiological tools in the 1980s for precise hemodynamic assessment [14].

The pathophysiological mechanism of EC-IC bypass in treating complex aneurysms and skull base tumors is more straightforward. Although very rare with the current advance of endovascular techniques and advancement of surgical skills, but in very special cases, such as recurrent nasopharyngeal carcinoma involving the ICA wall, the affected arteries must be sacrificed, and because of insufficient collaterals - primarily from the anterior communicating, artery (Acom a.) or posterior communicating artery (Pcom a.). EC-IC bypass becomes essential to replace blood flow [15–18]. Given that the arteries are occluded in a single-stage procedure, this results in acute cerebral ischemia, leaving no time for collateral establishment. Thus, medium- or high-flow bypass are typically required in these circumstances. Even in cases whose natural collaterals exist, and a balloon occlusion test (BOT) indicates no signs of acute ischemia, there remains a potential risk of delayed ischemia [19, 20] or aneurysm formation within the collateral pathways, such as the Acom a. Under such circumstances, EC-IC bypass remains valuable.

B. Xu (✉) · Y. Liao
Department of Neurosurgery, Huashan Hospital, Fudan University, National Center for Neurological Disorders, Shanghai, China

V. Beneš, D. Netuka (eds.), *Surgical and Interventional Treatment of Cerebral Ischemia*,
https://doi.org/10.1007/978-3-032-08934-2_20

1 Flow Augmentation Bypass

1.1 Moyamoya Vasculopathy (MMV)

MMV is a chronic, occlusive cerebrovascular disorder of unknown etiology, characterized by bilateral stenosis or occlusion at the terminal portion of the ICA and the presence of abnormal "moyamoya" vessels at the base of the brain [21]. One of the hallmark pathophysiological features of MMV is its extraordinary capacity for angiogenesis.

At our institution, MMV is a common clinical entity, encompassing both ischemic and hemorrhagic subtypes. Notably, there are no strict boundaries between these two clinical presentations in practice. Patients with hemorrhagic onset are often more susceptible to subsequent cerebral ischemia, including transient ischemic attacks (TIAs) or infarctions. Conversely, patients with ischemic symptoms may exhibit microbleeds on MRI susceptibility-weighted imaging (SWI). Currently, there are no effective medical therapies for MMV, and surgical revascularization is advocated as the primary treatment once a diagnosis is confirmed [22, 23].

Direct bypass, represented by superficial temporal artery (STA)-to-MCA anastomosis, is widely employed in the management of MMV. Following end-to-side anastomosis between the STA and an MCA cortical branch, blood flow is immediately introduced into the MCA network. In cases where a sufficient pressure gradient exists between the donor and recipient arteries, and the MCA network remains relatively intact, bypass flow can retrogradely perfuse the M1-M2 junction and the entire MCA territory, which is defined as Matsushima Grade A revascularization (Table 1) [24]. Over time, the STA diameter may continue to increase, sometimes exceeding 3.5 mm, approaching the caliber of the ICA (Fig. 1a–d). In rare cases, our experience indicates that bypass flow may exceed 100 ml/min as early as 1 week postoperatively. This form of revascularization can rapidly improve cerebral perfusion pressure (CPP), reversing ischemia. Additionally, blood flow redistribution facilitated by the bypass can alleviate hemodynamic stress on deep collaterals, potentially resulting in the regression or disappearance of peripheral aneurysms. This mechanism is considered key in reducing hemorrhagic risk following surgery.

In contrast, indirect bypass, typified by encephalo-duro-myo-synangiosis (EDMS), promotes large-scale angiogenesis between the temporal muscle, dura mater, and cerebral cortex. This process facilitates the introduction of external carotid artery (ECA) blood flow to the cortical surface through these extracranial tissues. Theoretically, this approach effectively addresses ischemia in the superficial brain regions. In pediatric patients [25–27] and adults with active angiogenesis, indirect bypass is both effective and safe, yielding satisfactory clinical and radiological outcomes (Fig. 1e–h).

Table 1 Matsushima grading system

Grade	Description
A	Area perfused by revascularization > 2/3 MCA territory
B	Area perfused by revascularization between 1/3 and 2/3 MCA territory
C	rea perfused by revascularization < 1/3 MCA territory

1.1.1 Routine Procedure for MMV in Author's Department

STA-MCA anastomosis combined with EDMS, is set as routine procedure for MMV in authors' department [28]. The patient is placed in the supine position, with the head rotated to the contralateral side at around 60°. A skin incision is curved posteriorly to the parietal branch of the STA and extends upward to the anterior by 1.5 cm above the superior temporal line. The temporal muscle is incised along the margin of the flap and separated from the temporal bone. A frontal-temporal craniotomy was performed. The dura is incised in a radial fashion for preservation of the middle meningeal artery (MMA) and its main branches. After hemostasis, the dura matter is flipped over for attachment of cortex. The MCA (M4) branch with a compatible diameter in the exposure is chosen as recipient. The parietal branch of the STA is dissected from the scalp flap. After penetration through the temporalis muscle, it is temporary clipped, dissected in the distal end, and irrigated with heparinized saline, prepared for anastomosis. We use two slightly curved mini-clips to temporarily occlude the recipient artery without sacrificing any perforators. The wall of the M4 recipient is cut open and flushed. The dissected STA is anastomosed with the M4 recipient in an end-to-side fashion using a 10–0 nylon suture. In closure, the margin of the temporal muscle was sutured with the dura mater at the fold of the flip-over and fixed to the bone window. The bone flap was trimmed into a compatible shape followed by reduction and fixation without compressing the STA, the inferior edge of the bone flap needed to be elevated a little to reduce the space-occupying effect of temporal muscle (Fig. 2).

1.1.2 Selection of Recipient Artery: Morphological Considerations

Traditionally, the angularis gyri artery is favorable recipient artery due to its relatively straight course, fewer branches, and size similarity to the STA. However, available options are often more limited than anticipated in MMV patients (Fig. 3a, b). In addition, cortical branch around subacute or old infarctions should be avoided (Fig. 3c, d). The spatial relationship between donor and recipient arteries should be optimized to facilitate the anastomosis process. This can help reduce the duration of temporal occlusion and improve long-term patency rate.

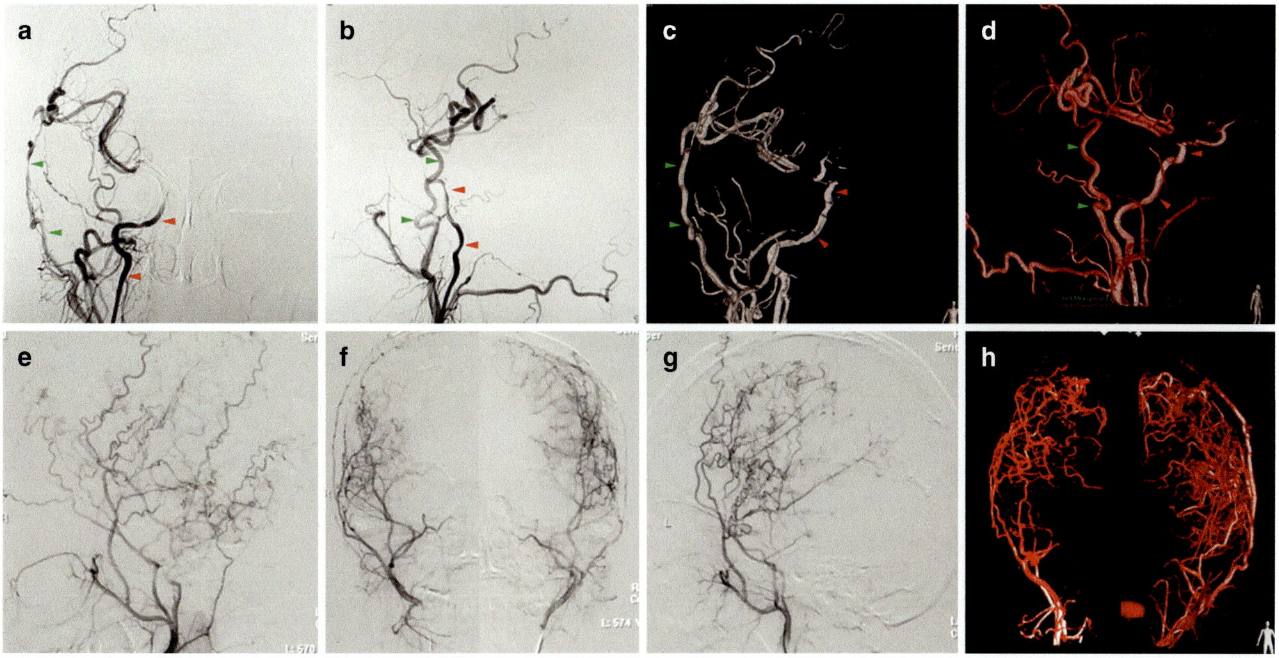

Fig. 1 Angiographic follow-up of direct and indirect bypass for MMV. (**a**, **b**), digital substructional angiography (DSA) demonstrated STA-MCA bypass flow retrogradely perfuse the M1-M2 junction and entire MCA territory (green arrowhead-STA, red arrowhead-ICA). (**c**, **d**), 3D-DSA demonstrated growing of STA with a diameter around 3.5 mm (green arrowhead-STA, red arrowhead-ICA). (**e**, **f**, **g**, and **h**), DSA follow-up in a 12-yo girl indicated well-established indirect anastomosis in bilateral MCA territory, mainly in superficial brain tissues. I, 3D-DSA in a 15-yo boy demonstrated Matsushima grade A revascularization bilaterally

Color and vessel wall condition of the recipient artery are critical factors. A pink cortical branch is considered the most suitable candidate, because of its relatively healthier vessel wall (Fig. 3e). While a pink-white or white cortical branch usually represents a feeding artery to distal infarcted brain region or a poorly preserved vessel network. The pathological change in vessel wall such as dissections, may significantly complicate the anastomosis procedure (Fig. 3d, e). In contrast, a dark red cortical branch is often indicative of congestion in extremely small perforators, with thin and fragile vessel walls. Such vessels pose not only technical challenges, but also a higher risk of postoperative rupture and long-term aneurysm formation at the anastomosis site (Fig. 3f).

Donor-to-recipient diameter ratio is ideally between 1.0 and 1.5. If the STA is too small, with a ratio below 0.8, it is advisable to shorten the STA to reduce resistance. Conversely, if the STA is significantly larger, with a ratio exceeding 2.0, dissecting a longer STA may be reasonable to increase resistance (Fig. 3g), reduce the pressure gradient between the donor and recipient arteries, and perform the anastomosis before a bifurcation (Fig. 3f). Narrowing of STA by absorbable sutures maybe an option. These methods aim to prevent hyperperfusion (Fig. 3h).

1.1.3 Vessel Network, Blood Flow Direction and Pressure Gradient in MCA Territory

Distal vessel networks are also critical. Cortical branches with more extensive branching and well-developed distal vessel networks are better suited to distribute STA blood flow rapidly and effectively to ischemic brain, which is also beneficial to the positive remodeling of bypass (Fig. 4a). While poor vessel network is commonly seen in MMV (Fig. 4b, c). It'll induce localized hyperperfusion while addressing hemispheric hypoperfusion, which is bad for prognosis of bypass patency (Fig. 4d). As mentioned before, anastomosis to a cortical branch with bifurcation maybe a reasonable solution (Fig. 4e).

Furthermore, from a hemodynamic perspective, the recipient artery should be selected to maximize the pressure gradient (δP) between donor and recipient arteries. Simply put, a cortical branch located downstream of the intracranial origin blood flow would be a better choice. However, in MMV patients, the origin blood flow is not always physiological due to presence of various collateral pathways. In the author's case series, retrograde flow in MCA territory in DSA images was observed in approximately half of MMV cases, where blood flows from the cortex toward the sylvian fissure

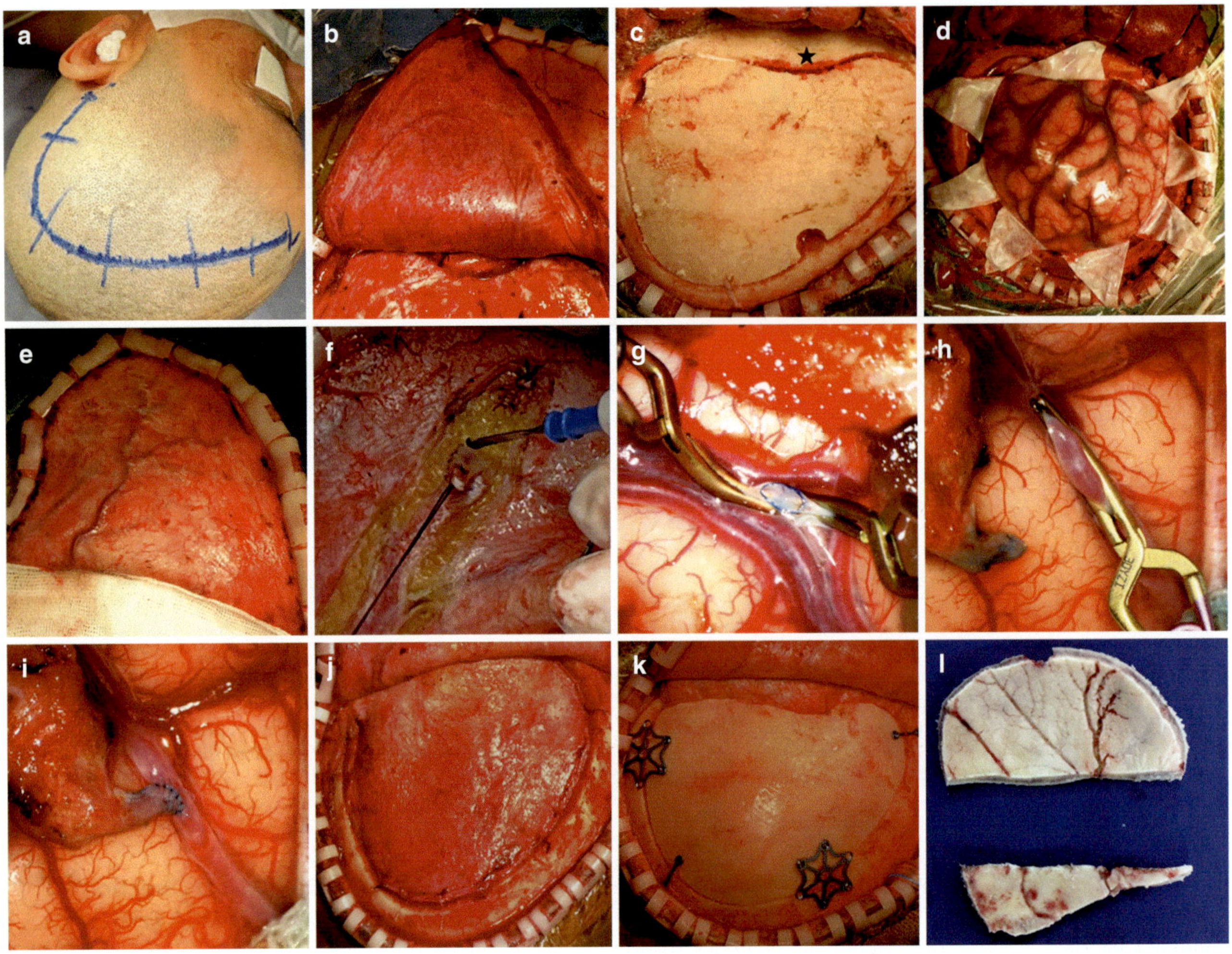

Fig. 2 Combined revascularization for MMV. (**a**), enlarged pterional skin incision covering large area of fronto-temporal lobe. (**b**), temporal muscle is incised along the margin of the flap and separated from the temporal bone. (**c**), bone flap. (**d**), dura is incised in a radial fashion, prepared to be flipped over for attachment to cortex (no spontaneous collaterals from MMA or main branches needed to be preserved in this area). (**e**, **f**), exposure, and dissection of STA from the inner surface of skin flap. (**g**), temporal occlusion of recipient artery on cortex with two mini-clips applied face-to-face. Ostia made on the recipient with micro scissor. (**h**), temporal occlusion with only one mini-clip. (**i**), stoma. (**j**), closure of temporal muscle for encephalo-myosynangiosis. (**k**), fixation of bone flap. (**l**), the lower part of bone flap is usually cut to relief compression to temporal muscle

(Fig. 4f–h). Identifying the blood flow direction is critical for distinguishing upstream and downstream arteries, as previously mentioned. Based on that, aligning the donor and recipient blood flow in the same direction is advisable to reduce flow competition and energy loss (Fig. 4i-l).

To verify the blood flow direction and further investigate pressure gradient, we have developed a method for intraluminal direct measurement of cortical branch. Conventional endovascular routes using pressure guidewires are impossible, as the guidewires cannot reach the cortical vessels to obtain pressure data. Instead, we employ a method of inserting the pressure housing probe into the harvested donor vessel side branch and measuring the pressure in the bypass conduits after completing the anastomosis. This deliberate approach allowed for accurately assessing the MAP and pressure gradients (δP) of donor, cortical recipient artery and different pathways. While the main donor artery was clipped, all obtained pressure data was referred to as pre-bypass baseline pressure. Conversely, when the main donor artery clip was removed, the pressure was referred to as post-bypass pressure (Fig. 5). A comprehensive elaboration of the entire measurement procedure is available in our recent publication [29].

1.1.4 Tailored EC-IC Bypass in Late-Stage MMV

Spontaneous collaterals are frequently observed in MMV patients, especially in Suzuki stage 5 and 6 (late-stage). The presence of collaterals is a reassuring sign of the brain's self-repair mechanism, but they also simultaneously pose significant technical challenges for EC-IC bypass surgery. These

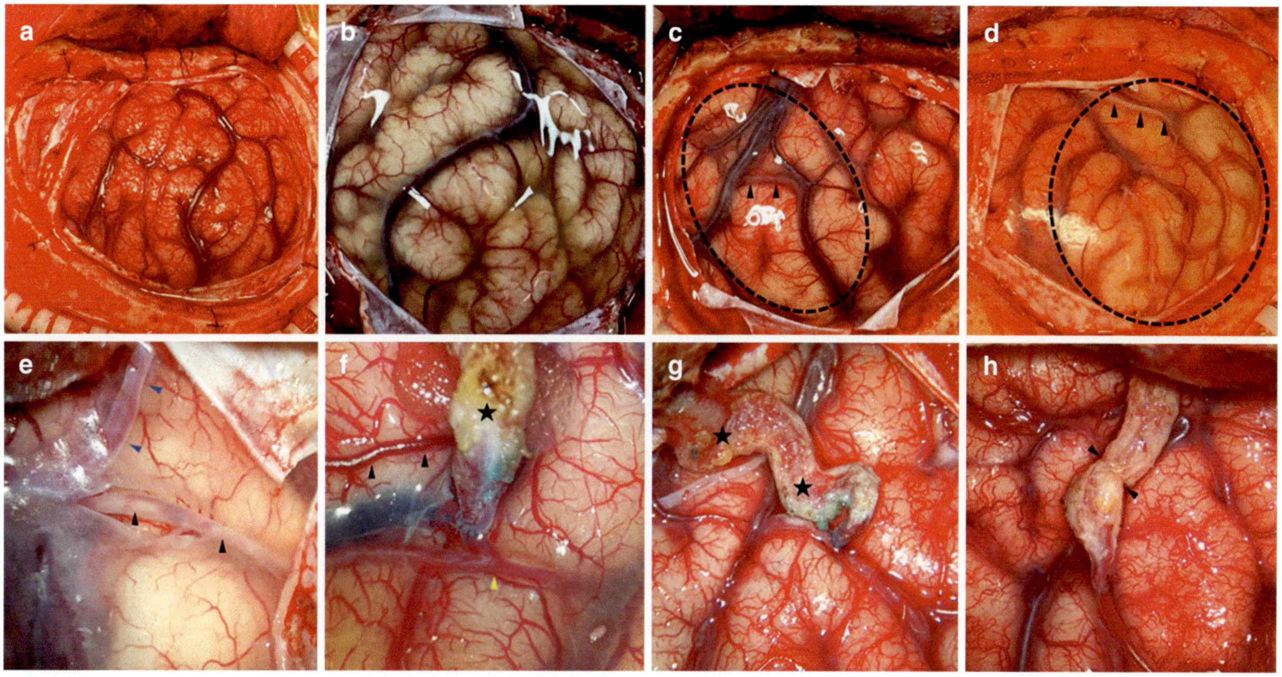

Fig. 3 Selection of recipient artery. (**a**), commonly seen cortex in MMV patients with congestion of small branches. (**b**), atrophic cortex with misery perfusion. (**c**), cortical branch (black arrowhead) within subacute infarcted gyrus (black dotted circle) should not be recipient artery, because of potential hemorrhagic risk. (**d**), subacute infarcted gyrus (black dotted circle) with pin-white partially thrombosed or occluded cortical branch (black arrowhead). (**e**), pink healthy (blue arrowheads) and pink-white thrombosed (black arrowheads) cortical branch. (**f**), a thick STA (black star) was anastomosed to a thin artery proximal to a bifurcation (yellow arrowhead). A dark red cortical branch (black arrowhead) nearby unsuited to be recipient. (**g**), long and tortuous STA (black stars) to increase resistance. (**h**), ligation of STA (black arrowhead) with absorbable suture for blood flow control

collateral vessels often develop in the pterional region, making them particularly vulnerable to injury during surgical procedure.

First is to recognize commonly seen collaterals. MMA is the most common source of spontaneous collaterals. Cutaneous arteries, such as the STA, occipital artery (OA), and, less commonly, the posterior auricular artery (PAA), can also serve as collateral sources, especially in patients with a prior history of cranial surgeries, such as cerebral hematoma evacuation or external ventricular drainage. To this end, super-selective ECA angiography is strongly recommended to acquire detailed information regarding collateral vessel distribution. Perfusion imaging can further aid in identifying ischemic regions most in need of revascularization.

The procedure must be meticulously tailored to the patient's individual vascular anatomy, encompass all critical surgical steps [30]. Skin incision should be adjusted forward or backward to avoid injury if collateral existed. In patients with severe ischemia in the territories of bilateral ACA, bilateral frontal lobe should be targeted so a coronal incision is a best option (Fig. 6).

The anterior branch of MMA provides collateral blood flow to the ACA territory through the falx cerebri, sometimes on the convexity. Preoperative localization of MMA is of paramount importance. Usually, the course of MMA is approximately parallel to that of STA parietal branch, by 2–3 cm anteriorly (Fig. 7a, b). A deep groove in the cranium compressed by the hypertrophic MMA could be identified clearly under X-ray (Fig. 7c), sometimes even from the outside of cranium during procedure (Fig. 7d). The relationship between MMA groove and coronal suture is of great help in localizing MMA in craniotomy (Fig. 7d). In case with hypertrophic MMA, divided bone flaps maybe a best option for preservation of collaterals, with bone bridge covering MMA (Fig. 7e, f). Hemostasis of middle meningeal vein poses potential risk of injury to accompany artery (Fig. 7g, h). It's proved to be an effective and safe method to suture the dura margin into a shape of barrel with the inner surface facing outside, containing meningeal arteries, accompanying veins, and some gelatin sponge, which is named as "Spring roll"-a traditional cuisine in China-by the author (Fig. 7i).

1.2 ACVD

Atherosclerotic occlusion of ICA and MCA (M1 or M2 segments) is common in the author's department. While many

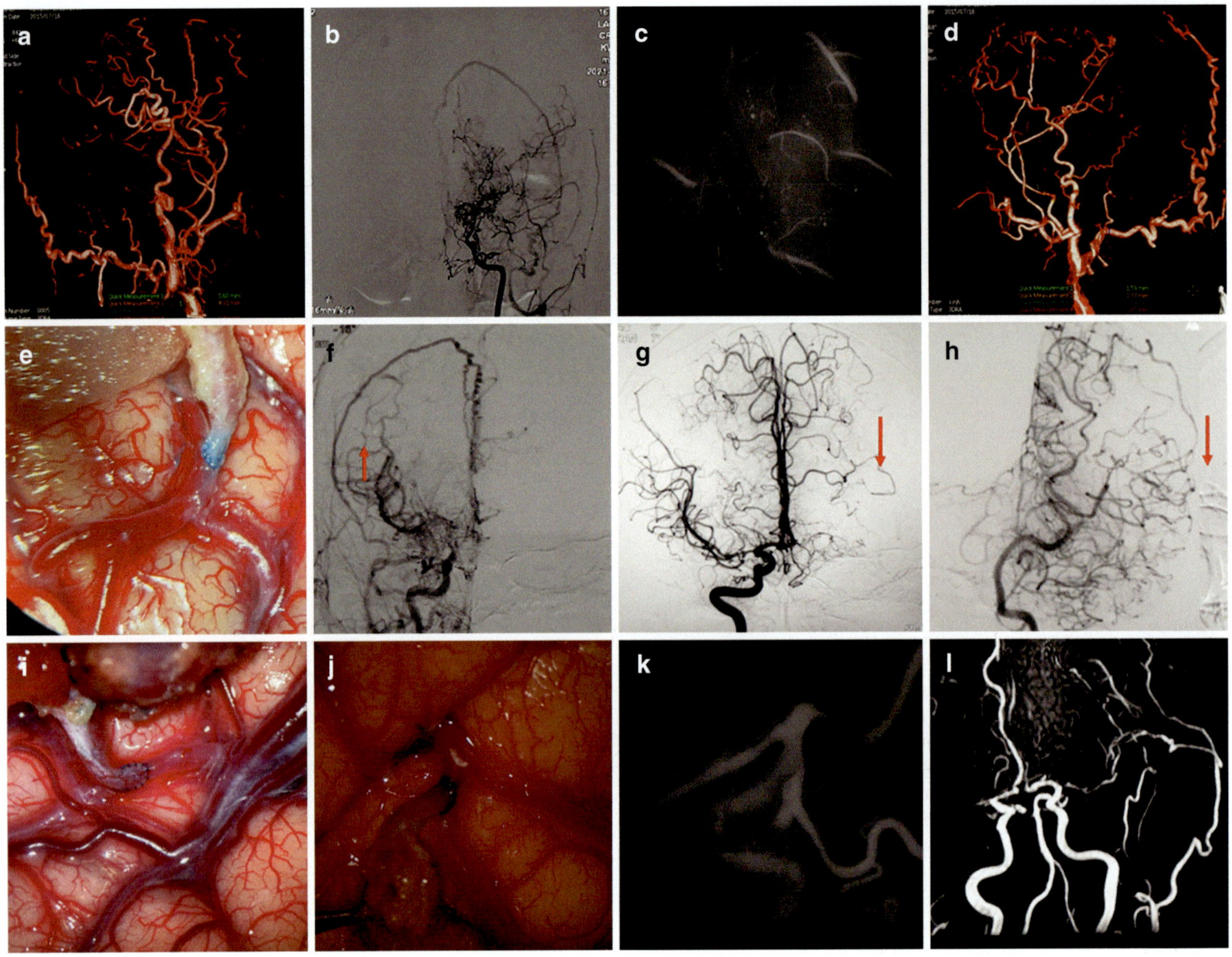

Fig. 4 MCA vessel network. (**a**), 3D-DSA showed an enlarged bypass with well-preserved MCA vessel network in an MMV patient. (**b**), Left ICA angiogram AP view demonstrated typical moyamoya change with atrophy MCA vessel network. (**c**), ICG videography showed atrophic cortical branches. (**d**), 3D-DSA showed an atrophic bypass (STA parietal branch) due to poor MCA vessel network in the same patient as figure a. (**e**), anastomose to a cortical branch with bifurcation maybe a reasonable solution. (**f**), right ICA angiogram AP view demonstrated antegrade flow (red arrow) in MCA territory despite of severe stenotic-occlude change in M1 segment. (**g**, **h**), angiogram demonstrated retrograde flow (red arrow) in MCA territory from anterior cerebral artery (ACA) and posterior cerebral artery (PCA). (**i**), retrograde bypass toward the sylvian fissure, aligning the donor and recipient blood flow in the same direction. (**j**, **k**), retrograde bypass to proximal of recipient artery in a patient with retrograde flow in MCA territory (under microscope and indocyanine green (ICG) videography). (**l**), postoperative CT angiogram confirmed the patency of bypass perfusing M1-2 junction retrogradely

randomized controlled trials (RCTs) have indicated no significant benefit of EC-IC bypass compared to medical therapy alone [31, 32], in highly selective cases with hemodynamic impairment unresponsive to maximal medical therapy, EC-IC bypass may remain the only viable option, especially treated in high-flow centers by experiential neurosurgeons [33]. Since indirect bypass could not promote adequate pial collateral in these patients [34], keyhole bypass is proved to be a better option [35, 36]. Due to its minimally invasive nature, reduced surgical trauma, and faster postoperative recovery, this technique is significantly more acceptable to patients compared to traditional large-incision EC-IC bypass.

To achieve satisfactory outcomes in bypass surgery, two critical factors must be considered: an adequate pressure gradient (ΔP) and a well-preserved vascular network. Inspired by these principles, we have also applied the keyhole bypass to selected MMV cases (Fig. 8). Our initial findings confirm that the procedure is both safe and effective. However, it is important to emphasize that this approach is suitable only for MMV patients with relatively intact MCA networks, as these cases provide the necessary hemodynamic foundation for successful bypass.

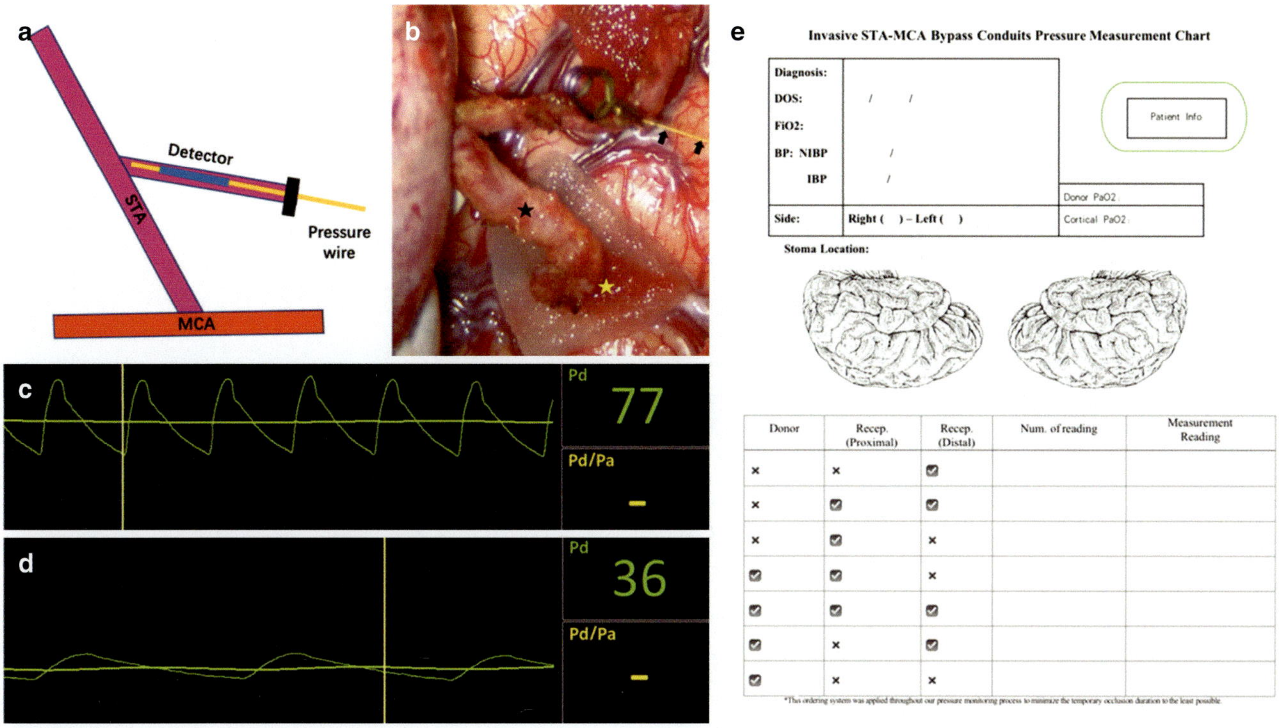

Fig. 5 Real-time pressure measurement. (**a**), Schematic drawing of pressure measurement in STA and cortical recipient artery. (**b**), a pressure wire (black arrows) was inserted to a side branch of STA (black star) after completing the stoma (yellow star). (**c**, **d**), pressure numerical value and wave form of STA and recipient artery. Notice the different wave form of intra- and extra-cranial arteries. (**e**), record chart for pressure measurement

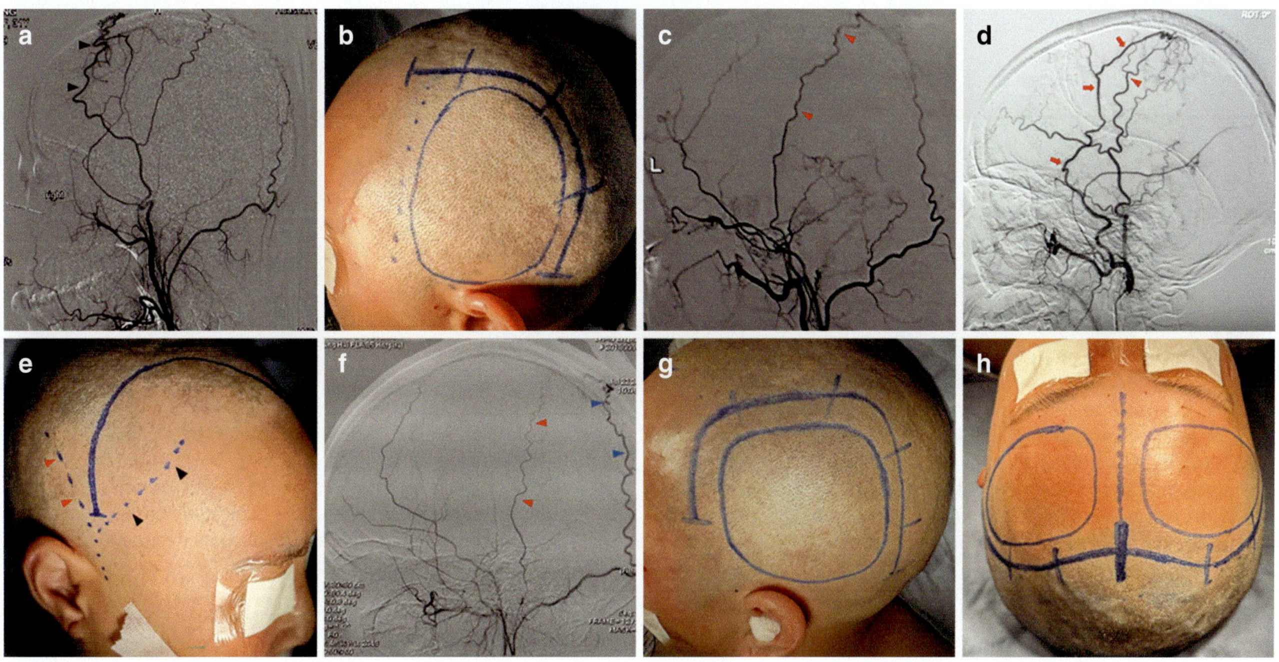

Fig. 6 Tailored adjustment of skin incision in late-stage MMV. (**a**), ECA angiogram lateral view demonstrated spontaneous collaterals from frontal branch of STA (f-STA, black arrowheads). (**b**), back warded incision to preserve f-STA. (**c**, **d**), ECA angiogram lateral view demonstrated spontaneous collaterals from parietal branch of STA (p-STA, red arrowheads), with a final anastomosed channel with blood flow from OA(c) and MMA (d, red arrows). (**e**), forwarded incision to preserve the p-STA. (**f**), ECA angiogram lateral view revealed an atrophic p-STA in a 38-yo female, and PAA becomes an substitute. (**g**), a horseshoe incision containing PAA was adopted. (**h**), a coronal incision for the revascularization of bifrontal lobe, in ACA territory

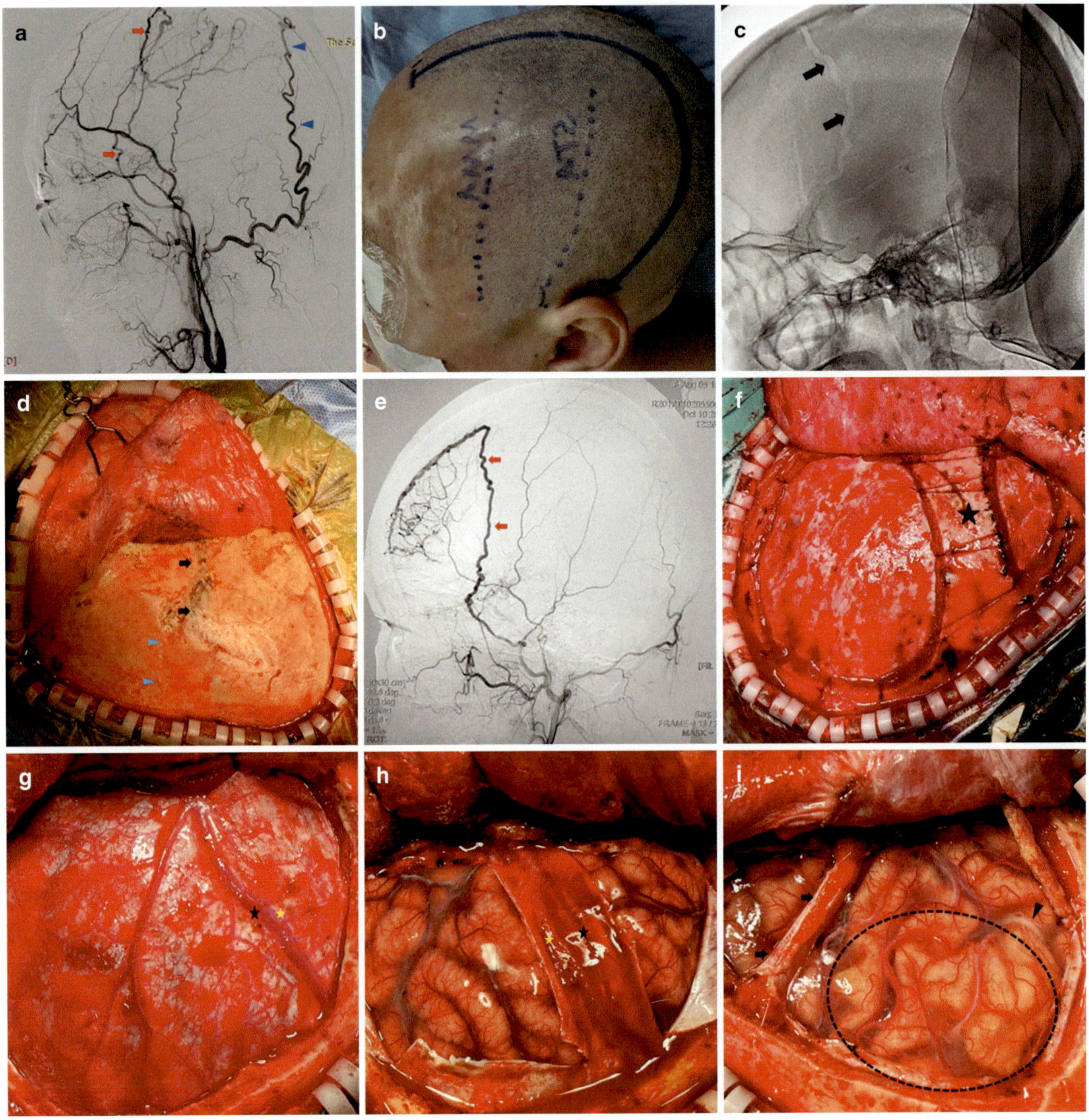

Fig. 7 Tailored process of dura and MMA branches in late-stage MMV. (**a**), ECA angiogram lateral view demonstrated spontaneous collaterals from MMA (red arrows) and occipital artery (blue arrowheads), the MMA is parallel to p-STA, about 2 cm anteriorly. (**b**), preoperative localization of MMA course's projections on the skin. (**c**, **d**), a deep MMA groove (black arrows) shown clearly under X-ray image (**c**), and identified from outer surface of skull, and coronal fissure (blue arrowheads). (**e**), hypertrophic MMA (red arrows). (**f**) divided bone flaps with bone bridge (black star) covering MMA. (**g**, **h**), hemostasis of meningeal vein (black star) accompanied by MMA (yellow star) is difficult. (**i**), "Spring roll" (black arrows) for the hemostasis of meningeal vein, note the subacute infarcted gyrus (black dotted circle) with white occluded cortical branch (black arrowhead)

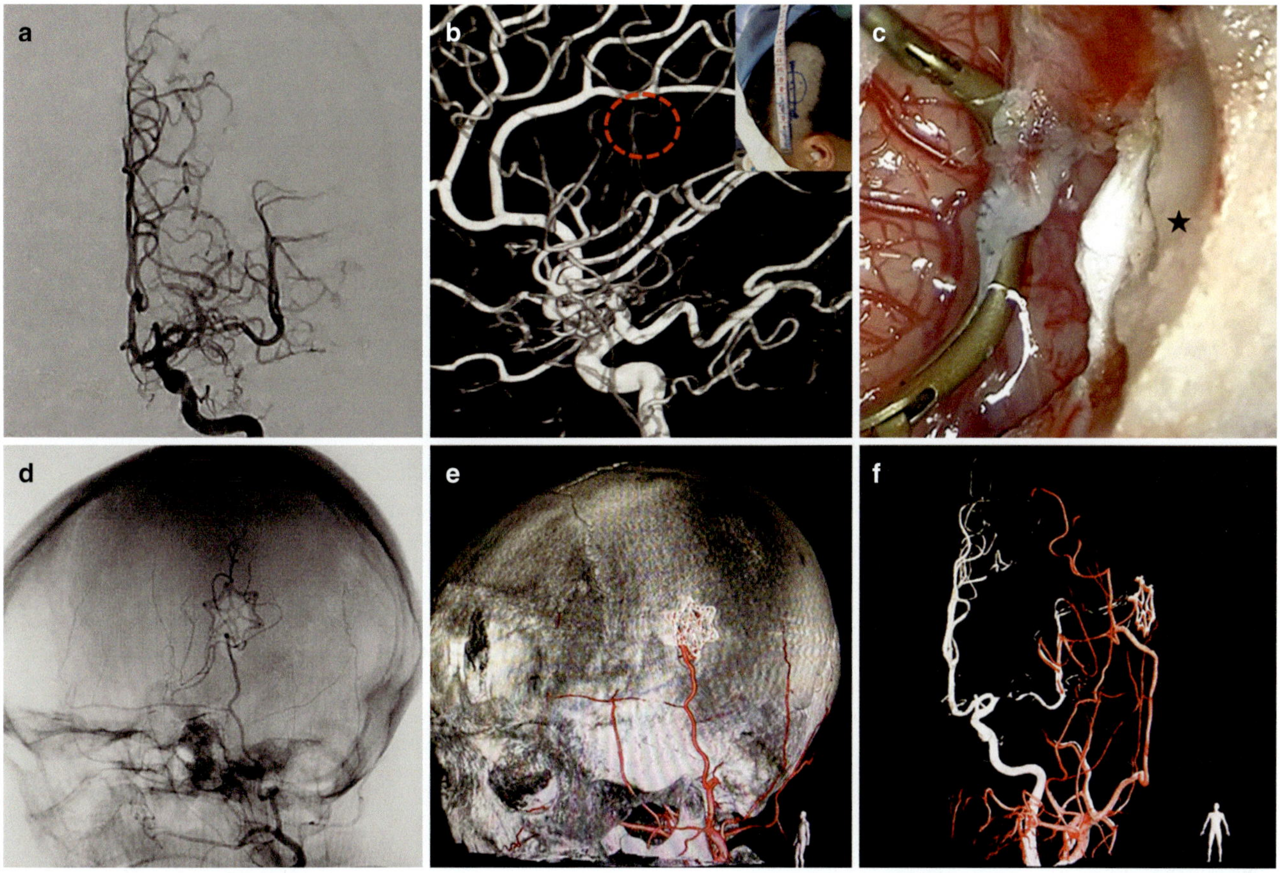

Fig. 8 Keyhole bypass and follow-up. (**a**), ICA angiogram AP view indicated moyamoya change with antegrade blood flow and relatively intact MCA vessel network. (**b**), donor, and recipient arteries were identified on 3D-DSA (red circle), upper right showed the skin incision. (**c**), stoma within a keyhole with a diameter of 2 cm, cranium (black star). (**d**, **e**), ECA angiogram lateral view confirmed the patency of bypass in a precise keyhole. (**f**), fused 3D-DSA demonstrated the blood flow redistribution between ECA (red) and ICA (white)

1.2.1 Different Collateral Pathways in ICA and MCA Occlusion

It is essential to recognize that IC-IC collateral pathways differ significantly between ICA occlusion and MCA occlusion, as they are driven by distinct pathophysiological mechanisms. In ICA Occlusion, the Acom a. and Pcom a. serve as the primary collateral pathways. These collaterals maintain a normal anterograde blood flow direction within the MCA territory, originating from the Sylvian fissure and perfusing the frontal and temporal lobes. While in MCA occlusion, in contrast, pial anastomoses from the ACA and PCA form the main collateral pathways. These anastomoses result in a retrograde blood flow direction, which is typically opposite to that observed in ICA occlusion. Recognizing these differences in blood flow direction is essential for identifying the optimal recipient artery and determining the flow direction of the STA during bypass.

1.2.2 Cortical Perfusion Pressure

Interestingly, we observed a significantly reduced cortical perfusion pressure in a patient with ICA occlusion, despite DSA showing robust compensation via the Acom a. and Pcom a. with no evident delay in contrast filling. This phenomenon suggests that perfusion pressure may be a more reliable indicator than the BOT for predicting delayed ischemia.

2 Flow Replacement Bypass

Traditionally, ECA-saphenous vein (SV)-MCA bypass is defined as high-flow bypass, ECA-radial artery (RA)-MCA is medium, and STA-MCA bypass is low-flow bypass However, as previously noted, we have observed STA diameters exceeding 3.5 mm in long-term follow-up, delivering blood flow exceeding 100 ml/min under adequate pressure gradients (ΔP) and favorable vessel networks. This observation challenges the conventional "low-flow" classification of STA-MCA bypass. A more appropriate term may be "dynamic flow bypass," which better reflects its adaptability based on individual hemodynamic conditions.

We can design tailored bypass procedures by combining existing techniques to meet the unique needs of each patient. In the first author's experience, ECA-RA-MCA combined with STA-MCA bypass holds the potential to provide high blood flow while avoiding the disadvantages of vein grafts. STA trunk-RA-MCA bypass is capable to deliver medium blood flow to the brain. Double-barreled STA-MCA bypass is enough to perfuse entire MCA territory, achieving medium-flow bypass as per traditional definitions (Table 2, Fig. 9).

2.1 Innovative Flow-Demand Based Classification and Surgical Strategy

A critical question is how to select appropriate bypass procedure for each patient. The first author has developed a straightforward and effective strategy for blood flow replacement in complex cases. Preoperative DSA imaging plays a pivotal role in determining the perfusion area and guiding surgical planning. When the affected artery perfuses bilateral ACAs and the ipsilateral MCA, the blood flow demand is defined as high level. When the perfusion area includes the ipsilateral ACA and MCA, the demand is medium. And the

Table 2 Blood flow delivered by different procedures

	Traditional	Newly combined
High-Flow	ECA-SV-MCA bypass	ECA-RA-MCA bypass + STA (1/2)
Medium-Flow	ECA-RA-MCA bypass	STA trunk-RA-MCA bypass Or STA (2)
Low-Flow	STA-MCA bypass (STA)	–

STA 1/2, STA-MCA single- or double-barrel bypass. STA (2), STA-MCA double-barrel bypass

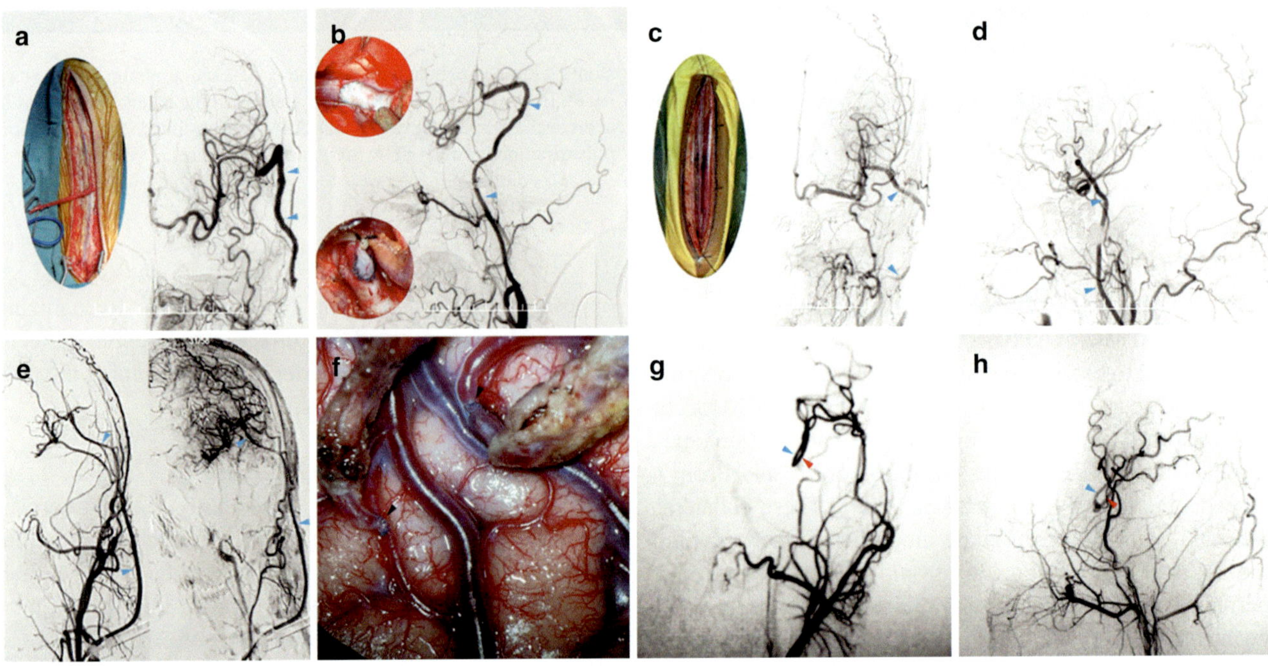

Fig. 9 Different types of bypasses and efficacy. (**a**, **b**), ECA-SV-MCA bypass (blue arrowheads) perfusing ipsilateral MCA and ACA territory, AP view and dissection of saphenous vein (**a**), oblique view and stomas (**b**). (**c**, **d**), ECA-RA-MCA bypass (blue arrowheads) and STA-MCA double barrel bypass perfusing ipsilateral MCA and ACA territory, providing high flow to brain. Dissection of radial artery (c, left). (**e**, **f**), ECA-RA-MCA bypass (blue arrowheads) alone acting as midum-flow bypass, perfusing ipsilateral MCA area. (**g**, **h**, and **i**), stomas of STA-MCA double barrel bypass (**g**), feeding two thirds of MCA areas, blue and red arrowheads indicated two M2 trunks

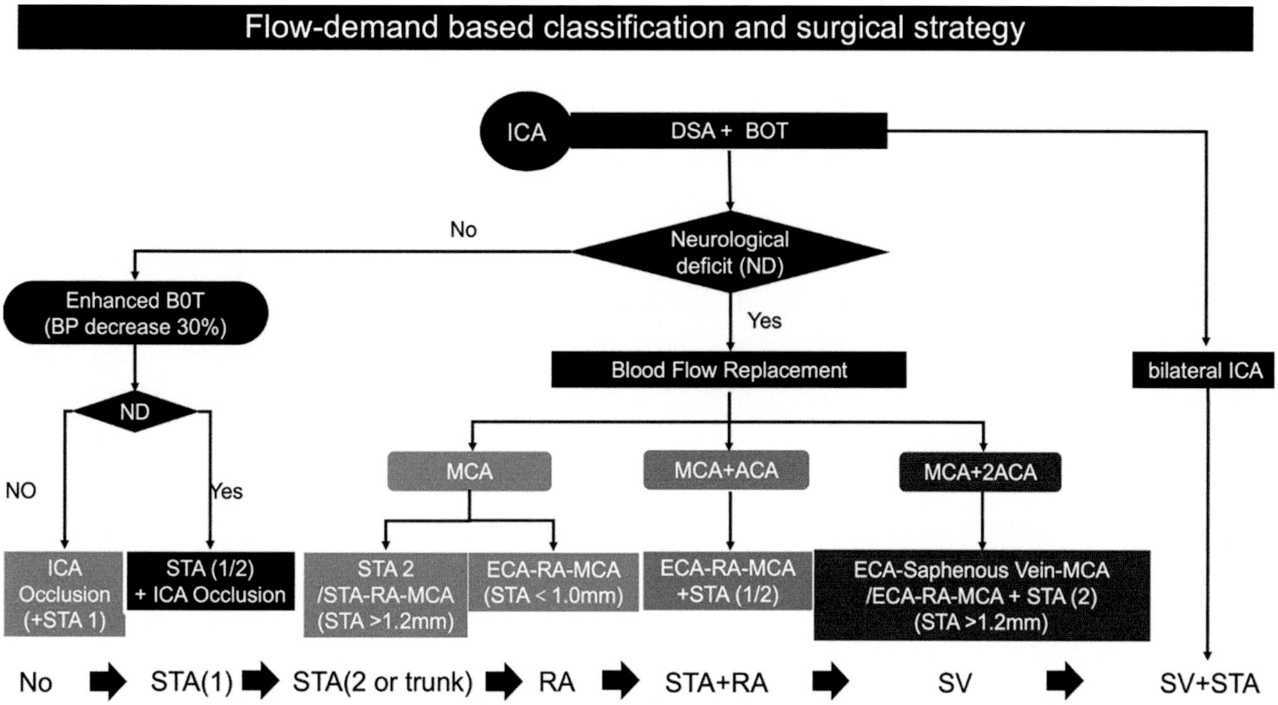

Fig. 10 flow demand-based classification and surgical strategy. ND, no deficit. BP, blood pressure. STA 1, STA-MCA single barrel bypass. STA 2, STA-MCA double barrel bypass. STA 1/2, STA-MCA single- or double-barrel bypass

demand is low level when only ipsilateral MCA area needed to be perfused. This flow demand-based classification system has proven to be an effective method for selecting appropriate bypass procedures to ensure optimal blood flow replacement (Fig. 10).

2.2 Staged Occlusion and EC-IC Bypass Strategy

Inspired by Selverstone clamp introduced in 1950s [37], it is reasonable to extend the occlusion phase from a one-stage acute process to a staged process. For instance, the first author has developed a clamp for controlling the cervical segment of the ICA, which facilitates staged occlusion within 1–2 weeks after the initial operation. It's symmetrical in structure, the opening of clamping blades is equal on both sides (Fig. 11).

In recent years, the treatment of these complex diseases has evolved alongside advancements in hybrid concepts and devices. A commonly employed method involves partial coiling of the aneurysm and parent artery, rather than complete occlusion. By creating proximal stenosis, subacute thrombosis can be induced, eventually resulting in total occlusion over weeks or months (Fig. 12). Another less commonly used method involves wrapping absorbable sutures around clip blades. This strategy prevents immediate occlusion due to the resistance of the sutures, instead causing a gradual occlusion as the sutures are absorbed. In essence, this strategy transforms acute ischemia into a chronic process, creating a time buffer for the development of IC-IC collaterals and enabling selective EC-IC bypass to deliver higher-level blood flow to the brain. This approach minimizes tissue trauma, simplifies the surgical process, and maintains safety and efficacy.

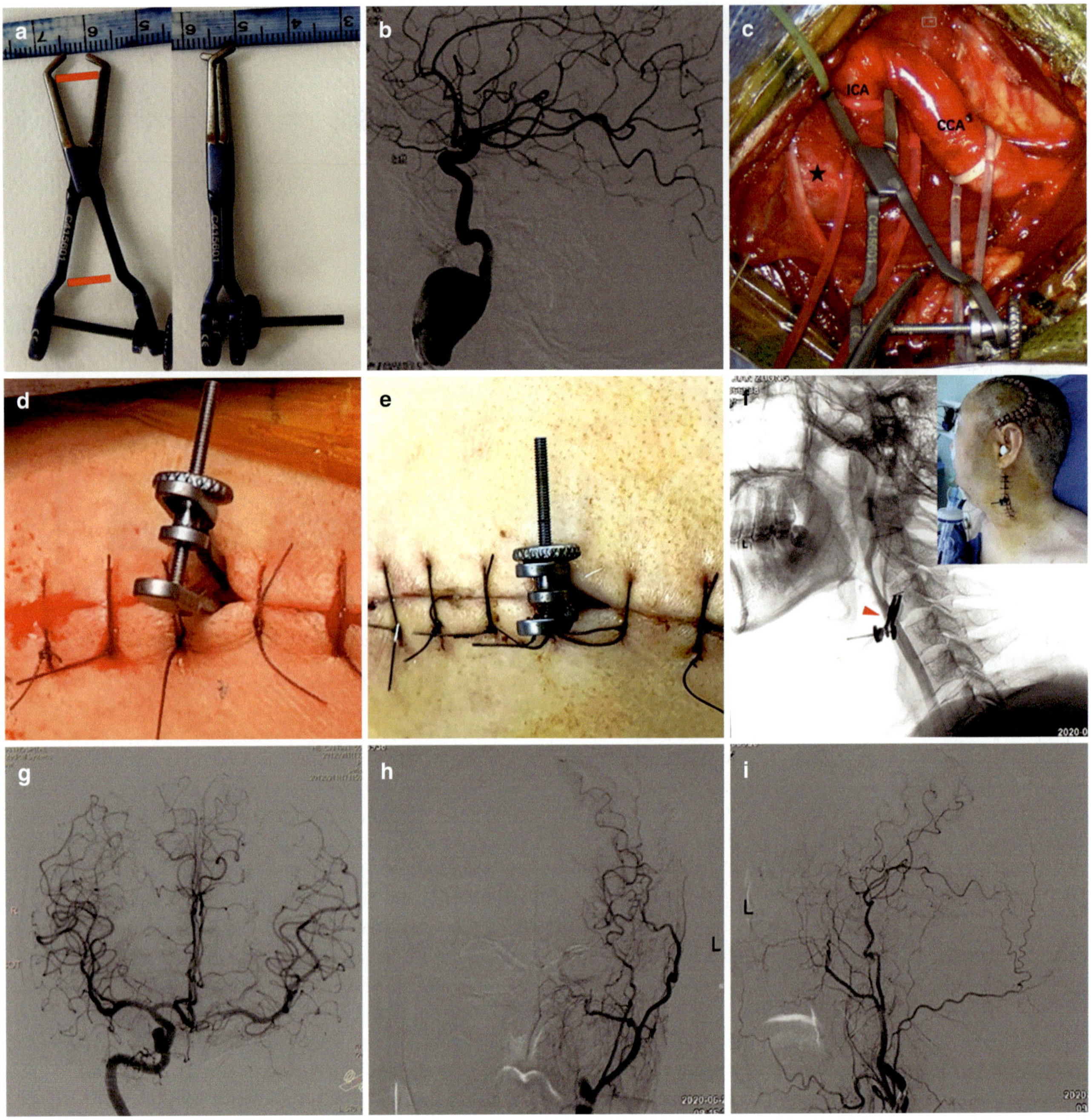

Fig. 11 Staged occlusion of ICA and EC-IC bypass in a giant ICA aneurysm. (**a**), Special-designed occlusion clamp for the staged occlusion of ICA, fully open (left) and closed (right). (**b**), DSA revealed a giant aneurysm in left ICA C1 segment in a 55-yo male complaining symptoms of chronic ischemia due to the turbulence inside the dome, in addition to thromboembolism. And it's impossible to perform BOT because of the special vascular architecture. (**c**), exposure, and control of ICA proximal to aneurysm (black star), STA-MCA double barrel bypass was performed firstly. (**d**, **e**), staged occlusion of proximal ICA by closure of clamp within a duration of 7 days, partially closed (**d**) and totally closed (**e**). F, DSA follow-up showed totally occlusion of diseased ICA and skin incisions (upper right). (**g**), angiogram of contralateral ICA showed some collateral via Acom a., with thin left A1 and slow flow in distal MCA area. (**h**, **i**), angiogram of left ECA, AP view (**h**) and lateral view (**i**), indicated the STA-MCA double barrel bypass perfused two thirds of MCA area. The diseased ICA was ligated permanently proximal to aneurysm and the clamp was removed, and the patient was discharged uneventfully 1 week after the second operation

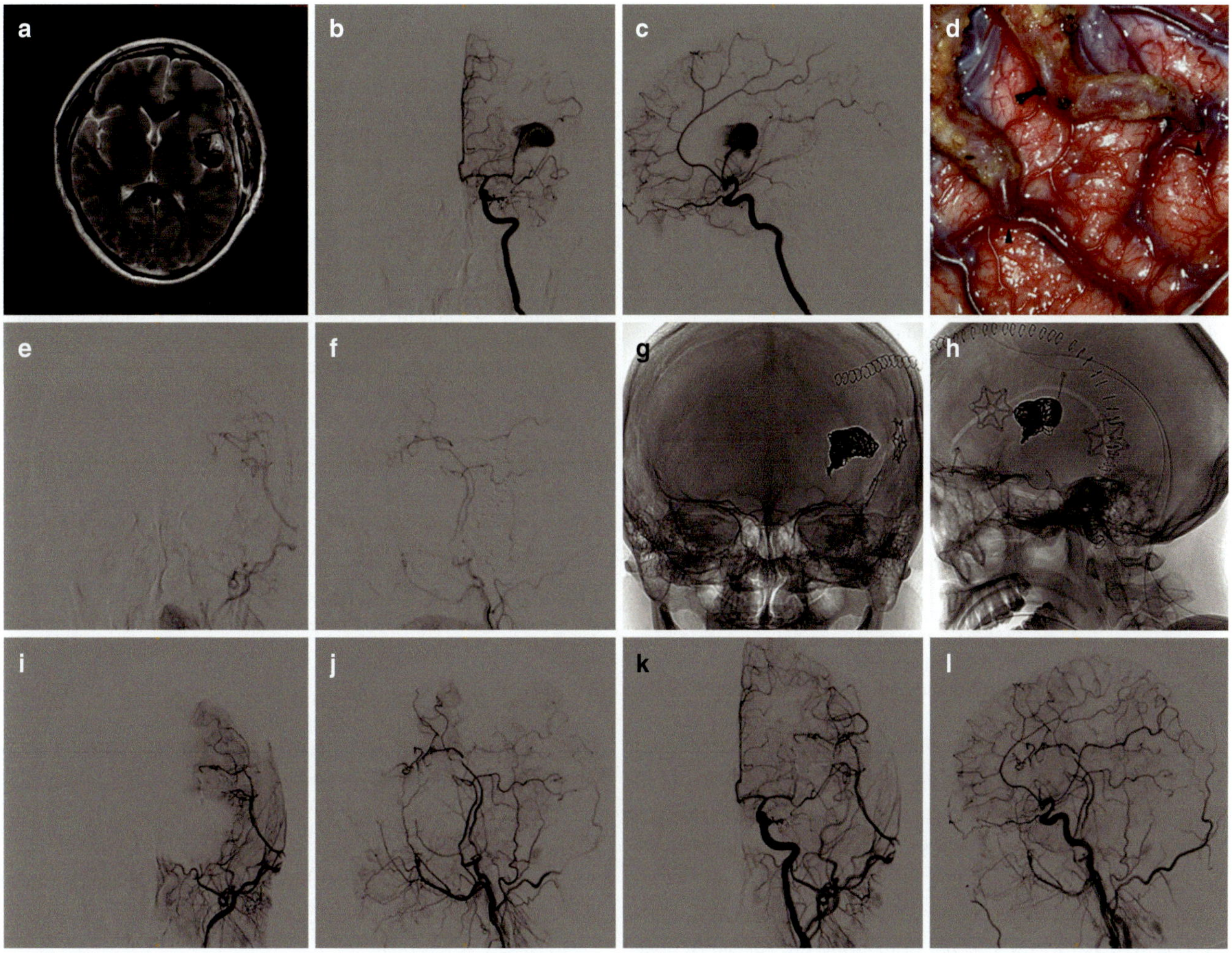

Fig.12 Hybrid treatment of large MCA aneurysm. (**a**), MRI revealed a lesion with flowing void effect in left sylvian fissure. (**b, c**), left ICA angiogram demonstrated a large aneurysm in superior M2. (**d**), left STA-MCA double barrel bypass (black arrowheads) was performed firstly. (**e, f**), hybrid DSA confirmed the patency of two bypasses. (**g, h**), the dome was partially coiled. (**i, j**), final angiogram of left ECA showed thicker bypasses feeding a larger territory, compared with pre-coiling. (**k, l**), final angiogram of left CCA showed obliteration of aneurysm and the superior M2 territory was fed by STA

3 Closure

Bypass surgery is fundamentally unique. Unlike other types of surgical interventions, it serves to increase the structural order of the vascular system, akin to an entropy-reduction process. This underlying philosophy underscores the necessity for bypass surgery to be precise, delicate, and sophisticated. A successful bypass procedure not only provides significant benefits to patients but also holds profound meaning for the operating neurosurgeon. However, it is a procedure that demands exceptional expertise and preparation. To execute bypass surgery perfectly, neurosurgeons must possess: profound theoretical knowledge, superb microsurgical skills, and essential character traits such as calmness, patience, and perseverance. Mastering bypass surgery represents the pinnacle of a neurosurgeon's skill set, as it combines art, science, and philosophy into one of the most demanding yet rewarding procedures in modern neurosurgery.

Declarations

Competing Interests The author(s) has no competing interests to declare that are relevant to the content of this manuscript.

Ethics Approval The author(s) declares that this manuscript does not include primary research with human participants.

References

1. Otani N, Yoshino A. Ischemic stroke revascularization. Adv Tech Stand Neurosurg. 2022;44:79–96. https://doi.org/10.1007/978-3-030-87649-4_4.
2. Mehdorn HM. Cerebral revascularization by EC-IC bypass–present status. Acta Neurochir Suppl. 2008;103:73–7. https://doi.org/10.1007/978-3-211-76589-0_13.
3. Yasargil MG, Yonekawa Y. Results of microsurgical extra-intracranial arterial bypass in the treatment of cerebral ischemia. Neurosurgery. 1977;1(1):22–4. https://doi.org/10.1227/00006123-197707000-00005.
4. Engel S, Ferraz H. Indications and results of extra-intracranial arterial bypasses. Int Surg. 1983;68(3):197–200.
5. Auer LM. EC-IC Bypass. Neurosurgery. 1985;16(3):436. https://doi.org/10.1097/00006123-198503000-00030.
6. Newell DW, Dailey AT, Skirboll SL. Intracranial vascular anastomosis using the microanastomotic system. Technical note. J Neurosurg. 1998;89(4):676–81. https://doi.org/10.3171/jns.1998.89.4.0676.
7. Newell DW, Vilela MD. Superficial temporal artery to middle cerebral artery bypass. Neurosurgery. 2004;54(6):1441–8. https://doi.org/10.1227/01.neu.0000124754.84425.48. discussion 1448-9. PMID: 15157302
8. Horn P, Scharf J, Peña-Tapia P, Vajkoczy P. Risk of intraoperative ischemia due to temporary vessel occlusion during standard extracranial-intracranial arterial bypass surgery. J Neurosurg. 2008;108(3):464–9. https://doi.org/10.3171/JNS/2008/108/3/0464.
9. Barnett HJ. Progress towards stroke prevention: Robert Wartenberg lecture. Neurology. 1980;30(11):1212–25. https://doi.org/10.1212/wnl.30.11.1212.hemo.
10. Derdeyn CP, Videen TO, Yundt KD, Fritsch SM, Carpenter DA, Grubb RL, Powers WJ. Variability of cerebral blood volume and oxygen extraction: stages of cerebral haemodynamic impairment revisited. Brain. 2002;125(Pt 3):595–607. https://doi.org/10.1093/brain/awf047.
11. Low SW, Teo K, Lwin S, Yeo LL, Paliwal PR, Ahmad A, Sinha AK, Teoh HL, Wong LY, Chong VF, Seet RC, Chan BP, Yeo TT, Chou N, Sharma VK. Improvement in cerebral hemodynamic parameters and outcomes after superficial temporal artery-middle cerebral artery bypass in patients with severe stenoocclusive disease of the intracranial internal carotid or middle cerebral arteries. J Neurosurg. 2015;123(3):662–9. https://doi.org/10.3171/2014.11.JNS141553. Epub 2015 May 29
12. Grubb RL Jr, Derdeyn CP, Fritsch SM, Carpenter DA, Yundt KD, Videen TO, Spitznagel EL, Powers WJ. Importance of hemodynamic factors in the prognosis of symptomatic carotid occlusion. JAMA. 1998;280(12):1055–60. https://doi.org/10.1001/jama.280.12.1055.
13. Fluri F, Engelter S, Lyrer P. Extracranial-intracranial arterial bypass surgery for occlusive carotid artery disease. Cochrane Database Syst Rev. 2010;2010(2):CD005953. https://doi.org/10.1002/14651858.CD005953.pub2. PMID: 20166076; PMCID: PMC6544774
14. EC/IC Bypass Study Group. Failure of extracranial-intracranial arterial bypass to reduce the risk of ischemic stroke. Results of an international randomized trial. N Engl J Med. 1985;313(19):1191–200. https://doi.org/10.1056/NEJM198511073131904.
15. Mohit AA, Sekhar LN, Natarajan SK, Britz GW, Ghodke B. High-flow bypass grafts in the management of complex intracranial aneurysms. Neurosurgery. 2007;60(2 Suppl 1):ONS105-22; discussion ONS122-3. https://doi.org/10.1227/01.NEU.0000249243.25429.EE.
16. Zhu W, Tian YL, Zhou LF, Song DL, Xu B, Mao Y. Treatment strategies for complex internal carotid artery (ICA) aneurysms: direct ICA sacrifice or combined with extracranial-to-intracranial bypass. World Neurosurg. 2011;75(3-4):476–84. https://doi.org/10.1016/j.wneu.2010.07.043.
17. Chen Y, Chen P, Duan G, Li R, Li Z, Guo G. Extracranial-intracranial bypass surgery for intracranial aneurysm of the anterior cerebral circulation: a systematic review and meta-analysis. Front Neurol. 2023;14:1174088. https://doi.org/10.3389/fneur.2023.1174088. PMID: 37064185; PMCID: PMC10102499
18. Wolfswinkel EM, Landau MJ, Ravina K, Kokot NC, Russin JJ, Carey JN. EC-IC bypass for cerebral revascularization following skull base tumor resection: current practices and innovations. J Surg Oncol. 2018;118(5):815–25. https://doi.org/10.1002/jso.25178. Epub 2018 Sep 9
19. Tomura N, Omachi K, Takahashi S, Sakuma I, Otani T, Watarai J, Ishikawa K, Kinouchi H, Mizoi K. Comparison of technetium Tc 99m hexamethylpropyleneamine oxime single-photon emission tomography with stump pressure during the balloon occlusion test of the internal carotid artery. AJNR Am J Neuroradiol. 2005;26(8):1937–42. PMID: 16155138; PMCID: PMC8148825
20. Kuribara T, Mikami T, Iihoshi S, Miyata K, Kim S, Kawata Y, Komatsu K, Kimura Y, Enatsu R, Akiyama Y, Hirano T, Mikuni N. Ischemic tolerance evaluated by computed tomography perfusion during balloon test occlusion. J Stroke Cerebrovasc Dis. 2020;29(6):104807. https://doi.org/10.1016/j.jstrokecerebrovasdis.2020.104807. Epub 2020 Apr 13
21. Suzuki J, Takaku A. Cerebrovascular "moyamoya" disease. Disease showing abnormal net-like vessels in base of brain. Arch Neurol. 1969;20(3):288–99. https://doi.org/10.1001/archneur.1969.00480090076012.
22. Research Committee on the Pathology and Treatment of Spontaneous Occlusion of the Circle of Willis, Health Labour Sciences Research Grant for Research on Measures for Infractable Diseases. Guidelines for diagnosis and treatment of moyamoya disease (spontaneous occlusion of the circle of Willis). Neurol Med Chir (Tokyo). 2012;52(5):245–66.
23. Kappel AD, Feroze AH, Torio E, Sukumaran M, Du R. Management of moyamoya disease: a review of current and future therapeutic strategies. J Neurosurg. 2024;141(4):975–82. https://doi.org/10.3171/2024.1.JNS221977.
24. Matsushima Y, Inaba Y. Moyamoya disease in children and its surgical treatment. Introduction of a new surgical procedure and its follow-up angiograms. Childs. Brain. 1984;11(3):155–70. https://doi.org/10.1159/000120172.
25. Matsushima Y, Aoyagi M, Fukai N, Tanaka K, Tsuruoka S, Inaba Y. Angiographic demonstration of cerebral revascularization after encephalo-duro-arterio-synangiosis (EDAS) performed on pediatric moyamoya patients. Bull Tokyo Med Dent Univ. 1982;29(1):7–17.
26. Matsushima T, Fujiwara S, Nagata S, Fujii K, Fukui M, Kitamura K, Hasuo K. Surgical treatment for paediatric patients with moyamoya disease by indirect revascularization procedures (EDAS, EMS, EMAS). Acta Neurochir (Wien). 1989;98(3-4):135–40. https://doi.org/10.1007/BF01407339.
27. Shen W, Xu B, Li H, Gao X, Liao Y, Shi W, Zhao R, Zhang Y. Enlarged Encephalo-Duro-Myo-Synangiosis Treatment for Moyamoya Disease in Young Children. World Neurosurg. 2017;106:9–16. https://doi.org/10.1016/j.wneu.2017.06.088. Epub 2017 Jun 20
28. Xu B, Song DL, Mao Y, Gu YX, Xu H, Liao YJ, Liu CH, Zhou LF. Superficial temporal artery-middle cerebral artery bypass combined with encephalo-duro-myo-synangiosis in treating moyamoya disease: surgical techniques, indications and midterm follow-up results. Chin Med J (Engl). 2012;125:4398–405.
29. Helmy M, Liao Y, Luo S, Xu B. How I do it: direct pressure measurement in moyamoya bypass. Acta Neurochir (Wien). 2023;165(12):3631–5. https://doi.org/10.1007/s00701-023-05842-w. Epub 2023 Oct 23

30. Bin X. Individualized Extracranial-intracranial revascularization in the treatment of late-stage Moyamoya disease. Surgical techniques in Moyamoya vasculopathy tricks of the trade. Peter Vajkoczy. Thieme; 2020.
31. Powers WJ, Clarke WR, Grubb RL Jr, Videen TO, Adams HP Jr, Derdeyn CP, COSS Investigators. Extracranial-intracranial bypass surgery for stroke prevention in hemodynamic cerebral ischemia: the Carotid Occlusion Surgery Study randomized trial. JAMA. 2011;306(18):1983–92. https://doi.org/10.1001/jama.2011.1610. Erratum in: JAMA. 2011 Dec 28;306(24):2672. Obviagele, Bruce [corrected to Ovbiagele, Bruce]. PMID: 22068990; PMCID: PMC3601825
32. Ma Y, Wang T, Wang H, Amin-Hanjani S, Tong X, Wang J, Tong Z, Kuai D, Cai Y, Ren J, Wang D, Duan L, Maimaitili A, Hang C, Yu J, Bai X, Powers WJ, Derdeyn CP, Wu Y, Ling F, Gu Y, Jiao L, CMOSS Investigators. Extracranial-intracranial bypass and risk of stroke and death in patients with symptomatic artery occlusion: the CMOSS randomized clinical trial. JAMA. 2023;330(8):704–14. https://doi.org/10.1001/jama.2023.13390. PMID: 37606672; PMCID: PMC10445185
33. Garrett MC, Komotar RJ, Starke RM, Merkow MB, Otten ML, Sciacca RR, Connolly ES. The efficacy of direct extracranial-intracranial bypass in the treatment of symptomatic hemodynamic failure secondary to athero-occlusive disease: a systematic review. Clin Neurol Neurosurg. 2009;111(4):319–26. https://doi.org/10.1016/j.clineuro.2008.12.012. Epub 2009 Feb 7
34. Komotar RJ, Starke RM, Otten ML, Merkow MB, Garrett MC, Marshall RS, Elkind MS, Connolly ES. The role of indirect extracranial-intracranial bypass in the treatment of symptomatic intracranial atheroocclusive disease. J Neurosurg. 2009;110(5):896–904. https://doi.org/10.3171/2008.9.JNS17658.
35. Coppens JR, Cantando JD, Abdulrauf SI. Minimally invasive superficial temporal artery to middle cerebral artery bypass through an enlarged bur hole: the use of computed tomography angiography neuronavigation in surgical planning. J Neurosurg. 2008;109(3):553–8. https://doi.org/10.3171/JNS/2008/109/9/0553.
36. Bin X, Liao Y, Helmy M. 3D DSA-guided Keyhole STA-MCA bypass in moyamoya vasculopathy. In: Kanaan IN, Beneš V, editors. Neuroanatomy guidance to successful neurosurgical interventions. Cham: Springer; 2024. https://doi.org/10.1007/978-3-031-59838-8_25.
37. Mount LA. Results of treatment of intracranial aneurysms using the Selverstone clamp. J Neurosurg. 1959;16:611–8. https://doi.org/10.3171/jns.1959.16.6.0611.

Vertebrobasilar System Bypasses

Laura Stone McGuire, Tatiana Abou-Mrad, Richard Bram, Gursant Atwal, Ali Alaraj, and Fady T. Charbel

1 Introduction

Bypasses of the vertebrobasilar system have generally been reserved for complex conditions of the posterior circulation. Specifically, the indications for these procedures may be divided into two categories: (1) flow replacement and (2) flow augmentation [3, 4, 23]. On one hand, bypasses for flow replacement supplant the normal blood supply when a disease requires occlusion and circumvention of the native vasculature for adequate treatment (e.g., giant, fusiform aneurysm of basilar and vertebrobasilar junction or a vessel-encasing tumor.). On the other hand, those for flow augmentation aim to supplement the blood supply to a circulation long suffering from poor cerebral blood flow (e.g., intracranial atherosclerotic disease). These bypass categories and technical details will be discussed in this chapter. Despite the clear differences in indication for bypasses of the vertebrobasilar system, the techniques tend to depend more on anatomic location and segment of the involved vertebral artery (VA), which will be detailed in the sections below. The anatomy of the VA has been covered in detail in a separate chapter in this book and should be referenced.

L. S. McGuire
Department of Neurosurgery, University of Illinois at Chicago, Chicago, IL, USA

Department of Neurological Surgery, University of Wisconsin-Madison, Madison, WI, USA
e-mail: mcguire@neurosurgery.wisc.edu

T. Abou-Mrad · R. Bram · G. Atwal · A. Alaraj · F. T. Charbel (✉)
Department of Neurosurgery, University of Illinois at Chicago, Chicago, IL, USA
e-mail: tamrad@uic.edu; rbram3@uic.edu; gatwal@uic.edu; alaraj@uic.edu; fcharbel@uic.edu

2 Complex Aneurysms of the Posterior Circulation

The treatment of complex, giant, and fusiform aneurysms of the VA, basilar artery, and vertebrobasilar junction remain challenging, despite technological advances in the endovascular space. The anatomic location, intimate association with numerous small and critical perforating vessels, and typically calcified or partially thrombosed morphology—all represent features contributing to the unique complexity of these lesions and their management.

Complex aneurysms of the vertebrobasilar system vary from those of the basilar apex that involve thalamoperforators to dolichoectatic or fusiform vertebrobasilar aneurysms [19]. Management of these aneurysms is not straight forward, and options range from endovascular and open surgical treatment (or a combination) to conservative. While flow-diverting stents have been described in the past two decades for the treatment of some of these aneurysms, outcomes remain highly variable [25, 26, 33, 42]. Direct surgical clipping of these lesions also carries risk [13, 27, 28] and may not offer a definitive solution. A recent systematic review and meta-analysis of treatment strategies for dolichoectatic vertebrobasilar aneurysms identified 41 cases treated with open cerebrovascular surgery, 61 treated endovascularly, and 47 managed conservatively [15]. The published outcomes of dolichoectatic vertebrobasilar aneurysms are striking, noting 51.9% with good outcome rate, 45.5% with poor outcomes, and 22.3% mortality.

Other treatment strategies focus on hemodynamic modification to facilitate aneurysm remodeling and resolution. Hunterian ligation of the basilar artery or VA - occlusion of the parent artery proximal to the aneurysm - was historically described in the treatment of complex vertebrobasilar aneurysms, particularly dolichoectatic lesions. Endovascular vessel sacrifice with coiling has become standard for most vessel take-downs (Fig. 1). However, when occluding the proximal basilar artery for this purpose, the brainstem perforators in

V. Beneš, D. Netuka (eds.), *Surgical and Interventional Treatment of Cerebral Ischemia*,
https://doi.org/10.1007/978-3-032-08934-2_21

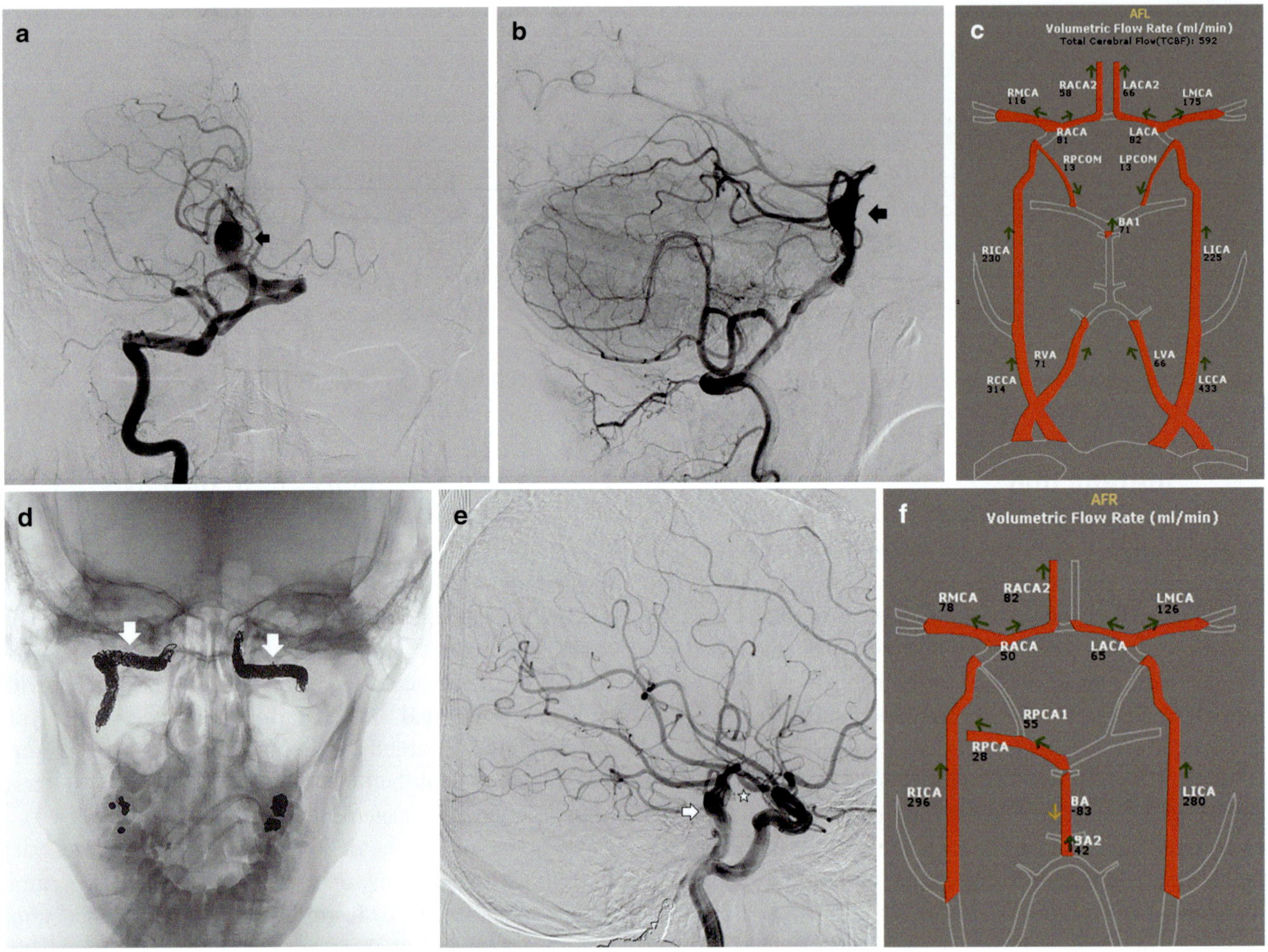

Fig. 1 Example of vertebral artery sacrifice with coil embolization to treat complex dolichoectatic basilar artery aneurysm, using flow reversal to aid in vessel remodeling. Diagnostic cerebral angiogram of right VA in AP (**a**) and lateral (**b**) views (black arrow points to basilar artery aneurysm). (**c**) Baseline NOVA. (**d**) Post-coil embolization of bilateral VA (white arrows point to coil mass). (**e**) Follow-up diagnostic cerebral angiogram showing retrograde flow through posterior communicating artery (white star) into top of basilar artery (white arrow). (**f**) Follow-up NOVA showing change in direction of blood flow

the vertebrobasilar system cannot be visualized or well accounted for endovascularly, and thus, surgical clip occlusion may offer another viable option [31]. Nonetheless, altering the flow in the brainstem may cause insufficiency or ischemic stroke [45], and authors have argued for combining ligation techniques with bypass, particularly in the absence of adequate posterior communicating arteries [30, 35]. Extracranial-to-intracranial (EC-IC) bypass combined with and prior to proximal parent vessel occlusion has been described, including superficial temporal artery (STA) to posterior cerebral artery (PCA) and also STA to superior cerebellar artery (SCA).

3 Vertebrobasilar Insufficiency

Posterior circulation strokes constitute about one-third of all ischemic strokes, with symptomatic vertebrobasilar disease posing a significant risk of recurrence [3, 4, 16, 39, 49]. A leading cause of vertebrobasilar insufficiency (VBI) is atherosclerotic disease, such that the development of plaque causes progressive narrowing and gradual symptom onset. Subsequent plaque rupture may cause acute ischemia due to occlusion or embolization.

A higher degree of stenosis confers a higher risk of recurrent stroke [39]. Thus, stroke risk in vertebrobasilar disease has been shown to be related to hemodynamic compromise [3, 4, 7–10, 41]. The risk of recurrent stroke due to vertebrobasilar stenosis over 50% has been previously estimated at 10–15% (38 [37, 49]). Stenosis of 80% or more generates the most significant lowering of cerebral blood flow, with tandem disease generating even more hemodynamic compromise [6].

Other diseases, such as dissection and fibromuscular dysplasia, may also compromise blood flow to the posterior circulation. Ultimately, this diminished flow can present with neurologic symptoms ranging from dizziness to severe stroke. While collateral circulation typically compensates for arterial stenosis, many patients lack sufficient anatomic redundancy due to conditions like incomplete Circle of Willis or generalized atherosclerosis.

Revascularization becomes an option for patients who remain symptomatic despite maximal medical management. Although endovascular solutions are often preferred, including balloon angioplasty with or without stenting, certain anatomical and pathological scenarios necessitate surgical approaches. The evolution of surgical techniques for VA revascularization began in the 1970s. Pioneers like Berguer and colleagues first described subclavian-to-vertebral artery bypass in 1976 in their case series of 4 patients [14]. Subsequent advancements by Carney and Anderson in 1978 introduced carotid-to-distal VA bypass method for carotid occlusion [17]. Carney et al. later published their series of 219 patients in 1986 who underwent VA revascularization surgery, and these approaches demonstrated efficacy and safety, with reported long-term graft patency rates of 87% and perioperative mortality and stroke rate of 3% [18]. For intracranial bypass surgery, Ausman et al. performed the first intracranial posterior revascularization procedure for vertebrobasilar insufficiency using an occipital artery to posterior inferior cerebellar artery bypass in 1976 and then using a STA to SCA bypass in 1979 [11, 12].

4 Preoperative Considerations

Preoperative evaluation includes advanced imaging modalities to visualize vascular anatomy and assess hemodynamic reserve.

4.1 Anatomic Assessment

Refer to the chapter on VA anatomy for more details. The VA generally originates from the subclavian artery and then enters the cervical transverse foramen at C6 level, although normal anatomical variation exists. The VA then exits C2 transverse foramen, enters the C1 transverse foramen, and subsequently loops around the C1 sulcus arteriosus prior to entering the foramen magnum. The sulcus arteriosus may be enclosed as a foramen, secondary to calcification of the atlanto-occipital ligament of C1, which is referred to as *ponticulus posticus* (meaning "little posterior bridge") or arcuate foramen.

The four segments of the VA are described in relation to the cervical spine:

1. V1 segment: from the origin (primarily at the subclavian artery) to its entry point at the cervical transverse foramen (usually at C6)
2. V2 segment: the VA course within the cervical transverse foramen (often described as C6-C2, although some include C1)
3. V3 segment: from its exit point at the cervical transverse foramen to entry point at the foramen magnum
4. V4 segment: intracranial, intradural component from the foramen magnum to its merge with the contralateral VA to form the basilar artery

Digital Subtraction Angiography (DSA) is essential for determining the extent of stenosis, collateral flow, and potential donor and recipient vessels. **Computed Tomography Angiography (CTA)** offers detailed views of surrounding bony and soft tissue structures. The path of the VA should be understood by the surgeon from its origin and then entrance in the cervical transverse foramen to its course around C1 and through the dura, and any aberrant anatomy should be duly noted and prepared for.

4.2 Hemodynamic Assessment

In steno-occlusive disease, evaluating the patient's hemodynamic reserve aids in decision-making. **Quantitative magnetic resonance angiography (QMRA)** may be used to measure blood flow, which not only detects regions of poor blood flow but also approximates the blood flow required to supplement or replace a particular vessel in suregry. With the addition of a vasodilatory challenge, such as administration of Diamox, the practitioner can assess the hemodynamic response and any impairment. This institution uses a multimodal MRI-based protocol that uses QMRA with and without Diamox, in addition to assessment of (1) local blood oxygenation level-dependent (BOLD) signal due to increased regional blood flow with task performance during functional MRI and (2) global BOLD signal response due to increased widespread cerebral blood flow after the vasodilatory challenge [21, 48, 50]. This protocol detects compromised hemodynamic reserve via an absence of the expected responses, which may support revascularization.

In preparation for surgery for complex aneurysms or tumors involving the vertebrobasilar system, a **balloon**

occlusion test (BOT) may be employed to evaluate collateral capacity and ensure cerebral perfusion during temporary vessel occlusion. The BOT procedure involves temporary balloon inflation intravascularly, under full heparinization, in the vessel of interest in an awake patient, allowing for continued monitoring of the patient's neurological exam. The blood pressure of the patient is maintained at normotensive for 10–15 min while the balloon is inflated. If the patient passes this normotensive phase, then the blood pressure is lowered chemically for an additional 10–15 min. During this hypotensive phase, 99 m technetium is administered, such that a **single photon emission computed tomography (SPECT)** may be completed immediately afterward. The balloon is deflated and removed, the blood pressure is normalized, and the patient is sent to complete the SPECT study. Asymmetries present on the SPECT study highlight different uptake of the 99 m technetium tracer and the affected vascular territory during the hypotensive phase.

5 Surgical Approaches

5.1 Segment-Specific Techniques

As mentioned above, the surgical approach varies per VA segment. In summary:

1. V1 Segment: Proximal vertebral artery lesions are often treated with transposition to the common carotid or subclavian artery.
2. V2 Segment: Due to its deep intraosseous location, direct access is rare. Lesions in this segment are typically bypassed to the more accessible V3 segment.
3. V3 Segment: Requires exposure through the posterior cervical triangle, with bypass grafting from donor arteries such as the occipital or carotid arteries.
4. V4 Segment: Intracranial bypass procedures may be required for distal lesions, often involving suboccipital or far-lateral craniotomies.
5. Other Extracranial-Intracranial Bypasses: Occipital artery (OA) to posterior inferior cerebellar artery (PICA), STA-SCA, and STA-PCA bypasses, have been described. These bypasses are usually performed via subtemporal or posterior transpetrosal approaches but may also be completed using a transsylvian or anterior temporal approach [46].

5.2 Technical Considerations

5.2.1 Donor Selection

The choice of donor artery depends on the location of the disease and the patient's anatomy.

- V1 Segment: If the origin is the diseased site, then the VA may be reimplanted to the subclavian artery or transposed carotid artery.
- V2–3 Segments: If the diseased segment involves V2 or V3, then an interposition graft may be necessary to connect the VA to its donor (common carotid artery, external carotid artery, cervical internal carotid artery, subclavian artery, or occipital artery).
- V4 Segment: If an intracranial bypass is required with the V4 segment, the donor vessel depends on the disease. The VA may serve as the donor in the setting of PICA reimplantation for aneurysm treatment [47].
- Other Extracranial-Intracranial Bypasses: Other bypasses described in the service of complex aneurysm treatment involve the superficial temporal artery as the donor vessel (e.g., STA-PCA or STA-SCA bypass) or the occipital artery (e.g., OA-PICA) [30, 35].

5.2.2 Graft Selection

If an interposition graft is required, autologous saphenous veins or radial arteries are commonly used, selected based on length and diameter compatibility. Of importance, in our institutional data, the STA may offer an average of approximately 60 mL/min, cadaveric vein graft 80 mL/min, and autologous vein graft 100 mL/min [40, 44].

5.2.3 Patient Positioning

Precise positioning ensures optimal exposure of both proximal and distal anastomosis sites. For surgeries involving the V1–3 segments, patients are generally placed supine with slight neck extension, with head turning contralateral direction to the operative site. To facilitate head turning and neck extension, a shoulder roll may be needed. For surgeries involving the V4 segment, often the far lateral approach is employed, and thus, the patient may be positioned prone with head maximally flexed and rotated ipsilaterally. Other intracranial approaches require different positioning based on the technique selected (e.g., subtemporal approach for STA-PCA bypass). Head fixation with head holders, such as the Mayfield, Doro, or Sugita frames, is optional for surgery of the V1–3 segments but mandatory for procedures of the V4 segment and other intracranial vessels.

5.3 Representative Techniques

5.3.1 V1 Transposition

For disease of the origin of the vertebral artery, the V1 transposition offers the best option for revascularization. In this procedure, the inflow artery can be either the subclavian artery or the common carotid artery; however, these vessels must also be carefully evaluated for disease, such that a disease-free segment is used for the transposition.

The patient may be positioned supine with the head turned contralaterally and with the neck extended, opening the targeted operative site. The head of the bed is usually elevated, which reduces venous pressure. The head does not require fixation. A transverse incision near the clavicle provides access and is planned 1–2 cm superior to the clavicle and over both heads of the sternocleidomastoid muscle.

After sharply opening the skin, the platysma muscle is dissected to aid in skin mobilization. Dissection proceeds between the two heads of the sternocleidomastoid muscle. If needed for additional exposure, the omohyoid muscle may be safely divided. The common carotid artery and neighboring vagus nerve should be retracted medially, and the jugular vein should be mobilized and then retracted laterally. When operating on the left, the thoracic duct will be encountered and can be ligated and divided.

During dissection, attention should be paid to identification of the prescalene fat pad, which rests over the anterior scalene muscle, and importantly, the phrenic nerve. Further dissection should be medial to the prescalene fat pad in order to protect the phrenic nerve.

At the angle of the anterior scalene muscle and the longus colli, the vertebral vein and vertebral artery will be seen. The vertebral vein may be ligated and divided for additional exposure and mobilization of the vertebral artery. The vertebral artery should be fully freed from its origin at the subclavian artery to the tendon of the longus colli. During this dissection, great care should be taken to identify the sympathetic chain, which travels on the anterior surface of the vertebral artery. The sympathetic trunk should be mobilized from the VA.

After isolating the VA from its surrounding structures, the artery is prepared for ligation and anastomosis to the implantation site of a healthy donor artery (subclavian artery or common carotid artery for this procedure). Weight-based systemic heparinization should be administered prior to VA ligation. Next, a clamp is placed on the distal V1. The proximal V1 is ligated and divided immediately above the diseased portion, ensuring both the transposed VA will be free of plaque but also adequate vessel length for the transposition.

The donor (inflow) vessel is then clamped. An aortic punch may be used for the arteriotomy—on the lateral wall of the common carotid artery or on the superior wall of the subclavian artery. Then, 7–0 Prolene sutures may be used at as anchors to bring the VA to the donor artery, followed by a running 7–0 Prolene suture to complete the anastomosis.

Attention is paid to avoid tension in the graft and to provide adequate slack in the VA, preserving neck mobility. Before cinching the final tie in the anastomosis, the VA should be flushed with heparinized saline, allowed to back bleed, and then reclamped, in order to flush out any debris and air from the vessel. The donor vessel should also be flushed with heparinized saline, after which the suture may be tightened and tied. Clamps are removed from the donor and recipient arteries.

5.3.2 V3 Bypass with Interposition Graft

For disease of the V2 or V3 segment, a V3 bypass with interposition graft may be used. The patient may be positioned supine with the head rotated contralaterally and the neck extended, fully opening the neck and operative corridor. If the inflow vessel is the carotid artery, a vertical incision is planned from the angle of the jaw and along the anteromedial border of the sternocleidomastoid, allowing exposure of the V3 segment superiorly and the carotid artery inferiorly. If the inflow vessel is the subclavian artery, two incisions may be planned: first, a transverse incision at the upper neck for the V3 segment and a transverse incision above the clavicle for the subclavian artery.

An interposition graft should be harvested and prepared prior to neck incision(s) and dissection. Suitable interposition grafts include the radial artery or saphenous vein (autologous or cadaveric) and should be measured for diameter and length.

Neck dissection is carried out anterior to the sternocleidomastoid muscle and posterior to the jugular vein. Once the spinal accessory nerve has been exposed, it is followed to the transverse process of C1. The origin of the levator scapulae muscle is seen at the transverse processes of C1 and C2, and the anterior ramus of the C2 nerve root can be seen at this level. Importantly, the anterior ramus of C2 nerve root may be followed to the VA.

The levator scapulae muscle is elevated with a right-angle clamp to disconnect it from the C2 transverse process. The anterior ramus of the C2 nerve root must be divided to visualize V3. Once the VA is in full view, it must be circumferentially dissected free from the surrounding venous plexus.

After dissection of the VA, the donor vessel should be dissected and prepared. The inflow vessel must be assessed preoperatively for the presence of any atherosclerotic disease or stenosis. If the carotid artery will serve as the inflow, a standard dissection used for carotid endarterectomy may be used to isolate the internal carotid artery and common carotid artery. After all vessels have been fully exposed, the patient should be systemically heparinized.

The distal V3 anastomosis with the interposition graft should be performed first. Note that the proximal VA will be permanently clipped. The distal VA is temporarily clamped. A longitudinal incision on the VA is performed to produce the arteriotomy. The interposition graft is brought into view and anchored with 8–0 Nylon suture. An end-to-side anastomosis between the graft and V3 segment is completed with running 8–0 Nylon suture.

Next, the proximal carotid anastomosis with the interposition graft is performed. The graft is brought to the lateral border of the common carotid artery. The common carotid artery is clamped, and if needed, additional clamps on the internal carotid artery and external carotid artery may be placed, based on the exposure achieved. An aortic punch is used to produce the arteriotomy in the carotid artery. Anchoring sutures with 7–0 Prolene are placed to bring the graft to the carotid artery, and then, an end-to-side anastomosis is completed using running 7–0 Prolene suture.

Prior to cinching the final suture in both anastomoses, the graft is flushed with heparinized saline, and the clamp is briefly released to allow back-bleeding and elimination of air and debris. This step must be performed at both anastomotic sites. The final suture may then be tied, and temporary clamps are removed.

Fig. 2 shows an example of the left V3 to common carotid artery bypass with interposition graft

5.3.3 PICA-VA Reimplantation

Preoperatively, the origin of the PICA on the VA should be determined, and CTA may be useful to determine the relationship of the vessels to the surrounding bony anatomy. The patient is prepared for a far-lateral craniotomy, and a hockey-stick incision is planned, which grants access to the V4 segment and the origin of the PICA on the VA.

Following skin incision, the superficial muscle layer, including the sternocleidomastoid and trapezius muscles, is identified. The sternocleidomastoid muscle is detached from the mastoid tip and reflected laterally. Then, the next layer of muscles comes to view, and the splenius capitis muscles is detached and reflected medially, followed by the longissimus capitis and semispinalis capitis muscles. The deepest muscles, including the superior and inferior oblique muscles, attach to the transverse process of C1 and can be released laterally and reflected medially.

The VA should be identified. The VA runs through the transverse foramen of C1, and the transverse process of C1 can be palpated. Also, the dorsal ramus of C2 can be followed to the C1–2 interspace, which will localize the VA. Note that the VA will be surrounded by a venous plexus. Subperiosteal dissection of C1 and C2 should be carried laterally.

A C1 hemilaminectomy is performed to fully mobilize the VA. A suboccipital craniotomy is completed, followed by occipital condylectomy. The posterior third of the occipital condyle is removed to facilitate access to the lateral cerebellomedullary space.

The VA is usually under the dentate ligament when it comes intracranially, and the dentate ligament can be cut from the foramen magnum and at C1 to widen the surgical corridor. The dura is opened, and CSF is allowed to egress for relaxation. The origin of the PICA is located by following its tonsillar loop proximally to the cistern. Any perforating vessels are identified and protected. Care is taken to gently dissect and mobilize the cranial nerve IX, X, and XI complex, which can obstruct the view of origin.

A clip is placed on the PICA, including a permanent clip at its origin and a temporary clip more distally. The PICA is disconnected and then dissected free within the subarachnoid space to fully mobilize it. The PICA is then brought to the VA to the site of planned reimplantation. The patient should be systemically heparinized. Temporary clips are placed on the vertebral artery. A linear arteriotomy is completed on the VA, and the PICA is brought into close approximation to the VA as an end-to-side bypass. Anchor sutures are placed using 8–0 Nylon, and then, the anastomosis may be completed using a running 8–0 Nylon suture.

5.3.4 Additional Bypasses and Procedures

While the following bypasses will not be covered in this chapter, they do relate to the vertebrobasilar system and should be noted. As discussed earlier in this chapter, the STA-SCA or STA-PCA bypass via a subtemporal approach may be combined with VA sacrifice for treatment of complex giant or dolichoectatic basilar artery aneurysms, when the patient lacks sufficient collateral supply through the posterior communicating artery. As shown in Fig. 1, the posterior communicating artery provided robust collateral supply to the top of the basilar artery following bilateral vertebral artery sacrifice, without requiring the addition of an STA-SCA or STA-PCA bypass.

The PICA-PICA bypass is another bypass for awareness in the setting of a complex PICA aneurysm. This procedure is typically performed with a suboccipital craniotomy, allowing a side-to-side bypass to be completed where the bilateral PICA vessels meet medially at their tonsillar loops.

Lastly, Bowhunter syndrome is a dynamic form of vertebrobasilar insufficiency, caused by rotation of the neck that compresses the vertebral artery. Following diagnostic imaging that demonstrates the exact point of compression of the vertebral artery, decompressive surgery can be planned. Bony decompression surrounding the vertebral artery usually suffices to alleviate the patient's symptoms.

Fig. 3 shows an example of Bowhunter syndrome treated with left C1 hemilaminectomy for decompression of the V3 segment

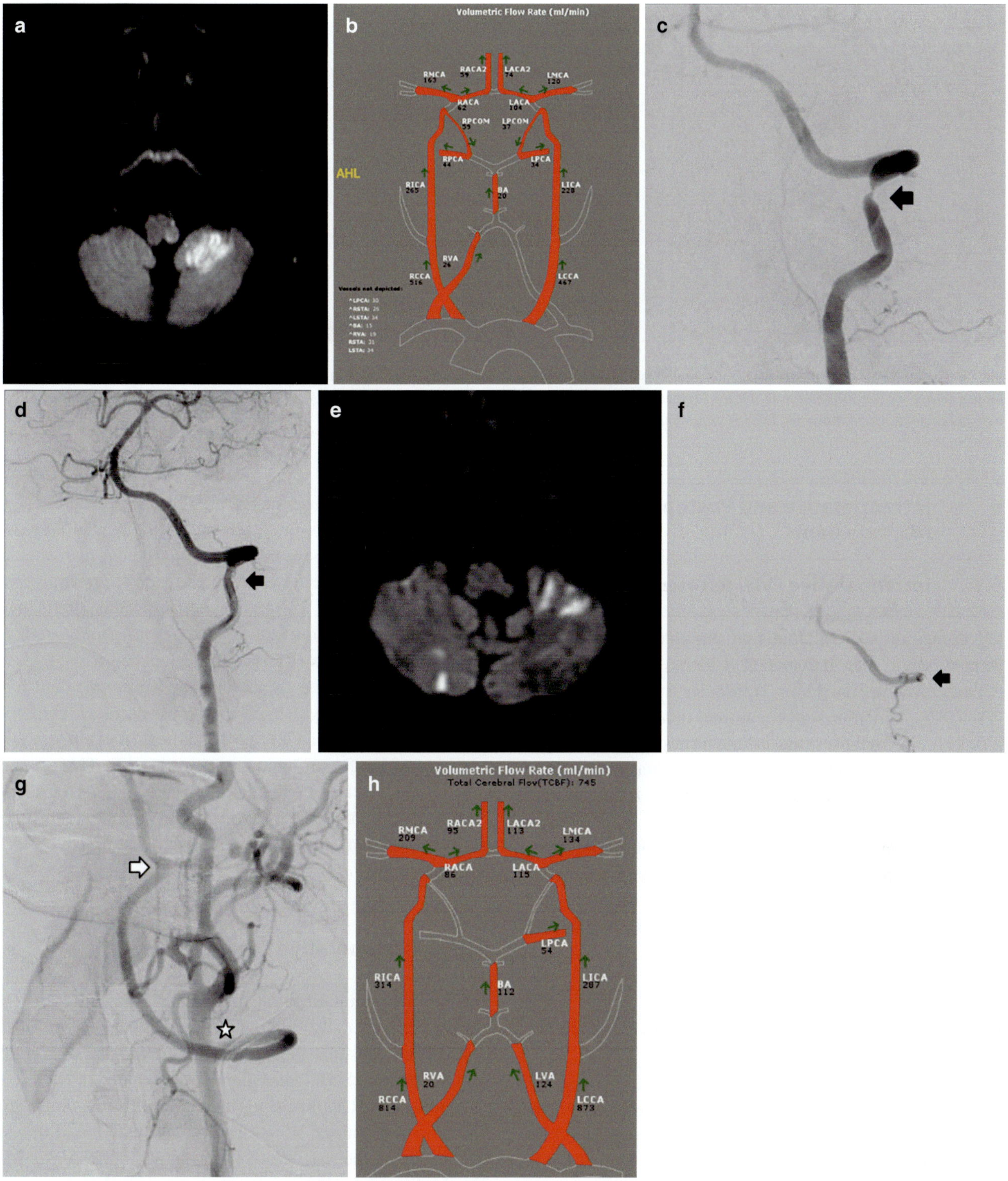

Fig. 2 Example of the left V3 to common carotid artery bypass with interposition graft. (**a**) Initial presentation with left PICA stroke and (**b**) poor vertebrobasilar flow on NOVA. Diagnostic cerebral angiogram of left VA with (**c**) pre- and (**d**) post-angioplasty of severe V3 stenosis (black arrows point to area of stenosis in left VA). (**e**) Follow-up NOVA with improved flow in left VA. (**f**) MRI with recurrent stroke and (**f**) follow-up angiogram with left VA occlusion on AP view (black arrow points to point of reconstitution via muscular branch). (**g**) Post-bypass angiogram with patent bypass from left common carotid artery (white star) to left V3 (white arrow) and (**h**) NOVA showing improved flow

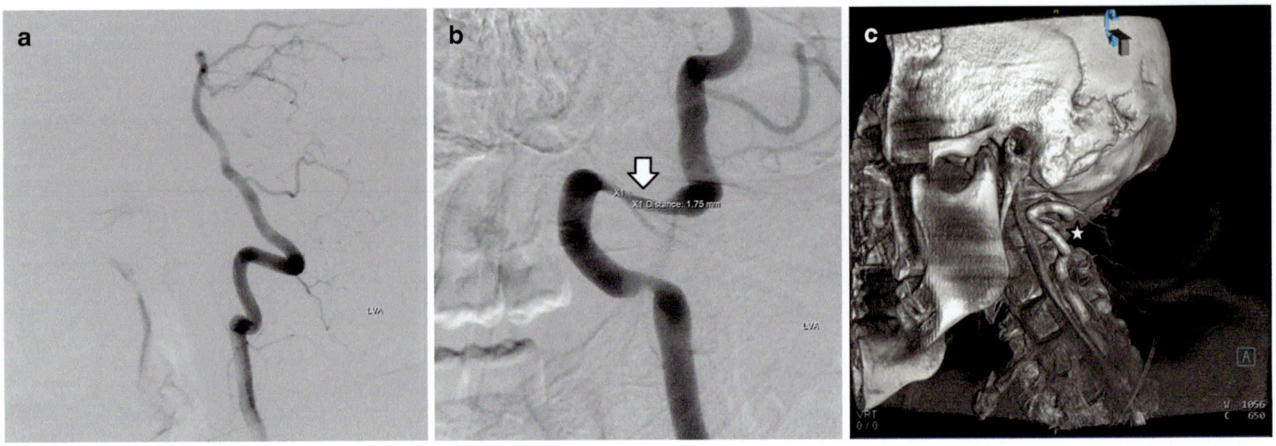

Fig. 3 Example of Bowhunter syndrome treated with left C1 hemilaminectomy for decompression of the V3 segment. Dynamic diagnostic cerebral angiogram shows the left VA in (**a**) neutral position and then (**b**) head turned to right (white arrow points to region of stenosis). (**c**) Post-operative Dyna CT with contrast shows the bony decompression surrounding the vertebral artery (white star)

6 Intraoperative and Postoperative Management

6.1 Intraoperative Flow Assessment

Direct measurement of blood flow through the bypass is performed using the intracranial Charbel micro-flowprobe (Charbel Micro-Flowprobe; Transonics System Inc., Ithica, NY, USA), which provides real-time quantitative feedback [20, 21]. This tool uses transit-time ultrasonic technology to quantifies blood flow, gives waveform data, and provides acoustic feedback. Because this probe utilizes transit-time ultrasound, the flow measurement is not influenced by turbulence, hematocrit, or flow velocity profile [36]. When ready to measure blood flow, the micro-flowprobe is gently placed around the vessel of interest, using either a small quantity of sterile ultrasound gel or saline irrigation as ultrasound couplant.

6.2 Cut Flow and Cut Flow Index

Metrics like the cut flow and cut flow index guide intraoperative decision-making, predicting long-term patency. The **cut flow** refers to the maximum carrying capacity of blood flow through an *in situ* graft, like the STA or OA [1, 3, 4]. After harvesting the donor vessel, the micro-flowprobe is used to determine the amount of flow that can be transferred through this vessel, when distal resistance has been removed. To illustrate this point, in the scalp, the proximal STA or OA flow ranges from 5–10 mL/min due to the high resistance of distal branches; however, once the STA or OA have been dissected and disconnected from the distal end during bypass preparation, the flow rises to 60 mL/min [40]. The cut flow should fall within 20% of the flow measured in the recipient to prevent ischemia [22, 24, 29], and larger interposition grafts may be needed if the cut flow falls beyond this threshold.

The **cut flow index (CFI)** can be calculated as the bypass flow (mL/min) divided by the cut flow (mL/min). CFI has been studied primarily in bypass for steno-occlusive cerebrovascular disease, and a CFI of >0.5 at the time of surgery is a predictor of long-term bypass patency [1, 43]. The general concept of CFI can be extended to bypass surgery for aneurysms, and a poor CFI may raise concern for the donor vessel, interposition graft, anastomosis, or recipient vessel intraoperatively.

6.3 Postoperative Care

Patients are maintained on antiplatelet therapy, typically aspirin 325 mg daily. Follow-up imaging, including DSA and QMRA, ensures graft patency and evaluates cerebral hemodynamics. Serial measurements of blood flow using quantitative MRA, such as that with NOVA software (Noninvasive Optimal Vessel Analysis; VasSol, Inc., Illinois, USA) follows the patency of the bypasss [41, 2, 5, 32, 34, 51]. Multimodal MRI protocols, as described above, may also monitor long-term vascular health, by combining the QMRA with regional and global BOLD imaging with task performance and vasodilatory challenge to check hemodynamic reserve.

7 Conclusion

Surgical revascularization remains a critical option for managing vertebral artery disease in patients unresponsive to medical therapy or endovascular interventions. Success hinges on meticulous preoperative planning, precise surgical execution, and robust postoperative monitoring. Advances in imaging and flow measurement continue to enhance the outcomes of these complex procedures.

Declarations

Competing Interests The author(s) has no competing interests to declare that are relevant to the content of this manuscript.

Ethics Approval The author(s) declares that this manuscript does not include primary research with human participants.

References

1. Amin-Hanjani S, Du X, Mlinarevich N, Meglio G, Zhao M, Charbel FT. The cut flow index: an intraoperative predictor of the success of extracranial-intracranial bypass for occlusive cerebrovascular disease. Neurosurgery. 2005;56(1 Suppl):75–85. discussion 75–85
2. Amin-Hanjani S, Shin JH, Zhao M, Du X, Charbel FT. Evaluation of extracranial-intracranial bypass using quantitative magnetic resonance angiography. J Neurosurg. 2007 Feb;106(2):291–8.
3. Amin-Hanjani S, Alaraj A, Charbel FT. Flow replacement bypass for aneurysms: decision-making using intraoperative blood flow measurements. Acta Neurochir. 2010a;152(6):1021–32. discussion 1032
4. Amin-Hanjani S, Rose-Finnell L, Richardson D, Ruland S, Pandey D, Thulborn KR, Liebeskind DS, Zipfel GJ, Elkind MS, Kramer J, Silver FL, Kasner SE, Caplan LR, Derdeyn CP, Gorelick PB, Charbel FT, VERiTAS Study Group. Vertebrobasilar flow evaluation and risk of transient Ischaemic attack and stroke study (VERiTAS): rationale and design. Int J Stroke. 2010b Dec;5(6):499–505.
5. Amin-Hanjani S, Singh A, Rifai H, et al. Combined direct and indirect bypass for moyamoya: quantitative assessment of direct bypass flow over time. Neurosurgery. 2013;73(6):962–7. discussion 967–8
6. Amin-Hanjani S, Du X, Rose-Finnell L, Pandey DK, Richardson D, Thulborn KR, Elkind MS, Zipfel GJ, Liebeskind DS, Silver FL, Kasner SE, Aletich VA, Caplan LR, Derdeyn CP, Gorelick PB, Charbel FT, VERiTAS Study Group. Hemodynamic features of symptomatic Vertebrobasilar disease. Stroke. 2015;46(7):1850–6.
7. Amin-Hanjani S, Pandey DK, Rose-Finnell L, Du X, Richardson D, Thulborn KR, Elkind MS, Zipfel GJ, Liebeskind DS, Silver FL, Kasner SE, Aletich VA, Caplan LR, Derdeyn CP, Gorelick PB, Charbel FT, Vertebrobasilar flow evaluation and risk of transient ischemic attack and stroke study group. Effect of hemodynamics on stroke risk in symptomatic atherosclerotic Vertebrobasilar occlusive disease. JAMA Neurol. 2016 Feb;73(2):178–85.
8. Amin-Hanjani S, Turan TN, Du X, Pandey DK, Rose-Finnell L, Richardson D, Elkind MS, Zipfel GJ, Liebeskind DS, Silver FL, Kasner SE, Gorelick PB, Charbel FT, Derdeyn CP, VERiTAS Study Group. Higher stroke risk with lower blood pressure in hemodynamic Vertebrobasilar disease: analysis from the VERiTAS study. J Stroke Cerebrovasc Dis. 2017 Feb;26(2):403–10.
9. Amin-Hanjani S, Stapleton CJ, Du X, Rose-Finnell L, Pandey DK, Elkind MSV, Zipfel GJ, Liebeskind DS, Silver FL, Kasner SE, Caplan LR, Derdeyn CP, Gorelick PB, Charbel FT, VERiTAS Study Group. Hypoperfusion symptoms poorly predict hemodynamic compromise and stroke risk in Vertebrobasilar disease. Stroke. 2019 Feb;50(2):495–7.
10. Amin-Hanjani S, See AP, Du X, Rose-Finnell L, Pandey DK, Chen YF, Elkind MSV, Zipfel GJ, Liebeskind DS, Silver FL, Kasner SE, Gorelick PB, Charbel FT, Derdeyn CP, VERiTAS Study Group. Natural history of hemodynamics in Vertebrobasilar disease: temporal changes in the VERiTAS study cohort. Stroke. 2020 Nov;51(11):3295–301.
11. Ausman JI, Diaz FG, de los Reyes RA, Pak H, Patel S, Mehta B, et al. Posterior circulation revascularization. Superficial temporal artery to superior cerebellar artery anastomosis. J Neurosurg. 1982;56:766–76.
12. Ausman JI, Diaz FG, Vacca DF, Sadasivan B. Superficial temporal and occipital artery bypass pedicles to superior, anterior inferior, and posterior inferior cerebellar arteries for vertebrobasilar insufficiency. J Neurosurg. 1990;72:554–8.
13. Batjer HH, Samson DS. Causes of morbidity and mortality from surgery of aneurysms of the distal basilar artery. Neuro Surg. 1989;25:904–16.
14. Berguer R, Andaya LV, Bauer RB. Vertebral artery bypass. Arch Surg. 1976 Sep;111(9):976–9.
15. Bin-Alamer O, Qedair J, Palmisciano P, Mallela AN, Nayar GM, Lu VM, Labib MA, Lang MJ, Gross BA, Langer DJ, Couldwell WT, Friedlander RM, Abou-Al-Shaar H. Dolichoectatic vertebrobasilar aneurysms: a systematic review and meta-analysis of management strategies and outcomes. Neurosurg Focus. 2023 May;54(5):E9.
16. Caplan LR, Wityk RJ, Glass TA, Tapia J, Pazdera L, Chang HM, Teal P, Dashe JF, Chaves CJ, Breen JC, Vemmos K, Amarenco P, Tettenborn B, Leary M, Estol C, Dewitt LD, Pessin MS. New England Medical Center posterior circulation registry. Ann Neurol. 2004 Sep;56(3):389–98.
17. Carney AL, Anderson EM. Carotid distal vertebral bypass for carotid occlusion: case report and technique. Clin EEG Neurosci. 1978;9(3):105–9.
18. Carney AL, Anderson EM, Martinez DM. Advances in vertebral artery surgery at the skull base. Tex Heart Inst J. 1986 Mar;13(1):83–90.
19. Charbel FT. Flow assisted aneurysm surgery-cerebral aneurysm handbook. New York: Transonic Systems; 2004.
20. Charbel FT, Hoffman WE, Misra M, Ostergren L. Ultrasonic perivascular flow probe: technique and application in neurosurgery. Neurol Res. 1998 Jul;20(5):439–42.
21. Charbel FT, Guppy KH, Zhao M, Clark ME. Computerized hemodynamic evaluation of the cerebral circulation for bypass. Neurosurg Clin N Am. 2001;12(3):499–508. viii
22. Charbel FT, Zhao M, Amin-Hanjani S, Hoffman W, Du X, Clark ME. A patient-specific computer model to predict outcomes of the balloon occlusion test. J Neurosurg. 2004 Dec;101(6):977–88.
23. Charbel FT, Guppy KH, Ausman JI. Cerebral revascularization: Superficial temporal middle cerebral artery anastomosis. In: Sekhar LN, Fessler RG, editors. Atlas of neurosurgical techniques. New York: Thieme; 2006.
24. Eckert B, Thie A, Carvajal M, Groden C, Zeumer H. Predicting hemodynamic ischemia by transcranial Doppler monitoring during therapeutic balloon occlusion of the internal carotid artery. AJNR Am J Neuroradiol. 1998 Mar;19(3):577–82.
25. Fiorella D, Kelly ME, Albuquerque FC, Nelson PK. Curative reconstruction of a giant midbasilar trunk aneurysm with the pipeline embolization device. Neurosurgery. 2009;64(2):212–7.

26. Fiorella D, Hsu D, Woo HH, Tarr RW, Nelson PK. Very late thrombosis of a pipeline embolization device construct: case report. Neurosurgery. 2010;67(3 suppl operative):onsE313–4.
27. Hernesniemi J, Vapalahti M, Niskanen M, Kari A. Management outcome for vertebrobasilar artery aneurysms by early surgery. Neurosurgery. 1992;31:857–62.
28. Heros RC, Lee SH. The combined pterional/anterior temporal approach for aneurysms of the upper basilar complex: technical report. Neurosurgery. 1993;33:244–51.
29. Jawad K, Miller D, Wyper DJ, Rowan JO. Measurement of CBF and carotid artery pressure compared with cerebral angiography in assessing collateral blood supply after carotid ligation. J Neurosurg. 1977 Feb;46(2):185–96.
30. Kalani MY, Zabramski JM, Nakaji P, Spetzler RF. Bypass and flow reduction for complex basilar and vertebrobasilar junction aneurysms. Neurosurgery. 2013;72(5):763–75. discussion 775–6
31. Kellner CP, Haque RM, Meyers PM, Lavine SD, Connolly ES Jr, Solomon RA. Complex basilar artery aneurysms treated using surgical basilar occlusion: a modern case series. Clin Article J Neurosurg. 2011;115(2):319–27.
32. Kim T, Bang JS, Kwon OK, et al. Hemodynamic changes after unilateral revascularization for Moyamoya disease: serial assessment by quantitative magnetic resonance angiography. Neurosurgery. 2017;81(1):111–9.
33. Klisch J, Turk A, Turner R, Woo HH, Fiorella D. Very late thrombosis of flow diverting constructs after the treatment of large fusiform posterior circulation aneurysms. AJNR Am J Neuroradiol. 2011;32(4):627–32.
34. Koch MJ, Stapleton CJ, Charbel FT, Russin J, Amin-Hanjani S. Intracranial-intracranial bypass for aneurysms: quantitative intraoperative assessment of flow preservation. Oper Neurosurg (Hagerstown). 2022;22(5):337–42.
35. Lawton MT, Abla AA, Rutledge WC, Benet A, Zador Z, Rayz VL, Saloner D, Halbach VV. Bypass surgery for the treatment of Dolichoectatic basilar trunk aneurysms: a work in Progress. Neurosurgery. 2016 Jul;79(1):83–99.
36. Lundell A, Bergqvist D, Mattsson E, Nilsson B. Volume blood flow measurements with a transit time flowmeter: an in vivo and in vitro variability and validation study. Clin Physiol. 1993 Sep;13(5):547–57.
37. Moufarrij NA, Little JR, Furlan AJ, Leatherman JR, Williams GW. Basilar and distal vertebral artery stenosis: long-term follow-up. Stroke. 1986;17(5):938–42.
38. Qureshi AI, Ziai WC, Yahia AM, Mohammad Y, Sen S, Agarwal P, Zaidat OO, Suarez JI, Wityk RJ. Stroke-free survival and its determinants in patients with symptomatic vertebrobasilar stenosis: a multicenter study. Neurosurgery. 2003 May;52(5):1033-9; discussion 1039-40. https://pubmed.ncbi.nlm.nih.gov/12699544/.
39. Qureshi AI, Qureshi MH, Lien LM, Lee JT, Jeng JS, Hu CJ, Lai TC, Liu CH, Chen CH, Chen PL, Chen TS, Li JY, Lin CL, Hsu CY, Taiwan Stroke Registry Investigators. One-year risk of recurrent stroke and death associated with Vertebrobasilar artery stenosis and occlusion in a cohort of 10,515 patients. Cerebrovasc Dis. 2019;47(1–2):40–7.
40. Rustemi O, Amin-Hanjani S, Shakur SF, Du X, Charbel FT. Donor selection in flow replacement bypass surgery for cerebral aneurysms: quantitative analysis of long-term native donor flow sufficiency. Neurosurgery. 2016;78(3):332–41. discussion 341–2
41. See AP, Pandey DK, Du X, Rose-Finnell L, Charbel FT, Derdeyn CP, Amin-Hanjani S, VERiTAS Study Group. Optimized hemodynamic assessment to predict stroke risk in vertebrobasilar disease: analysis from the VERiTAS Study. J Am Heart Assoc. 2020;9(12):e016406.
42. Siddiqui AH, Abla AA, Kan P, et al. Panacea or problem: flow diverters in the treatment of symptomatic large or giant fusiform vertebrobasilar aneurysms. J Neurosurg. 2012;116(6):1258–66.
43. Stapleton CJ, Atwal GS, Hussein AE, Amin-Hanjani S, Charbel FT. The cut flow index revisited: utility of intraoperative blood flow measurements in extracranial-intracranial bypass surgery for ischemic cerebrovascular disease. J Neurosurg. 2019;133:1396–400.
44. Stapleton CJ, Hussein AE, Behbahani M, Alaraj A, Amin-Hanjani S, Charbel FT. Comparative efficacy of autologous versus cadaveric saphenous vein grafts in cerebral revascularization surgery. J Neurosurg. 2020 May 22;134(5):1562–8.
45. Steinberg GK, Drake CG, Peerless SJ. Deliberate basilar or vertebral artery occlusion in the treatment of intracranial aneurysms. Immediate results and longterm outcome in 201 patients. J Neurosurg. 1993;79(2):161–73.
46. Takeuchi S, Tanikawa R, Tsuboi T, Noda K, Oda J, Miyata S, Ota N, Yoshikane T, Kamiyama H. Superficial temporal artery to proximal posterior cerebral artery bypass through the anterior temporal approach. Surg Neurol Int. 2015 Jun 1;6:95.
47. Tayebi Meybodi A, Lawton MT, Feng X, Benet A. Posterior inferior cerebellar artery reimplantation: buffer lengths, perforator anatomy, and technical limitations. J Neurosurg. 2016 Oct;125(4):909–14.
48. Thulborn K, McGuire LS, Charbel FT, Amin-Hanjani S. Magnetic resonance imaging methods for monitoring hemodynamic reserve in chronic steno-occlusive cerebrovascular disease, Cerebrovascular reactivity. Chapter 8. Berlin: Springer; 2021.
49. WASID Study Group. Prognosis of patients with symptomatic vertebral or basilar artery stenosis. The warfarin-aspirin symptomatic intracranial disease (WASID) study group. Stroke. 1998 Jul;29(7):1389–92.
50. Zhao M, Charbel FT, Alperin N, Loth F, Clark ME. Improved phase-contrast flow quantification by three-dimensional vessel localization. Magn Reson Imaging. 2000 Jul;18(6):697–706.
51. Zhu F, Qian Y, Xu B, et al. Quantitative assessment of changes in hemodynamics of the internal carotid artery after bypass surgery for moyamoya disease. J Neurosurg. 2018 Sep;129(3):677–83.

Rare Conditions: Moya-Moya, Fibromuscular Dysplasia, Dissections

Kikutaro Tokairin, Masaki Ito, and Miki Fujimura

1 Moyamoya Disease

1.1 Introduction

Moyamoya disease (MMD) is a rare idiopathic cerebrovascular disorder characterized by chronic, progressive stenosis or occlusion of the terminus of internal carotid arteries or its main branches around the circle of Willis [1–4]. This pathology is accompanied by the formation of an abnormal network of fine collateral blood vessels, which resemble "puffs of smoke" on cerebral angiography. MMD was initially reported in Japan during the 1950s as a unique cerebrovascular condition demonstrating these characteristic angiographic findings [3, 4]. The term "moyamoya," derived from a Japanese word meaning "hazy or puff of smoke," was first coined by Suzuki et al. in 1969 to describe this angiographic appearance [4]. Despite extensive research, the fundamental etiology of MMD remains unclear. While a subset of patients with similar vascular abnormalities secondary to underlying conditions are categorized under "quasi-MMD". Quasi-MMD refers to moyamoya-like vasculopathy associated with specific diseases or syndromes, such as Down syndrome, neurofibromatosis type 1, sickle cell disease, meningitis, or a history of cranial irradiation [2]. The strict definition of MMD is confined to patients in whom these associated conditions are absent, thereby distinguishing it as a primary, idiopathic entity [2]. Both bilateral and unilateral cases can be diagnosed as moyamoya Disease [2].

1.2 Epidemiology of Moyamoya Disease

The prevalence of MMD exhibits a marked ethnic and racial predisposition, with significantly higher incidences reported in East Asian countries such as Japan and South Korea compared to other regions globally such as United States of America and Europe. In Japan, the prevalence of MMD was reported as 6.03 per 100,000 individuals as of 2003, with an annual incidence of newly diagnosed cases ranging between 0.54 and 0.94 per 100,000 per year [5–7]. By comparison, the annual incidence in the United States has been estimated at 0.57 per 100,000, based on nationwide data collected between 2002 and 2008 [8]. MMD affects both pediatric and adult populations, with a characteristic bimodal age distribution [6, 9]. The first peak occurs in children under 10 years of age, while the second peak is observed in adults around 40 years of age [9]. Additionally, the proportion of MMD patients aged over 50 years has been increasing, accounting for 25.5% of cases in 2003 [6]. This trend likely reflects the impact of an aging society. The disease demonstrates a female predominance, with a reported male-to-female ratio of 1:1.8–2.0 [6, 7]. Familial occurrence of MMD is also recognized, comprising approximately 10–12% of all reported cases, further suggesting a potential genetic predisposition [6, 7].

1.3 Pathophysiology of Moyamoya Disease

1.3.1 Histopathological Feature of Moyamoya Disease

The pathophysiology of MMD remains unclear. Histopathological analyses have identified key vascular abnormalities, including medial thinness, waviness of the elastic lamina, and fibrocellular thickening of the intima in the terminal portions of the cerebral arteries [10, 11]. These abnormalities in the arterial wall of patients with MMD lead to the shrinkage of outer diameter and concentric luminal stenosis, and these vascular findings are called as negative remodeling. A reduction in the outer diameter of affected vessels is another characteristic finding of MMD, distinguishing it from atherosclerotic vascular disease [12–14].

K. Tokairin · M. Ito · M. Fujimura (✉)
Department of Neurosurgery, Hokkaido University Graduate School of Medicine, Sapporo, Japan
e-mail: fujimur@med.hokudai.ac.jp

V. Beneš, D. Netuka (eds.), *Surgical and Interventional Treatment of Cerebral Ischemia*,
https://doi.org/10.1007/978-3-032-08934-2_22

This feature is detectable using advanced imaging techniques, such as heavy T2-weighted imaging, as discussed in the next sub-section (1.5. Diagnosis criteria of Moyamoya disease) [2]. Multiple cell types, endothelial cells (ECs), vascular smooth muscle cells, endothelial and vascular smooth muscle progenitor cells (EPCs and VSMCs) as well as macrophages and T cells, are believed to play significant roles in the pathological process [15, 16]. Extensive histological studies have contributed to our understanding of these pathological features [11, 17, 18]. Recent advances include the use of induced pluripotent stem cells (iPSCs) derived from MMD patients. Studies suggest that EC dysfunction may play a more critical role in MMD pathogenesis compared to VSMCs [19, 20]. In MMD, the cerebral arteries, particularly those within the circle of Willis, undergo progressive stenosis, leading to the development of abnormal collateral vessels termed "basal moyamoya". To compensate for cerebral hypoperfusion, additional collateral pathways form via "ventriculofugal subependymal artery" and "ventriculopetal medullary artery" anastomoses, collectively described as "periventricular anastomoses". These anastomoses primarily involve lenticulo-striatal (at the caudate), thalamic (at medial thalamus or insular cortex), and choroidal (at the posterior body of lateral ventricle) channels [21]. Of note, choroidal periventricular anastomoses have been reported as a potential source of intracerebral hemorrhage (especially posterior hemorrhage) at high risk of rebleeding in MMD [22].

1.3.2 Genetics of Moyamoya Disease

From a genetic perspective, the *RNF213* (ring finger protein 213) gene, located on chromosome 17q25.3, has emerged as a key susceptibility factor. Identified in 2011 in Japan, the *RNF213* p.R4810K variant is the most prevalent mutation and is considered a founder mutation in East Asian MMD [23, 24]. This variant is present in 74–90% of MMD patients and in 93–100% of familial cases in East Asian race, with a low estimated penetrance of <1% [23–25]. Despite its strong association, the *RNF213* p.R4810K variant is found in 0.5–2.0% of healthy individuals in East Asian population [24]. Notably, no major susceptibility genes have been identified in Caucasian MMD patients, suggesting that additional genetic or environmental factors may underlie disease onset [26]. Emerging research highlights alterations in microRNA profiles and DNA methylation patterns in MMD patients, pointing to epigenetic contributions to pathogenesis [27, 28]. Although the mechanism underlying *RNF213* p.R4810K variant in MMD patients is undetermined, *in vivo* experiment using the *RNF213*-deficient mice and/or RNF213-knock-in mice may give clue to address this important question. The *RNF213*-deficient mice and/or RNF213-knock-in mice did not spontaneously develop MMD, indicating that not only the genetic factors but also the environmental factors play a role in the pathophysiology of MMD [29, 30]. In fact, the "two-hit" hypothesis has been proposed to explain MMD's etiology, and this theory suggests that a genetic predisposition, such as *RNF213* mutations, requires additional triggers, such as immune dysregulation, infection, or environmental factors, to manifest as MMD [31, 32]. Continued research into these factors is critical for elucidating the complex mechanisms underlying this enigmatic disease.

1.4 Clinical Presentation of Moyamoya Disease

1.4.1 Overview of Clinical Symptoms

The clinical manifestations of MMD vary depending on age and the type of vascular event. The most common presentations include transient ischemic attacks (TIAs), cerebral infarction, intracranial hemorrhage, and headache. Rare presentations such as seizures and involuntary movements have also been documented. Additionally, the detection of asymptomatic cases is increasing due to the widespread use of magnetic resonance imaging (MRI) for brain screening during routine health check-ups, especially in developed countries.

1.4.2 Pediatric Presentation

In pediatric patients, MMD typically presents with TIAs or cerebral infarctions. These ischemic events are often triggered by hyperventilation or physical activity, which exacerbate cerebral ischemia. TIAs are transient episodes of neurological dysfunction, commonly causing paresis or sensory disturbances in the limbs. Hemorrhagic onset is rare in pediatric cases.

1.4.3 Adult Presentation

In adults, MMD can present with either ischemic symptoms (TIAs or cerebral infarction) or intracranial hemorrhage. Hemorrhagic presentations result from the rupture of fragile, abnormal collateral vessels formed in response to chronic cerebral ischemia. Intracranial hemorrhages in MMD may take various forms, including intracerebral hematoma, subarachnoid hemorrhage, and intraventricular hemorrhage with severe neurological conditions and poorer prognosis compared with ischemic symptoms (TIAs or cerebral infarction). The anatomical basis for these hemorrhages lies in the periventricular anastomoses, which develop from the basal regions of the brain to the periventricular zone or basal ganglia or insular cortex [21, 22].

1.4.4 Other Symptoms

Headache is a symptom that affects both pediatric and adult MMD patients. Although the exact mechanism remains unclear, improvement of headache after revascularization surgery suggests that cerebral ischemia may play a role in its pathogenesis [33]. In pediatric cases, orthostatic hypotension has been reported as a symptom of MMD [34]. Cognitive dysfunction, observed in some MMD patients, is thought to result from cerebral infarct or atrophy, or chronic cerebral ischemia without apparent cerebral infarct or atrophy and may reflect long-term damage to critical brain regions involved in higher-order functions [35–37].

1.5 Diagnostic Criteria of Moyamoya Disease

1.5.1 Key Diagnostic Findings

The diagnostic approach to MMD is guided by the "Revised Version 2021 of the Guideline for the Diagnosis of Moyamoya Disease" published by the Research Committee on Moyamoya Disease under the Japanese Ministry of Health and Welfare in 2022 [3]. The diagnostic criteria emphasize the importance of catheter angiography as the gold standard. Key findings necessary for MMD diagnosis include (Fig. 1):

1. Stenosis or occlusion at the terminal portion of the intracranial internal carotid artery.
2. Abnormal vascular networks (moyamoya vessels) around the occlusive or stenotic regions during the arterial phase of angiography.

While bilateral involvement is a classic feature, unilateral cases can also be diagnosed as MMD under current guidelines [2].

1.5.2 Non-invasive Diagnostic Techniques

In pediatric (infants or toddler) and other cases where catheter angiography is contraindicated, diagnosis can be made using MRI and magnetic resonance angiography (MRA), provided the following criteria are met:

1. Stenosis or occlusion of the terminal portion of the intracranial internal carotid artery.
2. Reduction in outer vessel diameter of the terminal internal carotid artery and horizontal segment of the middle cerebral artery on heavy T2-weighted MRI.
3. Abnormal vascular networks in the basal ganglia or periventricular white matter observed on MRA.

The evaluation of outer vessel diameter using heavy T2-weighted MRI is critical for distinguishing MMD from atherosclerotic arterial stenosis [2].

1.5.3 Differentiation from Moyamoya Syndrome

A crucial aspect of diagnosis is differentiating MMD from Moyamoya syndrome (quasi-MMD), which involves similar cerebrovascular changes but is secondary to other conditions, such as: autoimmune diseases (e.g., systemic lupus erythematosus, antiphospholipid syndrome, polyarteritis nodosa, Sjögren syndrome), meningitis, brain tumors, prior cranial irradiation, genetic disorders (e.g., Down syndrome, neurofibromatosis type 1). An exception is hyperthyroidism, which may occasionally be diagnosed as MMD [2].

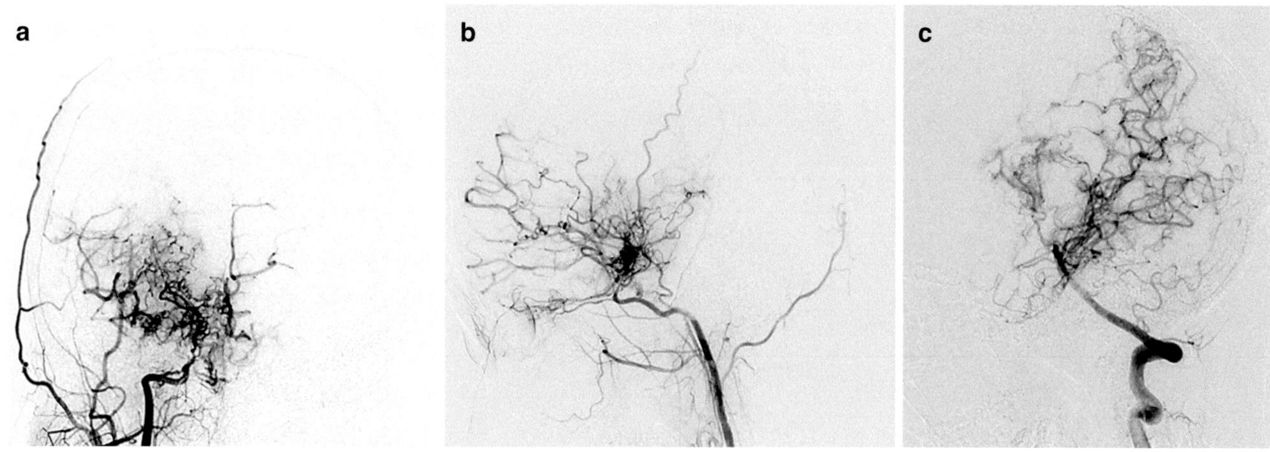

Fig. 1 Angiography of 14 y.o. female with moyamoya disease who presented transient ischemic attack. Suzuki's stage was judged as III. (**a**) and (**b**): Right internal carotid artery (ICA) angiogram (**a**: anteroposterior view, **b**: lateral view) showed stenosis of terminal of ICA and right middle and anterior cerebral artery was not depicted. Remarkable development of basal moyamoya was depicted as compensatory blood flow. (**c**): Left vertebral artery angiogram (lateral view) showed blood supply toward middle cerebral/anterior cerebral artery territory via leptomeningeal anastomosis

1.5.4 The Six-Stage Classification of the Findings of Cerebral Angiography

The Suzuki's angiographical staging system remains the gold standard for assessing cerebral angioarchitecture of MMD. Thus, MMD is known to have unique and dynamic nature to convert the vascular supply for the brain from internal carotid system to the external carotid system, as indicated by Suzuki's angiographic staging established in 1969 [38]. While considering the pathological condition of each patient, it is essential to go back to Suzuki's angiographical staging system and to consider the patients' angiographic and hemodynamic status. This system classifies MMD into six stages (I–VI) according to the regression of antegrade cerebral arterial flow and the development of moyamoya vessels and extracranial-intracranial anastomoses (e.g., transdural anastomoses) [39] (Fig. 2). Of note, advanced Suzuki's angiographical stage does not necessarily indicate clinical severity. Thus, as very recently demonstrated by Asymptomatic Moyamoya Registry (AMORE) from Japan, certain number of asymptomatic MMD patients demonstrated advanced Suzuki's angiographical stage (stage V or VI) [40]. Advancements in MRI/MRA technology have facilitated alternative staging methods, particularly for pediatric patients, where catheter angiography is less feasible. Several studies have proposed grading systems for MMD severity using MRA, providing practical diagnostic options [40–43].

1.5.5 Assessment of Cerebral Hemodynamics

In addition to vascular imaging, assessment of cerebral hemodynamic impairment is essential for evaluating disease severity and determining the need for surgical intervention. The gold standard for hemodynamic assessment is N-isopropyl-p-^{123}I-iodoamphetamine single-photon emission computed tomography (^{123}I-IMP-SPECT). Another option, ^{15}O-gas positron emission tomography (PET), has become less common due to concerns over radiation exposure from aerosolized isotopes. Quantitative measurements of cerebral blood flow (CBF) using ^{123}I-IMP SPECT offer detailed information on cerebral hemodynamic impairment. An acetazolamide challenge can further assess cerebrovas-

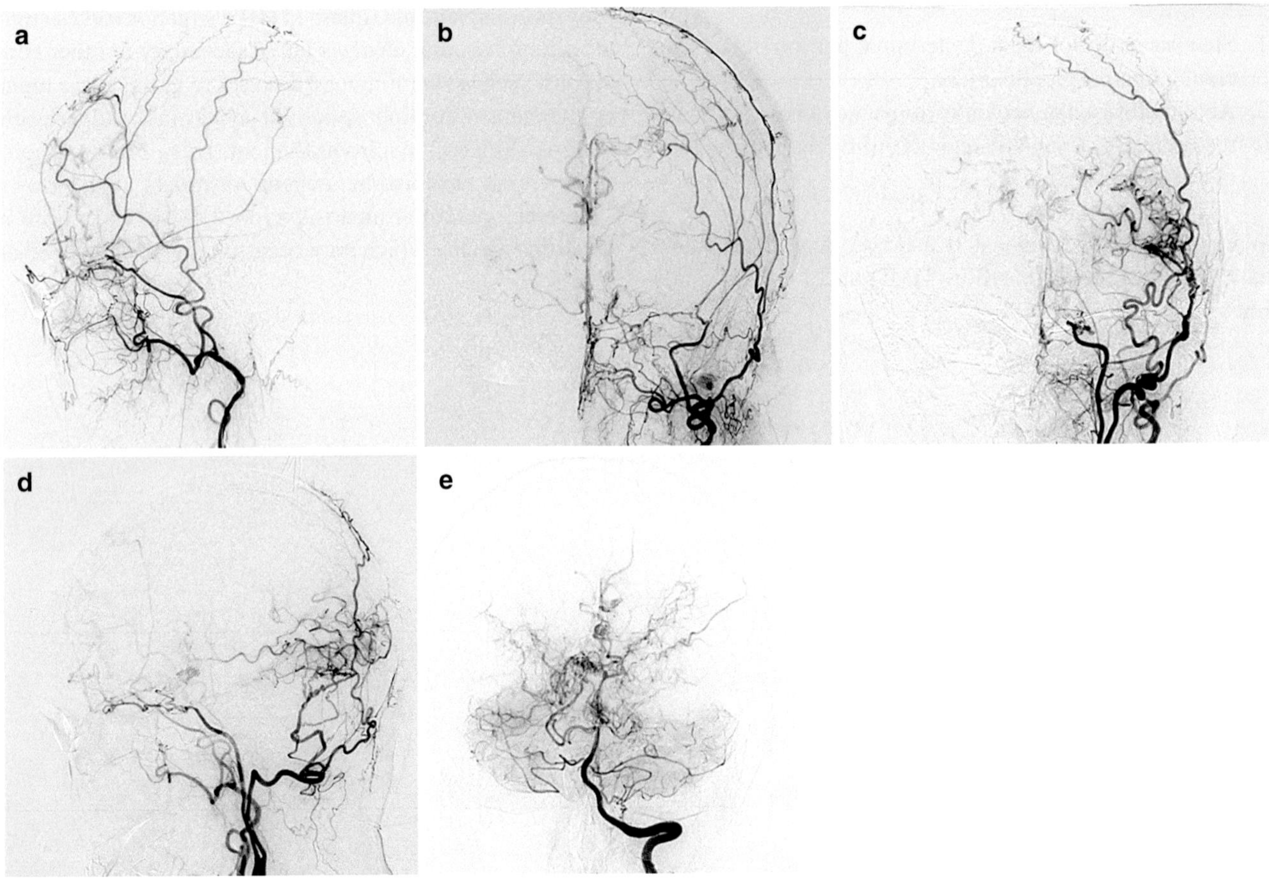

Fig. 2 Angiography of 58 y.o. female with moyamoya disease who presented cerebral infarct in left cerebral hemisphere. Suzuki's stage was judged as V. (**a**) and (**b**): Left external carotid artery angiogram (**a**: antero-posterior view, **b**: lateral view) showed transdural anastomosis from middle meningeal artery and ethmoidal artery. (**c**) and (**d**): left internal carotid artery (ICA) angiogram (**a**: antero-posterior view, **b**: lateral view) showed stenosis of terminal of ICA and left middle and anterior cerebral artery was not depicted. Occipital artery was branche from ICA and remarkable development of transosseous and transdural anastomosis was depicted as compensatory blood flow. (**e**): Left vertebral artery angiogram (lateral view) showed stenosis of left posterior cerebral artery

cular reserve, a critical parameter for identifying patients who would benefit from revascularization surgery (Fig. 3). A significant reduction in CBF or cerebrovascular reserve impairment is indicative of hemodynamic compromise and supports the need for revascularization surgery, as discussed in subsequent sections.

1.6 Surgical Indications for Moyamoya Disease

Treatment for MMD encompasses both medical and surgical approaches, with revascularization surgery being the only proven intervention to prevent stroke recurrence [1].

1.6.1 Medical Management

In ischemic-onset MMD, antiplatelet therapy may be utilized as a bridging strategy until surgical intervention. However, long-term administration of antiplatelet agents is generally discouraged due to the elevated risk of intracranial hemorrhage [1].

1.6.2 Indications for Surgical Treatment

Cerebral revascularization through extracranial-intracranial bypass is the most established surgical method for MMD, supported by substantial clinical evidence. This approach is strongly recommended for patients presenting with ischemic symptoms and documented hemodynamic compromise, as determined through imaging studies such as ^{123}I-IMP SPECT or ^{15}O-gas PET. Surgical revascularization has been shown to reduce recurrence of TIAs and cerebral infarctions and improve long-term cognitive function, attributed to postoperative improvements in CBF and metabolic activity. Revascularization surgery is also effective in preventing recurrent hemorrhages in hemorrhagic-onset MMD. The Japan Adult Moyamoya Trial (JAM Trial), a randomized controlled study, demonstrated that surgical intervention reduced the annual recurrence rate of intracranial hemorrhage to 3.2% in the surgical group compared to 8.2% in the non-surgical group (P = .048) [44]. The JAM trial and its planed supplementary analyses also analyzed hemorrhagic patterns, revealing that "posterior hemorrhages" had a higher recurrence rate (17.1% per year) than "anterior hemorrhages" (2.0% per year) in the non-surgical group (*P* = .001), preventive effects of surgery were significantly greater for patients with "posterior hemorrhage" (*P* = .013) [45]. Revascularization surgery is generally contraindicated in patients with: extensive ischemic or hemorrhagic scars in the cerebral hemispheres, significant disability, as indicated by a modified Rankin Scale score ≥ 3, suggesting dependency in activities of daily living.

1.6.3 Surgical Consideration for Asymptomatic Cases

The management of asymptomatic MMD remains controversial, as increasing MRI/MRA use has led to more incidental diagnoses. The AMORE study provided important insights: asymptomatic hemispheres carry a 1.0% annual risk of stroke over 5 years, with most being hemorrhagic strokes [40]. The presence of choroidal anastomoses is associated with a higher risk of hemorrhagic stroke. Asymptomatic cases exhibit a risk of disease progression, transient ischemic attacks, and de novo microbleeds at a rate of 5.9% per patient-year [46]. In summary, asymptomatic cases should be closely monitored with regular MRI/MRA imaging [40].

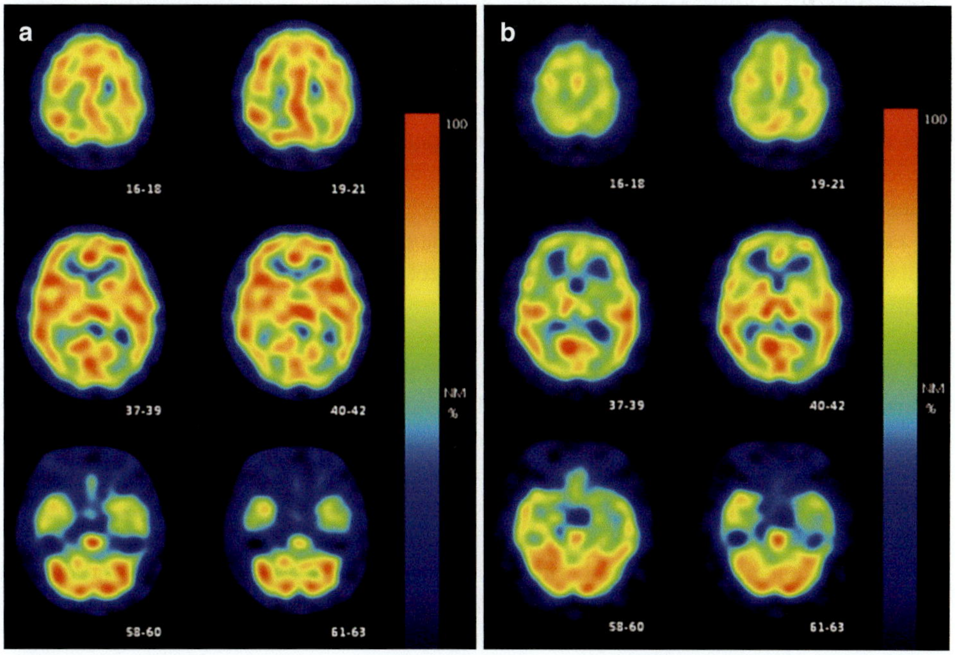

Fig. 3 ^{123}I-IMP-SPECT images of 14 y.o. female with moyamoya disease who presented transient ischemic attack. (**a**): ^{123}I-IMP-SPECT images at resting state showed mild cerebral blood flow (CBF) decrease in bilateral middle cerebral artery territory. (**b**): ^{123}I-IMP-SPECT images after acetazolamide challenge showed marked CBF decrease in bilateral middle and anterior cerebral artery territory, and it meant impaired cerebrovascular reserve in those territory

1.7 Surgical Procedures in Revascularization Surgery for Moyamoya Disease

Revascularization surgery, primarily through extracranial-intracranial (EC-IC) bypass, is a well-established surgical treatment for MMD. Revascularization techniques are broadly categorized into direct, indirect, and combined approaches.

1.7.1 Direct Revascularization

Direct revascularization involves creating an immediate bypass between the superficial temporal artery (STA) and the middle cerebral artery (MCA) to improve cerebral perfusion. Other direct anastomosis includes STA to anterior cerebral artery (ACA), and occipital artery (OA) to MCA or posterior cerebral artery (PCA). This approach restores blood flow directly and is associated with rapid postoperative improvement in hemodynamics.

1.7.2 Indirect Revascularization

Indirect revascularization involves the placement of vascularized tissue in proximity to the brain, stimulating angiogenesis over time. Common techniques include: *Encephalo-myo-synangiosis* (EMS): Placement of the temporalis muscle on the brain surface; *Encephalo-arterio-synangiosis* (EAS): Placement of the STA on the brain surface without direct anastomosis; *Encephalo-duro-synangiosis* (EDS): Attachment of the dura mater to the brain surface to encourage vascular ingrowth; *Encephalo-duro-myo-synangiosis* (EDMS): Attachment both of the dura mater and temporalis muscle to the brain surface to encourage vascular ingrowth; *Encephalo-duro-arterio-myo-synangiosis* (EDAMS): Attachment either the dura mater, temporalis muscle, and STA to the brain surface to encourage vascular ingrowth; *Encephalo-duro-myo-arterio-pericranio-synangiosis* (EDMAPS): Attachment either the dura mater, temporalis muscle, STA, and frontal pericranial flap to the brain surface to encourage vascular ingrowth [47]. Additional techniques, such as multiple burr-hole surgery, are employed to encourage indirect revascularization, particularly in pediatric patients or in cases where direct anastomosis is challenging.

1.7.3 Combined Revascularization

Combined revascularization integrates both direct and indirect techniques, providing immediate and long-term wider improvements in cerebral blood flow. Studies suggest that combined revascularization may achieve superior perfusion outcomes compared to indirect revascularization alone, particularly in adult patients [48, 49]. However, indirect-only revascularization is generally considered insufficient for adult MMD cases due to limited efficacy in this demographic [50].

1.8 Standard Surgical Techniques of Combined Revascularization in Moyamoya Disease

Herein, we present the standard surgical techniques of combined revascularization for MMD with our current clinical/practical considerations. Figure 4 are intra-operative photo(micro)graphs of right-side STA-MCA anastomosis with EDMS (combined revascularization) in 41 years old male who presented TIA. Under general anesthesia, clamp patient's skull with pins and hold the head at 80-degree (Fig. 4a). Skin incision is made along with the STA approximately 8 to 10 cm in length, and skin flap is inverted by "L-shape" incision in case of the using STA parietal branch, or by "question-marked" incision in case of the using STA frontal branch, so as to preserve another branch of STA (Fig. 4a, b). Craniotomy is performed around Sylvian fissure end, approximately 8 cm in diameter. The stump of donor STA is prepared as semi-fish mouse shape with the stump of 1.6 to 2.0 mm (Fig. 4c). Clamp recipient artery (M4 segment of MCA) using mini-clips and make incision on the recipient artery 0.8 to 1.2 mm in diameter (Fig. 4c). The stump of STA is anastomosed by 10–0 or 11–0 nylon monofilament suture to the recipient artery. It generally takes 3 to 4 sutures for each side (Fig. 4d, e). After reperfusion, the patency of STA-MCA anastomosis is confirmed by doppler ultrasonography and intra-operative indocyanine green (ICG) video angiography (arrows in Fig. 4f, g). The STA-MCA bypass is followed by indirect pial synangiosis with EDMS (Fig. 4h). The inner layer of the free bone flap is routinely drilled out for avoiding post-operative compression of the brain surface by the temporal muscle pedicle, and a wide bone window is made on the side of EDMS flap insertion [51, 52]. The temporal muscle is usually split out into two layers. The bone flap is fixed with titanium plates and/or bio-absorbable plates.

1.9 Surgical Complication and Peri-operative Management

Major surgical complications of the combined revascularization for MMD include cerebral infarction and CHP syndrome.

1.9.1 Cerebral Infarction

Perioperative ischemic stroke could be caused by various factors such as intra-operative hypotension and/or hypocapnia by inadequate general anesthesia, anemia, and surgical procedure [1]. Perioperative ischemic complications are categorized into three distinct mechanisms; thrombo-embolism at the site of the microvascular anastomosis, intrinsic hemodynamic ischemia by 'watershed shift phenomenon', and mechanical compression of the brain surface by swollen

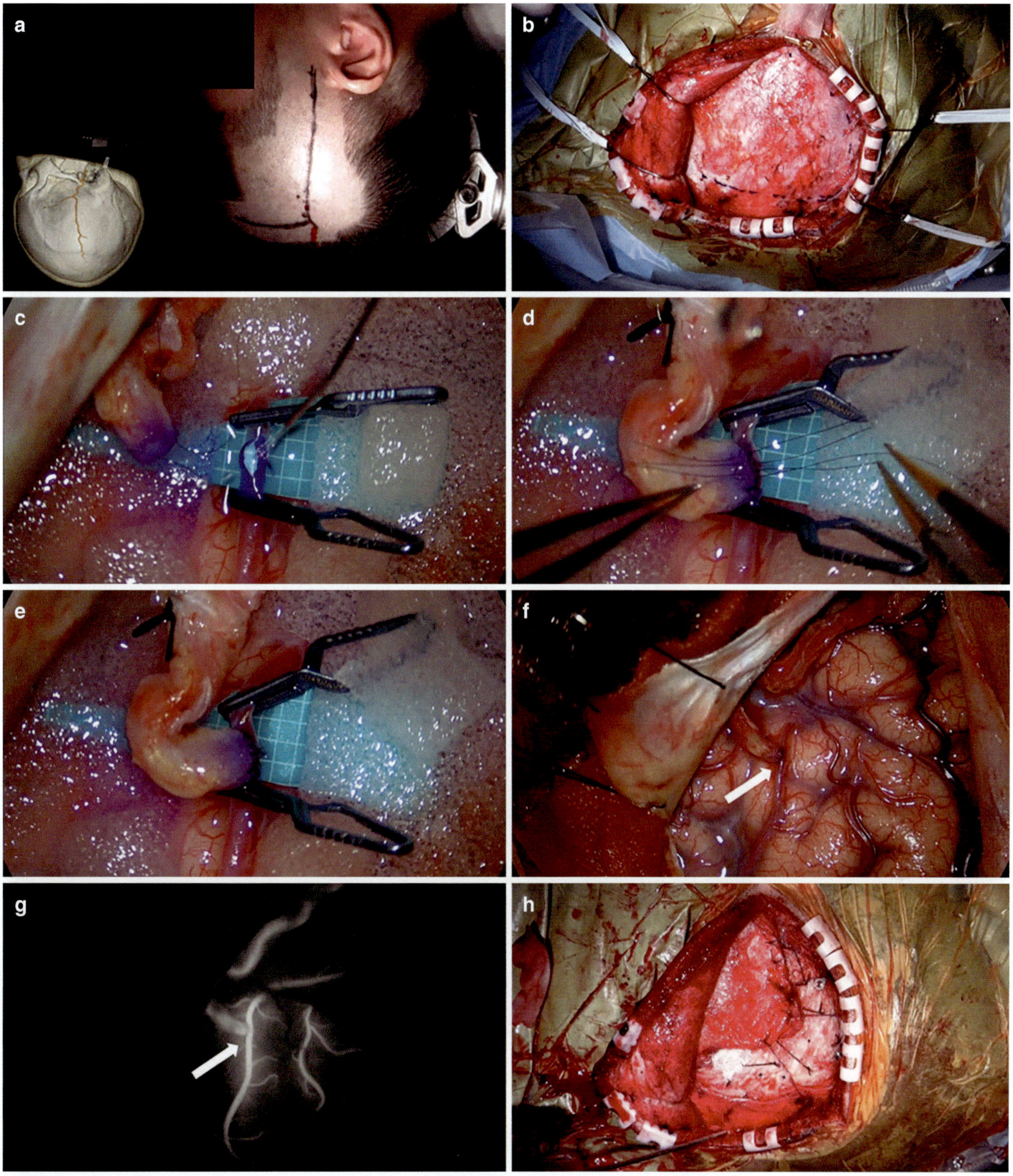

Fig. 4 Serial intraoperative images of 41 y.o. male with moyamoya disease who presented transient ischemic attack. He underwent right direct and indirect combined revascularization (superficial temporal artery-middle cerebral artery bypass with encephalo-duro-myo-synangiosis). (**a**): Patient's skull is clamped with pins and hold the head in 80-degree rotation and mild vertex-up position by using skull clamp system. Skin incision line is designed according to (superficial temporal artery) STA running. In this case, parietal branch of STAs is utilized and skin incision line should bend towards anterior direction in order to perform sufficient craniotomy STA. (**b**): Open the surgical field using skin hooks after harvesting STA, then cut the temporal muscle. (**c**): Clamp recipient artery using mini-clips, and make incision on the recipient artery using fine scalpel and cut appropriate length using microsurgical scissors (**d**): Perform anastomosis using 10–0 nylon. Make suture ligation for one side, followed by the other side. (**e**): It generally takes 3–4 sutures for each side. (**f**): Complete STA-MCA anastomosis, and check the patency by ultrasound doppler probe. It is important to observer there is no intraluminal thrombus in the anastomosed site. (**g**): Indocyanine green video angiography shows excellent patency of STA-MCA anastomosis. Check how the cortical blood flow is supplied from the donner STA. (**h**): Bone flap is fixed by titanium and absorbable plates. Blue arrowhead shows titanium plates, yellow arrowhead shows absorbable plate. Arrow shows cotton wool-like bioresorbable bone void filler. Lay superficial layer of split temporal muscle so as to cover the bone flap

temporal muscle pedicle used for additional indirect pial synangiosis [51, 53–56]. Among them, 'watershed shift phenomenon' is a characteristic pathophysiological condition after STA-MCA bypass for MMD, and is defined as a paradoxical CBF decrease at the adjacent cortex near the site of local CHP [55, 56]. Possible mechanism underling watershed shift phenomenon is that retrograde blood supply from STA-MCA bypass could conflict with the anterograde CBF from more proximal MCA, resulting in the transient CBF decrease at the cortex supplied by the adjacent branch of MCA [54]. Clinical outcome of watershed shift ischemia is generally favorable but its simultaneous occurrence with CHP could make the perioperative pathology more complex and difficult, since the management of each condition is contradictory [55, 56]. To avoid ischemic complications, it is essential to maintain proper perioperative hydration and blood pressure control with prompt hemoglobin concentration maintenance [1]. Efficacy of the anti-platelet agent during the peri-operative period is controversial among MMD patients, but recent multiple studies strongly suggested the advantage of aspirin administration to reduce the risk of perioperative complication after STA-MCA bypass for MMD [57, 58].

1.9.2 Cerebral Hyperperfusion in Adult MMD Patients

CHP syndrome is one of the most serious complications after STA-MCA bypass for MMD [59–64]. Excessive local increase in CBF at the site of the STA-MCA bypass is known to result in local hyperemia associated with vasogenic edema, which is called CHP. It is known that CHP basically does not occur in pediatric cases. The incidence rate of CHP is reported as 15%–50% in adult cases [60, 64, 65]. The mechanism for CHP after STA-MCA bypass remains undetermined, however, increased expression of serum matrix metalloproteinase-9, cytokines, angiogenic factors, and circulating endothelial progenitor cells are reportedly involved in the pathogenesis of MMD, and these factors are hypothesized to induce increasing BBB permeability and to develop CHP [66]. Most common clinical presentation of local CHP is transient neurological deteriorations, but it can also lead to epileptic seizure or intracerebral hemorrhage in a rare occasion [62, 67]. Blood pressure dependent worsening of the focal neurological sign has a diagnostic value for CHP syndrome. The gold standard modality of making diagnosis of CHP is ^{123}I-IMP-SPECT (Fig. 5.). Recent report discussed the pathological threshold of post-operative local CBF increase ratio in ^{123}I-IMP-SPECT for CHP syndrome and hemorrhagic CHP syndrome was 184.5% and 241.3%, respectively [68]. In order to avoid CHP after revascularization surgery in adult MMD patients, post-operative intensive management is required. The most critical point is strict blood pressure control, and systolic BP should be maintained under 130 mmHg [69]. We usually administrate minocycline hydrochloride which has protective effect of blood brain barrier in adult cases [66]. Edaravone infusion is another option

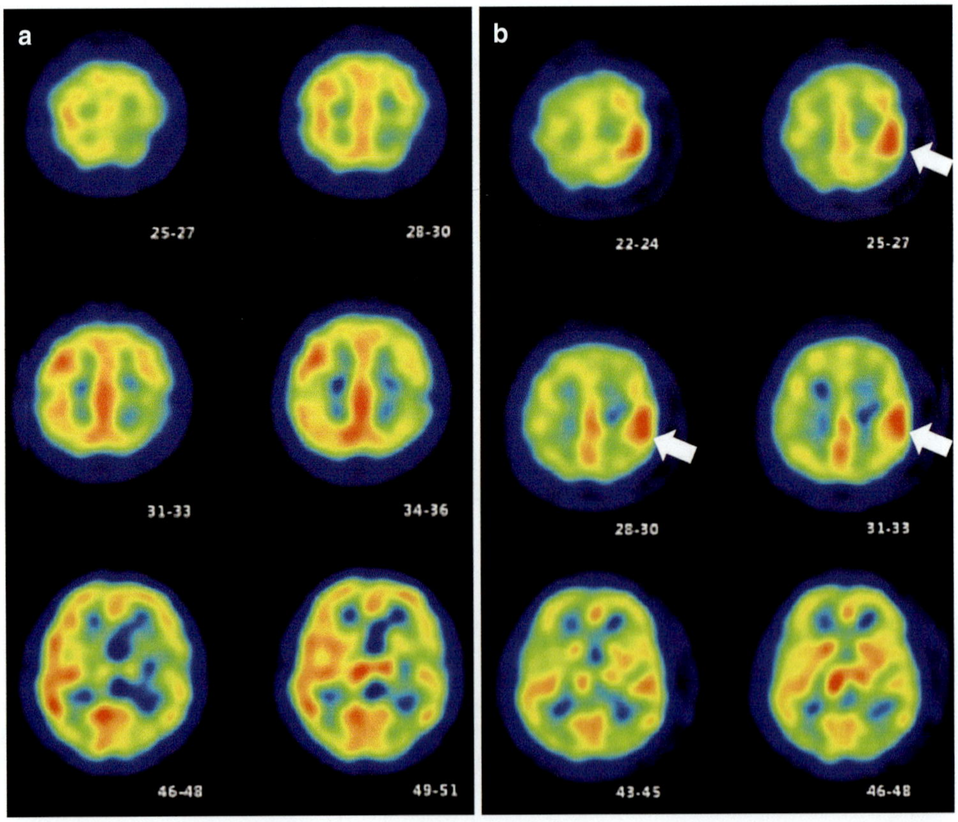

Fig. 5 Pre-and post-operative ^{123}I-IMP-SPECT images of 54 y.o. female with moyamoya disease who presented intracerebral hematoma. She underwent left direct and indirect combined revascularization. (**a**): ^{123}I-IMP-SPECT images at resting state before surgery showed mild cerebral blood flow (CBF) decrease in bilateral middle and anterior cerebral artery (MCA and ACA) territory. (**b**): ^{123}I-IMP-SPECT images at resting state taken postoperative day 1 showed focal CBF increase at anastomosed site of superior temporal artery-MCA bypass. She complained transient aphasia

in adult MMD cases to prevent CHP because it is anti-oxidant agent which shows neuroprotective effect by affecting neurovascular unit [64]. Anti-seizure drug (i.e. perampanel, lacosamide) administration is effective as well to avoid epileptic seizure and to expect neuroprotective effect [61, 70]. We usually take ^{123}I-IMP-SPECT scans on post-operative day (POD) 1 and 7 so as to monitor the CBF changes after revascularization in addition to these management. Representative finding of local CHP is shown in Fig. 5. ^{123}I-IMP SPECT 1 day after the left STA-MCA bypass with EDMS revealed intense focal increase of CBF at the site of the anastomosis (arrows in Fig. 5b). The patient complained transient aphasia at the same timing (POD 1). Under strict blood pressure control with the administration of minocycline hydrochloride and edaravone, the symptom disappeared, and local CHP was ameliorated by ^{123}I-IMP SPECT in POD7 (data not shown).

2 Fibromuscular Dysplasia

2.1 Etiology of Fibromuscular Dysplasia

Fibromuscular dysplasia (FMD) is a rare blood vessel disorder that causes the medium-sized arteries in the body to narrow or bulge. The exact prevalence of FMD and annual incidence of newly diagnosed FMD is unclear. The age prevalence of FMD shows peak in 50 s and sex ratio (male: female) is reported as 1:2–1:5 [71, 72]. Smoking is reported as a risk factor, and some connective tissue diseases are thought to have relation with FMD, such as neurofibromatosis Marfan's syndrome, and Ehlers Danlos Syndrome type IV [73]. Genetic background is considered, but fundamental cause of FMD is unknown.

2.2 Pathophysiology of FMD

The most frequent pathological type of FMD is dysplasia in medial layer of the artery which is characterized by alternative appearance of thickened and thinned of fibromuscular component including collagen along with medial layer of the artery. FMD affects medium size of arteries in the body. Cranio-cervical artery is affected in 25% of all FMD patients, which is second in frequency following renal artery (60%). Intraperitoneal arteries (10%) and external iliac arteries (5%) can be affected as well [72]. The important point is that atherosclerotic or inflammatory change is not typically observed in the affected lesion. Recently, relation between FMD and MMD are reported everywhere. Both are nonatherosclerotic vascular diseases and are common as fibromuscular hyperplasia in their vascular pathology. Very recently, Systemic vasculopathy is named as moyamoya-related systemic vasculopathy (MMRSV) with MMD [74]. MMRSV and FMD are reported to be seem to have similar histopathologic, clinicopathological, and genetic viewpoints. FMD predominantly exhibits proliferative reactions, not only in the intima but also in the media, with disruptive changes in the internal elastic lamina in advanced lesions. Recent genetic analysis reported a closer relationship between MMD and FMD as a nominal correlation with FMD and RNF213 and genetic variant of YY1AP1 or PHACTR1 was also reported not only in FMD cases but also in MMD cases [75]. Although pathological and genetic similarities seem to exist between MMD and FMD, the reason for the site predominance in the intracranial arteries of MMD and the systemic arteries of FMD remains unclear.

2.3 Clinical Presentation and Diagnosis of Fibrous Muscular Dysplasia

Most cases of FMD are asymptomatic, and symptoms of onset depend on the artery affected. FMD of renal artery sometimes develop renal hypertension, and claudication may occur in FMD around external iliac artery or peripheral artery of it [72]. Regarding neurosurgical area, most frequent presentation is cerebral ischemia symptoms brought by FMD around internal carotid artery. Patients are usually suspected as FMD by ultrasound scanning of the applicable artery, and the diagnosis of FMD is made by catheter angiography or CT angiography. The characteristic angiographical finding of FMD is called as "string of pearls" or "string of beads" sign of the affected artery (Fig. 6.).

2.4 Treatment Procedures of FMD in Internal Carotid Artery

Patients with FMD around internal carotid artery is usually asymptomatic, but may develop cerebral ischemia symptoms when the CBF is decreased due to the stenosis of internal carotid artery. The exact rate of symptomatic change from asymptomatic condition is unknown, and there are no consensuses about treatment methods for symptomatic FMD around internal carotid artery. When the affected artery develops severe stenosis, the anatomical etiology of the stenosis is dissection, so the treatment method would be considered according to the dissection of the ICA. See the next section of "dissection" for further treatment procedures.

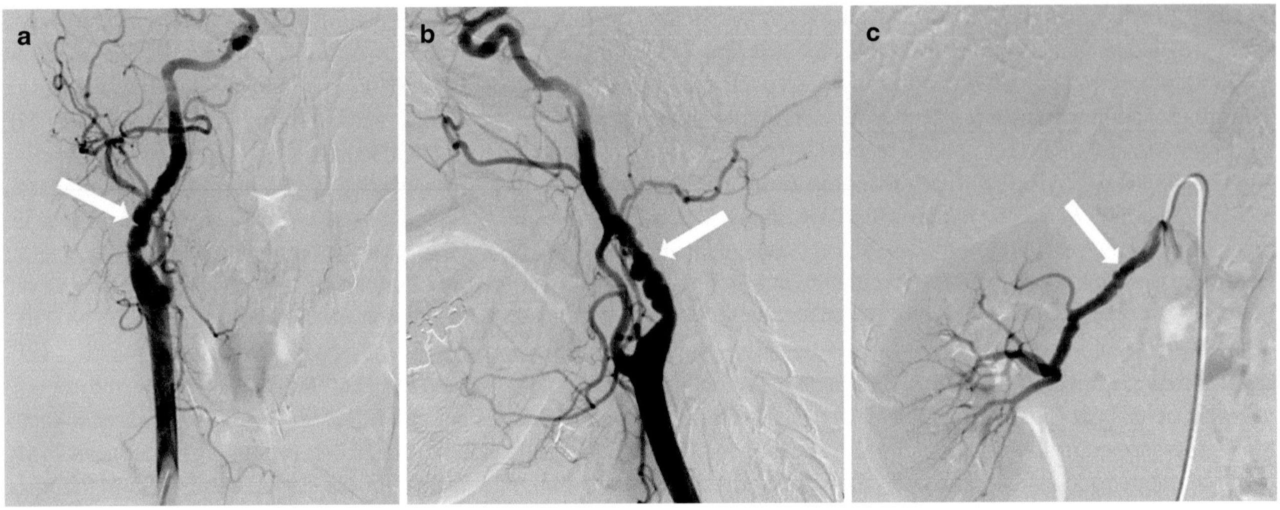

Fig. 6 Angiography of 43 y.o. female with fibromuscular dysplasia without any symptom. (**a**) and (**b**): Right common carotid artery angiogram (**a**: antero-posterior view, **b**: lateral view) showed "string of beads" sign of internal carotid. (**c**): Right renal artery angiogram (antero-posterior view) showed "string of beads" sign of right renal artery

3 Dissections

Arterial dissection is arterial disorder which shows a structural failure of an arterial wall that results in an intramural hemorrhage. It can cause stenosis of true lumen or dissecting aneurysm. Dissection occurs elsewhere in systemic artery, but internal carotid artery and vertebral artery are clinically important in neurosurgical field. It can cause not only pain but also cerebral ischemia or subarachnoid hemorrhage.

3.1 Epidemiology of Dissection

The spontaneous dissection without any medical history is observed frequently in young adults; the mean age at onset is reported 44–46 years old [76–78]. It accounts for approximately 20% of all ischemic stroke in young adults. According to observative study in Minnesota USA, the incidence rate of spontaneous dissection of ICA and VA is reported as 1.72 and 0.97 in 100,000, respectively [78]. However, the actual incidence rate of cervical artery dissection is estimated as higher when compared to those reports because many patients suffer relatively mild symptoms. Extracranial dissection is majority in Northern America and Europe, and intracranial dissection is reported as often seen in Asian population or pediatric cases [79, 80].

3.2 Pathophysiology of Dissection

Separation of arterial wall layers is fundamental histopathology of arterial dissection. Dissection forms a false lumen in the arterial wall, and subintimal disruption can cause true lumen stenosis or occlusion, and intimal tear can cause rupture of arterial rupture. A double channel of arterial flow is sometimes observed when false lumen runs back into true lumen. The common symptom of dissection in craniocervical region is pain; neck pain or headache. The mechanism of this pain is hypothesized that intramural hematoma cause expansion of arterial wall and activate nociceptor [81]. Frequent observed site of dissection in extracranial and intracranial ICA are approximately 20 mm distal from carotid bifurcation where ICA runs near skull base and supraclinoid segment, respectively [76, 82]. Dissection of extracranial ICA typically causes stenotic change and shows cerebral ischemic symptoms. The mechanism of cerebral ischemia is reported as thromboembolism from the stenotic site and/or cerebral hypoperfusion due to stenosis of true lumen where the blood flows. On the other hand, dissection of extracranial ICA sometimes forms "blood blister like aneurysm" which are different from intrinsic cerebral artery aneurysm. The characteristic phenomenon is the diameter of "blood blister like aneurysm" is typically small but is prone to rupture resulting in SAH.

Frequent observed site of dissection in VA is reported as V1 and V3 portion. Dissection of V1-V3 portion usually forms severe posterior neck pain or occipital pain with or without cerebral ischemia, and dissection of V4 portion can cause both cerebral ischemia and SAH. It is rare but MCA, ACA, or PCA can be affected by dissection, and it can also cause both cerebral ischemia and SAH. Observative study reported approximately 40% of cervical artery dissection is brought by prior mild neck trauma of dynamic neck flexion/extension [83]. Familial occurrence and heritable connective tissue disorders in cervical artery dissection is not common and its exact ratio is unclear, however, the most frequently reported disorder is FMD (15–20%), followed by Ehlers Danlos syndrome type IV (2%) [71, 84–86].

3.3 Clinical Presentation and Diagnosis of Dissection

The typical symptom of dissection around cranio-cervical region is sudden pain around the affected artery. If the dissected artery develops stenosis of normal blood vessel lumen, it can cause cerebral ischemia where the affected artery supplies. It sometimes leads to cerebral infarction due to low cerebral blood flow, occlusion of branch(es) which locate(s) around the dissected artery or thrombo-embolism from the abnormal blood vessel lumen [87, 88]. On the other hand, hemorrhagic presentation is observed when the dissected artery locates intradural portion and disrupts beyond outer membrane of vascular wall. Typically, it develops aneurysm first, and then the newly formed aneurysm develops rupture and results in subarachnoid hemorrhage. The frequently affected region is paraclinoid portion of ICA, so-called "blood blister like aneurysm", and V4 portion of VA. The gold standard examination for diagnosis of dissection is catheter angiography. Pearl and string sign is sometimes observed. CT with CTA or MRI with MRA is reported as useful to make diagnosis of dissection as well. However, these modalities just visualize the information of inner lumen of the vessels, so recently the vessel wall imaging (VWI) in MRI is emerging modality to visualize the dissection and attribute the appropriate diagnosis of arterial dissections [89]. VWI can visualize the intimal flap or intraluminal hematoma which are important histological findings in arterial dissection.

3.4 Treatment Procedure for Dissection

The treatment procedure is variously considered, according to the location of dissected artery and presentation types (hemorrhagic or ischemic), thus we describe the treatment procedure limited to frequent situation of dissection.

3.4.1 Ischemic Onset by the Dissection of the Internal Carotid Artery (Cervical Portion)

Carotid artery stenting is optimal treatment method for the dissection of the internal carotid artery. Patients usually suffer sudden symptoms of neck/head pain with or without cerebral ischemia, therefore the procedure is often performed emergently. Dual antiplatelet therapy including loading administration is essential before the procedure. When the location of dissection is limited to proximal portion of the internal carotid artery, the procedure is simple as same as CAS for atherosclerotic stenosis, and 6-10 mm diameter stent for CAS is utilized (i.e. Carotid Wall Stent, Precise Pro) (Fig. 7). However, if the dissection affects more distal portion of ICA such as petrous portion, choice of the stent is sometimes difficult because there is no specified stent for that potion of ICA in commercial base. We usually use stent which is normally used for stent assist coiling for aneurysm of intradural portion of ICA (i.e. Enterprise VRD). The difficult part of the actual procedure of CAS is the lesion cross of the dissected zone using micro-guidewire. The important tip is leading micro-guidewire through the true lumen of the affected artery. It is usually unnecessary to perform balloon angioplasty before and after deploying stent. Multiple stents are sometimes required for long lesion of dissection.

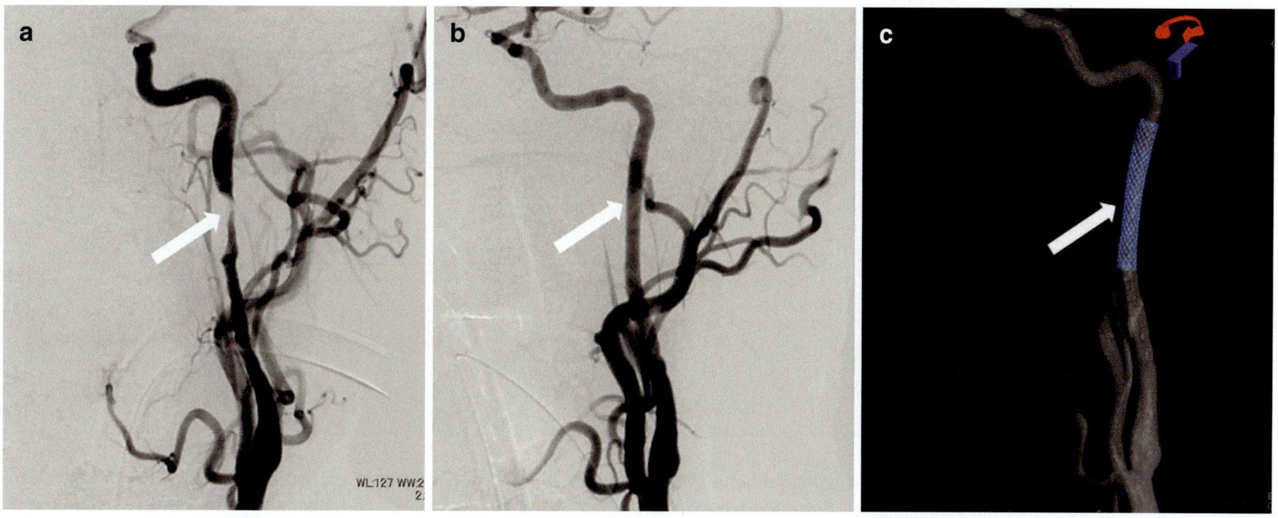

Fig. 7 Angiography of 45 y.o. male with internal carotid artery dissection with sudden headache and left amaurosis. He underwent emergent carotid artery stenting. (**a**): Preoperative right internal carotid artery angiogram (antero-posterior view) showed stenosis in extracranial portion of right ICA. (**b**): Postoperative right ICA angiogram (antero-posterior view) showed improvement of ICA stenosis by deployment of stent (Carotid Wall Stent 6 × 22 mm). (**c**): Three-dimensional rotational angiography showed good attachment of stent with ICA lumen

3.4.2 SAH Onset by the Dissection of the Internal Carotid Artery (Intradural Portion)

Dissection of intradural portion of ICA sometimes forms "blood blister like aneurysm" which results in rupture and SAH. It is usually difficult to apply aneurysmal clip for it because it is small and fragile in its histological nature. The treatment strategy for that type of dissection is trapping with bypass surgery or coiling with stent. Most cases are difficult to perform simple clipping or coiling.

Trapping with Bypass Surgery

Select the bypass scale according to the cerebral blood flow demand after trapping of ICA. It usually requires high flow bypass of ECA-radial artery-M2 bypass, but STA-MCA bypass can be applied for selective cases. Apply aneurysmal clips so as to interrupt the lesion preferably between proximal and distal portion of the lesion, but sometimes clip can be applied only in proximal portion of the lesion (proximal trapping). It is advantage for craniotomy surgery to check whether the lesion actually causes rupture by visual inspection because surgeons are suspicious to make diagnosis of that in its size by preoperative radiological findings. Wrap-clipping techniques are another method to treat "blood blister like aneurysm" if the conditions allow [90, 91].

Intervention

It depends on the shape of the "blood bister like aneurysm" whether stent assist coiling is available or not. VER (volume embolization rate) tends to be low because the neck-height aspect ratio of the aneurysm is low and small in its size. Should be careful for re-rupture in acute phase due to loose coil packing of aneurysm, however, stent assist coiling is optimal treatment option when the aneurysm locates near important branches and cannot be trapped (Fig. 8). Stent overlapping technique is reported to obtain flow diverter effect [92]. Recently, flow diverter stent is utilized to those cases, but there are several issues to perform flow diverter stent deployment in the acute phase [93]. For example, incomplete antiplatelet therapy results in stent occlusion by thrombus, or undetermined results of preventive effect for re-rupture in acute phase.

3.4.3 SAH Onset by the Dissection of the Vertebral Artery (Intradural Portion)

The treatment strategy differs according to the lesion involves PICA or other important branches/perforators. Internal trapping by intervention is optimal method when the lesion is apart from such important branches. Stent assist coiling is optimal when the lesion does not involve directly such important branches but is near from them. Trapping and bypass surgery is required in cases that the lesion involves PICA directly. OA-PICA bypass is performed prior to trapping. Trapping is performed either by internal trapping or direct clipping. Note that internal trapping cannot be applied in cases that both bilateral Pcom arteries and contralateral VA is aplastic or hypoplastic because BA flow is dependent on the ipsilateral VA.

Declarations The authors received no funding regarding this article.

Conflicts of Interest The authors have nothing to declare.

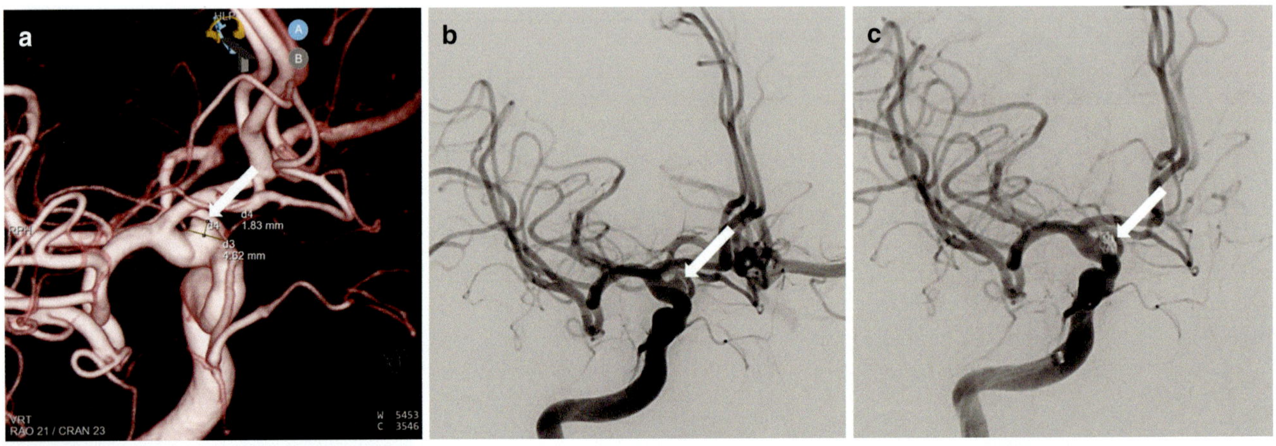

Fig. 8 Angiography of 42 y.o. female with subarachnoid hemorrhage due to ruptured "blood blister like aneurysm" in right internal carotid artery. She underwent emergent stent assist soil embolization because trapping was not feasible as anterior choroidal artery branched out from internal carotid artery at very near site of aneurysm. (**a**): Preoperative three-dimensional rotational angiography of right internal carotid artery (ICA) angiogram. (**b**): Intraoperative right ICA angiogram (working angle) before treatment. (**c**): Intraoperative right ICA angiogram (working angle after treatment. Coils were inserted into the aneurysm after deployment of stent. Stent was deployed from proximal segment of middle cerebral artery to ICA (C3 segment)

References

1. Fujimura M, Tominaga T, Kuroda S, Takahashi JC, Endo H, Ogasawara K, et al. 2021 Japanese guidelines for the management of Moyamoya disease: guidelines from the research committee on Moyamoya disease and Japan stroke society. Neurol Med Chir. 2022;62(4):165–70. https://doi.org/10.2176/jns-nmc.2021-0382.
2. Kuroda S, Fujimura M, Takahashi J, Kataoka H, Ogasawara K, Iwama T, et al. Diagnostic criteria for Moyamoya disease – 2021 revised version. Neurol Med Chir. 2022;62(7):307–12. https://doi.org/10.2176/jns-nmc.2022-0072.
3. Suzuki J, Kodama N. Moyamoya disease–a review. Stroke. 1983;14(1):104–9.
4. Suzuki J, Takaku A. Cerebrovascular "Moyamoya" disease. Disease showing abnormal net-like vessels in base of brain. Arch Neurol. 1969;20(3):288–99. https://doi.org/10.1001/archneur.1969.00480090076012.
5. Baba T, Houkin K, Kuroda S. Novel epidemiological features of Moyamoya disease. J Neurol Neurosurg Psychiatry. 2008;79(8):900–4. https://doi.org/10.1136/jnnp.2007.130666.
6. Kuriyama S, Kusaka Y, Fujimura M, Wakai K, Tamakoshi A, Hashimoto S, et al. Prevalence and clinicoepidemiological features of Moyamoya disease in Japan: findings from a nationwide epidemiological survey. Stroke. 2008;39(1):42–7. https://doi.org/10.1161/STROKEAHA.107.490714.
7. Wakai K, Tamakoshi A, Ikezaki K, Fukui M, Kawamura T, Aoki R, et al. Epidemiological features of Moyamoya disease in Japan: findings from a nationwide survey. Clin Neurol Neurosurg. 1997;99(Suppl 2):S1–5. https://doi.org/10.1016/s0303-8467(97)00031-0.
8. Starke RM, Crowley RW, Maltenfort M, Jabbour PM, Gonzalez LF, Tjoumakaris SI, et al. Moyamoya disorder in the United States. Neurosurgery. 2012;71(1):93–9. https://doi.org/10.1227/NEU.0b013e318253ab8e.
9. Sato Y, Kazumata K, Nakatani E, Houkin K, Kanatani Y. Characteristics of Moyamoya disease based on National Registry Data in Japan. Stroke. 2019;50(8):1973–80. https://doi.org/10.1161/STROKEAHA.119.024689.
10. Nanba R, Kuroda S, Ishikawa T, Houkin K, Iwasaki Y. Increased expression of hepatocyte growth factor in cerebrospinal fluid and intracranial artery in Moyamoya disease. Stroke. 2004;35(12):2837–42. https://doi.org/10.1161/01.STR.0000148237.13659.e6.
11. Takagi Y, Hermanto Y, Takahashi JC, Funaki T, Kikuchi T, Mineharu Y, et al. Histopathological characteristics of distal middle cerebral artery in adult and pediatric patients with Moyamoya disease. Neurol Med Chir. 2016;56(6):345–9. https://doi.org/10.2176/nmc.oa.2016-0031.
12. Kaku Y, Morioka M, Ohmori Y, Kawano T, Kai Y, Fukuoka H, et al. Outer-diameter narrowing of the internal carotid and middle cerebral arteries in Moyamoya disease detected on 3D constructive interference in steady-state MR image: is arterial constrictive remodeling a major pathogenesis? Acta Neurochir. 2012;154(12):2151–7. https://doi.org/10.1007/s00701-012-1472-4.
13. Liu S, Lu M, Gao X, Wen C, Sun B, Liu Y, et al. The diagnostic performance of high-resolution magnetic resonance-vessel wall imaging in differentiating atherosclerosis-associated Moyamoya vasculopathy from Moyamoya disease. Eur Radiol. 2023;33(10):6918–26. https://doi.org/10.1007/s00330-023-09951-z.
14. Yamamoto S, Kashiwazaki D, Akioka N, Kuwayama N, Noguchi K, Kuroda S. Progressive shrinkage of involved arteries in parallel with disease progression in Moyamoya disease. World Neurosurg. 2019;122:e253–e61. https://doi.org/10.1016/j.wneu.2018.10.001.
15. Kang HS, Moon YJ, Kim YY, Park WY, Park AK, Wang KC, et al. Smooth-muscle progenitor cells isolated from patients with Moyamoya disease: novel experimental cell model. J Neurosurg. 2014;120(2):415–25. https://doi.org/10.3171/2013.9.JNS131000.
16. Masuda J, Ogata J, Yutani C. Smooth muscle cell proliferation and localization of macrophages and T cells in the occlusive intracranial major arteries in Moyamoya disease. Stroke. 1993;24(12):1960–7. https://doi.org/10.1161/01.str.24.12.1960.
17. Bersano A, Guey S, Bedini G, Nava S, Herve D, Vajkoczy P, et al. Research progresses in understanding the pathophysiology of Moyamoya disease. Cerebrovasc Dis. 2016;41(3–4):105–18. https://doi.org/10.1159/000442298.
18. Achrol AS, Guzman R, Lee M, Steinberg GK. Pathophysiology and genetic factors in Moyamoya disease. Neurosurg Focus. 2009;26(4):E4. https://doi.org/10.3171/2009.1.FOCUS08302.
19. Hamauchi S, Shichinohe H, Uchino H, Yamaguchi S, Nakayama N, Kazumata K, et al. Cellular functions and gene and Protein expression profiles in endothelial cells derived from Moyamoya disease-specific iPS cells. PLoS One. 2016;11(9):e0163561. https://doi.org/10.1371/journal.pone.0163561.
20. Tokairin K, Hamauchi S, Ito M, Kazumata K, Sugiyama T, Nakayama N, et al. Vascular smooth muscle cell Derived from IPS cell of Moyamoya disease-comparative characterization with endothelial cell transcriptome. J Stroke Cerebrovasc Dis. 2020;29(12):105305. https://doi.org/10.1016/j.jstrokecerebrovasdis.2020.105305.
21. Funaki T, Takahashi JC, Yoshida K, Takagi Y, Fushimi Y, Kikuchi T, et al. Periventricular anastomosis in Moyamoya disease: detecting fragile collateral vessels with MR angiography. J Neurosurg. 2016;124(6):1766–72. https://doi.org/10.3171/2015.6.JNS15845.
22. Funaki T, Takahashi JC, Houkin K, Kuroda S, Takeuchi S, Fujimura M, et al. Angiographic features of hemorrhagic moyamoya disease with high recurrence risk: a supplementary analysis of the Japan adult Moyamoya trial. J Neurosurg. 2018;128(3):777–84. https://doi.org/10.3171/2016.11.JNS161650.
23. Kamada F, Aoki Y, Narisawa A, Abe Y, Komatsuzaki S, Kikuchi A, et al. A genome-wide association study identifies RNF213 as the first Moyamoya disease gene. J Hum Genet. 2011;56(1):34–40. https://doi.org/10.1038/jhg.2010.132.
24. Liu W, Morito D, Takashima S, Mineharu Y, Kobayashi H, Hitomi T, et al. Identification of RNF213 as a susceptibility gene for Moyamoya disease and its possible role in vascular development. PLoS One. 2011;6(7):e22542. https://doi.org/10.1371/journal.pone.0022542.
25. Kim EH, Yum MS, Ra YS, Park JB, Ahn JS, Kim GH, et al. Importance of RNF213 polymorphism on clinical features and long-term outcome in Moyamoya disease. J Neurosurg. 2016;124(5):1221–7. https://doi.org/10.3171/2015.4.JNS142900.
26. Guey S, Kraemer M, Herve D, Ludwig T, Kossorotoff M, Bergametti F, et al. Rare RNF213 variants in the C-terminal region encompassing the RING-finger domain are associated with Moyamoya angiopathy in Caucasians. Eur J Hum Genet. 2017;25(8):995–1003. https://doi.org/10.1038/ejhg.2017.92.
27. Uchino H, Ito M, Kazumata K, Hama Y, Hamauchi S, Terasaka S, et al. Circulating miRNome profiling in Moyamoya disease-discordant monozygotic twins and endothelial microRNA expression analysis using iPS cell line. BMC Med Genet. 2018;11(1):72. https://doi.org/10.1186/s12920-018-0385-3.
28. Tokairin K, Ito M, Lee AG, Teo M, He S, Cheng MY, et al. Genome-wide DNA methylation profiling reveals low methylation variability in Moyamoya disease. Transl Stroke Res. 2024; https://doi.org/10.1007/s12975-024-01299-w.
29. Kanoke A, Fujimura M, Niizuma K, Fujimura T, Kakizaki A, Ito A, et al. Temporal profile of magnetic resonance angiography and decreased ratio of regulatory T cells after immunological adjuvant administration to mice lacking RNF213, a susceptibility gene for Moyamoya disease. Brain Res. 2016;1642:1–9. https://doi.org/10.1016/j.brainres.2016.03.009.

30. Sonobe S, Fujimura M, Niizuma K, Nishijima Y, Ito A, Shimizu H, et al. Temporal profile of the vascular anatomy evaluated by 9.4-T magnetic resonance angiography and histopathological analysis in mice lacking RNF213: a susceptibility gene for Moyamoya disease. Brain Res. 2014;1552:64–71. https://doi.org/10.1016/j.brainres.2014.01.011.
31. Fujimura M, Sonobe S, Nishijima Y, Niizuma K, Sakata H, Kure S, et al. Genetics and biomarkers of Moyamoya disease: significance of RNF213 as a susceptibility gene. J Stroke. 2014;16(2):65–72. https://doi.org/10.5853/jos.2014.16.2.65.
32. Houkin K, Ito M, Sugiyama T, Shichinohe H, Nakayama N, Kazumata K, et al. Review of past research and current concepts on the etiology of Moyamoya disease. Neurol Med Chir. 2012;52(5):267–77.
33. Okada Y, Kawamata T, Kawashima A, Yamaguchi K, Ono Y, Hori T. The efficacy of superficial temporal artery-middle cerebral artery anastomosis in patients with Moyamoya disease complaining of severe headache. J Neurosurg. 2012;116(3):672–9. https://doi.org/10.3171/2011.11.JNS11944.
34. Uchino H, Kazumata K, Ito M, Nakayama N, Houkin K. Novel insights into symptomatology of Moyamoya disease in pediatric patients: survey of symptoms suggestive of orthostatic intolerance. J Neurosurg Pediatr. 2017;20(5):485–8. https://doi.org/10.3171/2017.5.PEDS17198.
35. Kikuchi T, Takagi Y, Nakagawara J, Ueno T, Ubukata S, Houkin K, et al. Neuronal loss in the bilateral medial frontal lobe revealed by (123)I-iomazenil single-photon emission computed tomography in patients with Moyamoya disease: the first report from cognitive dysfunction survey of Japanese patients with Moyamoya disease (COSMO-Japan study). Neurol Med Chir. 2023;63(8):334–42. https://doi.org/10.2176/jns-nmc.2023-0041.
36. Nakagawara J, Osato T, Kamiyama K, Honjo K, Sugio H, Fumoto K, et al. Diagnostic imaging of higher brain dysfunction in patients with adult Moyamoya disease using statistical imaging analysis for [123I]iomazenil single photon emission computed tomography. Neurol Med Chir. 2012;52(5):318–26. https://doi.org/10.2176/nmc.52.318.
37. Kusano Y, Funaki T, Ueda K, Nishida N, Tanaka K, Miyamoto S, et al. Characterizing the neurocognitive profiles of children with Moyamoya disease using the das Naglieri cognitive assessment system. Sci Rep. 2022;12(1):3638. https://doi.org/10.1038/s41598-022-07699-y.
38. Fujimura M, Tominaga T. Current status of revascularization surgery for Moyamoya disease: special consideration for its 'internal carotid-external carotid (IC-EC) conversion' as the physiological reorganization system. Tohoku J Exp Med. 2015;236(1):45–53. https://doi.org/10.1620/tjem.236.45.
39. Mugikura S, Takahashi S, Higano S, Shirane R, Sakurai Y, Yamada S. Predominant involvement of ipsilateral anterior and posterior circulations in Moyamoya disease. Stroke. 2002;33(6):1497–500. https://doi.org/10.1161/01.str.0000016828.62708.21.
40. Kuroda S, Yamamoto S, Funaki T, Fujimura M, Kataoka H, Hishikawa T, et al. Five-year stroke risk and its predictors in asymptomatic Moyamoya disease: asymptomatic Moyamoya registry (AMORE). Stroke. 2023;54(6):1494–504. https://doi.org/10.1161/STROKEAHA.122.041932.
41. Uchino H, Ito M, Fujima N, Tokairin K, Tatezawa R, Sugiyama T, et al. Predictive value of the hemispheric magnetic resonance angiography score on the development of indirect pial synangiosis after combined revascularization surgery for adult Moyamoya disease. Acta Neurochir. 2024;166(1):181. https://doi.org/10.1007/s00701-024-06079-x.
42. Houkin K, Nakayama N, Kuroda S, Nonaka T, Shonai T, Yoshimoto T. Novel magnetic resonance angiography stage grading for Moyamoya disease. Cerebrovasc Dis. 2005;20(5):347–54. https://doi.org/10.1159/000087935.
43. Nishizawa T, Fujimura M, Katsuki M, Mugikura S, Tashiro R, Sato K, et al. Prediction of cerebral Hyperperfusion after superficial temporal artery-middle cerebral artery anastomosis by three-dimensional-time-of-flight magnetic resonance angiography in adult patients with Moyamoya disease. Cerebrovasc Dis. 2020;49(4):396–403. https://doi.org/10.1159/000509740.
44. Miyamoto S, Yoshimoto T, Hashimoto N, Okada Y, Tsuji I, Tominaga T, et al. Effects of extracranial-intracranial bypass for patients with hemorrhagic Moyamoya disease: results of the Japan adult Moyamoya trial. Stroke. 2014;45(5):1415–21. https://doi.org/10.1161/STROKEAHA.113.004386.
45. Takahashi JC, Funaki T, Houkin K, Inoue T, Ogasawara K, Nakagawara J, et al. Significance of the hemorrhagic site for recurrent bleeding: prespecified analysis in the Japan adult Moyamoya trial. Stroke. 2016;47(1):37–43. https://doi.org/10.1161/STROKEAHA.115.010819.
46. Kuroda S, Yamamoto S, Funaki S, Fujimura M, Kataoka H, Hishikawa T, et al. Disease progression, transient ischemic attack, and de novo parenchymal lesions in asymptomatic Moyamoya disease: results of a 5-year interim analysis of the AMORE study. J Neurosurg. 2024:1–9. https://doi.org/10.3171/2024.6.JNS24736.
47. Kuroda S, Houkin K, Ishikawa T, Nakayama N, Iwasaki Y. Novel bypass surgery for Moyamoya disease using pericranial flap: its impacts on cerebral hemodynamics and long-term outcome. Neurosurgery. 2010;66(6):1093–101.; discussion 101. https://doi.org/10.1227/01.NEU.0000369606.00861.91.
48. Jeon JP, Kim JE, Cho WS, Bang JS, Son YJ, Oh CW. Meta-analysis of the surgical outcomes of symptomatic Moyamoya disease in adults. J Neurosurg. 2018;128(3):793–9. https://doi.org/10.3171/2016.11.JNS161688.
49. Nguyen VN, Motiwala M, Elarjani T, Moore KA, Miller LE, Barats M, et al. Direct, indirect, and combined Extracranial-to-intracranial bypass for adult Moyamoya disease: an updated systematic review and meta-analysis. Stroke. 2022;53(12):3572–82. https://doi.org/10.1161/STROKEAHA.122.039584.
50. Mizoi K, Kayama T, Yoshimoto T, Nagamine Y. Indirect revascularization for Moyamoya disease: is there a beneficial effect for adult patients? Surg Neurol. 1996;45(6):541–8.; discussion 8–9. https://doi.org/10.1016/0090-3019(95)00475-0.
51. Fujimura M, Kaneta T, Shimizu H, Tominaga T. Cerebral ischemia owing to compression of the brain by swollen temporal muscle used for encephalo-myo-synangiosis in Moyamoya disease. Neurosurg Rev. 2009;32(2):245–9.; discussion 9. https://doi.org/10.1007/s10143-009-0184-6.
52. Mizushima M, Ito M, Fujima N, Uchino H, Sugiyama T, Fujimura M. Chronological volume changes of the temporal muscle pedicle used for Encephalo-myo-synangiosis in combined revascularization for Moyamoya disease: a prospective observational study. Neurol Med Chir. 2023;63(7):304–12. https://doi.org/10.2176/jns-nmc.2023-0008.
53. Fujimura M, Kaneta T, Tominaga T. Efficacy of superficial temporal artery-middle cerebral artery anastomosis with routine postoperative cerebral blood flow measurement during the acute stage in childhood Moyamoya disease. Childs Nerv Syst. 2008;24(7):827–32. https://doi.org/10.1007/s00381-007-0551-y.
54. Hayashi T, Shirane R, Fujimura M, Tominaga T. Postoperative neurological deterioration in pediatric Moyamoya disease: watershed shift and hyperperfusion. J Neurosurg Pediatr. 2010;6(1):73–81. https://doi.org/10.3171/2010.4.PEDS09478.
55. Tashiro R, Fujimura M, Kameyama M, Mugikura S, Endo H, Takeuchi Y, et al. Incidence and risk factors of the watershed shift phenomenon after superficial temporal artery-middle cerebral artery anastomosis for adult Moyamoya disease. Cerebrovasc Dis. 2019;47(3–4):178–87. https://doi.org/10.1159/000500802.
56. Tu XK, Fujimura M, Rashad S, Mugikura S, Sakata H, Niizuma K, et al. Uneven cerebral hemodynamic change as a cause of

neurological deterioration in the acute stage after direct revascularization for Moyamoya disease: cerebral hyperperfusion and remote ischemia caused by the 'watershed shift'. Neurosurg Rev. 2017;40(3):507–12. https://doi.org/10.1007/s10143-017-0845-9.
57. Schubert GA, Biermann P, Weiss C, Seiz M, Vajkoczy P, Schmiedek P, et al. Risk profile in extracranial/intracranial bypass surgery--the role of antiplatelet agents, disease pathology, and surgical technique in 168 direct revascularization procedures. World Neurosurg. 2014;82(5):672–7. https://doi.org/10.1016/j.wneu.2013.06.010.
58. Zhao Y, Zhang Q, Zhang D, Zhao Y. Effect of aspirin in postoperative Management of Adult Ischemic Moyamoya Disease. World Neurosurg. 2017;105:728–31. https://doi.org/10.1016/j.wneu.2017.06.057.
59. Fujimura M, Kaneta T, Mugikura S, Shimizu H, Tominaga T. Temporary neurologic deterioration due to cerebral hyperperfusion after superficial temporal artery-middle cerebral artery anastomosis in patients with adult-onset Moyamoya disease. Surg Neurol. 2007;67(3):273–82. https://doi.org/10.1016/j.surneu.2006.07.017.
60. Fujimura M, Mugikura S, Kaneta T, Shimizu H, Tominaga T. Incidence and risk factors for symptomatic cerebral hyperperfusion after superficial temporal artery-middle cerebral artery anastomosis in patients with Moyamoya disease. Surg Neurol. 2009;71(4):442–7. https://doi.org/10.1016/j.surneu.2008.02.031.
61. Fujimura M, Shimizu H, Inoue T, Mugikura S, Saito A, Tominaga T. Significance of focal cerebral hyperperfusion as a cause of transient neurologic deterioration after extracranial-intracranial bypass for Moyamoya disease: comparative study with non-moyamoya patients using N-isopropyl-p-[(123)I]iodoamphetamine single-photon emission computed tomography. Neurosurgery. 2011;68(4):957–64.; discussion 64–5. https://doi.org/10.1227/NEU.0b013e318208f1da.
62. Fujimura M, Shimizu H, Mugikura S, Tominaga T. Delayed intracerebral hemorrhage after superficial temporal artery-middle cerebral artery anastomosis in a patient with Moyamoya disease: possible involvement of cerebral hyperperfusion and increased vascular permeability. Surg Neurol. 2009;71(2):223–7.; discussion 7. https://doi.org/10.1016/j.surneu.2007.07.077.
63. Kim JE, Oh CW, Kwon OK, Park SQ, Kim SE, Kim YK. Transient hyperperfusion after superficial temporal artery/middle cerebral artery bypass surgery as a possible cause of postoperative transient neurological deterioration. Cerebrovasc Dis. 2008;25(6):580–6. https://doi.org/10.1159/000132205.
64. Uchino H, Kuroda S, Hirata K, Shiga T, Houkin K, Tamaki N. Predictors and clinical features of postoperative hyperperfusion after surgical revascularization for Moyamoya disease: a serial single photon emission CT/positron emission tomography study. Stroke. 2012;43(10):2610–6. https://doi.org/10.1161/STROKEAHA.112.654723.
65. Kim T, Oh CW, Bang JS, Kim JE, Cho WS. Moyamoya disease: treatment and outcomes. J Stroke. 2016;18(1):21–30. https://doi.org/10.5853/jos.2015.01739.
66. Fujimura M, Niizuma K, Inoue T, Sato K, Endo H, Shimizu H, et al. Minocycline prevents focal neurological deterioration due to cerebral hyperperfusion after extracranial-intracranial bypass for Moyamoya disease. Neurosurgery. 2014;74(2):163–70.; discussion 70. https://doi.org/10.1227/NEU.0000000000000238.
67. Tokairin K, Kazumata K, Uchino H, Ito M, Ono K, Tatezawa R, et al. Postoperative intracerebral hemorrhage after combined revascularization surgery in Moyamoya disease: profiles and clinical associations. World Neurosurg. 2018;120:e593–600. https://doi.org/10.1016/j.wneu.2018.08.132.
68. Kameyama M, Fujimura M, Tashiro R, Sato K, Endo H, Niizuma K, et al. Significance of quantitative cerebral blood flow measurement in the acute stage after revascularization surgery for adult Moyamoya disease: implication for the pathological threshold of local cerebral Hyperperfusion. Cerebrovasc Dis. 2019;48(3–6):217–25. https://doi.org/10.1159/000504835.
69. Fujimura M, Inoue T, Shimizu H, Saito A, Mugikura S, Tominaga T. Efficacy of prophylactic blood pressure lowering according to a standardized postoperative management protocol to prevent symptomatic cerebral hyperperfusion after direct revascularization surgery for Moyamoya disease. Cerebrovasc Dis. 2012;33(5):436–45. https://doi.org/10.1159/000336765.
70. Huang C, Huang C, Zhan X. Predictive factors for seizures after revascularization in patients with Moyamoya disease. World Neurosurg. 2024;182:e205–e9. https://doi.org/10.1016/j.wneu.2023.11.075.
71. Olin JW, Gornik HL, Bacharach JM, Biller J, Fine LJ, Gray BH, et al. Fibromuscular dysplasia: state of the science and critical unanswered questions: a scientific statement from the American Heart Association. Circulation. 2014;129(9):1048–78. https://doi.org/10.1161/01.cir.0000442577.96802.8c.
72. Van der Niepen P, Robberechts T, Devos H, van Tussenbroek F, Januszewicz A, Persu A. Fibromuscular dysplasia: its various phenotypes in everyday practice in 2021. Kardiol Pol. 2021;79(7–8):733–44. https://doi.org/10.33963/KP.a2021.0040.
73. Schievink WI, Bjornsson J, Piepgras DG. Coexistence of fibromuscular dysplasia and cystic medial necrosis in a patient with Marfan's syndrome and bilateral carotid artery dissections. Stroke. 1994;25(12):2492–6. https://doi.org/10.1161/01.str.25.12.2492.
74. Abumiya T, Fujimura M. Moyamoya vasculopathy and Moyamoya-related systemic vasculopathy: a review with histopathological and genetic viewpoints. Stroke. 2024;55(6):1699–706. https://doi.org/10.1161/STROKEAHA.124.046999.
75. Kiando SR, Barlassina C, Cusi D, Galan P, Lathrop M, Plouin PF, et al. Exome sequencing in seven families and gene-based association studies indicate genetic heterogeneity and suggest possible candidates for fibromuscular dysplasia. J Hypertens. 2015;33(9):1802–10; discussion 10. https://doi.org/10.1097/HJH.0000000000000625.
76. Chaves C, Estol C, Esnaola MM, Gorson K, O'Donoghue M, De Witt LD, et al. Spontaneous intracranial internal carotid artery dissection: report of 10 patients. Arch Neurol. 2002;59(6):977–81. https://doi.org/10.1001/archneur.59.6.977.
77. Arnold M, Kappeler L, Georgiadis D, Berthet K, Keserue B, Bousser MG, et al. Gender differences in spontaneous cervical artery dissection. Neurology. 2006;67(6):1050–2. https://doi.org/10.1212/01.wnl.0000237341.30854.6a.
78. Lee VH, Brown RD Jr, Mandrekar JN, Mokri B. Incidence and outcome of cervical artery dissection: a population-based study. Neurology. 2006;67(10):1809–12. https://doi.org/10.1212/01.wnl.0000244486.30455.71.
79. Kim BM, Kim SH, Kim DI, Shin YS, Suh SH, Kim DJ, et al. Outcomes and prognostic factors of intracranial unruptured vertebrobasilar artery dissection. Neurology. 2011;76(20):1735–41. https://doi.org/10.1212/WNL.0b013e31821a7d94.
80. Debette S, Compter A, Labeyrie MA, Uyttenboogaart M, Metso TM, Majersik JJ, et al. Epidemiology, pathophysiology, diagnosis, and management of intracranial artery dissection. Lancet Neurol. 2015;14(6):640–54. https://doi.org/10.1016/S1474-4422(15)00009-5.
81. Arnold M, Cumurciuc R, Stapf C, Favrole P, Berthet K, Bousser MG. Pain as the only symptom of cervical artery dissection. J Neurol Neurosurg Psychiatry. 2006;77(9):1021–4. https://doi.org/10.1136/jnnp.2006.094359.
82. Downer J, Nadarajah M, Briggs E, Wrigley P, McAuliffe W. The location of origin of spontaneous extracranial internal carotid artery dissection is adjacent to the skull base. J Med Imaging Radiat Oncol. 2014;58(4):408–14. https://doi.org/10.1111/1754-9485.12170.

83. Besselmann M, Vennemann B, Lowens S, Ringelstein EB, Stogbauer F. Internal carotid artery dissection. Neurology. 2000;54(2):442. https://doi.org/10.1212/wnl.54.2.442.
84. Schievink WI. Spontaneous dissection of the carotid and vertebral arteries. N Engl J Med. 2001;344(12):898–906. https://doi.org/10.1056/NEJM200103223441206.
85. Debette S, Markus HS. The genetics of cervical artery dissection: a systematic review. Stroke. 2009;40(6):e459–66. https://doi.org/10.1161/STROKEAHA.108.534669.
86. Grond-Ginsbach C, Debette S. The association of connective tissue disorders with cervical artery dissections. Curr Mol Med. 2009;9(2):210–4. https://doi.org/10.2174/156652409787581547.
87. Lucas C, Moulin T, Deplanque D, Tatu L, Chavot D. Stroke patterns of internal carotid artery dissection in 40 patients. Stroke. 1998;29(12):2646–8. https://doi.org/10.1161/01.str.29.12.2646.
88. Morel A, Naggara O, Touze E, Raymond J, Mas JL, Meder JF, et al. Mechanism of ischemic infarct in spontaneous cervical artery dissection. Stroke. 2012;43(5):1354–61. https://doi.org/10.1161/STROKEAHA.111.643338.
89. Kang DW, Kim DY, Kim J, Baik SH, Jung C, Singh N, et al. Emerging concept of intracranial arterial diseases: the role of high resolution Vessel Wall MRI. J Stroke. 2024;26(1):26–40. https://doi.org/10.5853/jos.2023.02481.
90. Hanihara M, Yoshioka H, Kanemaru K, Hashimoto K, Shimizu M, Nishigaya K, et al. Long-term clinical and angiographic outcomes of wrap-clipping for ruptured blood blister-like aneurysms of the internal carotid artery using advanced monitoring. World Neurosurg. 2019;126:e439–e46. https://doi.org/10.1016/j.wneu.2019.02.070.
91. Kim YB, Hong CK, Chung J, Joo JY, Huh SK. Long-term clinical and angiographic outcomes of wrap-clipping strategies for unclippable cerebral aneurysms. Yonsei Med J. 2014;55(2):401–9. https://doi.org/10.3349/ymj.2014.55.2.401.
92. Kim MJ, Chung J, Shin YS, Lim YC. Forward deployed coil embolization with multiple overlapping stents for ruptured blood blister-like aneurysms: technical considerations and outcomes. Neurol Res. 2019;41(6):562–8. https://doi.org/10.1080/01616412.2019.1584424.
93. Duangprasert G, Sukhor S, Ratanavinitkul W, Tantongtip D. Evaluation of flow diverter use in acutely ruptured vertebral artery dissecting aneurysms: a focus on safety and efficacy for rapid aneurysm obliteration. Clin Neurol Neurosurg. 2024;242:108345. https://doi.org/10.1016/j.clineuro.2024.108345.

Stroke Unit Organization

Tatiana Abou-Mrad, Megan Donlick, Ali Alaraj, and Fady T. Charbel

List of Abbreviations

AHA	American Heart Association
ASA	American Stroke Association
BAC	Brain Attack Coalition
BEST-MSU	Benefits of Stroke Treatment Delivered Using a Mobile Stroke Units
CDC	Centers for Disease Control and Prevention
CSC	Comprehensive Stroke Center
CT	Computed Tomography
DTN	Door-to-Needle
FDA	Food and Drug Administration
ED	Emergency Department
EMS	Emergency Medical Services
ESO	European Stroke Organization
GWTG-S	Get with the Guidelines—Stroke
ICP	Intracranial Pressure
ICU	Intensive Care Unit
IV	Intravenous
MSU	Mobile Stroke Unit
MRI	Magnetic Resonance Imaging
mRS	Modified Rankin Scale
NCCU	Neurocritical Care Unit
NCT	Neurocritical Care Team
NSA	National Stroke Association
OT	Occupational Therapy
PSC	Primary Stroke Centers
PT	Physician Therapy
rtPA	Recombinant Tissue Plasminogen Activator
ICH	Intracranial Hemorrhage
SLP	Speech Language Pathology
TJC	The Joint Commission
TXA	Tranexamic Acid

T. Abou-Mrad · M. Donlick · A. Alaraj · F. T. Charbel (✉)
Department of Neurosurgery, University of Illinois at Chicago, Chicago, IL, USA
e-mail: fcharbel@uic.edu

1 Introduction

All things heal with a tincture of time, as the adage goes. Yet, as it pertains to stroke, one is reminded of the widely held axiom "time is brain", which encapsulates the urgency of stroke care and emphasizes the critical importance of time to diagnosis, treatment, and rehabilitation. Since the 1930s, stroke has remained one of the leading causes of death in the United States, with the interval from ictus to treatment being a key determinant of both functional and clinical outcomes [1]. This race against the clock has been the impetus in the development of specialized stroke care models, including the modern stroke unit, where early identification and timely treatment serve as guiding principles [2].

In the early 1900s, a diagnosis of "brain attack" often carried a grim prognosis, as treatment options were largely limited to prevention, supportive care, and rehabilitation [3]. The landscape of care was transformed in the latter half of the twentieth century. As the demand for improved stroke outcomes intensified, the trajectory of research, clinical trials, and technological advancements accelerated. Imaging modalities such as magnetic resonance imaging (MRI), computed tomography (CT), and transcranial doppler revolutionized stroke diagnosis. Landmark vascular interventions like carotid endarterectomy, catheter angiography, and mechanical thrombectomy offered viable treatment options. Additionally, pharmacologic discoveries such as anticoagulants, antiplatelets, statins, and thrombolytics further reduced disease burden. Taken together, these innovations collectively reshaped stroke care, enabling physicians to adapt as stroke management evolved [2].

The foundation of dedicated, specialized stroke services emerged in the 1950s, with the pioneering efforts of Dr. Charles Miller Fisher at Massachusetts General Hospital [2]. Early units initially aimed to provide more intensive care, but lacked necessary standardized protocols and scope, limiting their impact on morbidity or mortality [4]. Taking cue from coronary care units, stroke units gradually developed into

V. Beneš, D. Netuka (eds.), *Surgical and Interventional Treatment of Cerebral Ischemia*,
https://doi.org/10.1007/978-3-032-08934-2_23

outcomes. The effectiveness of a stroke unit is dictated by three fundamental components: physical infrastructure, specialized medical equipment, and a multidisciplinary team dedicated to coordinated patient management.

3.1 Physical Infrastructure

The physical layout of a stroke unit must facilitate the efficient movement of patients from the ED to the diagnostic and treatment areas, ensuring that delays in acute stroke care are minimized. Ideally, stroke units should be situated in close proximity to emergency services, allowing for immediate access to neuroimaging and critical care resources. Since rapid neuroimaging is essential in differentiating between ischemic and hemorrhagic strokes, CT and MRI scanners should be immediately available within or near the unit, allowing for urgent assessment of vascular occlusions, hemorrhagic transformation, and ischemic tissue viability. The prompt acquisition of imaging is critical in determining eligibility for reperfusion therapies, particularly IV tPA and mechanical thrombectomy, which have well-defined therapeutic windows [24].

Beyond access to diagnostic facilities, the infrastructure of a stroke unit must support continuous monitoring of neurological and systemic parameters, as stroke patients are at significant risk for secondary complications, including intracranial hypertension, respiratory failure, and hemodynamic instability. The availability of non-invasive and invasive blood pressure monitoring, continuous electrocardiographic telemetry, and ICP monitoring is essential in patients requiring hemodynamic stabilization, particularly those with large vessel occlusions, subarachnoid hemorrhage, or post-thrombectomy status. In addition, pulse oximetry and capnography are necessary to detect hypoxia and respiratory depression, which are particularly relevant in patients with decreased consciousness or brainstem involvement [25].

Rehabilitation infrastructure must also be integrated within the stroke unit, ensuring that early mobilization and multimodal rehabilitation strategies can be initiated as soon as medically appropriate. The presence of dedicated physical therapy (PT) and occupational therapy (OT) areas allows for the implementation of individualized motor retraining programs, gait restoration exercises, and functional independence training [26]. Speech-language pathology (SLP) services are essential for patients with post-stroke dysphagia, aphasia, or cognitive-communication impairments, ensuring that interventions are provided to mitigate the risk of aspiration pneumonia and improve long-term communication outcomes. The inclusion of rehabilitation facilities within the stroke unit enables a seamless transition from acute care to recovery, reducing hospital-acquired complications and optimizing post-stroke functional recovery [27].

3.2 Medical Equipment

The availability of advanced medical equipment is fundamental to the timely and effective management of stroke. In the acute setting, stroke units must be equipped with the necessary infrastructure to facilitate immediate intervention, particularly in cases of ischemic stroke requiring IV thrombolysis or endovascular thrombectomy. rtPA must be readily available for rapid administration in eligible ischemic stroke patients, as early treatment within the established therapeutic window is associated with significantly improved functional outcomes [22, 28–31]. In CSCs, mechanical thrombectomy devices and angiographic suites should be accessible for patients with large vessel occlusion, ensuring that clot retrieval procedures can be performed without unnecessary delays. Additionally, point-of-care laboratory testing, including blood glucose assessment, coagulation studies, and metabolic panels, must be immediately available to facilitate rapid clinical decision-making in the hyperacute phase of stroke management.

Stroke units must also be equipped with supportive and preventive measures to address complications commonly encountered in the post-stroke period. Given the high prevalence of post-stroke dysphagia, bedside dysphagia screening tools and fiberoptic endoscopic evaluation of swallowing should be readily available to assess swallowing function and prevent complications [32]. Automated infusion pumps are necessary for the precise administration of IV thrombolytics, anticoagulants, antihypertensive agents, and supportive fluids, ensuring that pharmacological interventions are delivered in a controlled manner. By ensuring the immediate availability of these medical resources, stroke teams are ensured adequate resources to manage acute interventions, mitigate secondary complications, and optimize patient prognosis.

3.3 Stroke Unit Staffing and Multidisciplinary Care

The composition of the stroke unit team plays a central role in determining the quality and efficiency of care delivered to stroke patients. A multidisciplinary team of specialists with expertise in cerebrovascular disease, acute stroke management, and neurorehabilitation, ensures that patients receive comprehensive care throughout the acute and post-acute phases of their hospitalization [33]. The stroke team is typically led by neurologists and stroke specialists, who are responsible for diagnostic evaluations, therapeutic decision-making, and ongoing neurological assessments. Their role includes determining eligibility for IV tPA and mechanical thrombectomy, monitoring post-treatment complications, and overseeing the implementation of secondary stroke prevention strategies.

Stroke care nurses are vital to the management of acute stroke patients, and they require specialized training in stroke assessment, managing post-stroke complications, and supporting patient rehabilitation [34, 35]. Nurses are responsible for monitoring and assessing patients, administering medications, and providing support to families. Their role is critical in identifying stroke symptoms early and coordinating care.

Rehabilitation specialists, including PT, OT and SLP, are integral to the stroke team. Physiotherapists focus on early mobilization, motor retraining, and the prevention of complications such as deep vein thrombosis and joint contractures. Occupational therapists assist patients in regaining functional independence by implementing interventions that facilitate activities of daily living, including dressing, bathing, and feeding. Speech-language pathologists provide essential assessment and treatment for patients with post-stroke dysphagia, dysarthria, and cognitive-linguistic deficits, ensuring that communication and swallowing functions are addressed as part of the recovery process.

Neuropsychologists and rehabilitation specialists play a critical role in addressing the cognitive, emotional, and behavioral sequelae of stroke. Given that post-stroke depression, cognitive impairment, and personality changes are common, neuropsychologists assess cognitive function and implement individualized interventions aimed at improving attention, memory, and executive function. Social workers and case managers further enhance stroke recovery by assisting patients and their families in navigating rehabilitation planning, long-term care coordination, and psychosocial support systems. Their role extends beyond hospital discharge, ensuring that patients receive appropriate follow-up care, financial assistance, and access to community-based stroke rehabilitation programs.

Effective communication among stroke unit staff is paramount in ensuring the seamless coordination of care. Structured interdisciplinary rounds allow for real-time updates on patient status, ensuring that therapeutic plans are consistently adapted to each patient's evolving clinical condition. By fostering a collaborative and coordinated approach to stroke management, multidisciplinary stroke teams optimize clinical outcomes, reduce hospital length of stay, and enhance the overall quality of care delivered to patients with acute cerebrovascular disease [33, 36].

4 Certification & Quality Improvement in Stroke Units

4.1 Stroke Unit Certification & Accreditation

Stroke center certification falls under the umbrella of TJC. The American Heart Association (AHA)/American Stroke Association (ASA) and TJC endorse stroke centers through a Disease-Specific Certification Program in North America, with an international panel also overseeing certification standards. The primary goal of quality assurance and accreditation is to ensure that certified centers provide stroke care that meets evidence-based standards. As previously mentioned, tPA administration, outcome measurement, regulatory minimums, and quality improvement monitoring were among the initial selection criteria for PSC certification, established in 2005 and later revised with updated BAC recommendations in 2011 [25]. By 2012, certification for CSCs were underway. These certifications were duly resource-dependent, with a noted increase in the rigorous selection criteria set forth for PSC accreditation, requiring an established NCCU, minimum case volume thresholds, and 24/7 access to advanced services [2].

4.2 Performance Metrics & Continuous Improvement

Continuous quality improvement within accredited stroke centers and units is a function of evidence-based practice outcomes, where teams focus the lens on identification of process gaps and variances in practice, and design interventions. Centers participate in educational opportunities and conduct quality research, disseminating the findings to add to the available body of stroke care knowledge. Wang et al. suggested in their randomized clinical trial published in JAMA in 2018 that "*quality improvement interventions have demonstrated that stroke care quality can be improved by conducting interventions such as using clinical pathways, training physicians on evidence-based guidelines, auditing care delivery, and providing timely feedback*" [37]. The development of high-quality performance measures falls under the purview of several invested organizations that shape the professional standards for stroke care such as the AHA, ASA, TJC and Center for Disease Control and Prevention (CDC), which function both independently and collaboratively within The Stroke Performance Measure Consensus Group [38].

Current written protocols, industry standards, and evidence-based guidelines have emerged from these groups and associative national quality improvement projects, such as Target: Stroke, pioneered by the AHA in 2010, trailblazing the quintessential DTN time < 60 min (target <30 min for best centers) in Phase I [28]. This became the gold standard of care and was not only implemented at all GWTG-S hospitals but set guidelines for all stroke centers [30]. Thrombectomy workflow optimization has also adhered to quality improvement with the DAWN and DIFFUSE trials showing time to reperfusion is paramount [29, 39]. Delays in groin puncture time < 90 min, which stemmed from the

PROACT II trial, have been associated with worse outcomes, akin to the findings of delayed thrombolysis [5, 31].

A crucial component of stroke center performance measurement and continuous improvement is the establishment of stroke registries and data-driven quality assessment programs. The CDC outlined targeted objectives and initiatives for stroke research in Healthy People 2010, which set national benchmarks for stroke prevention and treatment [40]. In alignment with these efforts, the Paul Coverdell Stroke Registry, launched in 2001, was designed to track and analyze stroke outcomes and quality metrics across healthcare institutions [2]. Additional organizations have developed performance monitoring systems to enhance stroke care standards. The US Department of Veterans Affairs monitors metrics through the Stroke Quality Enhancement Research Initiative. Concurrently, the AHA/ASA developed initiatives such as the Metro Stroke Task Force, Operation Stroke, and GWTG-S, all of which collect data from all registered hospitals in the database to establish benchmarks, track adherence to evidence-base protocols, and provide performance feedback to involved centers. The American Academy of Neurology also collects data and collaborates with the American Medical Association to integrate stroke care metrics into physician quality reporting systems, ensuring that clinical performance aligns with national and international standards [38]. These independent registries are well maintained and contain a wealth of epidemiological data, serving as a compendium of stroke care from three decades of collection that will be utilized to inform future stroke guidelines and written protocols.

5 Future Directions in Stroke Unit Care

The future of stroke unit organization is being shaped by technological innovations aimed at enhancing diagnostic accuracy, treatment efficiency, and rehabilitation outcomes. Advances in neuroimaging, personalized medicine, and rehabilitation techniques are revolutionizing stroke care by enabling highly individualized, evidence-based management. Firstly, advances in neuroimaging techniques are expanding the diagnostic capabilities of stroke units, offering real-time insights into cerebral perfusion, metabolic activity, and tissue viability. Functional MRI, positron emission tomography, and diffusion tensor imaging are providing unprecedented detail on brain network connectivity, ischemic injury patterns, and microstructural damage, enhancing clinicians' ability to tailor treatment strategies [41]. These imaging modalities hold promise for identifying patients who may benefit from late-window thrombectomy and predicting long-term functional recovery based on lesion location and extent. Moreover, the integration of personalized medicine into stroke care is also gaining momentum, allowing for interventions tailored to an individual's genetic and molecular profile [42]. Advances in genomic sequencing and pharmacogenetics are improving the ability to predict a patient's response to antithrombotic therapy, antihypertensive agents, and neuroprotective drugs, thereby enabling more precise and effective treatment regimens. By leveraging genetic markers associated with stroke risk, clotting disorders, and drug metabolism, personalized medicine is expected to enhance secondary prevention strategies and minimize adverse drug reactions [43, 44]. Simultaneously, the evolution of minimally invasive stroke interventions continues to refine the standard of care [45]. The development of novel fibrinolytic agents and neuroprotective therapies is likely to enhance the efficacy of acute stroke treatment by promoting clot dissolution, reducing ischemic injury, and mitigating reperfusion damage. These pharmacological advancements are being explored in ongoing clinical trials, with the potential to expand the therapeutic window for ischemic stroke and improve functional outcomes [46]. In parallel, telemedicine and remote stroke care models are transforming stroke management, particularly in regions with limited access to specialized stroke centers [47]. The expansion of telestroke networks enables real-time consultation with stroke experts, facilitating remote assessment, thrombolysis decision-making, and post-acute care coordination. As telemedicine infrastructure continues to advance, its role in long-term stroke rehabilitation and secondary prevention programs is expected to grow, allowing patients to receive continuous care through virtual platforms and remote monitoring [48].

6 Conclusion

The evolution of stroke units has fundamentally transformed the landscape of stroke care, emphasizing rapid diagnosis, timely intervention, and coordinated multidisciplinary management. From early rudimentary monitoring units to the development of Primary and Comprehensive Stroke Centers, the structured organization of stroke care has significantly improved patient survival, functional recovery, and long-term outcomes. Standardized protocols, including thrombolysis guidelines, endovascular treatment pathways, and early rehabilitation strategies, have been pivotal in reducing stroke-related morbidity and mortality. As stroke units evolve into highly specialized, technology-driven centers, these innovations will enable a more integrated, personalized, and data-driven approach to stroke care. The convergence of precision medicine, advanced neuroimaging, and rehabilitative robotics will not only enhance diagnosis, treatment, and recovery strategies but also support preventive efforts aimed at reducing stroke incidence. By embracing these advancements, stroke units are poised to redefine the landscape of cerebrovascular medicine, ensuring that patients receive timely, individualized, and multidisciplinary care at every stage of their stroke journey.

Declarations
Competing Interests The author(s) has no competing interests to declare that are relevant to the content of this manuscript.

Ethics Approval The author(s) declares that this manuscript does not include primary research with human participants.

References

1. Centers for Disease Control and Prevention (CDC). Decline in deaths from heart disease and stroke–United States, 1900–1999. MMWR Morb Mortal Wkly Rep. 48(30):649–56.
2. Gorelick PB. Primary and comprehensive stroke centers: history, value and certification criteria. J Stroke. 2013;15(2):78–89.
3. Towner J, Pieters T, Schmidt T, Pilcher W, Bhalla T. A history of mobile stroke units and review of literature. Am J Interv Radiol. 2:9.
4. Indredavik B, Slørdahl SA, Bakke F, Rokseth R, Håheim LL. Stroke unit treatment. long-term effects. Stroke. 1997;28(10):1861–6.
5. Damani R. A brief history of acute stroke care. Aging (Albany NY). 2018;10(8):1797–8.
6. Bershad EM, Feen ES, Hernandez OH, Suri MF, Suarez JI. Impact of a specialized neurointensive care team on outcomes of critically ill acute ischemic stroke patients. Neurocrit Care. 2008;9(3):287–92.
7. Langhorne P, Dennis MS. Stroke units: the next 10 years. Lancet. 2004;363(9412):834–5.
8. Langhorne P, Pollock A. What are the components of effective stroke unit care? Age Ageing. 2002;31(5):365–71.
9. Alberts MJ, Hademenos G, Latchaw RE, Jagoda A, Marler JR, Mayberg MR, et al. Recommendations for the establishment of primary stroke centers. Brain Attack Coalition Jama. 2000;283(23):3102–9.
10. Alberts MJ, Latchaw RE, Selman WR, Shephard T, Hadley MN, Brass LM, et al. Recommendations for comprehensive stroke centers: a consensus statement from the brain attack coalition. Stroke. 2005;36(7):1597–616.
11. Caplan LR. Primary stroke centers vs comprehensive stroke centers with interventional capabilities: which is better for a patient with suspected stroke? JAMA Neurol. 2017;74(5):504–6.
12. Siegel J, Pizzi MA, Brent Peel J, Alejos D, Mbabuike N, Brown BL, et al. Update on Neurocritical Care of Stroke. Curr Cardiol Rep. 2017;19(8):67.
13. Langhorne P, de Villiers L, Pandian JD. Applicability of stroke-unit care to low-income and middle-income countries. Lancet Neurol. 2012;11(4):341–8.
14. Alberts MJ, Wechsler LR, Jensen ME, Latchaw RE, Crocco TJ, George MG, et al. Formation and function of acute stroke-ready hospitals within a stroke system of care recommendations from the brain attack coalition. Stroke. 2013;44(12):3382–93.
15. Fassbender K, Walter S, Liu Y, Muehlhauser F, Ragoschke A, Kuehl S, et al. "Mobile stroke unit" for hyperacute stroke treatment. Stroke. 2003;34(6):e44.
16. Menon BK, Sajobi TT, Zhang Y, Rempel JL, Shuaib A, Thornton J, et al. Analysis of workflow and time to treatment on Thrombectomy outcome in the endovascular treatment for small Core and proximal occlusion ischemic stroke (ESCAPE) Randomized, Controlled Trial. Circulation. 2016;133(23):2279–86.
17. Walter S, Zhao H, Easton D, Bil C, Sauer J, Liu Y, et al. Air-mobile stroke unit for access to stroke treatment in rural regions. Int J Stroke. 2018;13(6):568–75.
18. Wu TC, Parker SA, Jagolino A, Yamal JM, Bowry R, Thomas A, et al. Telemedicine can replace the neurologist on a mobile stroke unit. Stroke. 2017;48(2):493–6.
19. Ehntholt MS, Parasram M, Mir SA, Lerario MP. Mobile stroke units: bringing treatment to the patient. Curr Treat Options Neurol. 2020;22(2):5.
20. Turc G, Hadziahmetovic M, Walter S, Churilov L, Larsen K, Grotta JC, et al. Comparison of mobile stroke unit with usual care for acute ischemic stroke management: a systematic review and meta-analysis. JAMA Neurol. 2022;79(3):281–90.
21. Bowry R, Parker S, Rajan SS, Yamal JM, Wu TC, Richardson L, et al. Benefits of stroke treatment using a mobile stroke unit compared with standard management: the BEST-MSU study run-in phase. Stroke. 2015;46(12):3370–4.
22. Mackey J, Yamal JM, Parker SA, Silnes K, Rajan SS, Jacob AP, et al. Golden hour treatment with tPA (tissue-type plasminogen activator) in the BEST-MSU study. Stroke. 2023;54(2):415–25.
23. Walter S, Audebert HJ, Katsanos AH, Larsen K, Sacco S, Steiner T, et al. European Stroke Organisation (ESO) guidelines on mobile stroke units for prehospital stroke management. Eur Stroke J. 2022;7(1):Xxvii–lix.
24. Yu W, Jiang WJ. A simple imaging guide for endovascular Thrombectomy in acute ischemic stroke: from time window to perfusion mismatch and beyond. Front Neurol. 2019;10:502.
25. Dusenbury W, Mathiesen C, Whaley M, Adeoye O, Leslie-Mazwi T, Williams S, et al. Ideal foundational requirements for stroke program development and growth: a scientific statement from the American Heart Association. Stroke. 2023;54(4):e175–e87.
26. Li X, He Y, Wang D, Rezaei MJ. Stroke rehabilitation: from diagnosis to therapy. Front Neurol. 2024;15:1402729.
27. Rodgers H, Price C. Stroke unit care, inpatient rehabilitation and early supported discharge. Clin Med (Lond). 2017;17(2):173–7.
28. Fonarow GC, Smith EE, Saver JL, Reeves MJ, Hernandez AF, Peterson ED, et al. Improving door-to-needle times in acute ischemic stroke: the design and rationale for the American Heart Association/American Stroke Association's target: stroke initiative. Stroke. 2011;42(10):2983–9.
29. Albers GW, Marks MP, Kemp S, Christensen S, Tsai JP, Ortega-Gutierrez S, et al. Thrombectomy for stroke at 6 to 16 hours with selection by perfusion imaging. N Engl J Med. 2018;378(8):708–18.
30. Xian Y, Xu H, Smith EE, Saver JL, Reeves MJ, Bhatt DL, et al. Achieving more rapid door-to-needle times and improved outcomes in acute ischemic stroke in a Nationwide quality improvement intervention. Stroke. 2022;53(4):1328–38.
31. Sun CH, Zaidat OO, Castonguay AC, Veznedaroglu E, Budzik RF, English J, et al. A decade of improvement in door-to-puncture times for mechanical Thrombectomy but ongoing stagnation in prehospital care. Stroke: Vasc Interv Neurol. 2023;3(1):e000561.
32. González-Fernández M, Ottenstein L, Atanelov L, Christian AB. Dysphagia after stroke: an overview. Curr Phys Med Rehabil Rep. 2013;1(3):187–96.
33. Clarke DJ, Forster A. Improving post-stroke recovery: the role of the multidisciplinary health care team. J Multidiscip Healthc. 2015;8:433–42.
34. Tanlaka EF, McIntyre A, Connelly D, Guitar N, Nguyen A, Snobelen N. The role and contributions of nurses in stroke rehabilitation units: an integrative review. West J Nurs Res. 2023;45(8):764–76.
35. Babkair LA, Safhi RA, Balshram R, Safhei R, Almahamdy A, Hakami FH, et al. Nursing care for stroke patients: current practice and future needs. Nurs Rep. 2023;13(3):1236–50.

36. Heip T, Van Hecke A, Malfait S, Van Biesen W, Eeckloo K. The effects of interdisciplinary bedside rounds on patient centeredness, quality of care, and team collaboration: a systematic review. J Patient Saf. 2022;18(1):e40–e4.
37. Wang Y, Li Z, Zhao X, Wang C, Wang X, Wang D, et al. Effect of a multifaceted quality improvement intervention on hospital personnel adherence to performance measures in patients with acute ischemic stroke in China: a randomized clinical trial. JAMA. 2018;320(3):245–54.
38. Smith EE, Saver JL, Alexander DN, Furie KL, Hopkins LN, Katzan IL, et al. Clinical performance measures for adults hospitalized with acute ischemic stroke: performance measures for healthcare professionals from the American Heart Association/American Stroke Association. Stroke. 2014;45(11):3472–98.
39. Jovin TG, Saver JL, Ribo M, Pereira V, Furlan A, Bonafe A, et al. Diffusion-weighted imaging or computerized tomography perfusion assessment with clinical mismatch in the triage of wake up and late presenting strokes undergoing neurointervention with Trevo (DAWN) trial methods. Int J Stroke. 2017;12(6):641–52.
40. Health UDo. Services H. Healthy people 2010. 2000;
41. Włodarczyk L, Cichon N, Saluk-Bijak J, Bijak M, Majos A, Miller E. Neuroimaging techniques as potential tools for assessment of angiogenesis and neuroplasticity processes after stroke and their clinical implications for rehabilitation and stroke recovery prognosis. J Clin Med. 2022;11(9):2473.
42. Petersen NH, Sheth KN, Jha RM. Precision medicine in neurocritical care for cerebrovascular disease cases. Stroke. 2023;54(5):1392–402.
43. Dichgans M, Beaufort N, Debette S, Anderson CD. Stroke genetics: turning discoveries into clinical applications. Stroke. 2021;52(9):2974–82.
44. Ross S, Krebs K, Paré G, Milani L. Pharmacogenomics in stroke and cardiovascular disease: state of the art. Stroke. 2023;54(1):270–8.
45. Raha O, Hall C, Malik A, D'Anna L, Lobotesis K, Kwan J, et al. Advances in mechanical thrombectomy for acute ischaemic stroke. BMJ Med. 2023;2(1):e000407.
46. Frank D, Zlotnik A, Boyko M, Gruenbaum BF. The development of novel drug treatments for stroke patients: a review. Int J Mol Sci. 2022;23(10):5796.
47. Verma A, Towfighi A, Brown A, Abhat A, Casillas A. Moving towards equity with digital health innovations for stroke care. Stroke. 2022;53(3):689–97.
48. Eng JJ, Pastva AM. Advances in remote monitoring for stroke recovery. Stroke. 2022;53(8):2658–61.

Thrombolysis in Stroke

Roman Herzig and David Školoudík

1 Introduction

1.1 Definition and Importance of Intravenous Thrombolysis

Acute ischemic stroke (AIS) is a leading cause of mortality and long-term disability worldwide, significantly impacting healthcare systems and patients' quality of life. AIS caused by a sudden occlusion of a cerebral artery, leading to reduced blood flow and oxygen supply to the brain, with subsequent neuronal damage, accounts for the majority of strokes.

Rapid restoration of cerebral blood flow is crucial to minimize irreversible injury and improve patient outcomes. Intravenous thrombolysis (IVT) has become a cornerstone in the management of AIS, aiming to dissolve thrombi and re-establish perfusion.

The significance of IVT lies in its ability to:

- **Reduce disability**: Early thrombolysis is associated with better functional outcomes [3, 26].
- **Widen treatment eligibility**: Advanced imaging techniques and extended time windows have allowed more patients to benefit from IVT [22, 24].
- **Integrate with other therapies**: IVT may be used as a "bridging therapy" before mechanical thrombectomy (MT) in cases of large vessel occlusions (LVO) [29, 32].

R. Herzig (✉)
Department of Neurology, Faculty of Medicine in Hradec Králové, Charles University, Hradec Králové, Czech Republic

Department of Neurology, Comprehensive Stroke Center, University Hospital Hradec Králové, Hradec Králové, Czech Republic

D. Školoudík
Centre for Health Research, Department of Clinical Neurosciences, Faculty of Medicine, University of Ostrava, Ostrava, Czech Republic

1.2 Historical Development

The evolution of IVT in AIS reflects decades of innovation in stroke care and is marked by significant advancements and evolving guidelines that have shaped its application in clinical practice:

- **1933**: Isolation of **streptokinase**, the first known fibrinolytic agent, marked the beginning of thrombolytic therapy [28].
- **1979**: The discovery of **tissue plasminogen activator (t-PA)**, a naturally occurring enzyme capable of dissolving fibrin clots, provided a targeted approach to fibrinolysis [27].
- **1983**: Biotechnological advancements led to the large-scale production of **recombinant t-PA (rt-PA)**, commercially known as alteplase, revolutionizing treatment and enabling clinical testing [25].
- **1995**: The NINDS-2 trial demonstrated the efficacy of rt-PA (0.9 mg/kg) for AIS when administered intravenously within 3 h of symptom onset. Patients treated with rt-PA were 30% more likely to have minimal or no disability at 3 months compared to those receiving a placebo. This study established rt-PA as a safe and effective treatment for AIS, leading to its widespread adoption [20].
- **2011**: The therapeutic window for alteplase was extended to 4.5 h, based on meta-analyses showing continued benefit for carefully selected patients, making IVT accessible to more patients [15].
- **2019–2020**: Studies employing advanced imaging techniques (e.g., computed tomography [CT] perfusion and diffusion-weighted magnetic resonance imaging [DWI-MRI]) demonstrated the safety and efficacy of IVT in selected patients up to 9 h post-onset or with unknown onset times, significantly broadening treatment eligibility [7, 22].

V. Beneš, D. Netuka (eds.), *Surgical and Interventional Treatment of Cerebral Ischemia*,
https://doi.org/10.1007/978-3-032-08934-2_24

2 Key Thrombolytic Agents

2.1 Alteplase

Alteplase (rt-PA) is a second-generation fibrinolytic agent. It was the first fibrinolytic agent approved for AIS, has been the gold standard of IVT for AIS for over two decades, and remains the most widely used thrombolytic drug in this indication.

- **Mechanism of Action**: Alteplase binds to fibrin and activates plasminogen to plasmin, leading to clot dissolution. Its high fibrin specificity minimizes systemic fibrinolysis [5].
- **Dosage and Administration**: The recommended dose of alteplase is 0.9 mg/kg (with a maximum total dose of 90 mg). The administration protocol involves giving 10% of the total dose as an intravenous bolus over 1 min, followed by the remaining dose infused intravenously over 60 min (due to a short biological half-life of 4–8 min) [21, 26].
- **Advantages**:
  - Cost-effective.
  - Broad availability across healthcare settings.
  - Rapid treatment initiation without the need for specialized imaging equipment.
  - Proven efficacy through decades of use and research. Meta-analyses show alteplase improves outcomes in AIS patients treated within 4.5 h, with 10–15% more patients achieving functional independence (modified Rankin scale [mRS] ≤2).
- **Limitations**:
  - Increased risk of symptomatic intracerebral hemorrhage (sICH): 6.4% in clinical trials [12].
  - Limited efficacy in recanalizing LVO. Recanalization rates are suboptimal compared to mechanical interventions, reducing its effectiveness in severe strokes [4, 31].

2.2 Tenecteplase

Tenecteplase, a third-generation fibrinolytic agent, was developed through genetic modifications of t-PA, enhancing its pharmacokinetics.

- **Mechanism**: Higher fibrin specificity and increased resistance to inactivation [5, 22].
- **Dosage and Administration**: The recommended dose of tenecteplase is 0.25 mg/kg with its administration within 4.5 h from stroke onset. Its longer half-life (11–20 min) allows for administration as a single intravenous bolus, which simplifies treatment logistics and reduces delays [2, 5].
- **Advantages**:
  - Streamlined administration compared to alteplase [2, 5].
  - Superior efficacy in LVO and complex cases—trials showed higher recanalization rates and comparable functional outcomes in patients treated with tenecteplase versus alteplase [6, 22, 24].
  - Lower incidence of sICH at a dose of 0.25 mg/kg compared to alteplase [22, 33].
  - Recommended by the European Stroke Organization (ESO) and the American Heart Association/American Stroke Association (AHA/ASA) at a dose of 0.25 mg/kg as a first-line treatment for AIS patients with LVO within 4.5 h of symptom onset who are candidates for endovascular therapy (EVT) [3, 26].
- **Limitations**:
  - Higher cost and variable availability.
  - Less accessible in certain regions compared to alteplase.

3 Time-Sensitive Aspects of Treatment

3.1 The "Golden Hour" in Thrombolysis

The "golden hour" concept emphasizes the critical importance of initiating treatment as quickly as possible after the onset of AIS symptoms. IVT within the first hour of symptom onset has been shown to significantly improve outcomes:

- **Efficacy**: Meta-analyses report that patients treated within the first ("golden") hour have 30–50% higher odds of achieving excellent functional outcomes (mRS score of 0–1) at 90 days compared to later interventions [1].
- **Safety**: Meta-analyses confirm that earlier treatment was associated with decreased rates of significant disability or mortality at 90 days [1].
- **Clinical Implications**: Streamlined stroke protocols, prehospital notification systems, and rapid imaging are essential to maximize the benefits of early thrombolysis [3, 26].

3.2 Extended Time Windows

The traditional 4.5-h window for IVT has been extended for selected patients, based on advanced imaging techniques:

Table 1 Basic indication criteria for the administration of intravenous thrombolysis in the anterior circulation stroke

Time from symptoms onset	Age (years)	Pre-stroke mRS	NIHSS	Noncontrast CT	CTP Ischemic core volume (ml)	CTP Penumbra volume (ml)	CTP Hypoperfusion/ischemic core volume mismatch
0–4.5 h	≥16	0–3	≥2 *and/or* disabling neurologic deficits	negative *or* early ischemia <1/3 of the MCA territory *or* ASPECTS ≥7[a]			
4.5–9 h *or* unknown onset time	≥18	0–2	≥2 *and/or* disabling neurologic deficits *and* < 25		<70	>10	>1.2

ASPECTS Alberta Stroke Program Early CT Score, *CT* computed tomography, *CTP* CT perfusion, *MCA* middle cerebral artery, *mRS* modified Rankin Scale, *NIHSS* National Institutes of Health Stroke Scale

[a] IVT may still be considered in cases with extensive ischemic changes after careful risk-benefit analysis

- **Advanced Imaging**: Techniques such as CT perfusion and DWI-MRI identify salvageable brain tissue (penumbra), enabling IVT up to 9 h post-onset and in wake-up strokes or strokes with unknown onset time [3, 21, 26].
- **Tenecteplase in Extended Time Windows**:
  - The TWIST and TIMELESS randomized trials demonstrate the safety and efficacy of tenecteplase in patients treated up to 24 h after last seen well [22].
- **Clinical Benefits**:
  - Expands treatment eligibility to wake-up strokes and strokes of unknown onset [3, 21, 26].
  - Improves outcomes in patients with ischemic penumbra identified through imaging [3, 21, 26].

4 Indications

The indications for IVT in AIS stroke primarily revolve around timely intervention in patients with clear neurological deficits and appropriate imaging findings. Basic indication criteria for IVT administration in the anterior circulation stroke are presented in Table 1 [3, 21, 26].

5 Contraindications

Contraindications for IVT are crucial to prevent adverse events, particularly hemorrhagic complications. The issue of contraindications to IVT is complex and beyond the scope of this chapter. Major absolute contraindications include [21]:

- Known allergy to the drug substance or any formulation component.
- Imaging findings demonstrating intracranial hemorrhage, brain disease other than ischemia as a cause of acute neurological deficits, and the presence of extensive early ischemic lesions exceeding the indication criteria (Table 1).
- Clinical findings: clinical signs suggestive of subarachnoid hemorrhage, even with negative findings on imaging, active bleeding or bleeding diathesis, severe uncontrolled arterial hypertension (systolic blood pressure > 185 mm Hg or diastolic blood pressure > 110 mm Hg) that cannot be controlled before treatment.
- Anamnestic data and present serious diseases: craniocerebral and spinal injuries in the last 3 months (especially in patients with severe residual clinical or radiological findings), history of intracranial hemorrhage within the last 6 months, recent major surgery or trauma within the last 14 days, manifest or severe or dangerous bleeding within the last 21 days (including bleeding into the chest, gastrointestinal or urogenital tract), known arteriovenous malformation and known symptomatic aneurysm, known thoracic aortic, abdominal aortic or peripheral artery aneurysm, intracranial or intraspinal surgery within the last 4 weeks, arterial puncture at a non-compressible site within the last 7 days, delivery within the last 10 days or the third trimester with imminent delivery, known infective endocarditis, dissection of the aortic arch arteries, intracranial intrinsic (intraaxial) tumor or metastatic tumors of the central nervous system, treatment by unfractionated heparin or low-molecular-weight heparin at a therapeutic dose in the last 24 h, and other known serious conditions with a high risk of serious or life-threatening bleeding.
- Laboratory findings: INR >1.7, platelet count <100,000/μl, and aPTT above the upper limit of the laboratory.

6 Specific Clinical Scenarios

6.1 Large Vessel Occlusion

Large vessel occlusions pose unique challenges due to the size of the clot and the higher risk of poor outcomes. IVT remains an integral part of LVO management, as it can facilitate early reperfusion and serve as a bridging therapy to EVT:

- **Role of Advanced Imaging**: Perfusion imaging identifies patients who may benefit from IVT despite being candidates for endovascular thrombectomy (EVT) [3, 21, 26, 32].
- **Efficacy of Tenecteplase**:
  - Trials demonstrate that tenecteplase was superior to alteplase for patients with LVO stroke for both reperfusion and functional outcomes, with or without thrombectomy [6, 22–24]. In the EXTEND-IA TNK trial, recanalization was achieved in 46% of LVO patients undergoing EVT treated with tenecteplase versus 23% with alteplase [35].
  - IVT before EVT improves outcomes without increasing the complication rate [22].

6.2 Posterior Circulation Strokes

Posterior circulation strokes (PCS), involving ischemia in the vertebrobasilar territory (e.g., vertebral and basilar arteries), are less common (accounting for approximately 12–19% of all IVT-treated strokes) and present unique clinical challenges due to anatomical differences and less specific symptoms compared to anterior circulation strokes [8, 13]. In the case of basilar artery occlusion, they are often devastating.

- **Clinical Evidence**:
  - IVT in PCS improves functional outcomes, particularly when administered within the traditional 4.5-h window [16].
  - Clinical outcomes after IVT for PCS can be favorable, with studies showing that 38–49% of patients achieve a mRS score of 0–1, indicating an excellent functional outcome [8, 14]. Furthermore, patients with PCS may experience better outcomes than those with anterior circulation strokes at follow-up [30].
  - Subgroup analyses suggest IVT remains safe and effective in extended windows for well-selected patients [8, 16], as better collateral circulation in the posterior circulation likely contributes to reduced bleeding risk and smaller ischemic damage volumes [14].
- **Guideline Recommendations**:
  - IVT is strongly advised for patients with posterior circulation strokes without contraindications [3, 26, 29].
  - IVT may be administered for basilar artery occlusions within 24 h of symptoms onset, even without advanced imaging [29].

6.3 Patients on Anticoagulants

Treating AIS patients on direct oral anticoagulants (DOACs) involves a delicate balance between benefits and bleeding risk:

- **Safety Data**:
  - Cohort studies and meta-analyses indicate no significant difference in sICH rates between patients on DOACs and non-anticoagulated patients and also show that patients treated with IVT despite recent DOAC use may achieve favorable functional outcomes similar to those not on anticoagulants, suggesting that the benefits of timely IVT may outweigh the risks in certain scenarios after careful assessment of coagulation status [9, 18].
- **Clinical Guidance**:
  - Key considerations include the timing of the last DOAC dose, renal function, and the availability of reversal agents such as idarucizumab for dabigatran [21].

7 Risks and Complications

7.1 Intracerebral Hemorrhage

The most serious complication of IVT is sICH, which can negate the benefits of treatment, as it is associated with poor clinical outcomes, often leading to significant morbidity or mortality [36]:

- **Incidence**: sICH occurs in approximately 2–7% of patients treated with alteplase, depending on stroke severity and comorbidities [34].
- **Risk Factors** [17, 19, 36]:
  - Advanced age
  - Male sex
  - Severe initial stroke symptoms
  - Poorly controlled arterial hypertension
  - Atrial fibrillation
  - Diabetes and hyperglycemia
  - Recent anticoagulant use
  - Combination antiplatelet use and lower platelet count
  - Leukoariosis
- **Prevention**:
  - Strict adherence to inclusion criteria and diligent blood pressure management significantly reduces sICH risk [3, 21, 26].

7.2 Comparison of Tenecteplase and Alteplase

Emerging evidence suggests that tenecteplase may offer a safer profile in certain scenarios:

- **Efficacy and Safety**: Tenecteplase at a dose of 0.25 mg/kg is associated with lower sICH rates compared to alteplase. Lower incidence of sICH at a dose of 0.25 mg/kg compared to alteplase [22, 33].
- **Higher Doses**: Tenecteplase at a 0.4 mg/kg dose has been linked to increased sICH risk, emphasizing the importance of dose selection [22, 37].

7.3 Other Complications

- **Reocclusion**: Reocclusion of treated vessels may occur, particularly in cases with high thrombus burden.
- **Major Systemic Bleeding**: Although rare, severe systemic bleeding can complicate IVT in anticoagulated patients [9]. This complication occurs in about 2% of patients treated with IVT and includes bleeding events outside the central nervous system, such as gastrointestinal or urinary tract bleeding [19].
- **Angioedema:** It can manifest as swelling of the face, tongue, or throat, and occurs in approximately 5% of patients. This condition can complicate airway management and may require immediate intervention [19].
- **Peripheral Hemorrhages:** These include bleeding from mucous membranes (gums, nasal cavity), skin, or other sites. While often less severe than intracranial hemorrhages, they can indicate an increased risk for more serious complications [17, 36].
- **Reperfusion Injury:** Following successful IVT, some patients may experience reperfusion injury characterized by edema or hemorrhagic transformation of the infarcted area. This can complicate recovery and impact overall outcomes [17].

8 Combined Approaches

8.1 Intravenous Thrombolysis and Mechanical Thrombectomy

The combination of IVT and MT is the standard of care for patients with LVO. This integrated approach leverages the strengths of both modalities to optimize outcomes:

- **Sequential Therapy**:
  - IVT serves as a "bridging therapy" to MT [3, 21, 26], increasing the likelihood of early reperfusion. Studies show higher rates of successful revascularization when IVT precedes MT compared to MT alone [29, 32].
  - The decision to use "bridging therapy" should involve a multidisciplinary team, including neurologists and interventionalists, who evaluate the risks and benefits based on individual patient characteristics and clinical presentation.

8.2 Guideline Recommendations

- Both ESO and AHA/ASA advocate for IVT in eligible patients with LVO, even if MT is planned [3, 26, 32].

9 Conclusion and Future Perspectives

Intravenous thrombolysis remains a pivotal intervention in the management of AIS. Ongoing research continues to refine patient selection criteria, optimal timing, and the choice of thrombolytic agents to enhance efficacy and safety. The integration of advanced imaging and combined therapeutic approaches holds promise for improving outcomes in a broader patient population. Key trends include:

- **Extended Treatment Windows**: Advances in imaging technologies, such as CT perfusion and MRI, have enabled the safe application of IVT in extended time frames, beyond the traditional 4.5-h window, using imaging criteria to select patients with salvageable brain tissue and exploring combination therapies that enhance the efficacy of thrombolytics [22, 24]. These innovations are critical for addressing wake-up strokes and cases with unknown onset times.
- **Increased Use of Tenecteplase**: Emerging evidence supports tenecteplase as a first-line thrombolytic in select scenarios. Its ease of administration, superior efficacy in LVO, and favorable safety profile make it a promising alternative to alteplase [3, 6, 22, 24, 26, 33].
- **Integrated Treatment Strategies**: The combination of IVT with MT continues to improve outcomes, particularly for patients with LVO. Research on optimizing the sequencing and timing of these therapies is ongoing.

9.1 Future Directions

- **Personalized Medicine**: Developing algorithms to tailor IVT regimens based on individual patient-specific factors, such as age, infarct size, and comorbidities, holds the potential to further refine outcomes.
- **Global Accessibility**: Addressing geographic disparities in access to thrombolytic agents, advanced imaging, and

stroke care infrastructure is critical for equitable treatment worldwide.

- **Mobile Stroke Units:** Innovations like mobile stroke units aim to deliver thrombolytic therapy rapidly at the site of care, reinforcing the principle that "time is brain" and potentially improving outcomes by reducing delays in treatment initiation [11].
- **Research Innovations**: Ongoing research is focused on optimizing treatment protocols, exploring new thrombolytic agents, and integrating advanced imaging techniques to better identify candidates for IVT beyond conventional time limits. Large-scale, randomized controlled trials and meta-analyses will continue to shape guidelines and clinical practice and expand the evidence base for IVT in stroke management.

In summary, IVT has evolved from a novel treatment into a cornerstone of AIS management. Continued research and adaptation of guidelines are essential to maximize its accessibility, and benefits while minimizing risks for patients.

Declarations

Competing Interests The authors have no competing interests to declare that are relevant to the content of this manuscript.

Ethics Approval The authors declares that this manuscript does not include primary research with human participants.

References

1. Al-Ajlan FS, Alkhiri A, Alamri AF, et al. Golden hour intravenous thrombolysis for acute ischemic stroke: a systematic review and meta-analysis. Ann Neurol. 2024;96:582–90.
2. Alamowitch S, Turc G, Palaiodimou L, et al. European stroke organisation (ESO) expedited recommendation on tenecteplase for acute ischaemic stroke. Eur Stroke J. 2023;8:8–54.
3. Berge E, Whiteley W, Audebert H, et al. European stroke organisation (ESO) guidelines on intravenous thrombolysis for acute ischaemic stroke. Eur Stroke J. 2021; https://doi.org/10.1177/2396987321989865.
4. Bhatia R, Hill MD, Shobha N, et al. Low rates of acute recanalization with intravenous recombinant tissue plasminogen activator in ischemic stroke: real-world experience and a call for action. Stroke. 2010;41(10):2254–8. https://doi.org/10.1161/STROKEAHA.110.592535.
5. Bivard A, Lin L, Parsonsb MW. Review of stroke thrombolytics. J Stroke. 2013;15(2):90–8. https://doi.org/10.5853/jos.2013.15.2.90.
6. Campbell BCV, Mitchell PJ, Churilov L, et al. Tenecteplase versus alteplase before thrombectomy for ischemic stroke. N Engl J Med. 2018;378:1573–82.
7. Donaldson J, Winders J, Alamri Y, et al. The changing landscape of intravenous thrombolysis for acute Ischaemic stroke. J Clin Med. 2024;13:5826. https://doi.org/10.3390/jcm13195826.
8. Dorňák T, Král M, Šaňák D, Kaňovský P. Intravenous thrombolysis in posterior circulation stroke. Front Neurol. 2019;10:417. https://doi.org/10.3389/fneur.2019.00417.
9. Ghannam M, AlMajali M, Galecio-Castillo M, et al. Intravenous thrombolysis for acute ischemic stroke in patients with recent direct Oral anticoagulant use: a systematic review and meta-analysis. J Am Heart Assoc. 2023;12:e031669. https://doi.org/10.1161/JAHA.123.031669.
10. Goyal M, Menon BK, van Zwam WH, for the HERMES collaborators, et al. Endovascular thrombectomy after large-vessel ischaemic stroke: a meta-analysis of individual patient data from five randomised trials. Lancet. 2016;387:1723–31.
11. Grotta JC. Intravenous thrombolysis for acute ischemic stroke. Continuum (Minneap Minn). 2023;29(2):425–42. https://doi.org/10.1212/CON.0000000000001207.
12. Hacke W, Donnan G, Fieschi C, ATLANTIS Trials Investigators; ECASS Trials Investigators; NINDS rt-PA Study Group Investigators, et al. Association of outcome with early stroke treatment: pooled analysis of ATLANTIS, ECASS, and NINDS rt-PA stroke trials. Lancet. 2004;363(9411):768–74. https://doi.org/10.1016/S0140-6736(04)15692-4.
13. Halúsková S, Herzig R, Krajíčková D, et al. Acute management should be optimized in patients with less specific stroke symptoms. J Clin Med. 2021;10(5):1143. https://doi.org/10.3390/jcm10051143.
14. Halúsková S, Herzig R, Mikulík R, et al. Intravenous thrombolysis in posterior versus anterior circulation stroke: clinical outcome differs only in patients with large vessel occlusion. Biomedicine. 2024;12:404. https://doi.org/10.3390/biomedicines12020404.
15. Jauch EC, Saver JL, Harold P, on behalf of the American Heart Association Stroke Council, Council on Cardiovascular Nursing, Council on Peripheral Vascular Disease, and Council on Clinical Cardiology, et al. Guidelines for the early management of patients with acute ischemic stroke: a guideline for healthcare professionals from the American Heart Association/American Stroke Association. Stroke. 2013;44:870–947. https://doi.org/10.1161/STR.0b013e318284056a.
16. Knapen RRMM, Frol S, van Kuijk SMJ, et al. Intravenous thrombolysis for ischemic stroke in the posterior circulation: a systematic review and meta-analysis. J Stroke Cerebrovasc Dis. 2024;33:107641.
17. Liu L, Wang W. Risk factors for acute ischemic stroke following intravenous thrombolysis: a 2-center retrospective cohort study. Ann Palliat Med. 2022;11(1):185–200. https://doi.org/10.21037/apm-21-3652.
18. Meinel TR, Wilson D, Gensicke H, et al. Intravenous thrombolysis in patients with ischemic stroke and recent ingestion of direct oral anticoagulants. JAMA Neurol. 2023;80(3):233–43. https://doi.org/10.1001/jamaneurol.2022.4782.
19. Miller DJ, Simpson JR, Silver B. Safety of thrombolysis in acute ischemic stroke: a review of complications, risk factors, and newer technologies. Neurohospitalist. 2011;1(3):138–47. https://doi.org/10.1177/1941875211408731.
20. National Institute of Neurological Disorders and Stroke rt-PA Stroke Study Group. Tissue plasminogen activator for acute ischemic stroke. N Engl J Med. 1995;333(24):1581–7. https://doi.org/10.1056/NEJM199512143332401.
21. Neumann J, Šaňák D, Tomek A, et al. Doporučení pro intravenózní trombolýzu v léčbě akutního mozkového infarktu—verze 2021. Cesk Slov Neurol N. 2021;84/117(3):291–9. https://doi.org/10.48095/cccsnn2021291.
22. Palaiodimou L, Katsanos AH, Turc G, et al. Tenecteplase for the treatment of acute ischemic stroke in the extended time window: a systematic review and meta-analysis. Ther Adv Neurol Disord. 2024;17:1–12. https://doi.org/10.1177/17562864231221324.
23. Parsons M, Spratt N, Bivard A, et al. A randomized trial of tenecteplase versus alteplase for acute ischemic stroke. N Engl J Med. 2012;366:1099–107.
24. Parsons MW, Yogendrakumar V, Churilov L, for the TASTE Investigators, et al. Tenecteplase versus alteplase for thrombolysis in patients selected by use of perfusion imaging within 4·5 h of onset of ischaemic stroke (TASTE): a multicentre, ran-

domised, controlled, phase 3 non-inferiority trial. Lancet Neurol. 2024;23:775–86. https://doi.org/10.1016/S1474-4422(24)00206-0.
25. Pennica D, Holmes WE, Kohr WJ, et al. Cloning and expression of human tissue-type plasminogen activator cDNA in E. coli. Nature. 1983;301(5897):214–21. https://doi.org/10.1038/301214a0.
26. Powers WJ, Rabinstein AA, Ackerson T, et al. on behalf of the American Heart Association stroke council. Guidelines for the early management of patients with Acute Ischemic Stroke: 2019 update to the 2018 guidelines for the early management of acute ischemic stroke a guideline for healthcare professionals from the American Heart Association/American Stroke Association. Stroke. 2019;50:e344–418. https://doi.org/10.1161/STR.0000000000000211.
27. Rijken DC, Collen D. Purification and characterization of the plasminogen activator secreted by human melanoma cells in culture. J Biol Chem. 1981;256(13):7035–41.
28. Röther J, Ford GA, Thijs VNS. Thrombolytics in acute ischaemic stroke: historical perspective and future opportunities. Cerebrovasc Dis. 2013;35(4):313–9. https://doi.org/10.1159/000348705.
29. Strbian D, Tsivgoulis G, Ospel J, et al. European stroke organisation (ESO) and European Society for Minimally Invasive Neurological Therapy (ESMINT) guideline on acute management of basilar artery occlusion. J Neurointerv Surg. 2024;16:e7. https://doi.org/10.1136/jnis-2024-022053.
30. Taha NA, El Khawas H, Tork MA, et al. Intravenous thrombolysis outcome in posterior vs anterior circulation stroke in a tertiary stroke center in Egypt. Egypt J Neurol Psychiat Neurosurg. 2021;57:73. https://doi.org/10.1186/s41983-021-00325-0.
31. Tsivgoulis G, Katsanos AH, Schellinger PD, et al. Successful reperfusion with intravenous thrombolysis preceding mechanical thrombectomy in large-vessel occlusions. Stroke. 2018;49(1):232–5. https://doi.org/10.1161/STROKEAHA.117.019261.
32. Turc G, Tsivgoulis G, Audebert HJ, et al. European Stroke Organisation (ESO)–European Society for Minimally Invasive Neurological Therapy (ESMINT) expedited recommendation on indication for intravenous thrombolysis before mechanical thrombectomy in patients with acute ischemic stroke and anterior circulation large vessel occlusion. J Neurointerv Surg. 2024; https://doi.org/10.1136/neurintsurg-2021-018589.
33. Warach SJ, Ranta A, Kim J, et al. Symptomatic intracranial hemorrhage with Tenecteplase vs Alteplase in patients with acute ischemic stroke: the comparative effectiveness of routine Tenecteplase vs Alteplase in acute ischemic stroke (CERTAIN) collaboration. JAMA Neurol. 2023;80:732–8. https://doi.org/10.1001/jamaneurol.2023.1449.
34. Yaghi S, Willey JZ, Cucchiara B, et al. Treatment and outcome of hemorrhagic transformation after intravenous alteplase in acute ischemic stroke: a scientific statement for healthcare professionals from the American Heart Association/American Stroke Association. Stroke. 2017;48:e343–61.
35. Yogendrakumar V, Churilov L, Guha P, EXTEND-IA TNK Investigators, et al. Tenecteplase treatment and thrombus characteristics associated with early reperfusion: an EXTEND-IA TNK trials analysis. Stroke. 2023;54(3):706–14. https://doi.org/10.1161/STROKEAHA.122.041061.
36. Zhang X, Yu Y, Jiang L, et al. The risk factors of early hemorrhage after emergency intravenous thrombolysis in patients with acute ischemic stroke. Ann Palliat Med. 2021;10(5):5706–13. https://doi.org/10.21037/apm-21-1200.
37. Zhang X, Wan T-F, Chen J, et al. Tenecteplase versus alteplase for patients with acute ischemic stroke: a meta-analysis of randomized controlled trials. Aging. 2023;15(24):14889–99.

Endovascular Revascularization

Richard Bram, Tatiana Abou-Mrad, Laura Stone McGuire, Gursant S. Atwal, Ali Alaraj, and Fady T. Charbel

List of Abbreviations

ADAPT	Direct Aspiration First Pass
AHA	American Heart Association
AIS	Acute Ischemic Stroke
ASA	American Stroke Association
ASPECT	Alberta Stroke Program Early CT Score
BAO	Basilar Artery Occlusion
BGC	Balloon Guide Catheter
BMT	Best Medical Treatment
CBF	Cerebral Blood Flow
CBV	Cerebral Blood Volume
CT	Computed Tomography
CTA	Computed Tomography Angiography
CTP	Computed Tomography Perfusion
ESO	European Stroke Organisation
ESMINT	European Society for Minimally Invasive Neurological Therapy
FDA	Food and Drug Administration
IA	Intra-Arterial
ICA	Internal Carotid Artery
ICAD	Intracranial Atherosclerotic Disease
ID	Internal Diameter
INR	International Normalized Ratio
IVT	Intravenous Thrombolysis
ITT	Intention to Treat
LKW	Last Known Well
LVO	Large Vessel Occlusion
MCA	Middle Cerebral Artery
MR	Magnetic Resonance
mRS	Modified Ranking Scale
MT	Mechanical Thrombectomy
MTT	Mean Transit Time
NIHSS	National Institutes of Health Stroke Scale
PCS	Posterior Circulation Stroke
RAPID	Rapid Processing of Perfusion and Diffusion
RCT	Randomized Clinical Trial
sICH	Symptomatic Intracranial Hemorrhage
TICI	Thrombolysis in Cerebral Infarction
tPA	Tissue Plasminogen Activator
TTP	Time to Peak
US	United States

R. Bram · T. Abou-Mrad · L. S. McGuire · G. S. Atwal · A. Alaraj
F. T. Charbel (✉)
Department of Neurosurgery, University of Illinois at Chicago, Chicago, IL, USA
e-mail: fcharbel@uic.edu

1 What Does Emergency Revascularization Add to Best Medical Therapy?

A discussion of stent retriever technology and pivotal clinical trials governing the implementation of MT begins with an understanding of best medical Therapy (BMT) alone. Intravenous thrombolysis (IVT) with the "clot-buster", tissue plasminogen activator (tPA) was first approved in the setting of myocardial infarction in 1987. In 1995, the pivotal National Institutes of Neurological Disorder and Stroke (NINDS) rt-PA Stroke Trial results were released and U.S. Food and Drug Administration (FDA) approval for use in AIS was obtained shortly thereafter in 1996 [1]. At 3 months, a favorable outcome as define by mRS scale score less than or equal to one was achieved by 39% in the tPA group and 26% in the placebo group (p = .019). Treated patients were 30% more likely to have a favorable outcome compared to placebo when considering multiple clinical assessment scales.

While undeniably promising, these clinical results must be considered in the context of real-world application of the treatment modality. At the current time, IVT administration remains a U.S. FDA approved standard of care for AIS within 3 h of last known well (LKW) time. Moreover, the American Heart Association (AHA)/American Stroke Association (ASA) and European Stroke Organization (ESO) have

V. Beneš, D. Netuka (eds.), *Surgical and Interventional Treatment of Cerebral Ischemia*,
https://doi.org/10.1007/978-3-032-08934-2_25

approved the extension of the time window to 4.5 h owing to the results of the European Cooperative Acute Stroke Study (ECASS) III [2–4]. Notably, this trial excluded patients with the following criteria: Age > 80 years, oral anticoagulant use irrespective of international normalized ratio (INR), severe stroke, and combination of both previous ischemic stroke and diabetes mellitus. Due to a combination of healthcare access limitations, delays in medical care, strict exclusion criteria and a brief window for administration, the percent of eligible patients who receive IVT is remarkably low: one early registry-based study determined that 3%–8.5% of potentially eligible patients receive IVT and < 20% of those who received it did so within 60 min [5].

Apart from the aforementioned limitations concerning inclusion and exclusion criteria, the efficacy of IVT in achieving recanalization is suboptimal, particularly in the setting of more proximal occlusions. A meta-analysis conducted in 2016 determined the rate of early recanalization to be 33% with lower rates in more proximal occlusions [6]. A more recent study examining factors associated with arterial recanalization during interhospital transfer for MT corroborated this value, finding recanalization rates to be 35% in patients receiving IVT with lower values in proximal LVO [7]. With this background, one can understand that MT in the modern era first provides substantial improvement over BMT on the basis of inclusivity: time windows for MT are significantly longer than that for IVT which substantially increases the pool of eligible patients. Secondly, rates of successful recanalization with MT are nearly double than that of IVT alone: these values ranged from 65.7–88% in the early window MT trials and as high as 76–84% in the late-window trials.

Advancements in interventional stroke treatment, namely MT, have brought into question the utility of IVT when MT is readily available . Some concerns surrounding the utilization of both treatment modalities sequentially include a subpar lytic effect of IVT in proximal LVO, clot fragmentation with distal embolization, and an increased risk of hemorrhagic complications. Several RCTs have examined the safety and efficacy of foregoing IVT when MT can be readily performed. Unfortunately, results were conflicting: while some trials demonstrated noninferiority of MT alone, others could not demonstrate the same finding [8–12]. A recent meta-analysis which assessed these aforementioned RCTs concluded that MT is non-inferior to MT and IVT and skipping IVT in centers where MT can be accomplished in a timely manner is reasonable [13]. The following chapters provide a more detailed overview beginning with MT technology before transitioning to the aforementioned clinical trials. In the latter parts of the chapter, the most recent data concerning MT for large core and posterior circulation LVO is discussed.

2 The Beginning of Mechanical Thrombectomy: Stent Retriever Technology and Early Window Trials

Functional outcome and mortality rates are directly correlated to recanalization, and as such, significant effort has been put towards achieving better means of recanalization. In the late 1990s, the Prolyse in Acute Cerebral Thromboembolism (PROACT) and PROACT II trials were the first RCTs investigating the efficacy of catheter-delivered intra-arterial (IA) thrombolysis [14]. Although the PROACT II trial demonstrated improved functional outcomes and recanalization rates with IA therapy, IA thrombolysis never gained FDA approval. Nevertheless, PROACT II paved the way for further research into device development and specifically, mechanical clot extraction.

The Mechanical Embolus Removal in Cerebral Ischemia (MERCI) trial was a non-randomized single-armed trial investigating recanalization rates with the Merci device up to 8 h in patients ineligible for IVT [15]. Using the spontaneous recanalization group of the PROACT II trial as a control, MERCI showed the device to be successful in restoring vascular patency for patients ineligible for IVT: recanalization was achieved in 46% of subjects in the intention to treat (ITT) analysis compared to the control rate of 18% in PROACT II. In 2007, a suction/aspiration system obtained FDA approval and the Penumbra Pivotal Stroke Trial demonstrated promising results: revascularization rates were as high as 82% which was markedly improved compared to the rate of 68% achieved by the latest generation Merci device at the time [16]. This device used contact aspiration with a separator which resolved the issue of aspiration catheter blockage by morselizing the clot via a back-and-forth motion under continuous aspiration. The use of this separator would eventually fall out of favor due to the risk of vascular perforation, especially in curved branching points of blood vessels.

In the same year the suction/aspiration device was approved, several cases of successful stent-assisted recanalization were also described [17, 18]. Self-expanding stents designed specifically for the cerebral vasculature offered the benefit of deployment under lower pressures and improved trackability. Although originally intended for applications in stent-assisted aneurysm coiling or intracranial atherosclerotic disease (ICAD), these devices could be used for cerebrovascular occlusion not adequately treated with IVT and proved to have significant efficacy in this regard [19]. The principal limitation of intracranial stenting was the requirement for antiplatelet therapy and the associated risk of hemorrhagic complications. Stent Retrievers, termed "Stentrievers" for short, circumvented the need for permanent implantation via a design which joined the stent with the microwire. In such a way, the stent could be temporarily deployed and embedded into the thrombus with subsequent retrieval from the intracranial circulation.

Released in 2012, the Solitaire (Medtronic) was the first stentriever engineered for the purpose of MT. In the same year, the Trevo (Stryker) stentriever was also approved. These second generation MT devices were pivotal as they demonstrated a notable improvement in clinical outcome when compared to the Merci device [20, 21]. The Solitaire and Trevo stentrievers were the primary devices employed in the interventional treatment arms of five Class 1 RCTs published in 2015: Multicenter Randomized Clinical Trial of Endovascular Treatment for Acute Ischemic Stroke in the Netherlands (MR CLEAN), Endovascular Treatment for Small Core and Anterior Circulation Proximal Occlusion with Emphasis on Minimizing CT to Recanalization Times (ESCAPE), Randomized Trial of Revascularization with Solitaire FR Device versus Best Medical Therapy in the Treatment of Acute Stroke Due to Anterior Circulation Large Vessel Occlusion (REVASCAT), Solitaire with the Intention for Thrombectomy as Primary Endovascular Treatment (SWIFT PRIME), Extending the Time for Thrombolysis in Emergency Neurological Deficits — Intra-Arterial (EXTEND IA) [22–26]. Table 1 summarizes the results of the early window trials.

Although inclusion criteria varied, the target population for the early window trials included adults ≥18 years old with good premorbid functional status (Modified Ranking Scale (mRS) Score ≤ 1) and LVO of the anterior circulation as demonstrated by CT angiography or MR angiography. In three of five trials, patients were required to present within 6 h, while the remaining two included patients up to 8 or 12 h. Patients with large infarct cores (Alberta Stroke Program Early CT Score (ASPECT) <6)or mild stroke symptoms (National Institutes of Health Stroke Scale (NIHSS) score < 6) were generally excluded with some variation between studies. Combining the data into a meta-analysis, the Highly Effective Reperfusion evaluated in Multiple Endovascular Stroke Trials (HERMES) study demonstrated an undeniable clinical benefit across the diverse patient populations of all studies [27]. At 90 days, a mRS score of 0–2 was achieved by 46% of the interventional group compared to 26.5% of the control group and the number needed to treat for one patient to have reduced disability of at least one point was 2.6. Importantly, the positive effect was demonstrated for several subgroups of specific interest to practitioners at the time: octogenarians, patients randomized over 300 min after symptom onset and those not receiving IVT.

In response to the positive findings of these studies, the AHA/ASA published an update to the previous guideline in 2015 [28]. This included a Class I recommendation for endovascular therapy with a stent retriever given the following criteria: Prestroke mRS score 0–1, AIS receiving IVT within 4.5 h, internal carotid artery (ICA) or M1 segment of the middle cerebral artery (MCA) occlusion, Age ≥ 18 years, NIHSS score ≥ 6, and groin puncture that can be initiated within 6 h of symptoms onset. At the present time, MT is routinely offered to patients presenting with LVO within 6 h even in the absence of advanced vascular or perfusion imaging. Although the subgroup of patients randomized over 300 min after symptom onset maintained a statistically significant clinical benefit in the HERMES analysis, the degree of benefit was less pronounced compared to patients with earlier intervention. The next phase of advancement in the field of endovascular revascularization would focus on the concept of the "Penumbra" and perfusion-based imaging studies which are paramount in identifying patients deriving the most clinical benefit from MT.

Table 1 Landmark early window trials of 2015

	Revascat	Mr Clean	Escape	Extend-IA	Swift prime
Study location	Spain	Netherlands	Multiple	Australia, New Zealand	USA, Europe
Number of patients	206 Total 103 EV 103 BMT	500 Total 233 EV 267 BMT	316 Total 120 EV 118 BMT	70 Total 35 EV 35 BMT	196 Total 98 EV 98 BMT
Time criteria	8 h	6 h	12 h	6 h	6 h
Imaging exclusion criteria	ASPECT <7 ASPECT<9 in patients 81–85 years	No ASPECT Score Cut-Off	**CT:**ASPECT <6 **CTA:** Poor Collateral Circulation **CTP:** Low CBF ASPECTS<6 or low CBF in >1/3 of the symptomatic MCA territory	**CTP:** Infarct Core >70 cc, Mismatch Ratio ≤ 1.2, Mismatch Volume ≤ 10 cc	**CT:** ASPECT <6 **CTP:** Core infarct >50, >100 cc lesion with T_{max} > 10 sec, Mismatch ratio ≤ 1.8, Mismatch Volume < 15 cc
TICI 2b-3 (%)	65.7	58.7	72.4	86	88
Favorable outcome (%)	43.7 EV 28.2 BMT Treatment Effect 2.1 (95% CI 1.1–4.0)	32.6 EV 19.1 BMT Treatment Effect 2.16 (95% CI 1.39–3.38)	53.0 EV 29.3 BMT Treatment Effect 1.7 (95% CI 1.3–2.2)	71 EV 40 BMT $p = .0009$	60 EV 35 BMT $p < 0.001$
NNT for favorable outcome	6.5	7.4	4.2	3.2	4
sICH (%)	1.9 EV 1.9 BMT[a] Treatment Effect 1.0 (95% CI 0.1–7.)	7.7 EV 6.4 BMT No statistically significant difference. treatment effect not reported.	3.6 EV 2.7 BMT Treatment Effect 1.2 (95% CI 0.3–4.6)	0 EV 6 BMT $p = 0.49$	0 EV 3 BMT $p = 0.12$
Mortality (%)	18.4 EV 15.5 BMT Treatment Effect 1.2 (95% CI 0.6–2.2) At 90 days	18.9 EV 18.4 BMT No statistically significant difference. treatment effect not reported. At 30 days	10.4 EV 19 BMT Treatment Effect 0.5 (95% CI 0.3–0.8) At 90 days	9 EVT 20 BMT $p = 0.18$ Any time point	9 EVT 12 BMT $p = 0.50$ At 90 days
Device(s)	Solitaire stent retriever	Multiple	Multiple	Solitaire stent retriever	Solitaire stent retriever

Abbreviations: *EV* Endovascular Treatment, *BMT* Best Medical Treatment, *TICI* Thrombolysis in Cerebral Infarction, *ASPECT* Alberta Stroke Program Early CT Score, *NNT* Number Needed to Treat, *sICH* Symptomatic Intracranial Hemorrhage, *CI* Confidence Interval, *mRS* Modified Rankin Scale

Favorable outcome defined as mRS ≤ 2

[a]sICH reported using SITS-MOST Criteria

3 Extending the Window: The Advent of Perfusion Imaging and Late Window Trials

Although perfusion imaging is not indicated in the 6 h window, the extended time window requires an interpretation of physiologic parameters derived from perfusion studies. By extrapolating physiologic information as intravenous contrast passes through the cerebral vasculature, this modality allows for the reliable identification of patients who benefit from intervention. The term "Penumbra" refers to reversibly injured brain tissue around an ischemic core, which is precisely the target of interventional stroke therapy [29]. The concept of penumbra facilitated a paradigm shift, departing from a strict adherence to time-based therapy and changing focus to a physiological understanding of infarcted versus salvageable brain. This advancement paved the way for treating patients in what is referred to as the late window of 6–24 h., provided certain imaging and exclusion criteria were met.

A CT-Perfusion (CTP) scan can generate a time attenuation curve from which physiologic parameters can be derived. The mean transit time (MTT) represents the average time required for blood to pass through a capillary network. Related to MTT is time to peak (TTP) which is a measure of the time from contrast administration to maximum enhancement. T_{MAX} reflects the TTP after it has been subjected to a deconvolution algorithm. Cerebral blood volume (CBV) reflects the volume of blood (mL) in 100 g of brain tissue. Cerebral blood flow (CBF) which is calculated by dividing CBV by MTT, represents the amount of blood flowing through a region per unit time. Both relative CBV and relative CBF can be used to estimate the ischemic core while measures of delay such as MTT or T_{MAX} approximate the area of tissue at risk. Perfusion imaging can therefore identify patients with an ischemic penumbra who would benefit the most from revascularization [30]. A widely accepted threshold for demarcating the ischemic core and area at risk respectively are relative CBF <30% compared to the contralateral hemisphere and $T_{max} > 6$ s. These thresholds are currently employed by the rapid processing of perfusion and diffusion (RAPID) software.

With perfusion-based imaging, there existed a way to identify patients with salvageable ischemic penumbra presenting past the traditional 6 h window. The DWI or CTP Assessment with Clinical Mismatch in the Triage of Wake-Up and Late Presenting Strokes Undergoing Neurointervention with Trevo (DAWN) and Endovascular Therapy Following Imaging Evaluation for Ischemic Stroke (DEFUSE 3) trials focused heavily on this and expanded the window to 24 h and 16 h, respectively [31, 32]. The results of both late window trials are summarized in Table 2. An illustrative case of a patient presenting in the late window successfully treated with MT is detailed in Fig. 1.

Table 2 Late-window trial summary

	Defuse III	Dawn
Study location	USA	Multiple
Publication year	2018	2017
Number of patients	182 Total 92 EV 90 BMT	206 Total 107 EV 99 BMT
Time criteria	6–16 h	6–24 h
Inclusion criteria	CTP: Ischemic core <70 cc	Group A: Age > 80 years, NIHSS ≥10, Core <21 cc
	Mismatch ratio ≥ 1.8	Group B: Age < 80, NIHSS≥10, Core <31 cc
	Penumbra ≥15 cc	Group C: Age < 80, NIHSS ≥20, Core 31–50 cc
TICI 2b-3 (%)	76	84
Favorable outcome (%)	45 EV 17 BMT $p < 0.001$ At 90 days	49 EV 13 BMT Posterior probability of superiority >0.999 At 90 days
NNT for favorable outcome	3.6	2.8
sICH (%)	7 EV 4 BMT $p = .075$	6 EV 3 BMT Risk Ratio 2 (95% CI 1–7)
Mortality (%)	14 EV 26 BMT $p = 0.05$ At 90 days	19 EV 18 BMT Risk ratio 1 (95% CI 1–2) At 90 days

Abbreviations: *EV* Endovascular Treatment, *BMT* Best Medical Treatment, *TICI* Thrombolysis in Cerebral Infarction, *NNT* Number Needed to Treat, *sICH* Symptomatic Intracranial Hemorrhage, *CI* Confidence Interval, *mRS*, Modified Rankin Scale
Favorable outcome defined as mRS ≤ 2

The DEFUSE III trial randomized 182 patients to MT vs. best medical treatment (BMT) at 6–16 h from LKW. Imaging criteria required the core infarct to be less than 70 cc and the ratio of ischemic tissue to infarct core to be ≥1.8. Patients in the MT group had significantly better clinical outcomes with 45% achieving functional independence (defined as mRS 0–2) compared to 17% in the medical group. 90 day mortality was 14% with MT and 26% with BMT with no difference in rates of symptomatic intracranial hemorrhage (sICH). In contrast to the DEFUSE III trial, the DAWN trial emphasized a mismatch between the clinical deficit and infarct volume. Selection criteria were strict, necessitating a pre-intervention mRS of 0–1. Moreover, patients with NIHSS <10 were ineligible as were patients >80 years old with larger core infarcts. The three eligible groups included the following: patients ≥80 years old with NIHSS ≥10 and infarct volume < 21 cc; patients <80 years old with NIHSS ≥10 and infarct volume < 31 cc; patients <80 years old with NIHSS ≥20 with an infarct volume 31–50 cc. In total, 206

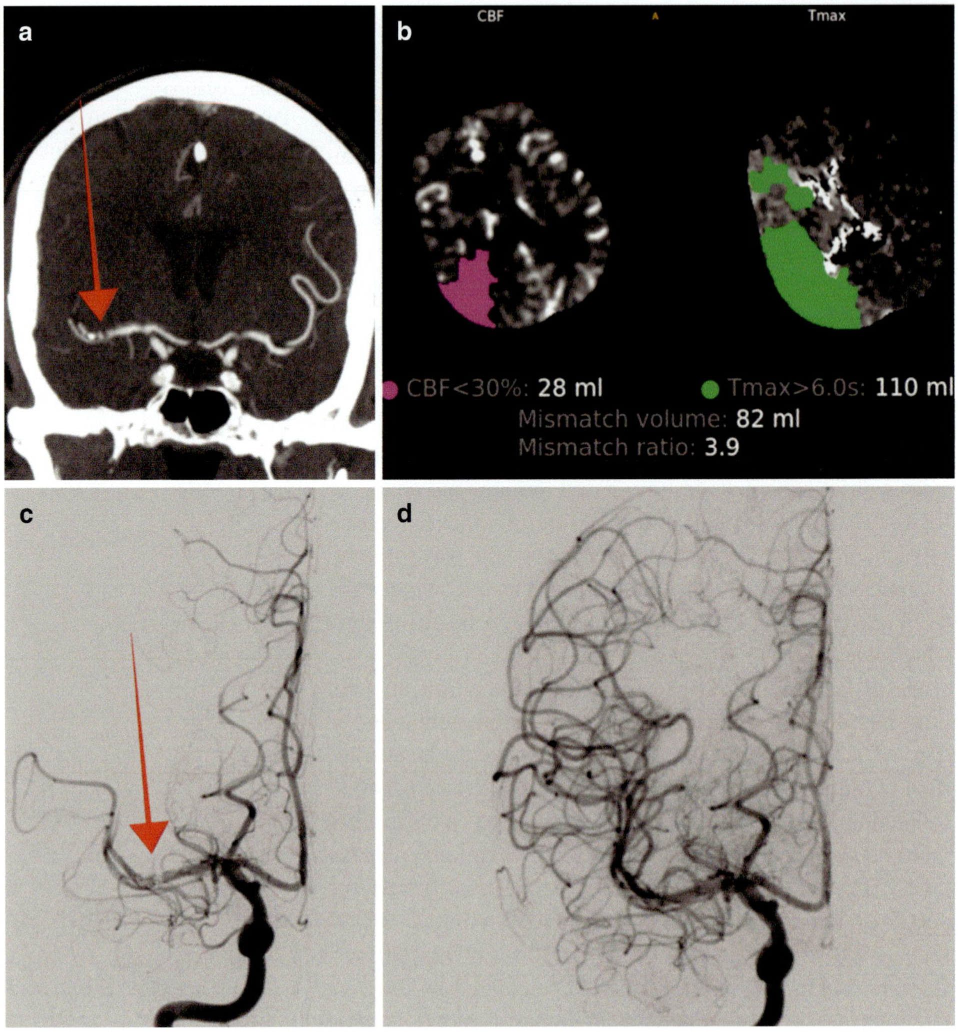

Fig. 1 **Illustrative Case of Middle Cerebral Artery Occlusion.** A 68 year-old female with a history of congestive heart failure, hypertension, hyperlipidemia, diabetes mellitus and atrial fibrillation on apixaban presented with left hemiparesis. She was ineligible for IVT due to active anticoagulant use and a LKW of 8 h prior to arrival. Initial NIHSS was 10 and CTA revealed a partial filling defect of the right M1 segment of the MCA (**a**, Red Arrow). CT perfusion demonstrated a 28 cc core infarct, 110 cc penumbra and mismatch ratio of 3.9 which met DAWN and DEFUSE III criteria (**b**). An initial right ICA injection demonstrated a subocclusive thrombus at the M1 segment of the right MCA with delayed filling of the MCA territory (**c**, Red Arrow). TICI3 revascularization was achieved after a single pass using direct aspiration only (**d**)

patients were enrolled. The rate of functional independence was 49% in the intervention group compared to 13% in the control group with no statistically significant difference in sICH nor mortality.

Beyond time and imaging inclusion criteria, an important distinction between the two late window trials concerns the inclusivity of the DEFUSE III trial. In DEFUSE III, patients with larger core infarcts, those with milder stroke symptoms, and those with pre-intervention mRS scores of up to 2 were eligible for MT. In 2019, based on evidence established by these late window trials, the AHA/ASA released new guidelines pertaining to endovascular revascularization [33]. Provided patients met eligibility criteria, MT is now recommended in the 6–16 h window and has been determined to be reasonable in the 16–24 h window. This represented a dramatic change in stroke care, offering treatment to patients who just several years prior may have been ineligible.

4 Mechanical Thrombectomy in Large Core Ischemic Infarcts

Although the DAWN and DEFUSE III trials significantly altered clinical practice, it is widely understood that selection criteria were stringent and restrictive. A substantial proportion of patients presenting to stroke centers around the world who do not meet DAWN/DEFUSE III eligibility criteria are still offered MT. In a meta-analysis of 9 studies exploring outcomes in MT for DAWN/DEFUSE III eligible versus ineligible patients, Morsi et al. concluded that both cohorts achieved similar rates of functional independence despite larger core infarct volumes in latter group [34]. However, ineligible patients suffered from greater rates of sICH and mortality. While initial pivotal RCTs focused on the early and late time windows, a subsequent series of six RCTs would shift attention to extending eligibility for patients with large core infarcts (Table 3).

Table 3 Summary of the six large core trials

	Rescue Japan limit	Tension	Laste	Angel aspect	Select 2	TESLA
Study location	Japan	Canada, Europe	Europe, USA	China	Canada, USA, Europe	USA
Publication year	2022	2023	2024	2023	2023	2024
Number of patients	203 Total 102 EV 101 BMT	253 Total 128 EV 125 BMT	333 Total 165 EV 159 BMT	456 Total 225 EV 230 BMT	352 Total 174 EV 178 BMT	300 Total 148 EV 152 BMT
Time criteria	6 h 24 h if MRI FLAIR negative	12 h	6.5 h 24 h if MRI FLAIR negative	24 h	24 h	24 h
Imaging inclusion criteria	ASPECT 3–5	ASPECT 3–5	ASPECT 0–5 ASPECT 4–5 For 80 years or Older	CT:ASPECT 3–5 CTP: Core 70–100 cc	ASPECT 3–5 CTP/MRI: Core ≥50 cc	ASPECT 2–5
Favorable outcome (%)	31 EV 12.7 BMT $p = .002$ At 90 days	34 EV 17 BMT $p = .0035$ At 12 months	33.5 EV 12.2 BMT Treatment effect 2.62 (95% CI 1.72–4.36) At 90 days	47 EV 33.3 BMT Treatment effect 1.50 (95% CI 1.17–1.91) At 90 days	37.9 EV 18.7 BMT Treatment effect 2.06 (95% CI 1.43–2.96) At 90 days	29.8 EV 19.9 BMT $p = .03$ At 90 days
sICH (%)	9 EV 4.9 BMT $p = .25$	Not reported	9.6 EV 5.7 BMT Treatment effect 1.73 (95% CI 0.78–4.68)	6.1 EV 2.7 BMT $p = .012$	0.6 EV 1.1 BMT Treatment effect 0.49 (95% CI 0.04 to 5.36)	4.0 EV 1.3 BMT Treatment effect 2.96 (95% CI 0.61–14.43)
Mortality (%)	18 EV 23.5 BMT $p = .33$ At 90 days	45 EV 56 BMT $p = .048$ At 12 months	36.1 EV 55.5 BMT Treatment effect 0.65 (0.50–0.84) At 90 days	21.7 EV 20.0 BMT $p = 0.99$ At 90 days	38.4 EV 41.5 BMT Treatment effect 0.91 (0.71–1.18) At 90 days	35.3 EV 33.3 BMT Treatment effect 1.06 (0.77–1.45) At 90 days

Abbreviations: *EV* Endovascular Treatment, *BMT* Best Medical Treatment, *TICI* Thrombolysis in Cerebral Infarction, *ASPECT* Alberta Stroke Program Early CT Score, *NNT* Number Needed to Treat, *sICH* Symptomatic Intracranial Hemorrhage, *CI* Confidence Interval, *mRS* Modified Rankin Scale

Favorable outcome defined as mRS ≤ 3

The Recovery by Endovascular Salvage for Cerebral Ultra-Acute Embolism–Japan Large Ischemic Core Trial (RESCUE-Japan LIMIT) was the first of the large core RCTs and commenced recruitment in 2018 with publication of results in 2022 [35]. Patients were required to have an ASPECTS score of 3–5 and be within 6 h of LKW. If an MRI was obtained and demonstrated no Fluid Attenuated Inversion Recovery (FLAIR) changes, patients could be enrolled up to 24 hrs from LKW. At 90 days, 31% of patients in the endovascular group and 12.7% in the BMT group achieved an mRS score of 0–3. Although the endovascular group had more ICH of any kind, rates of sICH were not significantly different. The positive results of two similar trials were published in 2024: The Efficacy and Safety of Thrombectomy in Stroke with extended lesion and extended time window (TENSION) trial randomized patients with an ASPECTS score of 3–5 within 12 h of LKW while the Large Stroke Therapy Evaluation(LASTE) trial had no lower limit on infarct size and recruited patients with an ASPECTS score ≤ 5 within 6.5 h of LKW. Both trials showed a significant benefit in mortality rates and long-term functional outcomes in the interventional treatment arms [36, 37]. Importantly, the TENSION trial also demonstrated improved outcomes on patient-reported quality of life measures.

While the aforementioned RCTs solely utilized CT or MRI for inclusion, two additional trials applied more advanced perfusion imaging modalities for patient selection. The Trial of Endovascular Therapy for Acute Ischemic Stroke With Large Infarct (ANGEL-ASPECT) randomized patients within 24 hrs if they had either an ASPECTS score 3–5 or if the core infarct was 70–100 mL [38]. In the Randomized Controlled Trial to Optimize Patient's Selection for Endovascular Treatment in Acute Ischemic Stroke (SELECT2) patients were also required to present within 24 hrs of last known well and to have an ASPECTS score of 3–5 or core infarct >50 mL with no upper limit [39]. Both trials were terminated early due to positive results demonstrating improved functional outcomes with MT. Although 5 RCTs showed significant benefit with MT for this population of patients, the Thrombectomy for Emergent Salvage of

Large Anterior Circulation Ischemic Stroke (TESLA) trial did not achieve the same results.

The TESLA trial was conducted in the USA and randomized a total of 300 patients with anterior circulation LVO to endovascular treatment or BMT [40]. Patients were required to have an ASPECTS score of 2–5 and present within 24 h of LKW. Although point estimates were directionally favorable (UW-mRS at 90 days 2.93(+/− 3.39) thrombectomy vs. 2.27 (+/− 2.98) BMT), the trial failed to show a statistically significant difference in the primary outcome measure. The authors emphasized long times from stroke onset to randomization with an average of 10.9 h for the interventional group and 44.7% of patients in this treatment arm undergoing randomization in the 12–24 h period. This would potentially explain the less favorable outcomes compared to the aforementioned RCTs.

Although there are currently no updated guidelines from professional societies governing MT in large-core ischemia, the results of these 6 RCTs can help inform a tailored approach to treatment [41]. Offering MT for these patients must entail a discussion of realistic expectations for patient outcomes: rates of functional independence at 90 days (mRS 0–2) in the 6 aforementioned RCTs ranged from 14–30% which is substantially lower than that of patients in the early and late window MT trials. Moreover, the phrase "time is brain" remains relevant in large-core ischemia where patients who underwent earlier randomization with shorter door-to-puncture times achieved better outcomes. Similarly, the RESCUE JAPAN LIMIT and LASTE trials required negative FLAIR on MRI prior to inclusion of patients past 6 or 6.5 h respectively. The benefit of MT in the subgroup of patients with the largest ischemic cores, namely ASPECTS 0–2 and/or core volume > 100 cc, remains less clear with some data from the ANGEL-ASPECT and SELECT2 trials demonstrating reduced efficacy in this population [42]. Lastly, inclusion criteria in nearly all of these trials required a pre-intervention mRS of 0–1.

5 Mechanical Thrombectomy for Basilar Artery Occlusion

Basilar artery occlusion (BAO) comprises only 10% of LVO in AIS yet is associated with a disproportionately high degree of morbidity and mortality [43]. Moreover, posterior circulation stroke (PCS) can be more challenging to diagnose, often resulting in treatment delays. Patients with PCS were largely excluded from the pivotal trials of MT in both the early and late time windows. Despite overwhelming evidence demonstrating the benefit of MT in anterior circulation stroke, high-quality evidence for MT in the posterior circulation has been lacking until very recently. Initially, the Basilar Artery Occlusion Endovascular Intervention vs Standard Medical Treatment (BEST) trial and Basilar Artery International Cooperation Study (BASICS) failed to establish superiority of MT [44, 45]. These two initial studies set the foundation for the Endovascular Treatment for Acute Basilar-Artery Occlusion (ATTENTION) and Basilar Artery Occlusion Chinese Endovascular Trials (BAOCHE) which demonstrated positive results in due time [46, 47]. The results of these four BAO RCTs are summarized in Table 4.

In the BASICS and BEST trials, methodological issues concerning clinical equipoise, patient recruitment, crossover and treatment outside the trials were thought to contribute to negative results despite a trend towards improved outcomes in the interventional arms. The BEST trial sought to enroll 288 patients to either MT or medical treatment within 8 h of vertebrobasilar occlusion yet only 131 were recruited: a third of qualified patients refused trial participation, the crossover rate was 22%, and a significant drop in the per-center recruitment ultimately lead to termination of the trial. In the as-treated analysis, patients receiving intervention had more favorable clinical outcomes (47% versus 24%) defined as mRS 0–3 at 90 days. Although the BASICS trial managed to recruit 300 patients, nearly 80% of subjects in both treatment arms received IVT within 4.5 hrs. As such, outcomes in the medical treatment arm may have been better than expected. Moreover, 29.2% of eligible patients were treated outside of the trial of which a majority (79%) went on to receive MT. Although functional outcomes trended in favor of intervention (90-day mRS 0–3 44.2% intervention vs. 37.7% BMT), this was not statistically significant. Authors of both studies acknowledged the respective limitations and the results would not dissuade practitioners from offering intervention to patients with BAO.

In contrast to BASICS and BEST, the ATTENTION trial more efficiently performed consecutive enrollment while both ATTENTION and BAOCHE trials minimized patient cross-over [48]. Rates of IVT (30% ATTENTION, 14% BAOCHE) aligned more closely with historical values in the Acute Basilar Artery Occlusion Study (BASILAR) registry which prospectively studied 1254 patients with BAO treated with either medical therapy or thrombectomy [49]. The ATTENTION trial was conducted in China and randomized 340 patients with BAO to either MT or BMT within 12 h of LKW. At 90 days, the interventional group had a statistically

Table 4 Summary of trials for basilar occlusion

	Basics	Best	Attention	Baoche
Study location	Europe, Brazil	China	China	China
Publication year	2021	2020	2022	2022
Number of patients	300 Total 154 EV 146 BMT	131 Total 66 EV 65 BMT	340 Total 226 EV 114 BMT	217 Total 110 EV 107 BMT
Time criteria	6 h	8 h	12 h	6–24 h
Imaging exclusion criteria	Bilateral extended brainstem ischemia	Bilateral extended brainstem ischemia	PC-ASPECTS <6 if <80 years PC Aspects <8 if ≥80	PC-ASPECTS <6 Presence of large infarct in brainstem
Favorable outcome (%)	44.2 EV 37.7 BMT Treatment effect 1.18 (95% CI 0.92–1.50) At 90 days	42 EV 32 BMT $p = .0.23$ At 90 days	46 EV 23 BMT Treatment effect 2.06 (95% CI 1.46–2.91) At 90 days	46 EV 24 BMT Treatment effect 1.81 (95% CI 1.26–2.60) At 90 days
sICH (%)	4.5 EV 0.7 BMT Treatment effect 6.9 (95% CI 0.9–53.0)	8 EV 0 BMT $P = 0.06$	5 EV 0 BMT No estimate	6 EV 1 BMT Treatment effect 5.18 (95% CI 0.64–42.18)
Mortality (%)	38.3 EV 43.2 BMT Treatment effect 0.87 (0.68–1.12) At 90 days	33 EV 38 BMT $p = 0.54$ At 90 days	37 EV 55 BMT Treatment effect 0.66 (95% CI 0.52–0.82) At 90 days	31 EV 42 BMT Treatment effect 0.75 (95% CI 0.54–1.04) At 90 days

Abbreviations: *EV* Endovascular Treatment, *BMT* Best Medical Treatment, *PC-ASPECT* Posterior Circulation Alberta Stroke Program Early CT Score, *sICH* Symptomatic Intracranial Hemorrhage, *CI* Confidence Interval, *mRS* Modified Rankin Scale
Favorable outcome defined as mRS ≤ 2

significant improvement in rates of good functional outcome defined as mRS 0–3 (46% Intervention vs. 23% BMT) and decreased mortality (37% Intervention vs. 55% BMT). The BAOCHE trial, which was also conducted in China, randomized 217 patients with BAO 6 to 24 h from stroke onset. At 90 days, good functional status (mRS 0–3) was significantly higher in the interventional arm (46% vs. 24%) with a trend towards improved mortality rates. Intracranial and/or extracranial stent deployment was performed in nearly 50% of patients in the ATTENTION trial and in 60% of patients in the BAOCHE trial which is reflective of the high prevalence of ICAD in this patient population. Despite the increased technical complexity of such cases and slightly higher rates of sICH, these trials demonstrated high-quality evidence in favor of MT for BAO.

Owing to the positive results in favor of MT from the ATTENTION and BAOCHE trials, new guidelines for treatment of BAO have since been released. The ESO and European Society for Minimally Invasive Neurological Therapy (ESMINT) now recommend MT for patients presenting with BAO and moderate-to-severe stroke symptoms (NIHSS ≥10) without extensive ischemic changes (pc-ASPECTS 7–10) [50]. The Society of Vascular and Interventional Neurology as well as the Society of Neurointerventional Surgeons have also published updated guidelines [51, 52] Areas for further investigation include MT for BAO in patients with milder stroke symptoms as well as in those with more severe ischemic changes on pre-procedural imaging. Moreover, the benefit of MT for BAO past 24 h remains less clear as does MT for occlusion of more distal posterior circulation vasculature such as the posterior cerebral artery. An illustrative case of basilar artery occlusion successfully treated with mechanical thrombectomy is detailed in Fig. 2.

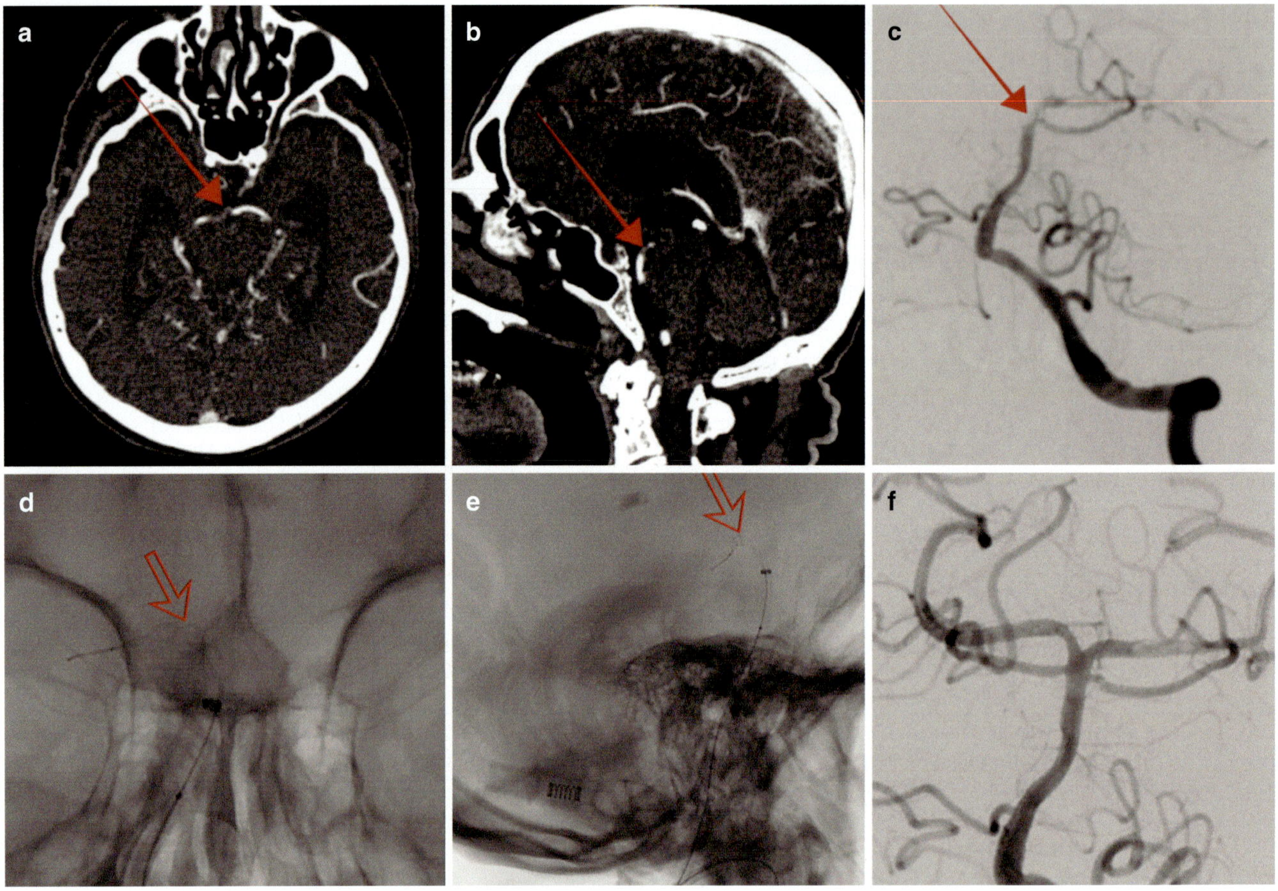

Fig. 2 **Illustrative Case of Basilar Artery Occlusion.** An 83 year-old male with a history of hypertension, diabetes mellitus, and atrial fibrillation off anticoagulation presented with progressively worsening ataxia and dysarthria upon awakening. His LKW was 15 hours prior to arrival, rendering him ineligible for IVT and initial NIHSS was 6. A CTA demonstrated thrombus at the top of the basilar artery with extension into the right P1 segment of the PCA (**a**&**b** Red Arrows). He was taken for mechanical thrombectomy where a left vertebral artery injection confirmed the presence of an occlusive thrombus at the top of the basilar artery with absent filling of the right PCA and SCA (**c**, Red Arrow). AP and lateral unsubtracted views demonstrate the stent retriever deployed from the top of the basilar artery into the right P1 segment of the PCA with the aspiration catheter positioned at the face of the thrombus (**d**&**e**, Red Arrows). TICI3 revascularization was achieved after a single pass with combined contact aspiration and stent-retrieval (f)

Declarations

Competing Interests The author(s) has no competing interests to declare that are relevant to the content of this manuscript.

Ethics Approval The author(s) declares that this manuscript does not include primary research with human participants.

References

1. National Institute of Neurological Disorders and Stroke rt-PA Stroke Study Group. Tissue plasminogen activator for acute ischemic stroke. N Engl J Med. 1995;333(24):1581–7.
2. Jauch EC, Saver JL, Adams HP, Bruno A, Connors JJB, Demaerschalk BM, et al. Guidelines for the early management of patients with acute ischemic stroke: a guideline for healthcare professionals from the American Heart Association/American Stroke Association. Stroke. 2013;44(3):870–947.
3. Hacke W, Kaste M, Bluhmki E, Brozman M, Davalos A, Guidetti D, et al. Thrombolysis with Alteplase 3 to 4.5 Hours after Acute Ischemic Stroke. N Engl J Med. 2011;365:687–96.
4. Berge E, Whiteley W, Audebert H, De Marchis GM, Fonseca AC, Padiglioni C, et al. European Stroke Organisation (ESO) guidelines on intravenous thrombolysis for acute ischaemic stroke. Eur Stroke J. 2021;6:I–LXII.
5. Arora S, Broderick JP, Frankel M, Heinrich JP, Hickenbottom S, Karp H, et al. Acute stroke care in the US: results from 4 pilot prototypes of the Paul Coverdell National Acute Stroke Registry. Stroke. 2005;36(6):1232–40.
6. Seners P, Turc G, Maïer B, Mas JL, Oppenheim C, Baron JC. Incidence and predictors of early recanalization after intravenous thrombolysis: a systematic review and meta-analysis. Stroke. 2016;47(9):2409–12.
7. Seners P, Wouters A, Ter Schiphorst A, Yuen N, Mlynash M, Arquizan C, et al. Arterial recanalization during interhospital transfer for thrombectomy. Stroke. 2024;55(6):1525–34.
8. LeCouffe NE, Kappelhof M, Treurniet KM, Rinkel LA, Bruggeman AE, Berkhemer OA, et al. A randomized trial of intravenous

alteplase before endovascular treatment for stroke. N Engl J Med. 2021;385(20):1833–44.
9. Zi W, Qiu Z, Li F, Sang H, Wu D, Luo W, et al. Effect of endovascular treatment alone vs intravenous alteplase plus endovascular treatment on functional independence in patients with acute ischemic stroke: the DEVT randomized clinical trial. JAMA. 2021;325(3):234–43.
10. Suzuki K, Matsumaru Y, Takeuchi M, Morimoto M, Kanazawa R, Takayama Y, et al. Effect of mechanical thrombectomy without vs with intravenous thrombolysis on functional outcome among patients with acute ischemic stroke: the SKIP randomized clinical trial. JAMA. 2021;325(3):244–53.
11. Yang P, Zhang Y, Zhang L, Zhang Y, Treurniet KM, Chen W, et al. Endovascular thrombectomy with or without intravenous alteplase in acute stroke. N Engl J Med. 2020;382(21):1981–93.
12. Fischer U, Kaesmacher J, Strbian D, Eker O, Cognard C, Plattner PS, et al. Thrombectomy alone versus intravenous alteplase plus thrombectomy in patients with stroke: an open-label, blinded-outcome, randomised non-inferiority trial. Lancet. 2022;400(10346):104–15.
13. Sattari SA, Antar A, Sattari AR, Feghali J, Hung A, Lee RP, et al. Endovascular thrombectomy versus endovascular thrombectomy preceded by intravenous thrombolysis: a systematic review and meta-analysis. World Neurosurg [Internet]. 2023;177:39–58. https://doi.org/10.1016/j.wneu.2023.05.033.
14. Furlan A, Higashida RT, Wechsler L, Gent M, Rowley H, Kase C. Intra-arterial prourokinase for acute ischemic stroke. The PROACT II study: a randomized controlled trial. JAMA J Am Med Assoc. 1999;282(21):2003–11.
15. Smith WS, Sung G, Starkman S, Saver JL, Kidwell CS, Gobin YP, et al. Safety and efficacy of mechanical embolectomy in acute ischemic stroke: results of the MERCI trial. Stroke. 2005;36(7):1432–8.
16. Investigators PPST. The penumbra pivotal stroke trial: safety and effectiveness of a new generation of mechanical devices for clot removal in intracranial large vessel occlusive disease. Stroke. 2009;40(8):2761–8.
17. Levy EI, Ecker RD, Horowitz MB, Gupta R, Hanel RA, Sauvageau E, et al. Stent-assisted intracranial recanalization for acute stroke: early results. Neurosurgery. 2006;58(3):458–62.
18. Levy EI, Mehta R, Gupta R, Woo HH, Albuquerque FC, Hopkins LN. Self-expanding stents for recanalization of acute cerebrovascular occlusions. Ajnr. 2007;28:816–22.
19. Levy EI, Siddiqui AH, Crumlish A, Snyder KV, Hauck EF, Fiorella DJ, et al. First food and drug administration-approved prospective trial of primary intracranial stenting for acute stroke: SARIS (Stent-Assisted Recanalization in Acute Ischemic Stroke). Stroke. 2009;40(11):3552–6.
20. Nogueira RG, Lutsep HL, Gupta R, Jovin TG, Albers GW, Walker GA, et al. Trevo versus Merci retrievers for thrombectomy revascularisation of large vessel occlusions in acute ischaemic stroke (TREVO 2): a randomised trial. Lancet. 2012;380(9849):1231–40.
21. Saver JL, Jahan R, Levy EI, Jovin TG, Baxter B, Nogueira RG, et al. Solitaire flow restoration device versus the Merci Retriever in patients with acute ischaemic stroke (SWIFT): a randomised, parallel-group, non-inferiority trial. Lancet. 2012;380(9849):1241–9.
22. Berkhemer OA, Fransen PSS, Beumer D, van den Berg LA, Lingsma HF, Yoo AJ, et al. A randomized trial of intraarterial treatment for acute ischemic stroke. N Engl J Med. 2015;372(1):11–20.
23. Goyal M, Demchuk AM, Menon BK, Eesa M, Rempel JL, Thornton J, et al. Randomized assessment of rapid endovascular treatment of ischemic stroke. N Engl J Med. 2015;372(11):1019–30.
24. Saver JL, Goyal M, Bonafe A, Diener H-C, Levy EI, Pereira VM, et al. Stent-retriever thrombectomy after intravenous t-PA vs. t-PA alone in stroke. N Engl J Med. 2015;372(24):2285–95.
25. Campbell BCV, Mitchell PJ, Kleinig TJ, Dewey HM, Churilov L, Yassi N, et al. Endovascular therapy for ischemic stroke with perfusion-imaging selection. N Engl J Med. 2015;372(11):1009–18.
26. Molina CA, Chamorro A, Rovira À, de Miquel A, Serena J, Roman LS, et al. REVASCAT: a randomized trial of revascularization with SOLITAIRE FR® device vs. best medical therapy in the treatment of acute stroke due to anterior circulation large vessel occlusion presenting within eight-hours of symptom onset. Int J Stroke. 2015;10(4):619–26.
27. Goyal M, Menon BK, Van Zwam WH, Dippel DWJ, Mitchell PJ, Demchuk AM, et al. Endovascular thrombectomy after large-vessel ischaemic stroke: a meta-analysis of individual patient data from five randomised trials. Lancet. 2016;387(10029):1723–31.
28. Powers WJ, Derdeyn CP, Biller J, Coffey CS, Hoh BL, Jauch EC, et al. American Heart Association/American stroke association focused update of the 2013 guidelines for the early management of patients with acute ischemic stroke regarding endovascular treatment: a guideline for healthcare professionals from the American. Stroke. 2015;46(10):3020–35.
29. Astrup J, Siesjö BK, Symon L. Thresholds in cerebral ischemia — the ischemic penumbra. Stroke. 1981;12(6):723–5.
30. Nicolas-Jilwan M, Wintermark M. Automated brain perfusion imaging in acute ischemic stroke: interpretation pearls and pitfalls. Stroke. 2021;52(11):3728–38.
31. Albers GW, Marks MP, Kemp S, Christensen S, Tsai JP, Ortega-Gutierrez S, et al. Thrombectomy for stroke at 6 to 16 hours with selection by perfusion imaging. N Engl J Med. 2018;378(8):708–18.
32. Nogueira RG, Jadhav AP, Haussen DC, Bonafe A, Budzik RF, Bhuva P, et al. Thrombectomy 6 to 24 hours after stroke with a mismatch between deficit and infarct. N Engl J Med. 2018;378(1):11–21.
33. Powers WJ, Rabinstein AA, Ackerson T, Adeoye OM, Bambakidis NC, Becker K, et al. Guidelines for the early management of patients with acute ischemic stroke: 2019 update to the 2018 guidelines for the early management of acute ischemic stroke a guideline for healthcare professionals from the American Heart Association/ American Stroke A. Stroke. 2019;50:344–418.
34. Morsi S, Ghozy S, Elfil M, Tolba H, Rabenstein A, Kadirvel R, et al. Endovascular thrombectomy for DAWN- and DEFUSE-3 ineligible acute ischemic stroke patients: a systematic review and meta-analysis. J Neurol. 2024;271(5):2230–7.
35. Yoshimura S, Sakai N, Yamagami H, Uchida K, Beppu M, Toyoda K, et al. Endovascular therapy for acute stroke with a large ischemic region. N Engl J Med. 2022;386(14):1303–13.
36. Thomalla G, Cheng B, Jensen M, Schell M, Schlemm E, Fiehler J, et al. Endovascular thrombectomy for acute ischaemic stroke with established large infarct (TENSION): 12-month outcomes of a multicentre, open-label, randomised trial. Lancet Neurol. 2024;23(9):883–92.
37. Costalat V, Jovin TG, Albucher JF, Cognard C, Henon H, Nouri N, et al. Trial of thrombectomy for stroke with a large infarct of unrestricted size. N Engl J Med. 2024;390(18):1677–89.
38. Huo X, Ma G, Tong X, Zhang X, Pan Y, Nguyen TN, et al. Trial of endovascular therapy for acute ischemic stroke with large infarct. N Engl J Med. 2023;388(14):1272–83.
39. Sarraj A, Hassan AE, Abraham MG, Ortega-Gutierrez S, Kasner SE, Hussain MS, et al. Trial of endovascular thrombectomy for large ischemic strokes. N Engl J Med. 2023;388(14):1259–71.
40. The Writing Committee for the TESLA Investigators TI. Thrombectomy for Stroke With Large Infarct on Noncontrast CT The TESLA Randomized Clinical Trial. JAMA. 2024;332(16):1355–266.
41. Chen H, Lee JS, Michel P, Yan B, Chaturvedi S. Endovascular stroke thrombectomy for patients with large ischemic core a review. JAMA Neurol. 2024;21201(10):1085–93.

42. Sun D, Guo X, Nguyen TN, Pan Y, Ma G, Tong X, et al. Alberta stroke program early computed tomography score, infarct core volume, and endovascular therapy outcomes in patients with large infarct: a secondary analysis of the ANGEL-ASPECT trial. JAMA Neurol. 2024;81(1):30–8.
43. Mattle HP, Arnold M, Lindsberg PJ, Schonewille WJ, Schroth G. Basilar artery occlusion. Lancet Neurol. 2011;10(11):1002–14.
44. Langezaal LCM, van der Hoeven EJRJ, Mont'Alverne FJA, de Carvalho JJF, Lima FO, Dippel DWJ, et al. Endovascular therapy for stroke due to basilar-artery occlusion. N Engl J Med. 2021;384(20):1910–20.
45. Liu X, Dai Q, Ye R, Zi W, Liu Y, Wang H, et al. Endovascular treatment versus standard medical treatment for vertebrobasilar artery occlusion (BEST): an open-label, randomised controlled trial. Lancet Neurol. 2020;19(2):115–22.
46. Tao C, Nogueira RG, Zhu Y, Sun J, Han H, Yuan G, et al. Trial of endovascular treatment of acute basilar-artery occlusion. N Engl J Med. 2022;387(15):1361–72.
47. Jovin TG, Li C, Wu L, Wu C, Chen J, Jiang C, et al. Trial of thrombectomy 6 to 24 hours after stroke due to basilar-artery occlusion. N Engl J Med. 2022;387(15):1373–84.
48. Alemseged F, Nguyen TN, Alverne FM, Liu X, Schonewille WJ, Nogueira RG. Endovascular therapy for basilar artery occlusion. Stroke. 2023;54(4):1127–37.
49. Zi W, Qiu Z, Wu D, Li F, Liu H, Liu W, et al. Assessment of endovascular treatment for acute basilar artery occlusion via a nationwide prospective registry. JAMA Neurol. 2020;77(5):561–73.
50. Strbian D, Tsivgoulis G, Ospel J, Räty S, Cimflova P, Georgiopoulos G, et al. European Stroke Organisation (ESO) and European Society for Minimally Invasive Neurological Therapy (ESMINT) guideline on acute management of basilar artery occlusion. J Neurointerv Surg. 2024;16:e7.
51. Asif KS, Novakovic R, Nguyen TN, Mansour O, deHavenon A, Masoud HE, et al. Endovascular treatment in acute basilar artery occlusion stroke: a brief practice update from the society of vascular and interventional neurology. Stroke. 2023;3(6):1–16.
52. Heit JJ, Chaudhary N, Mascitelli JR, Al-Kawaz M, Baker A, Bulsara KR, et al. Focused update to guidelines for endovascular therapy for emergent large vessel occlusion: basilar artery occlusion patients. J Neurointerv Surg. 2024;16(8):752–5.

Rescue Procedures

Jiří Fiedler and Marek Grubhoffer

1 Introduction

Intravenous thrombolysis (IVT) and mechanical thrombectomy (MT) are the standard treatments for large vessel occlusion (LVO) in acute ischemic stroke [1–3]. The therapeutic windows for patients with preserved perfusion parameters have been extended to 16 hours and 24 hours for MT, respectively [4, 5]. In carefully selected patients with large core infarctions, these windows may be further extended [6–9]. Rapid advancements in endovascular technologies have facilitated successful treatment of distal arterial occlusions in both the anterior and posterior circulations [10–12]. However, these methods are not universally successful. The recanalization rate for middle cerebral artery (MCA) occlusions following IVT is approximately 30% [13]. Landmark endovascular studies published in 2015 demonstrated successful recanalization rates of 59–88% after MT [14–18]. However, MT failure with poor recanalization occurs in approximately 10% of cases [19].

Several factors contribute to MT failure, including unsuccessful femoral artery puncture, stenosis or elongation of extracranial arteries, embolus size or etiology, intracranial atherosclerosis, and endothelial damage sustained during the neurointervention process [19, 20]. Additional challenges include the lack of 24-hour availability of neurointerventional surgeons and the high financial cost of endovascular treatment, which poses a significant barrier, particularly in developing countries [21].

Persistent occlusion following failed MT is associated with unfavorable clinical outcomes [22]. Microsurgical intervention offers an alternative approach for revascularization through two primary rescue procedures: extracranial-intracranial bypass (EC-IC), which augments flow distal to the occlusion, and microsurgical embolectomy (ME), which involves the direct removal of the occlusion and restoration of flow to perforating arteries.

2 Historical Notes

The first embolectomy was described in 1956 by Welch, who performed the procedure in two patients with MCA occlusion using perioperative hypothermia. Emboli were removed via a transverse arteriotomy, which was subsequently closed with a figure-of-eight suture [23]. A major breakthrough occurred in the early 1960s with the introduction of the operating microscope. Donaghy performed the first microsurgical embolectomy (ME) of the MCA, establishing the foundation for vascular microsuturing techniques [24]. Later, in 1969, Yasargil published a series of 11 cases involving direct arteriotomy with embolectomy or thrombectomy of the MCA. In nine of these cases, surgery was performed more than a week after symptom onset [25].

To evaluate the safety and efficacy of restoring cerebral blood flow in the acute phase of MCA occlusion, experimental studies were conducted in various animal models throughout the 1970s and early 1980s. These studies demonstrated that embolectomy within 5 hours of MCA occlusion was relatively safe and effective; however, procedures performed after 6 hours were associated with increased morbidity and mortality [26–28]. A literature review by Meyer et al. identified 64 cases of ME for MCA occlusion published prior to 1985. Of these, only 24 cases were treated within 24 hours of symptom onset. Among these, 14 patients (58%) showed

J. Fiedler (✉)
Department of Neurosurgery, České Budějovice Hospital JSC, České Budějovice, Czech Republic

Department of Neurosurgery, Department of Neurosurgery, University Hospital Brno, Masaryk University Medical School Brno, Brno, Czech Republic

M. Grubhoffer
Department of Neurosurgery, České Budějovice Hospital JSC, České Budějovice, Czech Republic

Department of Neurosurgery, Charles University Faculty of Medicine in Pilsen, University Hospital Pilsen, Pilsen, Czech Republic

V. Beneš, D. Netuka (eds.), *Surgical and Interventional Treatment of Cerebral Ischemia*,
https://doi.org/10.1007/978-3-032-08934-2_26

improvement in neurological deficits post-surgery, one case remained unchanged, and six patients succumbed to surgical complications or ischemia [29]. Meyer et al. also reported on their own cohort of 20 emergent ME cases for MCA occlusion, finding that the presence of collateral circulation strongly predicted favorable clinical outcomes [29]. These findings reinforced the concept of collateral protection, first noted by Welch in 1956 [23]. Despite these insights, no prospective studies evaluating the efficacy of ME for acute LVO were published in subsequent years.

The concept of EC-IC microanastomosis between the superficial temporal artery (STA) and the MCA was developed collaboratively by Donaghy and Yasargil. In 1967, both surgeons successfully performed EC-IC bypass procedures in Zurich and Burlington [30]. Over the following years, EC-IC bypass became a widely adopted technique for treating cerebral ischemia caused by internal carotid artery (ICA) occlusion. However, the 1985 Extracranial-Intracranial Bypass Study Group failed to demonstrate the efficacy of EC-IC bypass in preventing cerebral ischemia in patients with atherosclerotic ICA and MCA disease [31]. Subsequent studies, including the Carotid Occlusion Surgery Study (COSS) in 2011 and the Carotid and Middle Cerebral Artery Occlusion Surgery Study (CMOSS) in 2023, similarly failed to show clinical benefit [32, 33]. As a result, these technically demanding microsurgical techniques fell out of favor, especially with the advent of intravenous thrombolysis in the 1990s and later, endovascular treatments [34].

3 Current Position of Microsurgery

Although COSS did not demonstrate a benefit of EC-IC bypass over optimal medical treatment, the trial did not specifically target acute high-risk patients [32]. Pressure-related neurological deficits are relatively common in the management of acute LVO, which shifts the consideration of EC-IC bypass from secondary prevention to the acute management of ischemic stroke. Significant advances in penumbra analysis, facilitated by the development of cerebral perfusion imaging and automated stroke imaging software, have improved patient selection for revascularization. Unlike the COSS trial, several smaller studies have demonstrated the benefit of early EC-IC bypass in preventing progressive neurological deficits in acute ischemic stroke caused by LVO [35–41]. A recent systematic review reported neurological improvement in 53.8% of patients and a good functional outcome in 74.5% at 3 months post-intervention [42]. Advanced neuroimaging techniques, including hemodynamic and flow measurements such as blood oxygenation level-dependent functional magnetic resonance imaging and quantitative magnetic resonance angiography, play an increasingly important role in selecting patients with persistent LVO who may benefit from microsurgical revascularization [43].

In Japan, over the past two decades, microsurgical embolectomy (ME) has re-emerged as a first- or second-line therapeutic option for LVO in the anterior circulation, particularly when endovascular treatment is unavailable or unsuccessful. Numerous case series have reported excellent recanalization success rates within 24 hours of occlusion [21, 44–52]. To reduce operative time, Park developed a minimally invasive and rapid surgical embolectomy technique using a superciliary keyhole approach. This approach involves a 4 cm eyebrow incision and supraorbital mini-craniotomy. After removing the occlusion from the MCA or carotid terminus, the arteriotomy can be closed with a curved aneurysm miniclip [51, 52]. A highly refined ME technique was presented by Ota et al., achieving a surgical recanalization time of only 32.5 minutes, with efficacy comparable to MT [21]. ME has also been employed in unique cases involving foreign body extraction, such as embolized shotgun pellets following gunshot wounds to the neck, complications of endovascular procedures (e.g., migrating coils, glue, or Onyx leakage during embolization of malformations), and cases of stuck balloons or stents during MT [53–59].

Recently, the prospective study Emergent Microsurgical Intervention for Acute Stroke after Mechanical Thrombectomy Failure (EMIAS) demonstrated that emergent microsurgical intervention for acute stroke and MCA occlusion is a safe and effective therapeutic option in patients after IVT and MT failure. In the surgical group, functional independence was achieved in 58.3% of patients at 3 months following ME, EC-IC bypass, or a combination of both within 24 hours of symptom onset. By contrast, only 12% of patients in the conservative treatment group achieved functional independence [22].

4 Illustrative Cases

ME can recanalize MCA occlusions if a patent watershed exists distal to the occlusion. However, a significant disadvantage of ME is its technical complexity compared to EC-IC bypass. This complexity arises from the need to operate at the depth of the sphenoidal segment of the MCA. In addition to the use of specialized microsurgical instruments, advanced microsurgical training is essential for performing deep suturing effectively.

The hemodynamic status of the MCA following emergent LVO depends on the baseline flow conditions prior to the occlusion. For instance, if significant atherosclerotic stenosis was already present, there may have been sufficient time for collateral development. In cases of MCA occlusion, three primary types of leptomeningeal collateral pathways are typically encountered: the ramus dorsalis corporis callosi, cortical arteries from the posterior cerebral artery and the anterior cerebral artery. The following scenarios can be defined:

- LVO in a premorbidly severely stenotic MCA is a challenging scenario. In such cases, leptomeningeal collaterals may have had time to develop due to chronically reduced MCA flow prior to the occlusion. ME may be technically challenging in this context, making EC-IC bypass a viable alternative. Although high-flow bypass may not be necessary, a conventional STA-M4 bypass could provide sufficient flow restoration.
- Emergent LVO in the MCA with healthy vessel wall; ME is an option.

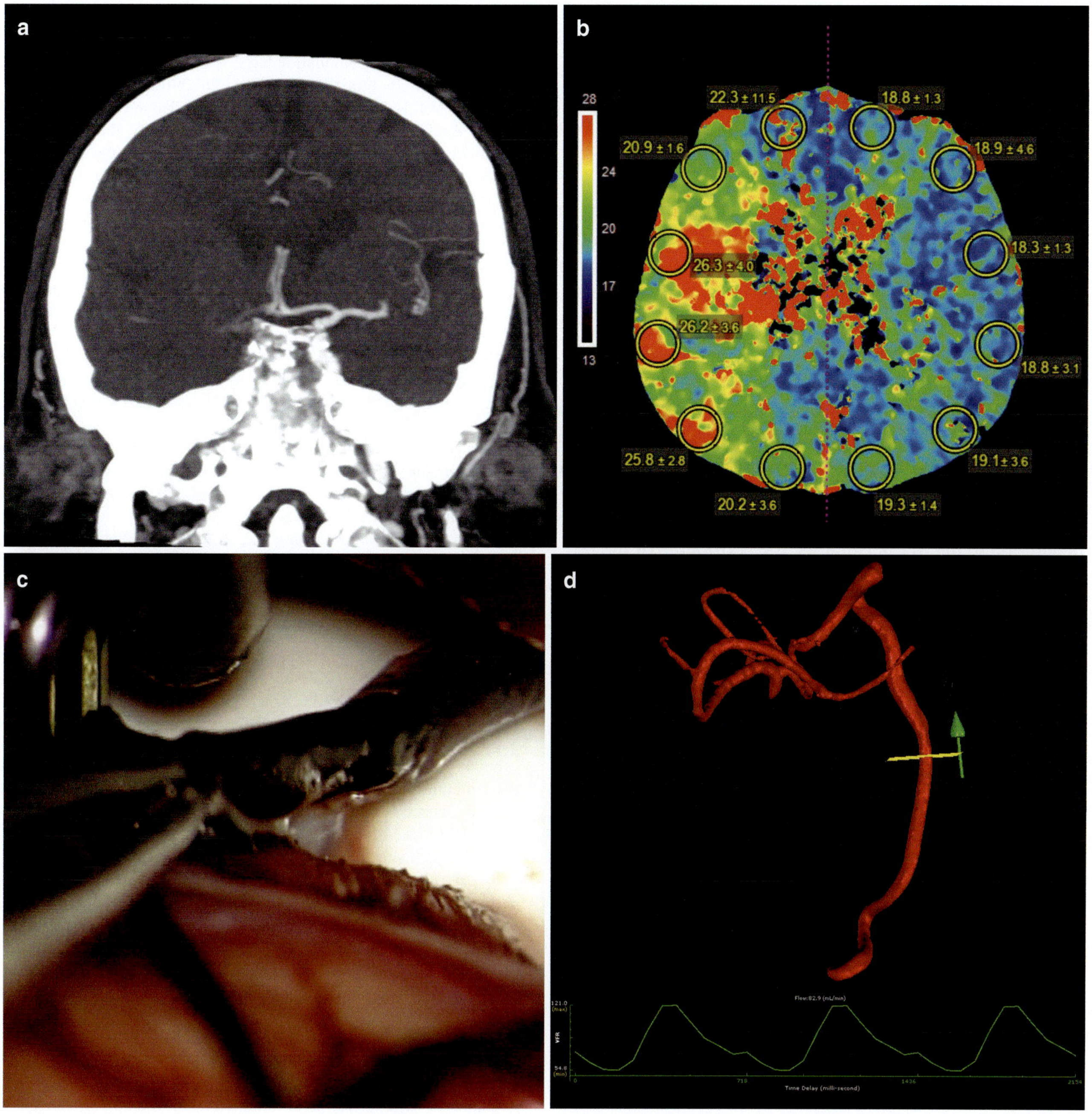

Fig. 1 (**a**) Occlusion of the right ICA and MCA on initial CT angiography. (**b**) Increase in time-to-peak in the right MCA territory on perfusion CT. (**c**) Removal of the residual thrombus from the M2 trunk using longitudinal arteriotomy after failure of MT. The retrograde flow in the artery was low and immeasurable using a intraoperative flowmetry. Therefore, a conventional STA-M2 bypass was performed using end-to-side technique, and it was sutured onto the arteriotomy. (**d**) Bypass flow of 83 mL/min on follow-up quantitative MR angiography at 3 months

- Emergent LVO in MCA associated with mural atherosclerosis in a region of severe pathology or concurrent ICA occlusion presents a complex clinical challenge. In such cases, ME with preparation for a potential EC-IC bypass, should be considered based on the hemodynamic status and flow dynamics following embolectomy (Fig. 1).

EC-IC bypass facilitates blood supply to MCA distal to the site of occlusion. However, even with successful revascularization, the neurological deficit resulting from occlusion of the lenticulostriate perforators remains unpredictable. This outcome is highly dependent on the anatomical specifics, particularly the extent to which one or more major M1 perforators are compromised. These variations give rise to two potential scenarios for the final clinical outcome.

1. Most major perforating arteries originate proximal to the bifurcation of MCA. While EC-IC bypass in the insular or opercular segments of the MCA may restore flow to the superior and inferior trunks, it is unlikely to provide clinical benefit as the lenticulostriate perforators will remain unperfused.
2. Significant perforating arteries may arise distal to the MCA bifurcation. In such cases, EC-IC bypass in the insular or opercular segments has the potential to restore perforator flow despite the presence of an M1 segment occlusion.

In addition to the M1 perforators, the perforators of the posterior communicating artery, Heubner's artery, and the anterior choroidal artery are anatomically close to this region. The anatomical variations within this group of perforators become particularly significant in cases of tandem occlusions involving both ICA and MCA.

Emergent microsurgery as a third-line treatment has been an integral part of the emergent LVO protocol at our comprehensive stroke center since 2016, with the outcomes detailed in the EMIAS study [22]. Key factors underpinning success include the availability of 24-hour services and seamless teamwork among the vascular neurologist coordinating acute treatment, the neurointerventional radiologist, the neurosurgeon, and the anesthesiologist. Furthermore, minimizing the time from patient admission to the procedure and optimizing the arrangement of stroke center resources—such as ensuring the proximity of the angiography suite and the operating room, ideally through the use of a hybrid operating room—are essential.

Declarations

Competing Interests The authors have no competing interests to declare that are relevant to the content of this manuscript.

Ethics Approval The author(s) declares that this manuscript does not include primary research with human participants.

References

1. Turc G, Bhogal P, Fischer U, Khatri P, Lobotesis K, Mazighi M, et al. European Stroke Organisation (ESO) – European Society for Minimally Invasive Neurological Therapy (ESMINT) guidelines on mechanical thrombectomy in acute ischemic stroke. J Neurointerv Surg. 2023;15(8):e8. https://doi.org/10.1136/neurintsurg-2018-014569.
2. Turc G, Tsivgoulis G, Audebert HJ, Boogaarts H, Bhogal P, De Marchis GM, et al. European Stroke Organisation – European Society for Minimally Invasive Neurological Therapy expedited recommendation on indication for intravenous thrombolysis before mechanical thrombectomy in patients with acute ischaemic stroke and anterior circulation large vessel occlusion. Eur Stroke J. 2022;7(1):1–26. https://doi.org/10.1177/23969873221076968.
3. Powers WJ, Rabinstein AA, Ackerson T, Adeoye OM, Bambakidis NC, Becker K, et al. Guidelines for the early management of patients with acute ischemic stroke: 2019 update to the 2018 guidelines for the early management of acute ischemic stroke: a guideline for healthcare professionals from the American Heart Association/American Stroke Association. Stroke. 2019;50(12):e344–418. https://doi.org/10.1161/STR.0000000000000211.
4. Albers GW, Marks MP, Kemp S, Christensen S, Tsai JP, Ortega-Gutierrez S, et al. Thrombectomy for stroke at 6 to 16 hours with selection by perfusion imaging. N Engl J Med. 2018;378(8):708–18. https://doi.org/10.1056/NEJMoa1713973.
5. Nogueira RG, Jadhav AP, Haussen DC, Bonafe A, Budzik RF, Bhuva P, et al. Thrombectomy 6 to 24 hours after stroke with a mismatch between deficit and infarct. N Engl J Med. 2018;378(1):11–21. https://doi.org/10.1056/NEJMoa1706442.
6. Sarraj A, Hassan AE, Abraham MG, Ortega-Gutierrez S, Kasner SE, Hussain MS, et al. Trial of endovascular thrombectomy for large ischemic strokes. N Engl J Med. 2023;388(14):1259–71. https://doi.org/10.1056/NEJMoa2214403.
7. Huo X, Ma G, Tong X, Zhang X, Pan Y, Nguyen TN, et al. Trial of endovascular therapy for acute ischemic stroke with large infarct. N Engl J Med. 2023;388(14):1272–83. https://doi.org/10.1056/NEJMoa2213379.
8. Yoshimura S, Sakai N, Yamagami H, Uchida K, Beppu M, Toyoda K, et al. Endovascular therapy for acute stroke with a large ischemic region. N Engl J Med. 2022;386(14):1303–13. https://doi.org/10.1056/NEJMoa2118191.
9. Thomalla G, Fiehler J, Subtil F, Bonekamp S, Aamodt AH, Fuentes B, et al. Endovascular thrombectomy for acute ischaemic stroke with established large infarct (TENSION): 12-month outcomes of a multicentre, open-label, randomised trial. Lancet Neurol. 2024;23(9):883–92. https://doi.org/10.1016/S1474-4422(24)00278-3.
10. Meyer L, Stracke CP, Jungi N, Wallocha M, Broocks G, Sporns PB, et al. Thrombectomy for primary distal posterior cerebral artery occlusion stroke: the TOPMOST study. JAMA Neurol. 2021;78(4):434–44. https://doi.org/10.1001/jamaneurol.2021.0001.
11. Anadani M, Alawieh A, Chalhoub R, Jabbour P, Starke RM, Arthur A, et al. Mechanical thrombectomy for distal occlusions: efficacy, functional and safety outcomes: insight from the STAR collaboration. World Neurosurg. 2021;151:e871–e9. https://doi.org/10.1016/j.wneu.2021.04.136.
12. Nogueira RG, Mohammaden MH, Haussen DC, Budzik RF, Gupta R, Krajina A, et al. Endovascular therapy in the distal neurovascular territory: results of a large prospective registry. J Neurointerv Surg. 2021;13(11):979–84. https://doi.org/10.1136/neurintsurg-2020-016851.
13. Bhatia R, Hill MD, Shobha N, Menon B, Bal S, Kochar P, et al. Low rates of acute recanalization with intravenous recombinant tissue plasminogen activator in ischemic stroke: real-world experi-

ence and a call for action. Stroke. 2010;41(10):2254–8. https://doi.org/10.1161/STROKEAHA.110.592535.
14. Berkhemer OA, Fransen PS, Beumer D, van den Berg LA, Lingsma HF, Yoo AJ, et al. A randomized trial of intraarterial treatment for acute ischemic stroke. N Engl J Med. 2015;372(1):11–20. https://doi.org/10.1056/NEJMoa1411587.
15. Jovin TG, Chamorro A, Cobo E, de Miquel MA, Molina CA, Rovira A, et al. Thrombectomy within 8 hours after symptom onset in ischemic stroke. N Engl J Med. 2015;372(24):2296–306. https://doi.org/10.1056/NEJMoa1503780.
16. Goyal M, Demchuk AM, Menon BK, Eesa M, Rempel JL, Thornton J, et al. Randomized assessment of rapid endovascular treatment of ischemic stroke. N Engl J Med. 2015;372(11):1019–30. https://doi.org/10.1056/NEJMoa1414905.
17. Campbell BC, Mitchell PJ, Kleinig TJ, Dewey HM, Churilov L, Yassi N, et al. Endovascular therapy for ischemic stroke with perfusion-imaging selection. N Engl J Med. 2015;372(11):1009–18. https://doi.org/10.1056/NEJMoa1414792.
18. Saver JL, Goyal M, Bonafe A, Diener HC, Levy EI, Pereira VM, et al. Stent-retriever thrombectomy after intravenous t-PA vs. t-PA alone in stroke. N Engl J Med. 2015;372(24):2285–95. https://doi.org/10.1056/NEJMoa1415061.
19. Leischner H, Flottmann F, Hanning U, Broocks G, Faizy TD, Deb-Chatterji M, et al. Reasons for failed endovascular recanalization attempts in stroke patients. J Neurointerv Surg. 2019;11(5):439–42. https://doi.org/10.1136/neurintsurg-2018-014060.
20. Maingard J, Phan K, Lamanna A, Kok HK, Barras CD, Russell J, et al. Rescue intracranial stenting after failed mechanical thrombectomy for acute ischemic stroke: a systematic review and meta-analysis. World Neurosurg. 2019;132:e235–e45. https://doi.org/10.1016/j.wneu.2019.08.192.
21. Ota N, Benet A, Kusdiansah M, Miyoshi N, Haraguchi K, Noda K, et al. Microsurgical thrombectomy: where the ancient art meets the new era. Neurosurg Rev. 2024;47:49. https://doi.org/10.1007/s10143-024-02281-8.
22. Fiedler J, Roubec M, Grubhoffer M, Ostry S, Prochazka V, Langova K, et al. Emergent microsurgical intervention for acute stroke after mechanical thrombectomy failure: a prospective study. J Neurointerv Surg. 2023;15(5):439–45. https://doi.org/10.1136/neurintsurg-2022-018643.
23. Welch K. Excision of occlusive lesions of the middle cerebral artery. J Neurosurg. 1956;13(1):73–80. https://doi.org/10.3171/jns.1956.13.1.0073.
24. Jacobson JH 2nd, Wallman LJ, Schumacher GA, Flanagan M, Suarez EL, Donaghy RM. Microsurgery as an aid to middle cerebral artery endarterectomy. J Neurosurg. 1962;19:108–15. https://doi.org/10.3171/jns.1962.19.2.0108.
25. Yasargil MG. Occlusions of the middle cerebral artery. In: Yasargil MG, editor. Microsurgery applied to neurosurgery. New York: Thieme; 1969. p. 101–5.
26. Sundt TM Jr, Grant WC, Garcia JH. Restoration of middle cerebral artery flow in experimental infarction. J Neurosurg. 1969;31(3):311–21. https://doi.org/10.3171/jns.1969.31.3.0311.
27. Dujovny M, Osgood CP, Barrionuevo PJ, Hellstrom R, Laha RK. Middle cerebral artery microneurosurgical embolectomy. Surgery. 1976;80(3):336–9.
28. Okada Y, Shima T, Oki S, Uozumi T. Experimental microsurgical embolectomy after middle cerebral artery embolization in the dog. J Neurosurg. 1983;58(2):259–66. https://doi.org/10.3171/jns.1983.58.2.0259.
29. Meyer FB, Piepgras DG, Sundt TM Jr, Yanagihara T. Emergency embolectomy for acute occlusion of the middle cerebral artery. J Neurosurg. 1985;62(5):639–47. https://doi.org/10.3171/jns.1985.62.5.0639.
30. Hayden MG, Lee M, Guzman R, Steinberg GK. The evolution of cerebral revascularization surgery. Neurosurg Focus. 2009;26(5):E17. https://doi.org/10.3171/2009.3.FOCUS0931.
31. EC/IC Bypass Study Group. Failure of extracranial-intracranial arterial bypass to reduce the risk of ischemic stroke. Results of an international randomized trial. N Engl J Med. 1985;313(19):1191–200. https://doi.org/10.1056/NEJM198511073131904.
32. Powers WJ, Clarke WR, Grubb RL Jr, Videen TO, Adams HP Jr, Derdeyn CP, et al. Extracranial-intracranial bypass surgery for stroke prevention in hemodynamic cerebral ischemia: the carotid occlusion surgery study randomized trial. JAMA. 2011;306(18):1983–92. https://doi.org/10.1001/jama.2011.1610.
33. Ma Y, Wang T, Wang H, Amin-Hanjani S, Tong X, Wang J, et al. Extracranial-intracranial bypass and risk of stroke and death in patients with symptomatic artery occlusion: the CMOSS randomized clinical trial. JAMA. 2023;330(8):704–14. https://doi.org/10.1001/jama.2023.13390.
34. Ansari S, Rahman M, Waters MF, Hoh BL, Mocco J. Recanalization therapy for acute ischemic stroke, part 1: surgical embolectomy and chemical thrombolysis. Neurosurg Rev. 2011;34(1):1–9. https://doi.org/10.1007/s10143-010-0293-2.
35. Horiuchi T, Nitta J, Ishizaka S, Kanaya K, Yanagawa T, Hongo K. Emergency EC-IC bypass for symptomatic atherosclerotic ischemic stroke. Neurosurg Rev. 2013;36(4):559–64; discussion 64–5. https://doi.org/10.1007/s10143-013-0487-5.
36. Burkhardt JK, Winklhofer S, Fierstra J, Wegener S, Esposito G, Luft A, et al. Emergency extracranial-intracranial bypass to revascularize salvageable brain tissue in acute ischemic stroke patients. World Neurosurg. 2018;109:e476–e85. https://doi.org/10.1016/j.wneu.2017.10.005.
37. Sugiyama T, Kazumata K, Asaoka K, Osanai T, Shimbo D, Uchida K, et al. Reappraisal of microsurgical revascularization for anterior circulation ischemia in patients with progressive stroke. World Neurosurg. 2015;84(6):1579–88. https://doi.org/10.1016/j.wneu.2015.07.053.
38. Park HS, Kim SH, Nah HW, Choi JH, Kim DH, Kang MJ, et al. Patient selection and clinical efficacy of urgent superficial temporal artery-middle cerebral artery bypass in acute ischemic stroke using advanced magnetic resonance imaging techniques. Oper Neurosurg (Hagerstown). 2017;13(5):552–9. https://doi.org/10.1093/ons/opx041.
39. Hwang G, Oh CW, Bang JS, Jung CK, Kwon OK, Kim JE, et al. Superficial temporal artery to middle cerebral artery bypass in acute ischemic stroke and stroke in progress. Neurosurgery. 2011;68(3):723–9; discussion 29–30. https://doi.org/10.1227/NEU.0b013e318207a9de.
40. Nussbaum ES, Janjua TM, Defillo A, Lowary JL, Nussbaum LA. Emergency extracranial-intracranial bypass surgery for acute ischemic stroke. J Neurosurg. 2010;112(3):666–73. https://doi.org/10.3171/2009.5.JNS081556.
41. Kim JH, Yoon W, Kim CK, Roh H, Bae HJ, Kwon TH, et al. Efficacy and safety of timely urgent superficial temporal artery-to-middle cerebral artery bypass surgery in patients with acute ischemic stroke: a single-institutional prospective study and a pooled analysis. Cerebrovasc Dis. 2021;50(1):34–45. https://doi.org/10.1159/000512106.
42. Sabouri M, Aminmansour B, Sourani A, Sharafi M, Sahraei A, Rahimi A, et al. The role of early superficial temporal to middle cerebral artery bypass revascularization surgery in middle cerebral artery-territory strokes: a systematic review study. Stroke Vasc Interv Neurol. 2022;2:281. https://doi.org/10.1161/SVIN.121.000281.
43. Sebok M, Hobner LM, Fierstra J, Schubert T, Wegener S, Kulcsar Z, et al. Flow-augmentation STA-MCA bypass for acute and subacute ischemic stroke due to internal carotid artery occlusion and

the role of advanced neuroimaging with hemodynamic and flow-measurement in the decision-making: preliminary data. Quant Imaging Med Surg. 2024;14(1):777–88. https://doi.org/10.21037/qims-23-876.
44. Horiuchi T, Nitta J, Sakai K, Tanaka Y, Hongo K. Emergency embolectomy for treatment of acute middle cerebral artery occlusion. J Neurosurg. 2007;106(2):257–62. https://doi.org/10.3171/jns.2007.106.2.257.
45. Sakai K, Nitta J, Horiuchi T, Ogiwara T, Kobayashi S, Tanaka Y, et al. Emergency revascularization for acute main-trunk occlusion in the anterior circulation. Neurosurg Rev. 2008;31(1):69–76. https://doi.org/10.1007/s10143-007-0116-2.
46. Horiuchi T, Nitta J, Ogiwara T, Sakai K, Hongo K. Outcome predictors of open embolectomy in middle cerebral artery occlusion. Neurol Res. 2009;31(9):892–4. https://doi.org/10.1179/174313209X382494.
47. Inoue T, Tamura A, Tsutsumi K, Saito I, Saito N. Surgical embolectomy for large vessel occlusion of anterior circulation. Br J Neurosurg. 2013;27(6):783–90. https://doi.org/10.3109/02688697.2013.793286.
48. Inoue T, Tamura A, Tsutsumi K, Saito I, Saito N. Surgical embolectomy for internal carotid artery terminus occlusion. Neurosurg Rev. 2015;38(4):661–9. https://doi.org/10.1007/s10143-015-0640-4.
49. Hino A, Oka H, Hashimoto Y, Echigo T, Koseki H, Fujii A, et al. Direct microsurgical embolectomy for acute occlusion of the internal carotid artery and middle cerebral artery. World Neurosurg. 2016;88:243–51. https://doi.org/10.1016/j.wneu.2015.12.069.
50. Horiuchi T, Nitta J, Miyaoka Y, Nagm A, Tsutsumi K, Ito K, et al. Open embolectomy of large vessel occlusion in the endovascular era: results of a 12-year single-center experience. World Neurosurg. 2017;102:65–71. https://doi.org/10.1016/j.wneu.2017.02.108.
51. Park J, Hwang YH, Kim Y. Extended superciliary approach for middle cerebral artery embolectomy after unsuccessful endovascular recanalization therapy: technical note. Neurosurgery. 2009;65(6):E1191–4. https://doi.org/10.1227/01.NEU.0000351783.00831.BB.
52. Park J, Hwang YH, Huh S, Kang DH, Kim Y. Minimally invasive and rapid surgical embolectomy (MIRSE) as rescue treatment following failed endovascular recanalization for acute ischemic stroke. Acta Neurochir. 2014;156(11):2041–9. https://doi.org/10.1007/s00701-014-2179-5.
53. Haninec P, Houstava L, Klener J. Shotgun pellet embolus of the middle cerebral artery treated by emergency embolectomy. Br J Neurosurg. 1996;10(3):311–4. https://doi.org/10.1080/02688699650040214.
54. Spetzger U, Reul J, Thron A, Warnke JP, Gilsbach JM. Microsurgical embolectomy and removal of a migrated coil from the middle cerebral artery. Cerebrovasc Dis. 1997;7(4):226–31. https://doi.org/10.1159/000108196.
55. Kim YB, Lee KC, Lee JW, Huh SK, Yoon PH, Kim DI. Rescue microsurgery in coil herniation causing thromboembolic occlusion of parent artery. Acta Neurochir. 2009;151(12):1609–16. https://doi.org/10.1007/s00701-009-0437-8.
56. Ibrahim GM, Abou-Hamden A, Shankar JJ, Bharatha A, Brugge K, Tymianski M. Microsurgical glue embolectomy of the middle cerebral artery following embolization of a maxillofacial arteriovenous malformation. J Clin Neurosci. 2011;18(12):1733–6. https://doi.org/10.1016/j.jocn.2011.04.020.
57. Oh JS, Kim DS, Shim JJ, Yoon SM. Surgical removal of embolic material after its unexpected migration through extracranial-intracranial anastomosis in the treatment of Barrow Type D carotid-cavernous fistula: case report. J Neurosurg. 2018;128(3):731–4. https://doi.org/10.3171/2016.9.JNS152677.
58. Tranmer BI, Humphreys RP, Chuang SH. Microsurgical recovery of a migrated balloon from the internal carotid artery of a child. Neurosurgery. 1985;16(3):381–6. https://doi.org/10.1227/00006123-198503000-00017.
59. Kang DH, Park J, Hwang YH, Kim YS. Inadvertent self-detachment of Solitaire AB stent during the mechanical thrombectomy for recanalization of acute ischemic stroke: lessons learned from the removal of stent via surgical embolectomy. J Korean Neurosurg Soc. 2013;53(6):360–3. https://doi.org/10.3340/jkns.2013.53.6.360.

Small Vessel Disease

David Školoudík and Petra Kešnerová

1 Introduction

Small vessel disease (SVD), also known as microvascular disease, cerebral small vessel disease or small vessel ischemic disease, is a pathological condition affecting the small blood vessels in the brain, including small arteries, arterioles, capillaries and small veins. It is one of the common cerebrovascular pathologies that leads to various clinical syndromes and contributes to cognitive decline and physical disability. SVD is the cause of a significant proportion of stroke and vascular dementia. Brain parenchyma lesions resulting from pathological vessel changes are adopted as a marker of SVD and often is used as a synonym of SVD. However, it is a dynamic disease process that is not limited to the cerebral vasculature, but ultimately affects the entire organism.

2 Epidemiology

SVD is prevalent worldwide, especially among older adults. Its incidence and prevalence increases with age, the presence of arterial hypertension, diabetes mellitus and other cardiovascular risk factors. Studies have shown that SVD-related changes can be detected in up to 95% of people over 60 years of age, with important public health implications. SVD is the leading cause of age-related cognitive decline and contributes to up to 45% of dementia, 20% of all strokes worldwide, and 25% of ischemic strokes (lacunar strokes). And, about 20% of patients after a lacunar stroke remain disabled [29]. However, the incidence of SVD is about ten times more common than the incidence of stroke [24]. It is estimated that for every symptomatic stroke, there are about 10 silent brain changes [35]. These silent strokes are often detected incidentally, especially in the elderly, with up to 25% of persons over 80 years of age having experienced ≥1 silent stroke [5].

3 Etiology and Pathophysiology

The pathophysiological mechanisms underlying SVD involve a complex interaction of vascular and neurodegenerative processes. The pathological changes primarily affect small vessels of 50–400 μm in diameter and lead to white matter damage in subcortical structures of the brain. The key pathological processes include endothelial dysfunction, disruption of the blood-brain barrier and chronic hypoperfusion leading to ischemic brain damage. The main pathological features of SVD include lipid and hyaline deposits within the vessel walls (lipohyalinosis and fibrohyalinosis) lead to thickening and narrowing of small cerebral vessels, reducing blood flow and causing lacunar infarcts, white matter hyperintensities (WMH), cerebral microbleeds, hemorrhages and damage to the blood-brain barrier, which can lead to leakage of blood components into brain tissue, contributing to inflammation and further damage to blood vessels [10].

The two most common vessel pathologies underlying SVD are arteriolosclerosis caused by aging, hypertension, and other conventional vascular risk factors and cerebral amyloid angiopathy (CAA) caused by vascular deposition of β-amyloid. Other rarer causes include monogenetic diseases, venous collagenosis or postradiation angiopathy [25]. Special subcategory is heterogeneous group of inflammatory and immunologically mediated small vessel disease [29].

Although diffuse arteriolosclerosis affecting small cerebral vessels is thought to play the most important role in the development of SVD, lacunar infarcts can also be caused by microatheromas at or near the outflow of perforating cerebral arterioles. This hypothesis is supported by C. Miller Fisher

D. Školoudík (✉)
Centre for Health Research, Department of Clinical Neurosciences, Faculty of Medicine, University of Ostrava, Ostrava, Czech Republic

P. Kešnerová
Department of Neurology, 2nd Medical Faculty, Charles University and Motol Hospital, Praha, Czech Republic

V. Beneš, D. Netuka (eds.), *Surgical and Interventional Treatment of Cerebral Ischemia*,
https://doi.org/10.1007/978-3-032-08934-2_27

in the 1960s is supported by both CVS risk factors and in vivo findings using high-resolution 7T-MRI [16, 21, 23]. Arteriolosclerosis changes characterized by loss of smooth muscle cells from the tunica media also lead to segmental arterial disorganization and microaneurysms. Cerebral amyloid angiopathy affects cortical and leptomeningeal vessels and is pathologically characterized by progressive deposition of amyloid-β in the vessel wall. Except lacunar infarcts and microbleeds, it is also a primary cause of lobar intracerebral hemorrhages and an independent contributor to age-related cognitive impairment [14, 33].

4 Risk Factors

Small vessel intrinsic pathology remains the most common cause of lacunar ischemic stroke although the underlying mechanism is unclear and this clinical unit is heterogenous. In most cases, the cause of SVD is likely to be multifactorial, with several contributing factors:

- Age. The risk of SVD increases with age, partly because blood vessels are naturally more susceptible to damage. The prevalence of white matter hyperintensities increases from approximately 5% in people aged 50 years to almost 100% in people aged 90 years, and the incidence of cerebral microbleeds from 6.5% in people aged 50 years to approximately 36% in people aged 80 years and over [31].
- Hypertension. Chronic high blood pressure leads to damage and thickening of the small blood vessel walls. Fisher attributes lipohyalinosis in small arteries to hypertension [17]. Also, the Beijing Stroke Registry showed a higher proportion of hypertension in lacunar (acute stroke symptoms plus subcortical lesions <2 cm in diameter on acute CT/MRI) than in non-lacunar strokes after adjustment for age and sex [15]. However, recent epidemiological data show that hypertension is equally common in both nonlacunar and lacunar ischemic stroke; and many patients with lacunar stroke are normotensive [20].
- Diabetes mellitus (DM): DM type II is an established risk factor for lacunar stroke. The pathogenesis of DM-related stroke is complex and still not completely understood. Morphological changes of the cerebral microcirculation include basement membrane thickening and increased angiogenesis. Published studies showed also increased blood-brain permeability, altered blood flow regulation increased occurrence of cerebral microbleeds in DM patients. Lacunar stroke patients with DM type II have higher mortality, poorer functional recovery, and higher stroke recurrence risk compered to non-DM patients [40].
- Hyperlipidemia: Elevated levels of cholesterol and other lipids can lead to atherosclerosis in vascular system including small vessels. Highest total cholesterol is associated with an increased risk of ischemic stroke, especially in patients with large vessel disease and lacunar stroke [38].
- Smoking: Tobacco use exacerbates vascular damage and increases the risk of SVD. But similarly to arterial hypertension, also diabetes mellitus, hypercholesterolemia, and smoking were in recent epidemiological studies as common in lacunar stroke as in other ischemic strokes [20]. However, most studies have been conducted in hospitals, and there is a lack of population scale data on lacunar stroke.
- Obstructive sleep apnoea.
- Chronic kidney disease.
- Branch atheromatous disease [21].
- Genetic Factors: Family history and certain genetic predispositions can increase susceptibility to SVD.

The most common genetically determined disease characterized by the involvement of small cerebral blood vessels is cerebral autosomal-dominant arteriopathy with stroke and ischemic leukoencephalopathy (CADASIL) linked to mutations in NOTCH3 gene [7, 22]. A similar condition is the cerebral autosomal recessive arteriopathy with subcortical infarcts and leukoencephalopathy (CARASIL), which is more common in Asian regions [18].

Mutations in genes encoding collagen type IV α1 (Col4A1) and α2 (Col4A2) associated with microangiopathies may be sporadic or genetically bound. The abnormal structure of collagen IV is associated with the fragility of the blood vessels and a diverse clinical picture. The spectrum of type IV collagen comprises autosomal dominant type I porencephaly, CSVD with hemorrhage, cerebral microangiopathy with Axenfeld–Rieger anomaly, and hereditary angiopathy with nephropathy, aneurysms and muscle cramps (HANAC).

Mutations in the *TREX-1* gene may result in retinal vasculopathy with cerebral leukodystrophy (RVCL) which manifests around the age of 40 years and is associated with ischemic strokes, transient cerebral ischemia and psychiatric symptoms. One of the most common mitochondrial diseases—mitochondrial encephalopathy with lactic acidosis and stroke-like episodes (MELAS)—is also associated with involvement of small vessels. About 80% of all cases occur in childhood; the clinical picture is dominated by stroke-like symptoms, increasing dementia, migraine headaches, myopathy, epilepsy and lactic acidosis. Lacunar strokes are observed also in the patients with Fabry disease—X-linked inherited disorder of glycosphingolipid metabolism. The disease is associated with frequent strokes and myocardial infarctions, renal insufficiency, painful peripheral neuropathy, dysfunction of the autonomic nervous system, angiokeratomas and corneal disorders. Fabry disease is responsible for 0.5% of vascular events at a young age. Ischemic strokes occur in 76%, transient ischemic attacks in 16% and hemorrhagic strokes in 8% of the cases. However, involvement of cerebral small vessels occurs also in asymptomatic patients [8].

5 Clinical Manifestations

SVD has usually been asymptomatic for many years and is only manifested by randomly detected changes in radiological examinations [32, 34, 42]. In its acute form, CSVD progresses as lacunar stroke or a focus of intracerebral hemorrhage [30]. Nevertheless, SVD can present with a wider range of clinical symptoms, often dependent on the extent and location of the vascular damage. Common manifestations include:

- Transient Ischemic Attack (TIA) and Stroke. A lacunar clinical syndrome could be due to either ischemia or a small hemorrhage [28]. Many hemorrhagic strokes in older people are also due to SVD pathology [29]. According to the classification of the Oxfordshire Community Stroke Project, lacunar stroke proceeds in the form of 1 of 5 syndromes. In more than 50% of cases it begins as pure motor stroke (PMS)—isolated, purely motor paresis or paralysis. Other clinical manifestations of this stroke include pure sensory stroke, sensorimotor stroke, ataxic hemiparesis, and dysarthria-clumsy hand syndrome [2]. However, lacunar symptoms and signs may overlap with cortical stroke syndromes in 15%–20% of cases and may be difficult to recognize in the acute stages.
- Other motor symptoms as gait disturbances, balance issues, and parkinsonism, typically presented as difficulty walking, frequent falls, and a shuffling gait. Damage to the white mass of the brain can lead to extrapyramidal syndrome with dominant posture and gait disorders, early and symmetrical involvement of the lower limbs, slight tremor of the limbs, pseudobulbar syndrome, and sphincter dysfunctions, as well as depression [19, 39].
- Cognitive Impairment. Chronic CSVD is mainly associated with progressive cognitive impairment, from mild cognitive impairment to subcortical dementia. It is characterized by slowed thinking, executive dysfunction, and mood disturbances. Neuropathological studies have shown that lacunes of vascular origin are related to cognitive functions decline, especially in DM patients [1].
- Mood Disorders: Depression and apathy are common in SVD, often preceding cognitive symptoms. Longitudinal subgroup analyses revealed that overall white matter hyperintensities significantly associated with depression but not deep lesions. A significant, but weak association between white matter hyperintensities and depression was found [41].

6 Diagnostics

SVD diagnosis is based on clinical assessment, detailed history and neurological examination to assess cognitive function, motor skills, and mood. The final diagnosis relies strongly on neuroimaging techniques. All patients with suspect or expected lacunar ischemic stroke should undergo brain imaging, where MRI is a gold standard superior to the brain CT (Fig. 1). Brain MRI allows a visualization of white matter hyperintensities, lacunar infarcts (Fig. 2a–c), and cerebral microbleeds. The use of advanced imaging modalities such as Diffusion Tensor Imaging (DTI) and susceptibility-weighted imaging (SWI) enhances the detection of subtle microstructural changes and microhemorrhages. Other standard examination methods include neck artery imaging (duplex sonography of carotid and vertebral arteries, transcranial Doppler or duplex sonography/CTA/MRA), screening for atrial fibrillation, and other routine stroke examinations as blood pressure monitoring, blood glucose, lipids, or markers of renal functions. It may be considered to identify treatable causes of the stroke, relevant comorbidities and preventable causes of future stroke. Echocardiography, cerebral artery imaging and additional tests, including ambulatory ECG may be indicated depending on age and initial findings [34].

Elevation in vascular resistance in intracranial arteries is typical for SVD (Fig. 3). Increased pulsatility and/or resistive indices measured by transcranial Doppler (TCD) show strong correlation with MRI evidence of SVD. TCD and transcranial duplex sonography are able also to detect intra-

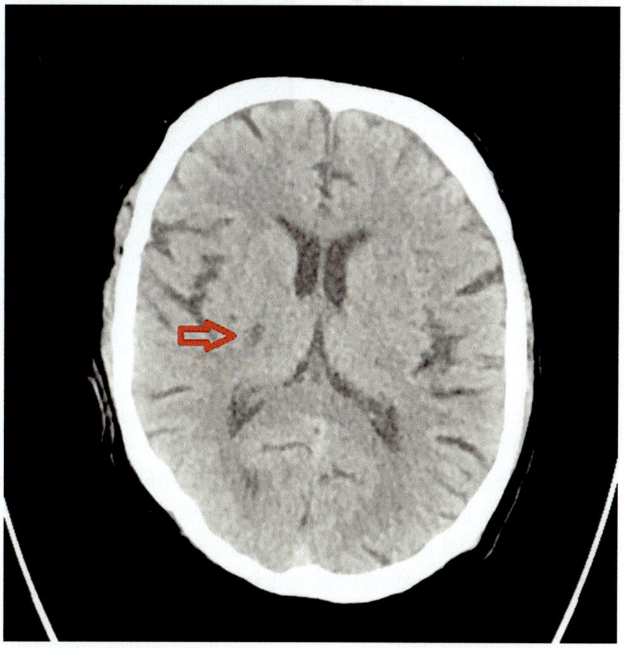

Fig. 1 Native brain CT: Lacunar infarction (arrow) in dorsal part of right internal capsule

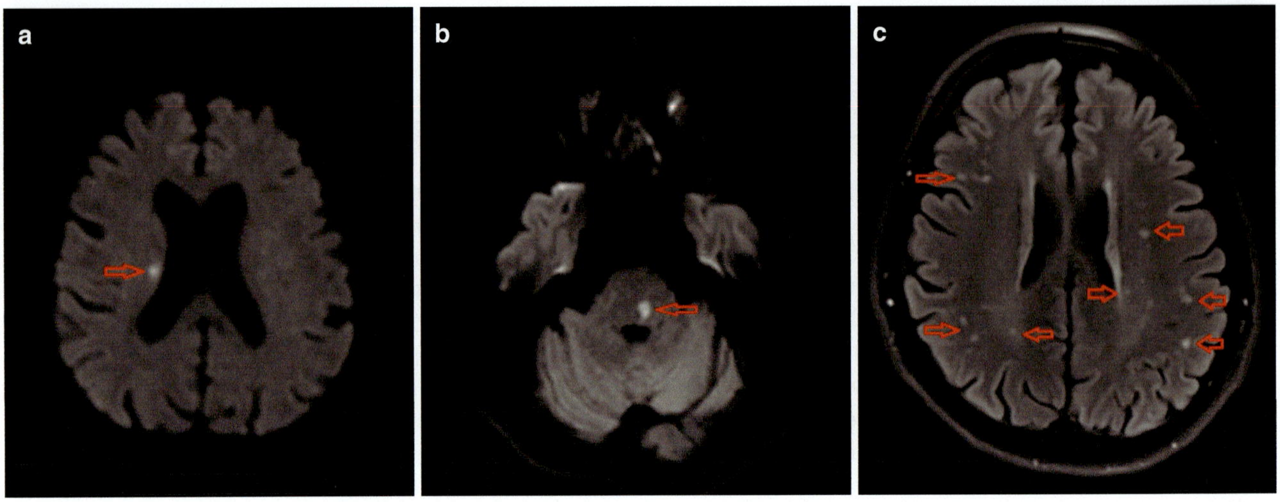

Fig. 2 Brain MRI: Periventricular lacunar infarct (arrow) in the right hemisphere (**a**) and lacunar infarct (arrow) in the brainstem (**b**) in diffusion-weighted images (DWI). Multiple lacunar infarcts (arrows) in both hemispheres (**c**) in T2-fluid-attenuated inversion recovery (FLAIR) sequences

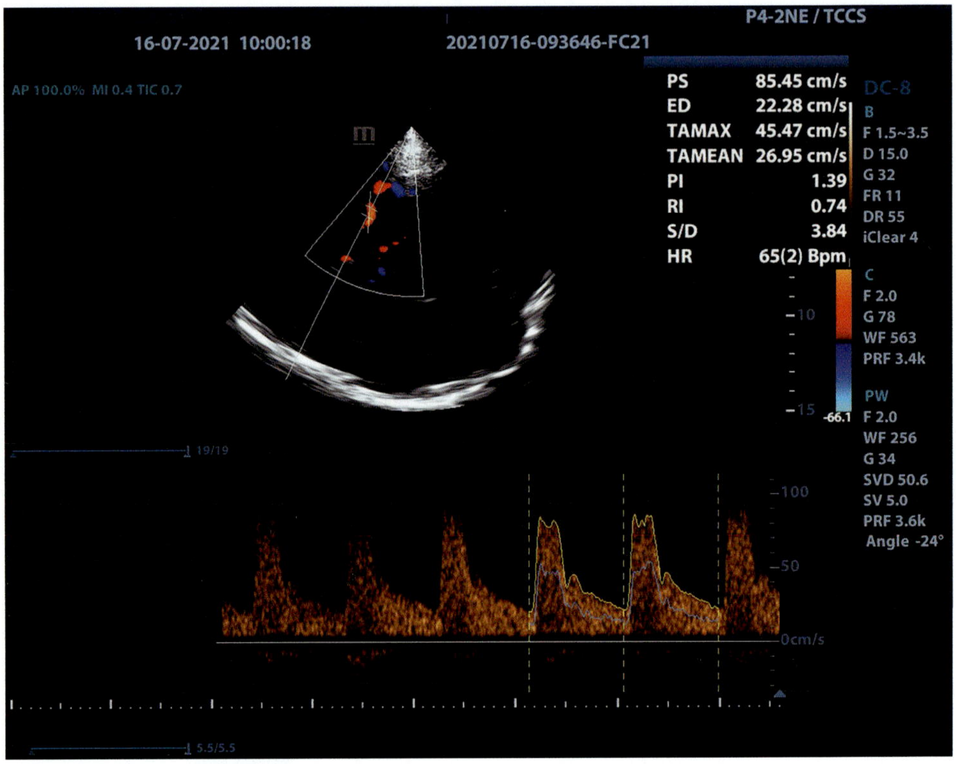

Fig. 3 Transcranial color-coded duplex sonography: Exaggerated pulsatile flow with increased pulsatility index (PI = 1.39) and resistive index (RI = 0.74) in middle cerebral artery in patient with small vessel disease

cranial stenoses or decrease blood flow velocities in patients with SVD [27].

Typical neuroimaging findings in SVD are changes in the white matter and subcortical grey matter, including recent small subcortical infarct, lacunes, white matter hyperintensities, prominent perivascular spaces, cerebral microbleeds and atrophy [43]. Different types of cerebral small vessel disease are in the Table 1.

Lacunar ischemic stroke is defined as a stroke that is attributable to a recent small infarct <1.5 (or <2.0) cm diameter in axial plane in the white matter, basal ganglia, pons or brainstem, and is consistent with a lacunar clinical syndrome [42, 43]. Main possible etiologies for lacunar ischemic stroke are atheroma of the main cerebral arteries (usually MCA) or perforating arterioles, embolism from the heart or carotid arteries, and intrinsic small vessel disease (lipohyalinosis or

Table 1 Types of cerebral small vessel disease according to STRIVE after Wardlaw et al. [43]

Type of cerebral small vessel disease	Description
Recent subcortical infarcts	Fresh, small (<20 mm in axial section) ischemic lesions with respect to perforating arteries, whose radiological features or clinical signs and symptoms indicate their formation in the few weeks before the test; best seen in the DWI sequence; these changes are hypointense in the T1 sequence, hyperintense in the T2 and FLAIR sequences, and isointense in the GRE-T2 sequence
Lacunae of presumed vascular origin	Round and oval subcortical lesions 3–15 mm in diameter, filled with fluid, with cerebrospinal fluid-like signal; these lacunae correspond to history of acute cerebral infarction or bleeding from the area of vascularization of the perforating artery; the lesions are characterized by a distinctive image in the FLAIR examination; each lesion is a cavity filled with cerebrospinal fluid and surrounded by a hyperintense rim; they are isointense in the DWI sequence, hypointense in the FLAIR and T1 sequences, and hyperintense in the T2 sequence
White matter hyperintensities	Symmetric regardless of size; hyperintense in the T2, FLAIR and GRE-T2 (gradient-echo T2) sequences; isointense in DWI; and hypointense in T1
Widened perivascular spaces (Virchow-Robin perivascular spaces)	Mostly seen in basal ganglia <2 mm in size; they usually accompany hyperintense lesions of the white matter and lacunar condition but not brain atrophy; the lesions are hyperintense in T2 sequences, hypointense in FLAIR and T1 sequences, and isointense in the GRE-T2 sequence
Cerebral microbleeds	Small, homogenous lesions <10 mm in diameter, characterized by the "blooming effect"; the lesions are best seen in the gradient-echo T2 sequence(hypointense lesions); in the T2, T1 and FLAIR, sequences they are isointense; microbleeds correspond to hemosiderin-loaded macrophages that are present in the perivascular space
Brain atrophy	Brain atrophy in the context of cerebral small vessel disease is considered only when the patient has not suffered a stroke or head injury

From Chojdak-Łukasiewicz et al. [9]
DWI diffuse-weighted imaging, *FLAIR* fluid-attenuated inversion recovery

fibrinoid necrosis). Except of SVD, cardioembolic, large artery atherothromboembolism, arterial dissection, intracranial atheromatous stenosis and rare monogenic disease may cause lacunar infarcts. The results of two studies suggest that it is not possible to identify the cause of a particular recent lacunar ischemic stroke based on its size, shape or location [3, 11].

7 Management Strategies and Treatment

There is no cure for SVD, but several strategies can help manage the condition and slow its progression. Management of SVD is multifaceted, focusing on the control of vascular risk factors, symptomatic treatment, and the prevention of disease progression. Key strategies include:

- Risk Factor Modification. Aggressive management of hypertension, diabetes, hyperlipidemia, and smoking cessation is still the main approach for treating or preventing SVD, despite the fact that most of these treatments have not yet shown ideal effects on long-term outcome:
  - Blood Pressure Control. Maintaining optimal blood pressure levels is crucial. Medications like ACE inhibitors, ARBs, and calcium channel blockers are commonly used. BP should be appropriately monitored and well controlled. BP <130/80 mmHg as generally recommended [44].
  - Diabetes Mellitus Management. Keeping blood sugar levels under control with medications, diet, and lifestyle changes might be beneficial but there is no clear evidence. Some glucose-lowering agents, e.g. glucagon-like-peptide-1 agonists or dipeptidyl peptidase-4-inhibitors may improve cerebral microvascular function through non-glucose pathways. However, the clinical benefit in patients with SVD remains unclear [40].
  - Cholesterol Lowering. Statins and other lipid-lowering agents can help reduce the risk of further vascular damage. But here is continued uncertainty regarding the effect of lipid lowering specific to SVD and lacunar stroke [44].
  - Lifestyle Modifications. Smoking cessation, regular physical activity, a healthy diet, and limiting alcohol intake. It is advisable to support a healthy lifestyle modifications and interventions (e.g. smoking cessation, dietary interventions, weight reduction, physical exercise, cognitive/behavioural or social interventions, sleep disorder/sleep apnoea interventions, or a mixture of these) [44].
- Pharmacotherapy. Antiplatelet agents, statins, and antihypertensive medications are commonly used.
  A systematic review of randomized trials found that any single antiplatelet appeared beneficial for secondary prevention of lacunar stroke, but the SPS3 trial showed that long-term dual antiplatelet treatment doubled the risk of bleeding without reducing the risk of stroke recurrence in patients with recent lacunar stroke [34, 36].

Also the most studies with lipid-lowering treatment in preventing white matter hyperintensities had neutral results [34, 37]. Post hoc analysis of a 2-year follow-up study showed that statins might be able to delay white matter hyperintensities progression in patients with severe baseline white matter hyperintensities [26]. Statins might also have other therapeutic effects including anti-inflammatory and pro-endothelial activities [4]. Antihypertensive treatment have still contradictory results because it might reduce white matter hyperintensities progression in some observational studies but demonstrated only little or no effects in randomized controlled trials [12, 13, 45].

- Vitamins. Likewise, subgroup analysis of the VITAmins TO Prevent Stroke (VITATOPS) MRI substudy shows that vitamin B supplementation may reduce WMH progression in patients with severe baseline CSVD [6].
- Cognitive and Physical Rehabilitation. Interventions aimed at improving cognitive function and mobility.

Nowadays, European Stroke Organization Guidelines, have no recommendations for patients with suspected acute lacunar ischemic stroke on the use of agents, such as phosphodiesterase-3 (e.g. cilostazol, pentoxifylline), anti-inflammatory agents (e.g. minocycline), anticoagulants, nitric oxide donors (e.g. transdermal glyceryl trinitrate), phosphodiesterase-5 inhibitors (sildenafil, tadalafil, dipyridamole) for acute treatment, to reduce any recurrent stroke, recurrent ischemic stroke, dependency, death, cognitive impairment or dementia, hemorrhagic stroke, MACE, mobility or gait disorder and mood disorder [44].

8 Future Directions

Research into the molecular mechanisms of SVD is ongoing, with a focus on identifying biomarkers for early detection and targets for novel therapies. Advances in neuroimaging and genetic studies hold promise for enhancing our understanding of SVD and improving patient outcomes.

Ongoing research is focused on:

- Biomarkers: Identifying biomarkers for early detection and monitoring of SVD progression.
- Neuroprotective Therapies: Developing treatments that can protect the brain from ischemic damage.
- Genetic Studies: Understanding the genetic basis of SVD to develop targeted therapies.

The endothelium of the brain, the blood -brain barrier and the microvascular function are potential targets for the prevention and treatment of SVD in the future. There are multiple potential endothelial targets: the prostacyclin/cyclic AMP (cAMP) system and the nitric oxide/cyclic guanylate monophosphate (cGMP) system. Interventions inducing cAMP or cGMP or reducing their degradation seem to be promising. Drugs that have these properties are nitric oxide donors, phosphodiesterases-3 and phosphodiesterases-5 inhibitors. And others are still in development [4, 25].

9 Conclusion

SVD is a significant cause of morbidity and mortality, with profound implications for stroke and dementia. A comprehensive approach to diagnosis and management, coupled with ongoing research, is essential for addressing the challenges posed by this complex disease.

Small Vessel Disease is a prevalent yet under-recognized condition that significantly impacts brain health. Understanding its pathology, risk factors, and clinical presentation is essential for timely diagnosis and management. While current treatments focus on managing risk factors and symptoms, ongoing research holds promise for more targeted and effective interventions in the future. By addressing SVD comprehensively, we can improve the quality of life for many individuals and reduce the burden of neurological diseases associated with this condition.

Declarations

Competing Interests The author(s) has no competing interests to declare that are relevant to the content of this manuscript.

Ethics Approval The author(s) declares that this manuscript does not include primary research with human participants.

References

1. Abner EL, Nelson PT, Kryscio RJ, et al. Diabetes is associated with cerebrovascular but not Alzheimer's disease neuropathology. Alzheimers Dement. 2016;12(8):882–9.
2. Asdaghi N, Jeerakathil T, Hameed B, et al. Oxfordshire community stroke project classification poorly differentiates small cortical and subcortical infarcts. Stroke. 2011;42(8):2143–8.
3. Asdaghi N, Pearce LA, Nakajima M, et al. Clinical correlates of infarct shape and volume in lacunar strokes: the Secondary Prevention of Small Subcortical Strokes trial. Stroke. 2014;45:2952–8.
4. Bath PM, Wardlaw JM. Pharmacological treatment and prevention of cerebral small vessel disease: a review of potential interventions. Int J Stroke. 2015;10:469–78.
5. Caruso P, Signori R, Moretti R. Small vessel disease to subcortical dementia: a dynamic model linking aging, cholinergic dysregulation and neurovascular drive. Vasc Health Risk Manag. 2019;15:259–81. https://doi.org/10.2147/VHRM.S190470.
6. Cavalieri M, Schmidt R, Chen C, et al. B vitamins and magnetic resonance imaging-detected ischemic brain lesions in patients with recent transient ischemic attack or stroke: the VITAmins TO Prevent Stroke (VITATOPS) MRI-substudy. Stroke. 2012;43:3266–70.

7. Chabriat H, Joutel A, Dichgans M, Tournier-Lasserve E, Bousser MG. Cadasil. Lancet Neurol. 2009;8(7):643–53.
8. Choi JC. Genetics of cerebral small vessel disease. J Stroke. 2015;17(1):7–16.
9. Chojdak-Łukasiewicz J, Dziadkowiak E, Zimny A, Paradowski B. Cerebral small vessel disease: a review. Adv Clin Exp Med. 2021;30(3):349–56.
10. Cuadrado-Godia E, Dwivedi P, Sharma S, et al. Cerebral small vessel disease: a review focusing on pathophysiology, biomarkers, and machine learning strategies. J Stroke. 2018;20(3):302–20.
11. Del Bene A, Makin SD, Doubal FN, et al. Variation in risk factors for recent small subcortical infarcts with infarct size, shape, and location. Stroke. 2013;44:3000–6.
12. Dufouil C, de Kersaint-Gilly A, Besancon V, et al. Longitudinal study of blood pressure and white matter hyperintensities: the EVA MRI Cohort. Neurology. 2001;56:921–6.
13. Dufouil C, Chalmers J, Coskun O, et al. Effects of blood pressure lowering on cerebral white matter hyperintensities in patients with stroke: the PROGRESS (Perindopril Protection Against Recurrent Stroke Study) Magnetic Resonance Imaging Substudy. Circulation. 2005;112:1644–50.
14. Durrani R, Wang M, Cox E, et al. Mediators of cognitive impairment in cerebral amyloid angiopathy. Int J Stroke. 2022;18:78–84.
15. Fang XH, Wang WH, Zhang XQ, et al. Incidence and survival of symptomatic lacunar infarction in the Beijing population: a 6-year prospective study. Eur J Neurol. 2012;19:1114–20.
16. Fisher CM. The arterial lesions underlying lacunes. Acta Neuropathol. 1968;12:1–15.
17. Fisher CM. Lacunar strokes and infarcts: a review. Neurology. 1982;32:871–6.
18. Haffner C, Vinters HV. CADASIL, CARASIL, CARASAL: the linguistic subtleties of cerebral small vessel disease. Neurology. 2016;87(17):1752–3.
19. Hatate J, Miwa K, Matsumoto M, et al. Association between cerebral small vessel diseases and mild parkinsonian signs in the elderly with vascular risk factors. Parkinsonism Relat Disord. 2016;26:29–34.
20. Jackson C, Sudlow C. Are lacunar strokes really different? A systematic review of differences in risk factor profiles between lacunar and nonlacunar infarcts. Stroke. 2005;36:891–901.
21. Khan U, Porteous L, Hassan A, Markus HS. Risk factor profile of cerebral small vessel disease and its subtypes. J Neurol Neurosurg Psychiatry. 2007;78:702–6.
22. Kim H, Lim YM, Lee EJ, Oh YJ, Kim KK. Clinical and imaging features of patients with cerebral autosomal dominant arteriopathy with subcortical infarcts and leukoencephalopathy and cysteine-sparing NOTCH3 mutations. PLoS One. 2020;15(6):e0234797.
23. Kong Q, Zhang Z, Yang Q, et al. 7T TOF-MRA shows modulated orifices of lenticulostriate arteries associated with atherosclerotic plaques in patients with lacunar infarcts. Eur J Radiol. 2019;118:271–6.
24. Leary MC, Saver JL. Annual incidence of first silent stroke in the United States: a preliminary estimate. Cerebrovasc Dis. 2003;16(3):280–5.
25. Markus HS, de Leeuw FE. Cerebral small vessel disease: recent advances and future directions. Int J Stroke. 2023;18(1):4–14.
26. Mok VC, Lam WW, Fan YH, et al. Effects of statins on the progression of cerebral white matter lesion: post hoc analysis of the ROCAS (Regression of Cerebral Artery Stenosis) study. J Neurol. 2009;256:750–7.
27. Mok V, Ding D, Fu J, Xiong Y, Chu WW, Wang D, Abrigo JM, Yang J, Wong A, Zhao Q, Guo Q, Hong Z, Wong KS. Transcranial Doppler ultrasound for screening cerebral small vessel disease: a community study. Stroke. 2012;43(10):2791–3.
28. Mori E, Tabuchi M, Yamadori A. Lacunar syndrome due to intracerebral hemorrhage. Stroke. 1985;16:454–9.
29. Pantoni L. Cerebral small vessel disease: from pathogenesis and clinical characteristics to therapeutic challenges. Lancet Neurol. 2010;9:689–701.
30. Park YS, Chung MS, Choi BS. MRI assessment of cerebral small vessel disease in patients with spontaneous intracerebral hemorrhage. Yonsei Med J. 2019;60(8):774–81.
31. Poels MM, Vernooij MW, Ikram MA, et al. Prevalence and risk factors of cerebral microbleeds: an update of the Rotterdam scan study. Stroke. 2010;41(10 Suppl):S103–6.
32. Saini M, Ikram K, Hilal S, Qiu A, Venketasubramanian N, Chen C. Silent stroke: not listened to rather than silent. Stroke. 2012;43(11):3102–4.
33. Schwarz G, Banerjee G, Hostettler IC, et al. MRI and CT imaging biomarkers of cerebral amyloid angiopathy in lobar intracerebral hemorrhage. Int J Stroke. 2022;18:85–94.
34. Shi Y, Wardlaw JM. Update on cerebral small vessel disease: a dynamic whole-brain disease. Stroke Vasc Neurol. 2016;1(3):83–92.
35. Smith E, Saposnik G, Biessels GJ, American Heart Association Stroke Council; Council on Cardiovascular Radiology and Intervention; Council on Functional Genomics and Translational Biology; and Council on Hypertension, et al. Stroke prevention in patients with silent cerebrovascular disease: a scientific statement for healthcare professionals from the American Heart Association/American Stroke Association. Stroke. 2017;48(2):e44–71.
36. SPS3 Study Group, Benavente OR, Coffey CS, et al. Blood-pressure targets in patients with recent lacunar stroke: the SPS3 randomised trial. Lancet. 2013;382:507–15.
37. Ten Dam VH, van den Heuvel DM, van Buchem MA, et al. Effect of pravastatin on cerebral infarcts and white matter lesions. Neurology. 2005;64:1807–9.
38. Tirschwell DL, Smith NL, Heckbert SR, Lemaitre RN, Longstreth WT Jr, Psaty BM. Association of cholesterol with stroke risk varies in stroke subtypes and patient subgroups. Neurology. 2004;63(10):1868–75.
39. van der Holst HM, van Uden IW, Tuladhar AM, et al. Cerebral small vessel disease and incident parkinsonism: the RUN DMC study. Neurology. 2015;85(18):1569–77.
40. van Sloten TT, Sedaghat S, Carnethon MR, Launer LJ, Stehouwer CDA. Cerebral microvascular complications of type 2 diabetes: stroke, cognitive dysfunction, and depression. Lancet Diabetes Endocrinol. 2020;8(4):325–36.
41. Wang L, Leonards CO, Sterzer P, Ebinger M. White matter lesions and depression: a systematic review and meta-analysis. J Psychiatr Res. 2014;56:56–64.
42. Wardlaw JM, Smith C, Dichgans M. Mechanisms of sporadic cerebral small vessel disease: insights from neuroimaging. Lancet Neurol. 2013;12(5):483–97.
43. Wardlaw JM, Smith EE, Biessels GJ, et al. Neuroimaging standards for research into small vessel disease and its contribution to ageing and neurodegeneration. Lancet Neurol. 2013;12:822–38.
44. Wardlaw JM, Chabriat H, de Leeuw FE, Debette S, Dichgans M, Doubal F, Jokinen H, Katsanos AH, Ornello R, Pantoni L, Pasi M, Pavlovic AM, Rudilosso S, Schmidt R, Staals J, Taylor-Rowan M, Hussain S, Lindgren AG. European Stroke Organisation (ESO) guideline on cerebral small vessel disease, part 2, lacunar ischaemic stroke. Eur Stroke J. 2024;9(1):5–68.
45. Weber R, Weimar C, Blatchford J, et al. Telmisartan on top of antihypertensive treatment does not prevent progression of cerebral white matter lesions in the prevention regimen for effectively avoiding second strokes (PRoFESS) MRI substudy. Stroke. 2012;43:2336–42.

Cardioembolic Stroke

David Školoudík, Michal Král, and Jiří Pudich

1 Introduction

Cardioembolic stroke, also known as cardiogenic stroke, is a subtype of ischemic stroke caused by cardioembolism. The primary etiopathological factor is the formation of emboli within the heart, which subsequently travel to the cerebral circulation, causing occlusion of cerebral arteries and leading to ischemic damage of the brain.

Cardioembolic stroke is a significant cause of morbidity and mortality worldwide, accounting for approximately 20–30% of all ischemic strokes. The incidence of cardiogenic stroke is closely linked to the prevalence of atrial fibrillation (AF), which is the most common sustained cardiac arrhythmia. AF affects about 1–2% of the general population, with the prevalence increasing significantly with age. The incidence of cardiogenic stroke is expected to rise due to the increasing prevalence of AF and other cardiac conditions, driven by demographic changes such as aging and the rising prevalence of risk factors like hypertension, diabetes, and obesity [15, 26, 33].

The recognition and management of cardiogenic stroke are critical due to its high recurrence risk and the severe disability it can cause. Understanding the etiopathology of cardiogenic stroke is crucial for developing effective prevention and treatment strategies.

D. Školoudík (✉)
Centre for Health Research, Department of Clinical Neurosciences, Faculty of Medicine, University of Ostrava, Ostrava, Czech Republic

M. Král
Department of Neurology, University Hospital Olomouc, Olomouc, Czech Republic

J. Pudich
Department of Internal Medicine, University Hospital Ostrava, Ostrava, Czech Republic

2 Pathophysiological Mechanisms

In the pathophysiology of cardioembolic stroke, thrombus formation in the heart (Figs. 1, 2, and 3), or in the venous system in cased of paradoxical embolization through the patent foramen ovale, plays an important role. The release of these thrombi flying subsequently through the arterial system to the brain leads to occlusion of the cerebral arteries, causing ischemia and infarction of brain tissue. The risk factors for cardioembolic stroke are largely those that predispose individuals to atrial fibrillation and other heart diseases including age, arterial hypertension, diabetes mellitus, lifestyle factors as smoking, alcohol consumption, and physical inactivity, and cardiac pathologies as valvular heart disease, acute or previous myocardial infarction, heart failure, etc. [15].

Ethnicity, geographic locations and socioeconomic factors also play a role, with individuals from lower socioeconomic backgrounds having higher rates of risk factors and poorer access to healthcare, leading to higher incidence and worse outcomes of cardioembolic stroke [14].

In patients with various cardiac pathologies, especially atrial fibrillation, impaired atrial contractility causes blood stasis, which, together with other factors acting as the Virchow triad, leads to thrombus formation and subsequent embolism to the brain. This is even more pronounced in patients with a coexisting atrial septal aneurysm.

However, it should always be kept in mind that all three conditions of Virchow's triad should be fulfilled in order to form a thrombus [31]:

- *Endothelial/endocardium damage (vessel wall injury).* A healthy endothelium/endocardium contains an anticoagulant and antiplatelet surface with a specific cell surface glycoproteins and the release of various molecules. However, various pathological processes can cause the detachment or exclusion of these molecules from the cell surface, which may tip hemostasis towards procoagulation.

V. Beneš, D. Netuka (eds.), *Surgical and Interventional Treatment of Cerebral Ischemia*,
https://doi.org/10.1007/978-3-032-08934-2_28

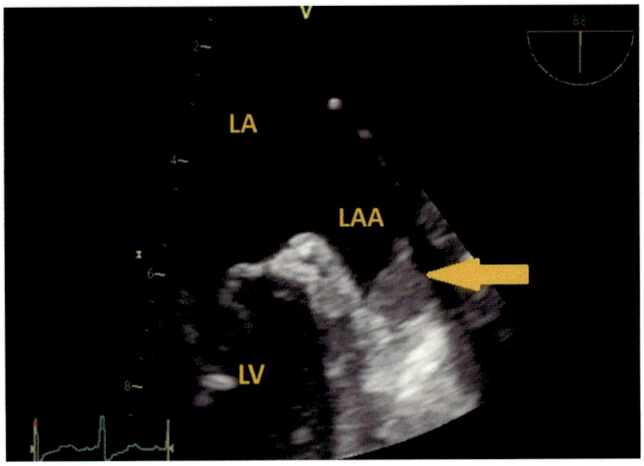

Fig. 1 Transesophageal echocardiography: Left atrial appendage thrombus (yellow arrow). LAA—left atrial appendage; LA—left atrium; LV—left ventricle

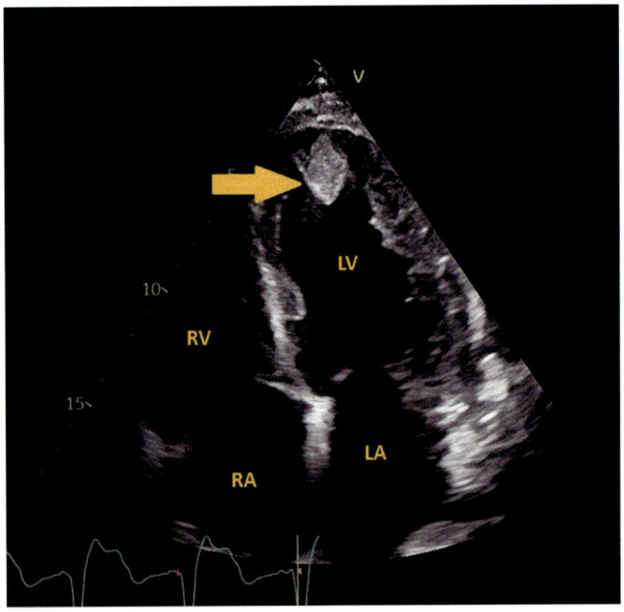

Fig. 2 Transthoracic echocardiography: Apical left ventricular thrombus (yellow arrow) in a patient with severe left ventricular systolic dysfunction complicated by an acute ischemic stroke. LA—left atrium. RA—right atrium. LV—left ventricle. RV—right ventricle

- *Alteration in blood flow in the vessels (turbulent blood flow and/or stasis).* As the central laminar blood flow is disrupted, numerous red blood cells, leucocytes, and platelets get concentrated near the vessel wall for adhesion and activation. High shear forces at the vessel wall further activate platelets and promote their adhesion to the exposed subendothelium. Therefore, stasis is required (i.e. in case of atrial fibrillation, atrial septal aneurysm or turbulent blood flow) to allow fibrin formation and secondary haemostasis.

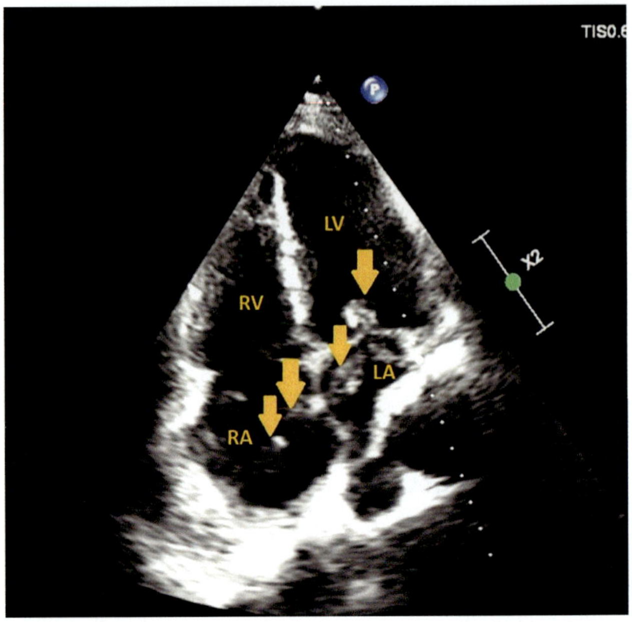

Fig. 3 Transthoracic echocardiography: An entrapped in flagranti thrombus (yellow marks) in-transit within the right atrium traversing the interatrial septum and protruding into the left atrium and to the left ventricle. RA—right atrium; RV—right ventricle; LV—left ventricle; LA—left atrium

- *Hypercoagulability of blood.* Soluble coagulation factors (such as fibrinogen and tissue factors) and cells (such as platelets) are implicated in thrombosis. However, a continuum exists between healthy state and hemostatic abnormalities in prothrombotic or hypercoagulable states.

3 Sources of Cardiac Embolism

To the high-risk sources of cardiac embolism belong atrial fibrillation or flutter, mechanical prosthetic valve, left atrial or ventricular thrombus, recent myocardial infarction, infective endokarditis, dilated cardiomyopathy, rheumatic heart disease, regional left ventricular akinesis, atrial myxoma and patent foramen ovale with thrombus in situ.

Risk factors for cardioembolic stroke includes:

1. *Atrial Fibrillation*
   Atrial fibrillation (paroxysmal and chronic atrial fibrillation) is the most common cause of cardioembolic stroke, especially in elderly individuals. It is found in up to 50% of all cardioembolic strokes Studies have shown that patients with AF have a fivefold increased risk of stroke compared to those without AF [21, 26, 33]. The irregular heart rhythm leads to stasis of blood in the atria and in combination with other cardiac pathologies increase the risk of thrombus formation, especially in the left atrial

appendage with subsequent potential embolization into the cerebral circulation. AF is the most common sustained cardiac arrhythmia, which affects approximately 1.0–1.5% of the general population, with increasing prevalence with age, ranging from 0.1% among adults <55 years of age to almost 10% among those >80 years of age. AF is associated with a three to fivefold increased risk of stroke [48]. The number of patients with AF has been steadily increasing in recent decades and it is assumed that number of patients with AF may double and the number of AF-related strokes may triple in the next few decades based on projections from high-income countries such as the U.S [20].

2. *Recent Myocardial Infarction*
   Acute myocardial infarction (MI) is one of the oldest established risk factors for ischemic stroke. The risk of stroke is highest in the first few weeks after MI, with a 2–3% incidence in the first 4 weeks [16]. Myocardial infarction can lead to the formation of left ventricular thrombi due to ventricular dyskinesis and endocardium damage, especially in cases of large anterior infarcts [47]. However, rates of stroke after acute MI are decreasing over time, perhaps due to acute reperfusion therapy, widespread use of antithrombotic medications, and improved long-term secondary prevention therapies [46].

   Another factors that increases the risk of ischaemic stroke in heart attack patients are percutaneous coronary interventions or other cardiac surgery, which are increasingly indicated in these patients and are associated with an increased risk of stroke [18, 37].
3. *Systolic Heart Failure*
   Heart failure is the most common reason for hospital admission in high-income countries. Regional stasis, a hypercoagulable state, and often present (undiagnosed) AF appear to predispose heart failure patients to cardiac thrombus. It results in at least three times higher risk of ischemic stroke than in the general population [29].
4. *Aortic Arch Atheroma*
   Atherosclerotic plaques are relatively prevalent in elderly, occurring in approximately 45% of individuals ≥45 years [35]. In particular, large, ulcerated, non-calcified or mobile atheromas might be associated with an increased risk of stroke [2, 12, 35]. Unfortunately, aortic atheromas may still be an underrecognized cause of stroke in routine clinical practice because necessary imaging modalities, such as transesophageal echocardiography, are not routinely performed in stroke patients [19]. The rate of stroke recurrence in patients with aortic atheromas varied between 2% and 12% per year [4, 26, 44].
5. *Prosthetic Heart Valves*
   Moderate to severe valvular heart disease is the predominant cardiac pathology, with surgical or endovascular valve replacement being the standard treatment for many of these patients, which is subsequently associated with an increased incidence of stroke. Patients with a mechanical aortic and mitral valves have even higher stroke risk than patients with bioprosthetic ones and use of long term anticoagulation with vitamin K antagonist (e.g. warfarin) significantly decrease the annual risk of stroke in patients with mechanical valve. Direct oral anticoagulants (DOACs) are contraindicated for mechanical valves due to inferior efficacy to a warfarin. On the other hand, patients with bioprosthetic valves are generally treated with long-term antiplatelet therapy unless other conditions (e.g. atrial fibrillation) require anticoagulation therapy [8, 39]. Although stroke risk has decreased over time, thromboembolic complications remain a significant cause of morbidity and mortality in patients with prosthetic heart valves [23].
6. *Patent Foramen Ovale*
   Patent foramen ovale (PFO) (Fig. 4) is a relatively rear cause of ischemic stroke except perhaps in very young stroke patients (<50 years). It affects between 8.6% and 42% of the general population [42], making it the most common passage for paradoxical embolism from the venous system to the cerebral arterial circulation. Patients with unexplained ischemic stroke are more likely to have a PFO than those with known causes, but the presence of a PFO is associated with a low risk of recurrent stroke comparable to overall recurrence rates [26, 42]. In a population-based study of stroke-free patients, the presence of a PFO was not significantly associated with the increased risk of clinically apparent stroke or silent cerebral infarction on magnetic resonance imaging [13].
7. *Infective Endocarditis*
   Infective endocarditis (Fig. 5) is a relatively rare but very strong risk factor for stroke. Approximately one in five patients with endocarditis is complicated by stroke, and

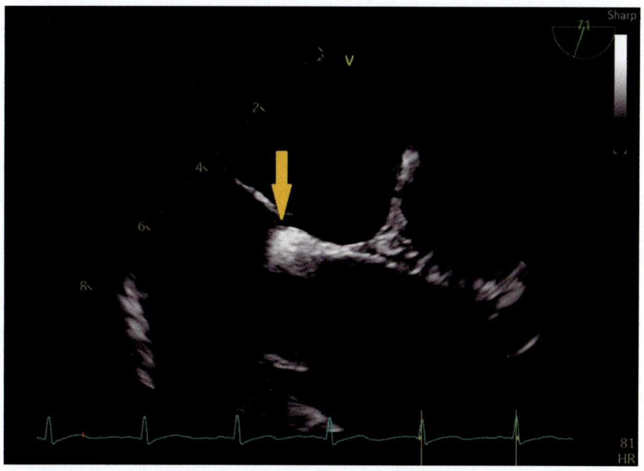

Fig. 4 Transesophageal echocardiography: Patent foramen ovale (yellow arrow)

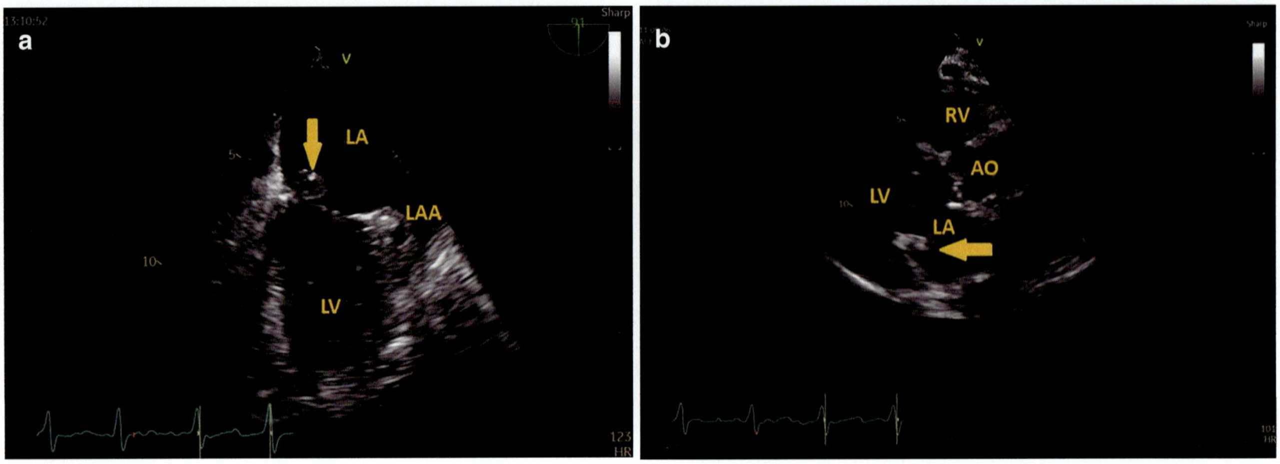

Fig. 5 Infective endocarditis of mitral valve shown on transesophageal echocardiography (5a) and transthoracic echocardiography (5b). Yellow arrow—vegetations; LA—left atrium; LAA—left atrial appendage; LV—left ventricle; RV—right ventricle; AO—aorta

there is a more than 20-fold relative increase in the risk of stroke within 1 month of the onset of bacteraemia or infective endocarditis [36].

8. *Cardiomyopathy*
   Dilated cardiomyopathy and other forms of cardiomyopathy can lead to thrombus formation in the heart due to reduced ejection fraction and blood stasis. Dilated cardiomyopathy and left ventricular dysfunction can lead to the formation of mural thrombi, which can embolize to the cerebral circulation [11].
9. *Atrial Septal Aneurysms*
   Atrial septal aneurysms have a high degree of association with other sources of embolism (mainly atrial fibrillation and PFO). However, there are insufficient data available to consider atrial septal aneurysm as an independent risk factor for stroke [25, 45].
10. *Other Causes*
    There are several rare causes of embolism, such as papillary fibroelastoma, myxoma (Fig. 6), lambl excrescences, nonbacterial thrombotic endocarditis, rheumatic mitral stenosis, mitral valve prolapse or stenosis, bicuspid aortic valves, mitral annular calcification, and atrial flutter. Each accounts for fewer than 1% of cardioembolic strokes [26].

Atherosclerosis of the aortic arch is also sometimes cited as a source of cardioembolism. Others include it among atherothrombotic sources and it is also frequently detected in patients with embolic stroke of undetermined source. But regardless of the classification, it is always necessary to think about this pathology when detecting the source of embolization into the brain [38].

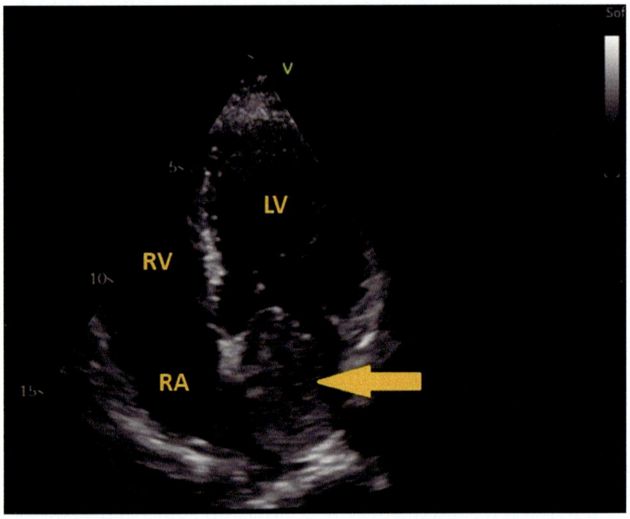

Fig. 6 Transthoracic echocardiography: Left atrial myxoma (yellow arrow). LV—left ventricle; RV—right ventricle; RA—right atrium

4 Clinical Presentation

The clinical picture of cardioembolic stroke is similar in many respects to other types of ischaemic stroke but may have specific features such as sudden onset, involvement of multiple vascular territories, a maximal deficit at the onset of the stroke and a neurological deficit with common symptoms that include hemiparesis, aphasia, visual disturbances and ataxia depending on the affected cerebral vascular territory.

5 Diagnostics

Acute diagnostics in cardioembolic stroke does not differ from other type of stroke. Neuroimaging methods such as CT/CTA or MRI (with diffusion-weighted imaging, DWI)/MRA are used to detect cerebral ischemia and acute cerebral artery occlusion (Figs. 7, 8, 9, and 10).

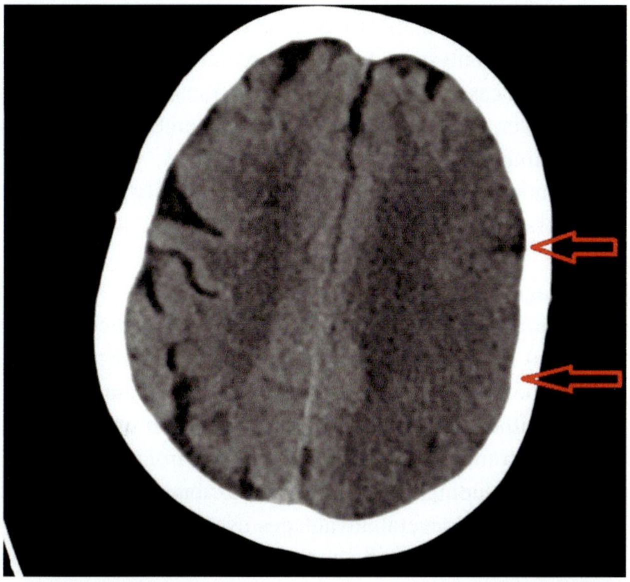

Fig. 7 Native brain CT: Acute ischemic stroke in left hemisphere (arrows) in patient with middle cerebral occlusion caused by cardioembolism

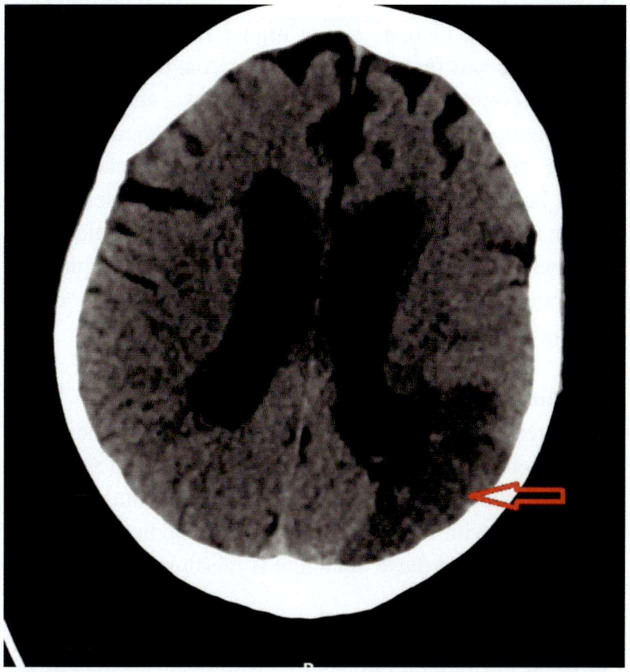

Fig. 8 Native brain CT: Subacute ischemic lesion (arrow) in left parietal lobe in patient with cardioembolic stroke

To establish cardiac pathology as a cardioembolic source, the following diagnostic methods should be used:

- Echocardiography: Transthoracic echocardiography (TTE) is the basic examination, however, when a cardioembolic cause is considered, transesophageal echocar-

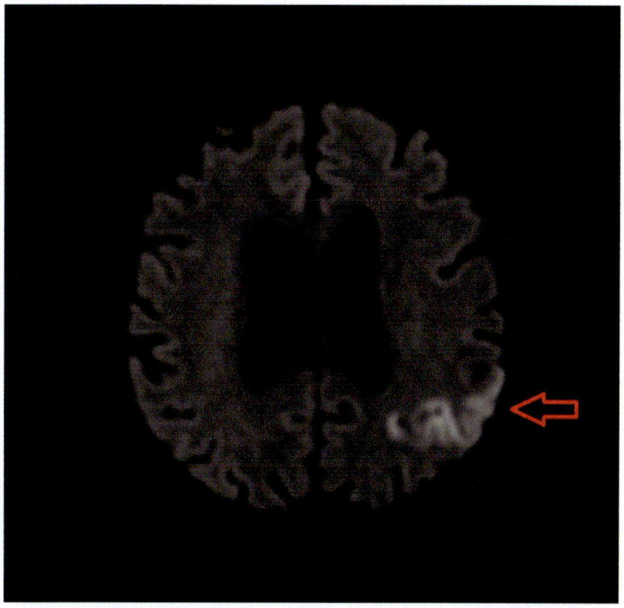

Fig. 9 Magnetic resonance imaging: Ischemic lesion (arrow) in left parietal lobe in patient with cardioembolic stroke imaged on diffusion-weighted images (DWI)

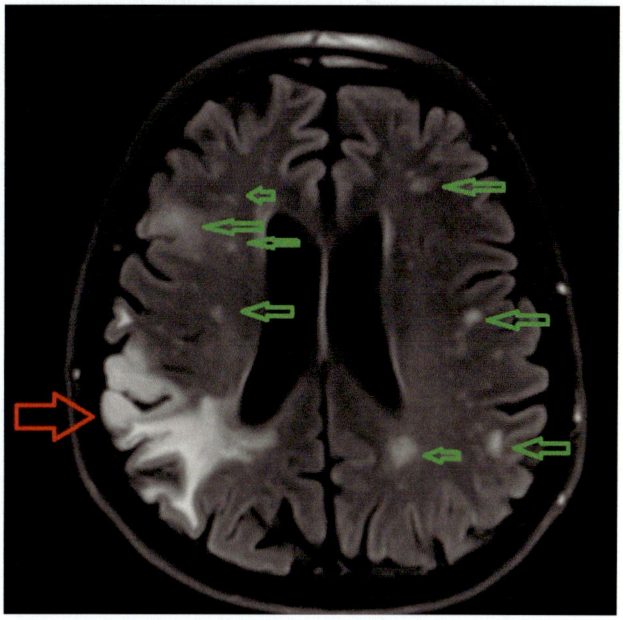

Fig. 10 Magnetic resonance imaging: Multiple ischemic lesions (arrows) caused by cardioembolism imaged on T2-fluid-attenuated inversion recovery (FLAIR) sequences

diography (TEE) is necessary due to its higher sensitivity to identify cardiac sources of embolism such as thrombi, vegetations or tumors [10].

- Electrocardiography (ECG) and Holter Monitoring—Short-term ECG, continuous heart monitoring during a hospital stay, or wearable or implanted Holter devices can detect atrial fibrillation or other arrhythmias. Long-term ECG monitoring can detect a greater number of specific arrhythmias with a high risk of recurrent stroke, allowing specific secondary preventive care to be deployed and reducing the risk of recurrent stroke [41].
- Cardiac MRI and CT: It provides a detailed view of cardiac structures and function, and allows the detection of structural abnormalities and thrombi that are not visible on echocardiography [9].
- Blood Tests: Coagulation profiles, cardiac biomarkers, and inflammatory markers help in identifying underlying conditions and risk factors [17].

There is still no gold standard for determining the etiology of stroke (including cardioembolic stroke). The TOAST (Trial of Org 10172 in the Acute Stroke Treatment) classification system, developed in the 1990s, remains the most widely used tool in routine clinical practice [1]. It categorizes stroke into five etiologic categories: (1) large vessel atherosclerosis, (2) cardioembolization, (3) small vessel disease, (4) other identifiable causes, and (5) stroke of "undetermined" etiology. However, with the development and increasing use of imaging and other diagnostic modalities and long-term cardiac rhythm monitoring, the proportion of patients with a combination of vascular, cardiac, and other abnormal findings is steadily increasing, increase up to 30% the proportion of "undetermined" etiology of stroke according to the TOAST classification based on the detection of multiple potential causes of stroke [30].

In an attempt to overcome these problems, a more sophisticated extension of the TOAST classification, the Causal Classification of Stroke (CCS), has been developed. This incorporates confidence levels for specific etiologies to successfully minimize the "indeterminate etiology" classification [5]. Also ASCOD phenotype classification system (as revised in 2013) more closely resembles this medical reasoning [3]. Although it is more complex than TOAST, it is less frequently used in clinical practice because its rather descriptive nature and does not serve well as a clinical decision-making tool [43].

There are several other classification systems: ASCO, SPARKLE, CISS, KOREAN-TOAST [40]. However, none of them has yet reached a wider use in common clinical practice. In addition to the aforementioned classification systems, the concept of embolic stroke of undetermined etiology (ESUS) was developed in 2014. ESUS defines a subgroup of patients with cryptogenic stroke with a nonlacunar course based on infarct topography and sufficient diagnostic testing to exclude the presence of a high-risk cardioembolic source or occlusive atherosclerosis [22].

6 Treatment

The acute treatment of patients with cardioembolic stroke does not differ from other types of ischemic stroke. Patients who meet the inclusion and exclusion criteria should be treated within a specifically defined time window with intravenous thrombolysis and/or endovascular mechanical thrombectomy in cases of large vessel occlusions.

However, the diagnosis of a cardioembolic source is mainly important for secondary prevention, when specific therapeutic procedures are indicated, especially anticoagulation therapy in patients with atrial fibrillation [24].

Anticoagulation

Long-term anticoagulation with direct oral anticoagulants (DOACs) or warfarin is recommended for patients with cardiac pathologies with a high-risk of stroke recurrence, i.e. atrial fibrillation, recent myocardial infarction with left ventricular thrombus, and other high-risk cardiac conditions. NOACs, including dabigatran, rivaroxaban, apixaban, and edoxaban, offer several advantages over warfarin, including fixed dosing and fewer dietary restrictions. They are increasingly used due to their favorable safety and efficacy profiles. However, in certain cases warfarin remains irreplaceable, for example in the case of mechanical valve replacement [7, 28].

A specific situation is represented by infective endocarditis, where, in addition to an increased risk of recurrent cerebral embolism, there is also a higher risk of intracererbal hemorrhage and therefore neither anticoagulation nor antiplatelet therapy is routinely indicated. However, anticoagulation or antiplatelet therapy should be considered if there is another factor coexisting with infective endocarditis that would benefit from anticoagulation or antiplatelet therapy (e.g. mechanical valve or atrial fibrillation for anticoagulation therapy, or high-grade stenosis of an extracranial or intracranial large artery for antiplatelet therapy) and thus outweigh the potential risk [6, 39].

Antiplatelet Therapy

Antiplatelet agents (Aspirin, clopidogrel, atc) may be used in cases where anticoagulation is contraindicated. In some specific case with high-risk of recurrent stroke, combination of antiplatelets with anticoagulants might be indicated. But the clear evidence for these treatment is missing [7].

Rate and Rhythm Control

For atrial fibrillation, rate control with beta-blockers or calcium channel blockers, and rhythm control with antiarrhythmic drugs, electrical cardioversion, or catheter ablation.

Treatment of Heart Failure

Optimal treatment in patients with heart failure may not only reduce mortality but also the risk of stroke [27].

Cardiac Surgery and Interventions

When indicated, valve replacement or repair for valvular heart disease, closure of PFO or removal of atrial myxomas, or left atrial appendage closure should be considered.

Other secondary prevention strategies as lifestyle modification, blood pressure control, lipid management and diabetes treatment are similar to other ischaemic strokes.

To stratify embolic risk in AF patients, the CHADS 2 scale was developed based on multiple clinical variables. It is widely employed due to its simplicity and ease of use [34]. More recently, the CHA 2 DS 2-VASc score was developed. This score considers patients with a prior stroke/TIA or patients >75 years as high-risk patients and therefore should receive oral anticoagulation (OAC) for stroke prevention. Furthermore, a combination of at least two risk factors from the following—hypertension, heart failure, diabetes, age 65–75, female gender, and pre-existing vascular disease—are also considered to be high risk [32].

A multidisciplinary approach, involving neurologists, cardiologists, radiologist/neuroradiologist, hematologists, surgeons and rehabilitation specialists, is essential in optimizing outcomes for patients with cardioembolic stroke. Comprehensive care plans should address both the cardiac source of embolism and the cerebral consequences of the stroke.

7 Public Health Impact

The public health burden of cardiogenic stroke is enormous. Patients with cardiogenic stroke often have worse outcomes compared to other types of ischemic stroke, with higher rates of recurrence, disability and mortality. The economic impact is substantial and includes direct costs of treatment, long-term care and lost productivity. Thus, prompt acute treatment and optimal early secondary prevention, particularly effective treatment of atrial fibrillation and optimal indication for anticoagulation therapy, are essential to reduce the negative public health impact of cardioembolic stroke.

8 Conclusion

Cardioembolic stroke is one of the most frequent cases of ischemic stroke with significant morbidity and mortality. However, it belongs to preventable and treatable disease. Timely diagnosis and appropriate management of the underlying cardiac conditions which requires a multidisciplinary approach are crucial in reducing the incidence and recurrence of stroke. Advances in diagnostic imaging, therapeutic interventions and secondary prevention approaches have improved outcomes, but ongoing research and adherence to clinical guidelines remain essential.

Declarations

Competing Interests The author(s) has no competing interests to declare that are relevant to the content of this manuscript.

Ethics Approval The author(s) declares that this manuscript does not include primary research with human participants.

References

1. Adams HP Jr, Woolson RF, Clarke WR, Davis PH, Bendixen BH, Love BB, et al. Design of the trial of org 10172 in acute stroke treatment (TOAST). Control Clin Trials. 1997;18:358–77.
2. Amarenco P, Cohen A, Tzourio C, Bertrand B, Hommel M, Besson G, Chauvel C, Touboul PJ, Bousser MG. Atherosclerotic disease of the aortic arch and the risk of ischemic stroke. N Engl J Med. 1994;331:1474–9.
3. Amarenco P, Bogousslavsky J, Caplan LR, Donnan GA, Wolf ME, Hennerici MG. The aSCOD phenotyping of ischemic stroke (updated ASCO phenotyping). Cerebrovasc Dis. 2013;36:1–5.
4. Amarenco P, Davis S, Jones EF, Cohen AA, Heiss WD, Kaste M, Laouenan C, Young D, Macleod M, Donnan GA. Aortic Arch Related Cerebral Hazard Trial I. Clopidogrel plus aspirin versus warfarin in patients with stroke and aortic arch plaques. Stroke. 2014;45:1248–57.
5. Ay H, Benner T, Arsava EM, Furie KL, Singhal AB, Jensen MB, et al. A computerized algorithm for etiologic classification of ischemic stroke: the causative classification of stroke system. Stroke. 2007;38:2979–84.
6. Baddour LM, Wilson WR, Bayer AS, Fowler VG Jr, Tleyjeh IM, Rybak MJ, Barsic B, Lockhart PB, Gewitz MH, Levison ME, Bolger AF, Steckelberg JM, Baltimore RS, Fink AM, O'Gara P, Taubert KA, American Heart Association Committee on Rheumatic Fever, Endocarditis, and Kawasaki Disease of the Council on Cardiovascular Disease in the Young, Council on Clinical Cardiology, Council on Cardiovascular Surgery and Anesthesia, and Stroke Council. Infective endocarditis in adults: diagnosis, antimicrobial therapy, and management of complications: a scientific statement for healthcare professionals from the American Heart Association. Circulation. 2015;132(15):1435–86.
7. Bhatia K, Ladd LM, Carr KH, Di Napoli M, Saver JL, McCullough LD, Hosseini Farahabadi M, Alsbrook DL, Hinduja A, Ortiz Garcia JG, Sabbagh SY, Jafarli A, Divani AA. Contemporary antiplatelet and anticoagulant therapies for secondary stroke prevention: a narrative review of current literature and guidelines. Curr Neurol Neurosci Rep. 2023;23(5):235–62.
8. Brennan JM, Edwards FH, Zhao Y, O'Brien S, Booth ME, Dokholyan RS, Douglas PS, Peterson ED. Long-term safety and effectiveness of mechanical versus biologic aortic valve prostheses in older patients: results from the Society of Thoracic Surgeons Adult Cardiac Surgery National Database. Circulation. 2013;127:1647–55.
9. Camen S, Haeusler KG, Schnabel RB. Cardiac imaging after ischemic stroke or transient ischemic attack. Curr Neurol Neurosci Rep. 2020;20(8):36.
10. Canali E, Serani M, Tarzia P, Ciampi P, Canestrelli S, Calò L. Echocardiography in cardioembolic stroke prevention. Eur Heart J Suppl. 2023;25(Suppl C):C212–7.

11. Deng Y, Chen Z, Hu L, Xu Z, Hu J, Ma J, Yu J, Hu J, Li J, Xiong Q, Hong K. Decreased eGFR is associated with ischemic stroke in patients with dilated cardiomyopathy. Clin Appl Thromb Hemost. 2019;25:1076029619866909.
12. Di Tullio MR, Sacco RL, Gersony D, Nayak H, Weslow RG, Kargman DE, Homma S. Aortic atheromas and acute ischemic stroke: a transesophageal echocardiographic study in an ethnically mixed population. Neurology. 1996;46:1560–6.
13. Di Tullio MR, Jin Z, Russo C, Elkind MSV, Rundek T, Yoshita M, DeCarli C, Wright CB, Homma S, Sacco RL. Patent foramen ovale, subclinical cerebrovascular disease and ischemic stroke in a population-based cohort. J Am Coll Cardiol. 2013;62:35–41.
14. Elkind MSV, Lisabeth L, Howard VJ, Kleindorfer D, Howard G. Approaches to studying determinants of racial-ethnic disparities in stroke and its sequelae. Stroke. 2020;51(11):3406–16.
15. Escudero-Martínez I, Morales-Caba L, Segura T. Atrial fibrillation and stroke: a review and new insights. Trends Cardiovasc Med. 2023;33(1):23–9.
16. Fonseca AC. Stroke and recent myocardial infarction, reduced left ventricular ejection fraction, left ventricular thrombus, and wall motion abnormalities. Curr Cardiol Rep. 2023;25(12):1687–97.
17. Fonseca AC, Coelho P. Update on biomarkers associated to cardioembolic stroke: a narrative review. Life (Basel). 2021;11(5):448.
18. Gaudino M, Angiolillo DJ, Di Franco A, Capodanno D, Bakaeen F, Farkouh ME, Fremes SE, Holmes D, Girardi LN, Nakamura S, Head SJ, Park SJ, Mack M, Serruys PW, Ruel M, Stone GW, Tam DY, Vallely M, Taggart DP. Stroke after coronary artery bypass grafting and percutaneous coronary intervention: incidence, pathogenesis, and outcomes. J Am Heart Assoc. 2019;8(13):e013032.
19. Giruparajah M, Bosch J, Vanassche T, Mattina K, Connolly SJ, Pater C, Hart RG. Global survey of the diagnostic evaluation and management of cryptogenic ischemic stroke. Int J Stroke. 2015;10:1031–6.
20. Go AS, Hylek EM, Phillips KA, Chang Y, Henault LE, Selby JV, Singer DE. Prevalence of diagnosed atrial fibrillation in adults: national implications for rhythm management and stroke prevention: the AnTicoagulation and Risk Factors in Atrial Fibrillation (ATRIA) Study. JAMA. 2001;285:2370–5.
21. Griñán K, Arboix A, Massons J, Díez L, Vergés E, Gil F, Arboix-Alió J, Sánchez-López MJ, García-Eroles L. Cardioembolic stroke: risk factors, clinical features, and early outcome in 956 consecutive patients. Rev Investig Clin. 2020;73(1):023–30.
22. Hart RG, Diener HC, Coutts SB, Easton JD, Granger CB. Embolic strokes of undetermined source: the case for a new clinical construct. Lancet Neurol. 2014;13:429–38.
23. Idrees JJ, Schiltz NK, Johnston DR, Mick S, Smedira NG, Sabik JF 3rd, Blackstone EH, Svensson LG, Soltesz EG. Trends, predictors, and outcomes of stroke after surgical aortic valve replacement in the United States. Ann Thorac Surg. 2016;101:927–35.
24. Jame S, Barnes G. Stroke and thromboembolism prevention in atrial fibrillation. Heart. 2020;106(1):10–7.
25. Janion M, Kurzawski J. Atrial fibrillation in patients with atrial septal aneurysm. Cardiol J. 2007;14(6):580–4.
26. Kamel H, Healey JS. Cardioembolic stroke. Circ Res. 2017;120(3):514–26.
27. Kato Y, Tsutsui K, Nakano S, Hayashi T, Suda S. Cardioembolic stroke: past advancements, current challenges, and future directions. Int J Mol Sci. 2024;25(11):5777.
28. Katsanos AH, Kamel H, Healey JS, Hart RG. Stroke prevention in atrial fibrillation: looking forward. Circulation. 2020;142(24):2371–88.
29. Kim W, Kim EJ. Heart failure as a risk factor for stroke. J Stroke. 2018;20(1):33–45.
30. Kolominsky-Rabas PL, Weber M, Gefeller O, Neundoerfer B, Heuschmann PU. Epidemiology of ischemic stroke subtypes according to TOAST criteria: incidence, recurrence, and long-term survival in ischemic stroke subtypes: a population-based study. Stroke. 2001;32:2735–40.
31. Kushner A, West WP, Khan Suheb MZ, et al. Virchow triad. In: StatPearls [Internet]. Treasure Island: StatPearls Publishing; 2024. Available from: https://www.ncbi.nlm.nih.gov/books/NBK539697.
32. Lip GYH, Nieuwlaat R, Pisters R, Lane DA, Crijins HJG. Refining clinical risk stratification for predicting stroke and thromboembolism in atrial fibrillation using a novel risk. Chest. 2010;137:263–72.
33. Markus A, Valerie S, Mira K. Promising biomarker candidates for cardioembolic stroke etiology. A brief narrative review and current opinion. Front Neurol. 2021;12:624930.
34. Marmagkiolis K, Nikolaidis IG, Politis T, Goldstein L. Approach to and management of the acute stroke patient with atrial fibrillation: a literature review. J Hosp Med. 2008;3(4):326–32.
35. Meissner I, Khandheria BK, Sheps SG, Schwartz GL, Wiebers DO, Whisnant JP, Covalt JL, Petterson TM, Christianson TJ, Agmon Y. Atherosclerosis of the aorta: risk factor, risk marker, or innocent bystander? A prospective population-based transesophageal echocardiography study. J Am Coll Cardiol. 2004;44:1018–24.
36. Merkler AE, Chu SY, Lerario MP, Navi BB, Kamel H. Temporal relationship between infective endocarditis and stroke. Neurology. 2015;85:512–6.
37. Messé SR, Acker MA, Kasner SE, Fanning M, Giovannetti T, Ratcliffe SJ, Bilello M, Szeto WY, Bavaria JE, Hargrove WC 3rd, Mohler ER 3rd, Floyd TF, Determining Neurologic Outcomes from Valve Operations (DeNOVO) Investigators. Stroke after aortic valve surgery: results from a prospective cohort. Circulation. 2014;129(22):2253–61.
38. Ntaios G, Pearce LA, Meseguer E, Endres M, Amarenco P, Ozturk S, Lang W, Bornstein NM, Molina CA, Pagola J, Mundl H, Berkowitz SD, Liu YY, Sen S, Connolly SJ, Hart RG. Aortic arch atherosclerosis in patients with embolic stroke of undetermined source: an exploratory analysis of the NAVIGATE ESUS trial. Stroke. 2019;50(11):3184–90.
39. Otto CM, Nishimura RA, Bonow RO, Carabello BA, Erwin JP 3rd, Gentile F, Jneid H, Krieger EV, Mack M, McLeod C, O'Gara PT, Rigolin VH, Sundt TM 3rd, Thompson A, Toly C. 2020 ACC/AHA guideline for the management of patients with valvular heart disease: a report of the American College of Cardiology/American Heart Association Joint Committee on clinical practice guidelines. Circulation. 2021;143(5):e35–71.
40. Radu RA, Terecoasă EO, Băjenaru OA, Tiu C. Etiologic classification of ischemic stroke: where do we stand? Clin Neurol Neurosurg. 2017;159:93–106. https://doi.org/10.1016/j.clineuro.2017.05.019. Epub 2017 May 24. PMID: 28609703.
41. Shafqat S, Kelly PJ, Furie KL. Holter monitoring in the diagnosis of stroke mechanism. Intern Med J. 2004;34(6):305–9.
42. Shehata A, Nasser A, Mohsen A, Anwar Samaan A, Mostafa A, Hassan M. Prevalence and characteristics of patent foramen ovale in a sample of Egyptian population: a computed tomography study. Egypt Heart J. 2024;76(1):73.
43. Sirimarco G, Lavallée PC, Labreuche J, Meseguer E, Cabrejo L, Guidoux C, et al. Overlap of diseases underlying ischemic stroke: the aSCOD phenotyping. Stroke. 2013;44:2427–33.

44. The French Study of Aortic Plaques in Stroke Group. Atherosclerotic disease of the aortic arch as a risk factor for recurrent ischemic stroke. N Engl J Med. 1996;334:1216–21.
45. Turc G, Lee JY, Brochet E, Kim JS, Song JK, Mas JL, CLOSE and DEFENSE-PFO Trial Investigators. Atrial septal aneurysm, shunt size, and recurrent stroke risk in patients with patent foramen ovale. J Am Coll Cardiol. 2020;75(18):2312–20.
46. Wang Y, Lichtman JH, Dharmarajan K, Masoudi FA, Ross JS, Dodson JA, Chen J, Spertus JA, Chaudhry SI, Nallamothu BK, Krumholz HM. National trends in stroke after acute myocardial infarction among Medicare patients in the United States: 1999 to 2010. Am Heart J. 2015;169:78–85.e74.
47. Weinreich DJ, Burke JF, Pauletto FJ. Left ventricular mural thrombi complicating acute myocardial infarction. Long-term follow-up with serial echocardiography. Ann Intern Med. 1984;100:789–94.
48. Wolf PA, Abbott RD, Kannel WB. Atrial fibrillation as an independent risk factor for stroke: the Framingham study. Stroke. 1991;22:983–8.

Summary of Guidelines for Surgical Interventions in the Management and Prevention of Ischemic Stroke

David Školoudík, Tomáš Hrbáč, and Martin Roubec

1 Introduction

In the following text, individual recommendations concerning surgical treatment in primary prevention, acute treatment and secondary prevention in patients with ischemic stroke are presented.

2 Primary Prevention of Ischemic Stroke

2.1 Carotid Endarterectomy

Several large clinical trials have shown that carotid artery revascularization in appropriately selected patients with asymptomatic carotid stenosis leads to a reduced risk of stroke compared with the best medical treatment. However, in the time since the publication of many of these studies, current medical therapy has improved significantly. Thus, new studies are needed to answer the question of which patients with an asymptomatic carotid stenosis will benefit from the best medical treatment and which will benefit from revascularization therapy. The current recommendations of various societies for the indication of carotid revascularization in patients with asymptomatic carotid stenosis are listed in Table 1. Practical guide for management of extracranial carotid artery disease is in the Fig. 1 [1].

D. Školoudík (✉)
Centre for Health Research, Department of Clinical Neurosciences, Faculty of Medicine, University of Ostrava, Ostrava, Czech Republic

T. Hrbáč
Department of Neurosurgery, University Hospital Ostrava, Ostrava, Czech Republic

Department of Anatomy, Faculty of Medicine, University of Ostrava, Ostrava, Czech Republic

M. Roubec
Department of Neurology, University Hospital Ostrava, Ostrava, Czech Republic

Current the American Heart Association/American Stroke Association (AHA/ASA) guidelines recommend [6]:

- In patients with asymptomatic carotid stenosis >70%, a joint decision between the patient and the medical team is recommended for the choice of treatment modality, which may be the best medical treatment, carotid endarterectomy or carotid artery stenting. **(class/strength of recommendation: 1; level of evidence: C—expert opinion)**
- Carotid revascularization (carotid endarterectomy or carotid artery stenting) may be indicated in addition to intensive medical therapy to reduce the risk of stroke in patients with asymptomatic atherosclerotic carotid stenosis >70% and low perioperative risk. **(class/strength of recommendation: 2b; level of evidence: B—randomized trial/s)**
- In patients with asymptomatic atherosclerotic carotid artery stenosis and high perioperative risk, the effectiveness of carotid revascularization to reduce risk of stroke is not established. **(class/strength of recommendation: 2b; level of evidence: B—non-randomized trial/s)**

2.2 Bariatric Surgery

Bariatric surgery, such as gastric bypass or sleeve gastrectomy, can lead to significant weight loss in obese patients.

Current AHA/ASA guidelines recommend [6]:

- In patients with obesity class II or higher (BMI $\geq$35.0 kg/m^2), bariatric surgery may be considered to promote weight loss and reduce the risk of stroke. Recent meta-analyses provide strong evidence that pharmacological treatments for diabetes that reduce both blood glucose and weight (i.e. glucagon-like peptide receptor agonists) and bariatric surgery in individuals with class II or III obesity, with or without diabetes, are associated with a reduction in the risk of cardiovascular events, including

V. Beneš, D. Netuka (eds.), *Surgical and Interventional Treatment of Cerebral Ischemia*,
https://doi.org/10.1007/978-3-032-08934-2_29

Table 1 Current societal guidelines for the use of CAS and CEA in asymptomatic carotid artery stenosis [1]

Organization (Ref. #)	Year of publication	CAS recommendation	"High risk for CEA" CAS recommendation	CEA recommendation	Multidisciplinary team recommendation
RACP [2]	2010	CAS should not be performed in the majority of patients	NA	CEA is gold standard	Determining suitability for procedures is often best done as a team approach
SVS [3]	2011	Insufficient data to recommend CAS	CAS should not be performed	I	No comment
AHA, ACCF [4]	2011	IIb	IIa	IIa	No comment
ESVS [5]	2017	IIb	IIb	IIa	I
ESC, ESVS [1]	2017	IIb	IIa	IIa	I

ACCF American College of Cardiology Foundation, *AHA* American Heart Association, *CAS* carotid artery stenting, *CEA* carotid endarterectomy, *ESC* European Society of Cardiology, *ESVS* European Society for Vascular Surgery, *RACP* Royal Australasian College of Physicians, *SVS* Society for Vascular Surgery

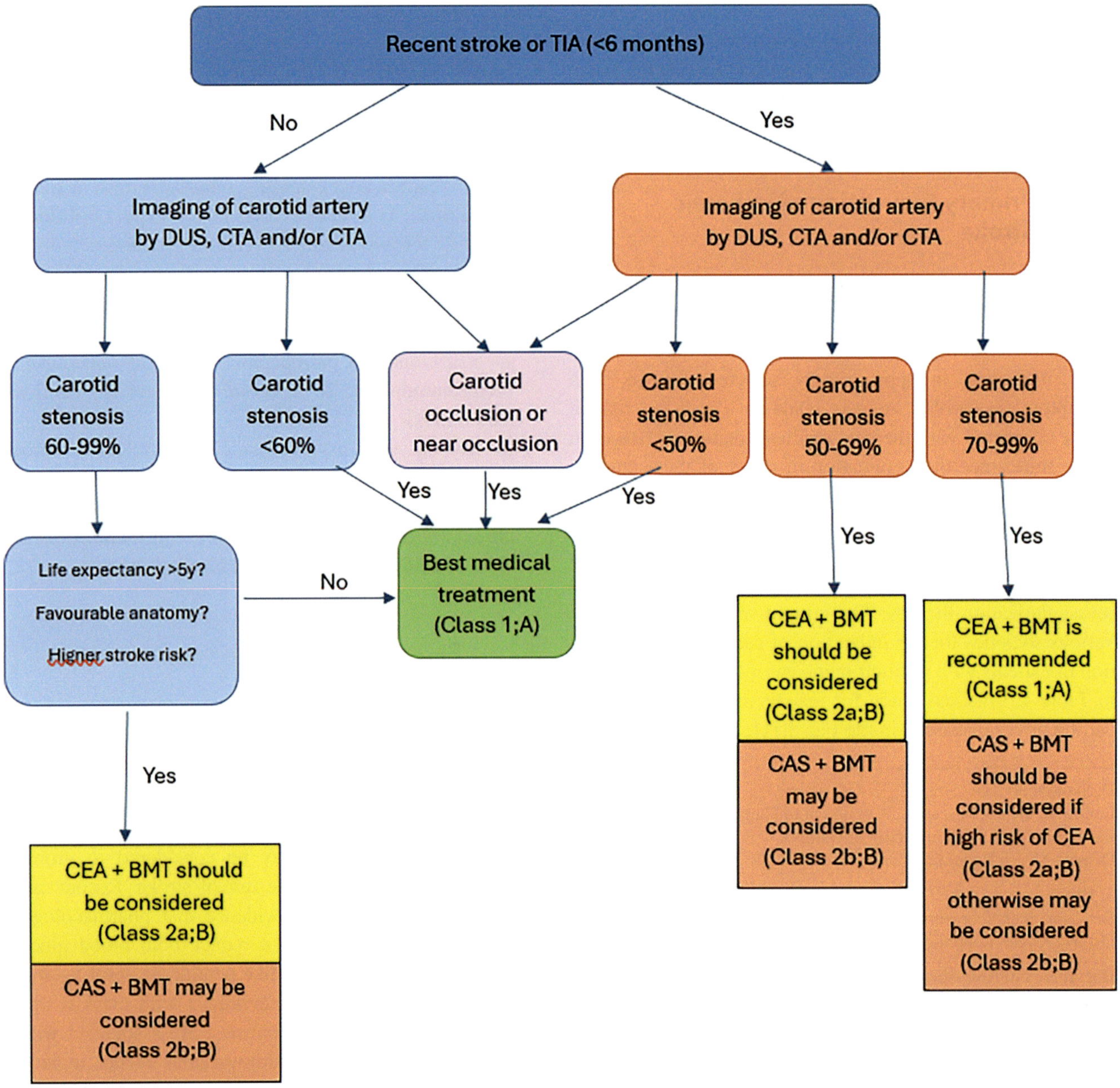

Fig. 1 Flowchart for managing patients with recent stroke or TIA (within six month after event) and extracranial carotid artery disease [1]. BMT—best medical treatment; CAS—carotid artery stenting; CEA—carotid endarterectomy; CTA—computed artery angiography; MRA—magnetic resonance angiography; TIA—transient ischemic attack

stroke, in selected patients. **(class/strength of recommendation: 2b; level of evidence: C—limited data)**

3 Acute Stroke

3.1 Decompressive Craniectomy

Brain swelling in patients with extensive territorial cerebral or cerebellar infarction can cause serious complications and even life-threatening conditions. Although less severe cerebral oedema can be managed medically, in very severe cases surgical treatment (early decompressive craniectomy) may be the only effective option which significantly reduces mortality. However, persistent morbidity is common and individual end-of-life decisions and levels of treatment should be considered in relation to the severity of neurological damage.

Current the American Heart Association/American Stroke Association (AHA/ASA) guidelines recommend [7]:

- Indication of decompressive craniectomy with dural expansion is reasonable in patients ≤60 years of age who develop neurological deterioration within 48 hours due to cerebral swelling (oedema) associated with unilateral middle cerebral artery infarction despite medical treatment. **(class/strength of recommendation: 2a; level of evidence: A)**
- Decompressive craniectomy with dural expansion may be considered in patients >60 years of age who develop neurological deterioration within 48 hours due to cerebral swelling associated with unilateral middle cerebral artery infarction despite medical treatment. **(class/strength of recommendation: 2b; level of evidence: B—randomized trial/s)**
- Ventriculostomy is recommended for the treatment of obstructive hydrocephalus in patients with cerebellar infarction. Simultaneous or subsequent decompressive craniectomy may or may not be necessary. Various factors such as infarct size, neurological status, degree of brainstem compression, and efficacy of medical treatment should be considered in making this decision. **(class/strength of recommendation: 1; level of evidence: C—limited data)**
- Decompressive suboccipital craniectomy with dural expansion should be performed in patients with cerebellar infarction who have deterioration in neurological status due to brainstem compression despite maximal medical therapy. Obstructive hydrocephalus should be treated concomitantly with ventriculostomy if deemed safe and indicated. **(class/strength of recommendation: 1; level of evidence: B—non-randomized trial/s)**

4 Secondary Prevention

4.1 Carotid Endarterectomy

Practical guide for management of extracranial carotid artery disease is in the Fig. 1 [1].

Current the American Heart Association/American Stroke Association (AHA/ASA) guidelines recommend [8]:

- Carotid endarterectomy is recommended to reduce the risk of future stroke in patients with an ipsilateral severe carotid artery stenosis 70%–99% and a transient ischemic attack or nondisabling ischemic stroke within the past 6 months; perioperative morbidity and mortality risk is estimated to be <6%. **(class/strength of recommendation: 1; level of evidence: A)**
- Carotid endarterectomy or carotid artery stenting should be performed in patients with ischemic stroke or transient ischemic attack and symptomatic extracranial carotid stenosis by operators with established periprocedural stroke and mortality rates of <6%. **(class/strength of recommendation: 1; level of evidence: A)**
- Carotid endarterectomy is recommended to reduce the risk of future stroke in patients with recent transient ischemic attack or ischemic stroke and ipsilateral moderate carotid stenosis 50%–69%, depending on patient-specific factors such as age, sex, and comorbidities, if the perioperative morbidity and mortality risk is estimated to be <6%. **(class/strength of recommendation: 1; level of evidence: B—randomized trial/s)**
- In patients ≥70 years of age with stroke or transient ischemic attack in whom carotid revascularization is being considered, it is reasonable to select carotid endarterectomy over carotid artery stenting to reduce the periprocedural stroke rate. **(class/strength of recommendation: 2a; level of evidence: B—randomized trial/s)**
- In patients in whom revascularization is planned within 1 week of the index stroke, it is reasonable to choose carotid endarterectomy over carotid artery stenting to reduce the periprocedural stroke rate. **(class/strength of recommendation: 2a; level of evidence: B—randomized trial/s)**
- When revascularization is indicated in patients with transient ischemic attack or nondisabling stroke, it is reasonable to perform the procedure within 2 weeks of the index event rather than delay surgery to increase the likelihood of stroke-free outcome. **(class/strength of recommendation: 2a; level of evidence: C—limited data)**
- In patients with symptomatic severe carotid stenosis ≥70% in whom anatomic or medical conditions probably increase the risk for surgery (such as radiation-induced stenosis or restenosis after carotid endarterectomy) it is

reasonable to choose carotid artery stenting to reduce the periprocedural complication rate. **(class/strength of recommendation: 2a; level of evidence: C—limited data)**

- Carotid artery stenting may be considered as an alternative to carotid endarterectomy for stroke prevention in patients with a symptomatic carotid stenosis ≥70% by non-invasive imaging or >50% by catheter-based imaging and average or low risk of complications associated with endovascular intervention and the anticipated rate of periprocedural stroke or death <6%, particularly in patients with significant cardiovascular comorbidities predisposing to cardiovascular complications with endarterectomy. **(class/strength of recommendation: 2b; level of evidence: A)**
- In patients with a recent stroke or transient ischemic attack in the past 6 months, the usefulness of transcarotid artery revascularization for prevention of recurrent stroke and transient ischemic attack is uncertain. **(class/strength of recommendation: 2b; level of evidence: B—nonrandomized trial/s)**
- Revascularization (carotid endarterectomy or carotid artery stenting) to reduce the risk of future stroke is not recommended in patients with recent transient ischemic attack or ischemic stroke and carotid artery stenosis <50%. **(class/strength of recommendation: 3—no benefit; level of evidence: A)**

4.2 Extracranial-Intracranial Bypass Surgery

Current the American Heart Association/American Stroke Association (AHA/ASA) guidelines recommend [8]:

- Extracranial-intracranial bypass surgery is not recommended in patients with stroke or transient ischemic attack in the territory of stenosis 50%–99% or occlusion of a major intracranial artery. **(class/strength of recommendation: 3—no benefit; level of evidence: B—randomized trial/s)**
- Extracranial-intracranial bypass surgery is not recommended in patients with a recent (within 120 days) transient ischemic attack or ischemic stroke ipsilateral to atherosclerotic stenosis or occlusion of the middle cerebral artery or carotid artery. **(class/strength of recommendation: 3—no benefit; level of evidence: A)**
- In patients with moyamoya disease and a history of ischemic stroke or transient ischemic attack, surgical revascularization with direct or indirect extracranial-intracranial bypass can be beneficial for the prevention of ischemic stroke or transient ischemic attack. **(class/strength of recommendation: 2a; level of evidence: C—limited data)**

4.3 Surgery for Vertebral Artery Stenosis

Current the American Heart Association/American Stroke Association (AHA/ASA) guidelines recommend [8]:

- In patients with ischemic stroke or transient ischemic attack in the territory of an extracranial vertebral artery stenosis who are having symptoms despite optimal medical treatment, the usefulness of open surgical procedures, including vertebral endarterectomy and vertebral artery transposition, is not well established. **(class/strength of recommendation: 2b; level of evidence: C—expert opinion)**

4.4 Bariatric Surgery

Current the American Heart Association/American Stroke Association (AHA/ASA) guidelines recommend [8]:

- In overweight or obese patients with ischemic stroke or transient ischemic attack, weight loss is recommended to improve the ASCVD risk factor profile. **(class/strength of recommendation: 2b; level of evidence: B—nonrandomized trial/s)**
- Obesity can be treated with intensive behavioural counselling to change eating patterns, medications that reduce appetite, and metabolic surgery. Observational research provides some evidence that weight loss after bariatric surgery may reduce risk for stroke [9, 10].

4.5 Cardiac Surgery

Current the American Heart Association/American Stroke Association (AHA/ASA) guidelines recommend [8]:

- In patients with ischemic stroke or transient ischemic attack and infective endocarditis who present with recurrent emboli and persistent vegetations despite appropriate antibiotic therapy, early surgery (during initial hospitalization before completion of a full therapeutic course of antibiotics) is reasonable to reduce the risk of recurrent embolism if there is no evidence of intracranial hemorrhage or extensive neurological damage. **(class/strength of recommendation: 2b; level of evidence: B—nonrandomized trial/s)**
- In patients with ischemic stroke or transient ischemic attack and native left-sided valve endocarditis who exhibit mobile vegetations >10 mm in length, early surgery (during initial hospitalization before completion of a full therapeutic course of antibiotics) may be considered to reduce the risk of recurrent embolism if there is no evidence of

intracranial hemorrhage or extensive neurological damage. **(class/strength of recommendation: 2b; level of evidence: B—non-randomized trial/s)**

- In patients with ischemic stroke or transient ischemic attack and infective endocarditis, early valve surgery (during initial hospitalization before completion of a full therapeutic course of antibiotics) may be considered in patients with an indication for surgery who have no evidence of intracranial hemorrhage or extensive neurological damage. **(class/strength of recommendation: 2b; level of evidence: B—non-randomized trial/s)**
- In patients with infective endocarditis and major ischemic stroke, delaying valve surgery for at least 4 weeks may be considered for patients with infective endocarditis and major ischemic stroke or intracranial hemorrhage if the patient is hemodynamically stable. **(class/strength of recommendation: 2b; level of evidence: B—non-randomized trial/s)**
- Indications and timing for surgical interventions in patients with infective endocarditis and stroke or transient ischemic attack depend on multiple factors, including recurrent events while on antibiotic therapy, size of the vegetation, and presence of associated intracranial hemorrhage [11].

In patients with stroke or TIA found to have a left-sided cardiac tumor, resection of the tumor can be beneficial to reduce the risk of recurrent stroke. **(class/strength of recommendation: 2a; level of evidence: C—limited data)**

Declarations

Competing Interests The author(s) has no competing interests to declare that are relevant to the content of this manuscript.

Ethics Approval The author(s) declares that this manuscript does not include primary research with human participants.

References

1. Aboyans V, Ricco J-B, Bartelink M-LEL, Björck M, Brodmann M, Cohnert T, Collet J-P, Czerny M, De Carlo M, Debus S, Espinola-Klein C, Kahan T, Kownator S, Mazzolai L, Naylor AR, Roffi M, Röther J, Sprynger M, Tendera M, Tepe G, Venermo M, Vlachopoulos C, Desormais I, ESC Scientific Document Group. 2017 ESC guidelines on the Diagnosis and Treatment of Peripheral Arterial Diseases, in collaboration with the European Society for Vascular Surgery (ESVS): document covering atherosclerotic disease of extracranial carotid and vertebral, mesenteric, renal, upper and lower extremity arteries. Endorsed by: the European Stroke Organization (ESO), the Task Force for the Diagnosis and Treatment of Peripheral Arterial Diseases of the European Society of Cardiology (ESC) and of the European Society for Vascular Surgery (ESVS). Eur Heart J. 2018b;39(9):763–816.
2. Carotid Stenting Guidelines Committee, Bladin C, Chambers B, New G, Denton M, Lawrence-Brown M. Guidelines for patient selection and performance of carotid artery stenting. ANZ J Surg. 2010;80(6):398–405.
3. Ricotta JJ, Aburahma A, Ascher E, Eskandari M, Faries P, Lal BK, Society for Vascular Surgery. Updated Society for Vascular Surgery guidelines for management of extracranial carotid disease. J Vasc Surg. 2011;54(3):e1–31.
4. Brott TG, Halperin JL, Abbara S, Bacharach JM, Barr JD, Bush RL, Cates CU, Creager MA, Fowler SB, Friday G, Hertzberg VS, McIff EB, Moore WS, Panagos PD, Riles TS, Rosenwasser RH, Taylor AJ, American College of Cardiology Foundation/American Heart Association Task Force on Practice Guidelines; American Stroke Association; American Association of Neuroscience Nurses; American Association of Neurological Surgeons; American College of Radiology; American Society of Neuroradiology; Congress of Neurological Surgeons; Society of Atherosclerosis Imaging and Prevention; Society for Cardiovascular Angiography and Interventions; Society of Interventional Radiology; Society of NeuroInterventional Surgery; Society for Vascular Medicine; Society for Vascular Surgery; American Academy of Neurology and Society of Cardiovascular Computed Tomography. 2011 ASA/ACCF/AHA/AANN/AANS/ACR/ASNR/CNS/SAIP/SCAI/SIR/SNIS/SVM/SVS guideline on the management of patients with extracranial carotid and vertebral artery disease. Stroke. 2011;42(8):e464–540.
5. Naylor AR, Ricco JB, de Borst GJ, Debus S, de Haro J, Halliday A, Hamilton G, Kakisis J, Kakkos S, Lepidi S, Markus HS, McCabe DJ, Roy J, Sillesen H, van den Berg JC, Vermassen F, ESVS Guidelines Committee, Kolh P, Chakfe N, Hinchliffe RJ, Koncar I, Lindholt JS, Vega de Ceniga M, Verzini F, ESVS Guideline Reviewers, Archie J, Bellmunt S, Chaudhuri A, Koelemay M, Lindahl AK, Padberg F, Venermo M. Editor's choice—Management of Atherosclerotic Carotid and Vertebral Artery Disease: 2017 clinical practice guidelines of the European Society for Vascular Surgery (ESVS). Eur J Vasc Endovasc Surg. 2018;55(1):3–81.
6. Bushnell C, Kernan WN, Sharrief AZ, Chaturvedi S, Cole JW, Cornwell WK 3rd, Cosby-Gaither C, Doyle S, Goldstein LB, Lennon O, Levine DA, Love M, Miller E, Nguyen-Huynh M, Rasmussen-Winkler J, Rexrode KM, Rosendale N, Sarma S, Shimbo D, Simpkins AN, Spatz ES, Sun LR, Tangpricha V, Turnage D, Velazquez G, Whelton PK. 2024 Guideline for the primary prevention of stroke: a guideline from the American Heart Association/American Stroke Association. Stroke. 2024;55(12):e344–424.
7. Powers WJ, Rabinstein AA, Ackerson T, Adeoye OM, Bambakidis NC, Becker K, Biller J, Brown M, Demaerschalk BM, Hoh B, Jauch EC, Kidwell CS, Leslie-Mazwi TM, Ovbiagele B, Scott PA, Sheth KN, Southerland AM, Summers DV, Tirschwell DL. Guidelines for the early management of patients with acute ischemic stroke: 2019 update to the 2018 guidelines for the early management of acute ischemic stroke: a guideline for healthcare professionals from the American Heart Association/American Stroke Association. Stroke. 2019;50(12):e344–418.
8. Kleindorfer DO, Towfighi A, Chaturvedi S, Cockroft KM, Gutierrez J, Lombardi-Hill D, Kamel H, Kernan WN, Kittner SJ, Leira EC, Lennon O, Meschia JF, Nguyen TN, Pollak PM, Santangeli P, Sharrief AZ, Smith SC Jr, Turan TN, Williams LS. 2021 Guideline for the prevention of stroke in patients with stroke and transient ischemic attack: a guideline from the American Heart Association/American Stroke Association. Stroke. 2021;52(7):e364–467.
9. Fisher DP, Johnson E, Haneuse S, Arterburn D, Coleman KJ, O'Connor PJ, O'Brien R, Bogart A, Theis MK, Anau J, et al. Association between bariatric surgery and macrovascular disease outcomes in patients with type 2 diabetes and severe obesity. JAMA. 2018;320:1570–82.

10. Sjöström L, Peltonen M, Jacobson P, Sjöström CD, Karason K, Wedel H, Ahlin S, Anveden Ĺ, Bengtsson C, Bergmark G, et al. Bariatric surgery and long-term cardiovascular events. JAMA. 2012;307:56–65.
11. Otto CM, Nishimura RA, Bonow RO, Carabello BA, Erwin JP 3rd, Gentile F, Jneid H, Krieger EV, Mack M, McLeod C, et al. 2020 ACC/AHA guideline for the management of patients with valvular heart disease: a report of the American College of Cardiology/American Heart Association Joint Committee on clinical practice guidelines. Circulation. 2021;143:e72–e227.

Decompressive Surgery in Ischemic Stroke

Jan Mraček and Vladimír Přibáň

Abbreviations

ACA	Anterior Cerebral Artery
ADC	Apparent Diffusion Coefficient
AHA	American Heart Association
ARR	Absolute Risk Reduction
ASA	American Stroke Association
ASPECTS	Alberta Stroke Program Early CT Score
ATP	Adenosine Triphosphate
CBF	Cerebral Blood Flow
CPP	Cerebral Perfusion Pressure
CSF	Cerebrospinal Fluid
CT	Computed Tomography
DC	Decompressive Craniectomy
DWI	Diffusion-Weighted Imaging
EEG	Electroencephalography
EVD	External Ventricular Drainage
GCS	Glasgow Coma Scale
ICG	Indocyanine-Green
ICP	Intracranial Pressure
IVT	Intravenous Thrombolysis
MCA	Middle Cerebral Artery
MCI	Malignant Cerebellar Infarction
MHI	Malignant Hemispheric Infarction
MRI	Magnetic Resonance Imaging
mRS	Modified Rankin Scale
MT	Mechanical Thrombectomy
NIHSS	National Institute of Health Stroke Scale
NNT	Number Needed to Treat
PCA	Posterior Cerebral Artery
QOL	Quality Of Life
RCTs	Randomized Controlled Trials
SDC	Suboccipital Decompressive Craniectomy
SSI	Surgical Site Infection
TBI	Traumatic Brain Injury
TCD	Transcranial Doppler Sonography
VP	Ventriculo-Peritoneal

J. Mraček (✉) · V. Přibáň
Faculty of Medicine in Pilsen, Charles University, University Hospital Pilsen, Department of Neurosurgery, Pilsen, Czech Republic
e-mail: mracek@fnplzen.cz; pribanv@fnplzen.cz

1 Introduction

Large vessel occlusion ischemic stroke, or large hemispheric infarction, or space-occupying middle cerebral artery (MCA) infarction accounts for approximately 10% of all ischemic strokes. It is defined as a stroke affecting the whole or most of the MCA territory, with or without involvement of the anterior cerebral artery (ACA) or posterior cerebral artery (PCA) territories. The term "malignant hemispheric infarction" (MHI) was introduced in 1996 and describes a severe hemispheric syndrome with a predictable fatal clinical course [1]. Characteristic symptoms of MHI include hemiplegia, hemianesthesia, hemianopia, eye and head deviation, pupillary dilatation, and unconsciousness [1]. The cause of clinical deterioration is space-occupying cerebral edema accompanying the infarcted area. Although MHI represents a minority of ischemic strokes, it is responsible for up to 96% of post-stroke mortality [2]. Malignant cerebral edema progresses over 2–5 days, with clinical deterioration typically occurring after 48 hours from the onset of the infarct [3, 4]. Despite aggressive nonoperative management, MHI has a mortality rate of up to 80% [1, 5]. Due to the failure of conservative therapy and the space-occupying effect of MHI, attention has turned to the historical technique of decompressive craniectomy (DC). The idea of decompressive craniectomy dates back to the early twentieth century, when Harvey Cushing described primary and secondary brain injuries occurring during the immediate (vascular injury), intermediate (lucid interval), and late (development of brain edema) phases of traumatic brain injury. He recommended performing DC under muscle cover in the subtemporal or suboccipital regions [6, 7]. One of the first to recognize the importance of DC in the management of intracranial

V. Beneš, D. Netuka (eds.), *Surgical and Interventional Treatment of Cerebral Ischemia*,
https://doi.org/10.1007/978-3-032-08934-2_30

hypertension was Theodor Kocher ("if there is no cerebrospinal fluid pressure, but brain pressure exists, then pressure relief must be achieved by opening the skull") [8]. In 1901, Joseph Babinski described the resolution of optic nerve papilledema after performing DC [9]. The parallel between the space-occupying manifestations of traumatic brain injury (TBI) described by Cushing and the space-occupying manifestations of MHI is evident. The first reports of using DC for extensive ischemic encephalomalacia, mimicking both clinical and radiological manifestations of a brain tumor, date back to the early 1950s [10, 11]. In the early 1970s, Ivamoto et al. demonstrated the convincing alleviating effect of DC on intracranial hypertension in MHI and published the first systematic review of DC in both hemispheric and cerebellar malignant infarctions [12].

Even though cerebellar infarction was initially described in 1938 [12], the first documented cases of suboccipital decompressive craniectomy (SDC) did not appear until 1956 [13, 14]. Since the 1970s, malignant cerebellar infarction (MCI) has been treated as a neurosurgical emergency, with SDC becoming a standard procedure [15].

DC has experienced a resurgence in both the treatment of traumatic brain injury and space-occupying ischemic stroke.

Despite compelling evidence of the benefits of DC, the procedure remains underutilized and does not match the incidence of MHI [16, 17]. However, the use of DC began to increase in the early 2000s, driven by randomized controlled trials (RCTs) that demonstrated its convincing benefits. This trend started to reverse in 2015 following a change in guidelines that established mechanical thrombectomy (MT) as the standard of care for patients with salvageable stroke tissue at risk [18–20]. Early revascularization should preserve viable brain tissue and reduce cerebral edema, which would thereby decrease the need for DC [18]. Surprisingly, the meta-analysis by Wo et al. demonstrated an association between the reduced risk of malignant edema and successful revascularization, but not with the administration of intravenous thrombolysis (IVT) or MT [21]. Large cohort studies, however, confirm a decrease in the incidence of malignant infarcts and a reduction of up to 50% in the need for DC due to the increasing use of MT [18, 20, 22, 23]. This discrepancy is explained by differences in baseline characteristics among the randomized, observational, and cohort studies.

2 Pathophysiology of Malignant Stroke

The occlusion of a major artery leads to a severe disruption of cerebral blood flow (CBF) throughout the affected vascular territory. The impairment of CBF results in neuronal death at the center of the lesion, occurring through necrosis, apoptosis, and autophagy [24]. This so-called ischemic core is surrounded by an area of tissue at critical risk [25]. This region, known as the penumbra, is characterized by the potential for functional recovery without morphological damage. The penumbral zone has reduced blood flow, and without timely reperfusion, it transforms into ischemic core tissue. While the ischemic core is beyond recovery, the penumbra represents potentially salvageable brain tissue, which is the focus of all therapeutic efforts.

In the core tissue, the restricted supply of glucose and oxygen forces cells to shift to anaerobic metabolism, leading to a shortage of adenosine triphosphate (ATP)—the primary energy source. This results in ischemia-induced energy failure. Simultaneously, excessive release of glutamate occurs, further worsening the ionic imbalance and contributing to excitotoxicity. As a result of hypoxia and subsequent reoxygenation, free radicals are generated, causing oxidative stress and ultimately the degradation of cellular molecules. The pathological process also involves an inflammatory response, with microglial activation leading to further neuronal damage. The failure of energy-dependent ion pumps leads to an influx of sodium and calcium into the cells, and an increase in extracellular potassium concentration. The physiological electrolyte balance is disturbed, water is drawn into the cells, and subsequent cytotoxic brain edema develops. In the next phase of brain infarction, proteolytic enzymes compromise the blood-brain barrier by degrading the basal lamina. The subsequent intake of serum proteins and additional fluids leads to the development of vasogenic brain edema. This late-phase edema reaches its peak 2–4 days after the onset of the stroke. A key factor in continuously stimulating this molecular-biochemical pathological cascade is likely cortical spreading depression, which may therefore also play an important role in secondary brain damage during malignant infarction [26–28].

The mass effect of a malignant stroke leads to a horizontal shift of midline structures, brain herniation with compression of the brainstem, and intracranial hypertension. Increased intracranial pressure can cause secondary brain ischemia by reducing CBF, leading to brain tissue hypoxia. Direct cerebrovascular compression may result in secondary infarctions, especially in the territory of the posterior and anterior cerebral arteries. The shift of the brainstem can cause stretching and tearing of the perforating arteries of the basilar artery, resulting in brainstem hemorrhage. These so-called Duret hemorrhages indicate irreversible brainstem damage and signify a fatal progression of the infarction [29].

3 Early Predictors of Malignant Brain Edema

Since the publication of key randomized studies, great emphasis has been placed on identifying early predictors of malignant brain edema, thus enabling the identification of high-risk patients who would benefit from decompressive craniectomy. These findings would be particularly helpful in medical centers where neurosurgical or neurocritical care services may not be readily available [30]. Predictors that have been tested include clinical, imaging, and laboratory characteristics.

Laboratory biomarkers that have been studied so far include glucose level, red and white blood cell counts, platelet count, hemoglobin level, creatinine, C-reactive protein, S-100B protein, and fibrinogen. No reliable correlation has yet been proven between any of these tested serum biomarkers and the development of malignant edema [30, 31].

MHI is characterized by severe neurological deficits. Consequently, it was expected that patients with more severe neurological deficits would be more likely to develop malignant cerebral edema [29]. A correlation was identified between malignant edema and clinical stroke features observed within 24 hours, including high National Institute of Health Stroke Scale (NIHSS) scores, impaired consciousness, gaze palsy, nausea, vomiting, and ventilation use [29]. The authors proposed a narrower range of NIHSS cutoff scores, specifically 15–17, to distinguish patients at risk for malignant edema from general stroke patients.

Another clear predictor of malignant edema is younger age. Age-related brain atrophy, which provides some buffering space for brain edema, is absent in younger patients. As a result, brain edema in younger patients tends to be malignant. However, a definitive cutoff age for predicting malignant edema has not been established [21, 32, 33].

Imaging plays an essential role in predicting the development of malignant stroke and in the early indication for DC. In most institutions, computed tomography (CT) is the first diagnostic procedure for patients with acute stroke. Early hypodensity occupying more than one half of the MCA territory is an important predictor of malignant edema [34]. Additional features include the appearance of edema within 6 hours, basal ganglia involvement, involvement of other vascular territories, carotid T occlusion, poor collateral blood flow, dens MCA sign, infarct volume >220 ml, and midline shift >5 mm within the first 48 hours [35, 36]. The risk of a malignant course can be estimated using ASPECTS (Alberta Stroke Program Early CT score), where a score of 7 was the cutoff for predicting the development of malignant infarction with 50% sensitivity and 86% specificity [37]. Along with CT angiography, perfusion CT offers robust capabilities for predicting edema. Early involvement of more than two-thirds of the MCA territory on CT perfusion maps predicts a malignant course with 92% sensitivity and 94% specificity [38].

Magnetic resonance imaging (MRI) is significantly more sensitive than CT in detecting early ischemic changes. A diffusion-weighted imaging (DWI) lesion volume greater than 145 ml within 14 hours of stroke predicts malignant infarction with 100% sensitivity and 94% specificity [39]. However, the determination of this volume depends on the threshold of apparent diffusion coefficient (ADC) reduction used for DWI evaluation [40].

Transcranial Doppler sonography (TCD) may also be used to assess brain edema and midline shift. A correlation between midline shift assessment via TCD and CT has been demonstrated. An elevated pulsatility index measured by TCD correlates with midline shift and intracranial hypertension [41, 42].

The systematic review and meta-analysis by Wu et al. demonstrated that younger age, higher NIHSS score, and larger parenchymal hypoattenuation on CT are reliable early predictors of malignant edema after ischemic stroke.

4 Medical Management of Malignant Stroke

Best medical treatment of patients with malignant infarction is not well defined and follows general measures for controlling intracranial pressure (ICP). Osmotherapy with Manitol or hypertonic saline, head elevation, neutral neck position, artificial ventilation and short-term hyperventilation, blood pressure control, treat seizures, maintenance of normal body temperature, blood glucose and intravascular volume are recommended to decrease ICP. Clinical trial evidence to support these strategies is, however, unavailable. Best medical management in deteriorating patients acts as a bridge to more definitive decompressive surgery [29, 43].

A phase III randomized controlled trial is currently underway to assess the effect of glibenclamide (glyburide) on functional outcomes in patients with MHI. Glibenclamide, a sulfonylurea initially approved for use in diabetes mellitus, is expected to have an inhibitory effect on brain edema formation. The phase II trial evaluating glibenclamide demonstrated a significant reduction in midline shift and significantly lower rates of neurological decline [44–46].

5 Technical Aspects of Decompressive Hemicraniectomy

Malignant MCA infarction typically affects one cerebral hemisphere, and the optimal surgical technique is therefore decompressive hemicraniectomy (Fig. 1a, b). The patient is usually operated on in the supine position with the head rotated contralaterally. A wide question mark-shaped incision is made from the rostral hairline near the middle of the forehead to the zygoma. The scalp, along with the temporal muscle, is dissected from the skull, thereby widely exposing it. Several burr holes are placed along the margins of the planned craniectomy. To achieve sufficient decompressive effect, it is necessary to perform temporal osteoclastic

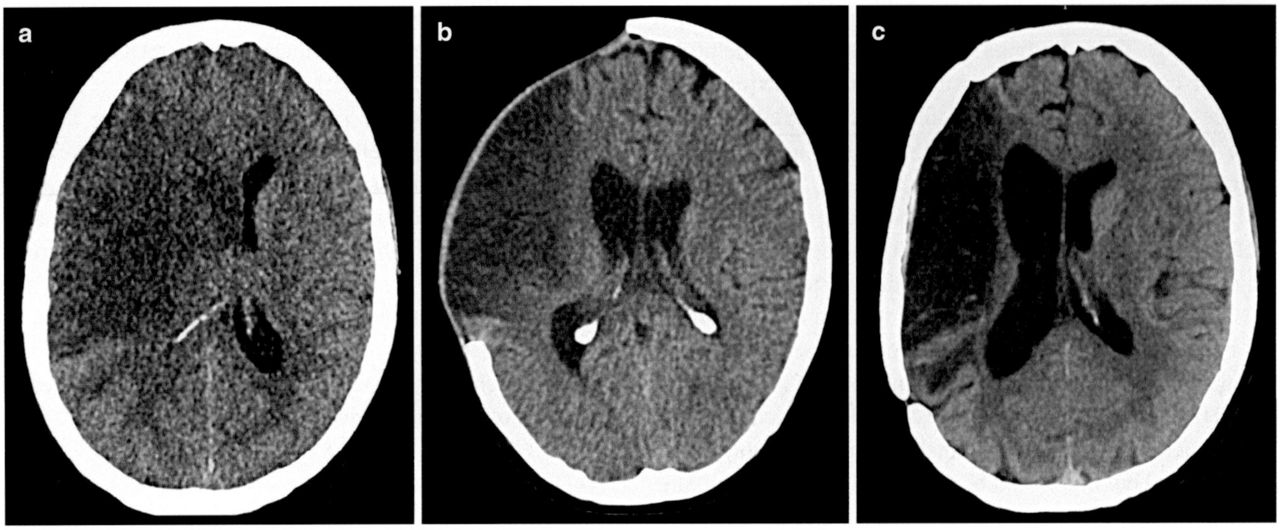

Fig. 1 CT scans documenting the surgical management of malignant hemispheric infarction. (**a**) Preoperative CT showing a partially demarcated malignant MCA infarction with a midline shift; (**b**) Postoperative CT showing the effect of decompressive hemicraniectomy. The cerebral hemisphere is decompressed, and the midline shift has resolved; (**c**) Postcranioplasty CT showing postischemic changes with atrophy of the left hemisphere and compensatory dilation of the lateral ventricle

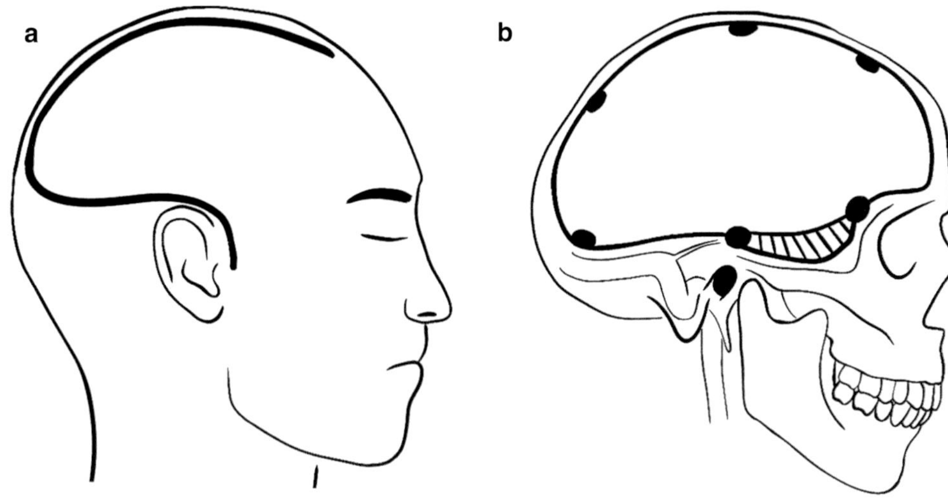

Fig. 2 An operative technique of decompressive hemicraniectomy. (**a**) A typical question mark-shaped skin incision; (**b**) The connections of burr holes for craniectomy, with additional osteoclastic decompression of the middle cranial fossa floor and the sphenoid wing

decompression to expose the entire temporal lobe down to the temporal cranial base (Fig. 2). Postoperative patency of the mesencephalic cisterns significantly correlates with the cranio-caudal diameter of the craniectomy [47].

The size of the craniectomy is recommended to be at least 15 cm from anterior to posterior and 12 cm from superior to inferior, as data support more reliable reduction of transtentorial herniation and improved outcomes with larger craniectomy [48, 49]. On the other hand, recent data have not shown that a larger craniectomy (>14 cm) improves long-term outcome in MHI [50]. The minimum size of the craniectomy, which guarantees the prevention of herniation damage to the brain, is 12 cm (Fig. 3). This threshold was also used in the methodology of RCTs [51–53].

The dura is opened in a C-shaped, U-shaped, or stellate pattern (Fig. 3). An expansile duraplasty using either a pericranial graft or dural substitutes should be performed. Meticulous hemostasis is essential. The temporal muscle is reapproximated and loosely placed over the duraplasty. A subgaleal drain is optional but preferred. The scalp is closed in two layers, with absorbable sutures for the galea and staples for the skin.

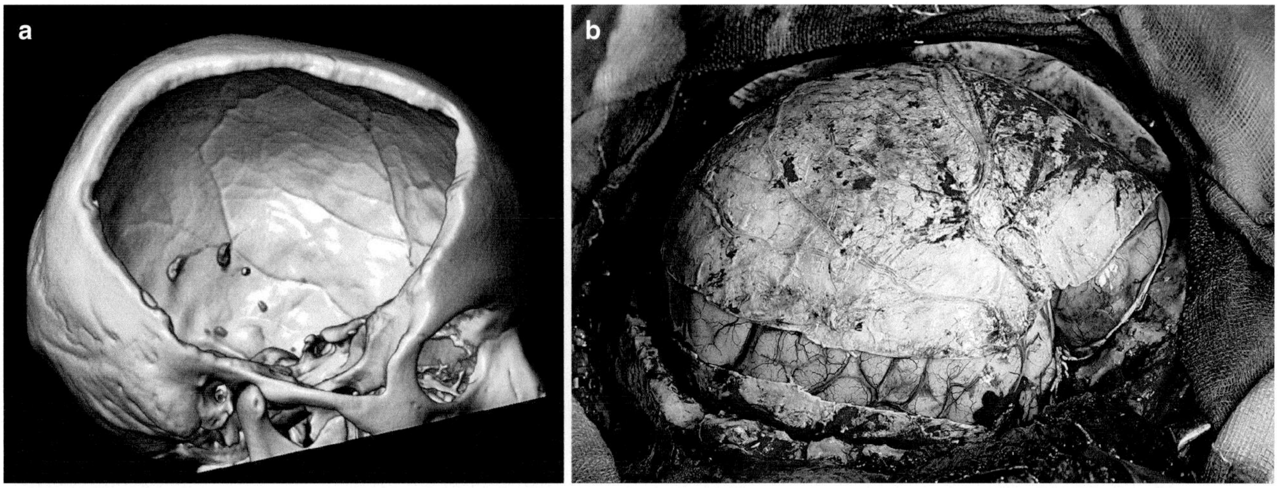

Fig. 3 An operative technique of decompressive hemicraniectomy. (**a**) Three-dimensional reconstruction of a skull showing a hemicraniectomy defect; (**b**) Intraoperative photograph illustrating an open "U"-shaped durotomy

6 Additional and Alternative Procedures to Decompressive Hemicraniectomy

Decompressive craniectomy alone may be inadequate in some cases. In these instances, it is necessary to use additional surgical techniques to reduce intracranial pressure [54]. One option is a resection of the temporal muscle, which creates additional space for the expanding edematous hemisphere. However, the benefit of this supportive technique has not been conclusively proven [22, 55].

Strokectomy, the resection of ischemic brain tissue, is another alternative technique for reducing intracranial pressure, which can be performed either as an adjuvant or alternative to DC. It is routinely used in cases of malignant cerebellar infarctions [13–15]. The rationale behind strokectomy is the resection of a sufficient amount of infarcted brain tissue, which should eliminate the deleterious mass effect of malignant edema. Strokectomy allows for the immediate replacement of the bone flap, thus avoiding cranioplasty. Additionally, partial resection of the temporal lobe immediately relieves brainstem compression. The disadvantage of strokectomy lies, on one hand, in the potential insufficient decompressive effect, and on the other hand, in the risk of resecting tissue within the penumbra that might still be salvageable. Intraoperative mapping with indocyanine-green (ICG) videoangiography and flow analysis of the penumbra region may assist in determining the indication and extent of strokectomy. Supratentorial resection of infarcted tissue, especially in the case of the dominant hemisphere, can also be risky with regard to eloquent areas. Nonetheless, a recent meta-analysis of current evidence showed that strokectomy for MHI may be non-inferior to hemicraniectomy [56]. Strokectomy has certain advantages, such as lower risk, cost savings, and the avoidance of bone reconstruction and its sequelae [56].

The influx of cerebrospinal fluid (CSF) from the cisterns into the brain tissue plays a major role in edema formation both in TBI and MHI patients. This so-called shift induces edema is the earliest contributor to edema formation. Spreading depolarization, which is triggered by the constriction of cerebral arteries and reduced cerebral blood flow, is a likely cause of this process [22]. Cisternostomy, a method that involves the opening of the frontobasal cisterns and the Sylvian fissure, has the potential to target this approach. It can be performed alone or in combination with decompressive craniectomy. While some studies have recommended cisternostomy for TBI, there is no data confirming its benefit for MHI [57, 58]. Moreover, the primary indication for an alternative surgical procedure, such as strokectomy or cisternostomy, when reliable evidence already supports the efficacy of DC, remains highly controversial.

A parenchymal ICP monitor or multimodal neuromonitoring are optional. There are some controversies surrounding ICP in MHI patients. ICP monitoring in stroke patients may not always be valid. Due to intracranial pressure gradients, the ICP may not reflect ongoing expansive processes, and global ICP can be underestimated. Pupillary abnormalities and signs of brain herniations are sometimes present despite normal ICP [59]. ICP monitoring may help guide treatment of intracranial hypertension in patients who are not indicated for surgery [22]. In patients who did not have significant consciousness impairment before surgery, early extubation without gagging is therefore preferred. In cases of ongoing sedation and mechanical ventilation, ICP monitoring is necessary, as it can alert to elevated ICP and the need for therapeutic intervention. Elevated ICP after DC is still an issue, occurring in 25–72% of malignant MCA strokes [54,

59–62]. Impaired cerebral autoregulation, which is common in MHI patients, is a reason for strict maintenance of cerebral perfusion pressure (CPP) within the physiological range. Both increases and decreases in CPP can have serious negative consequences.

7 Complications of Decompressive Hemicraniectomy

Although DC is considered a simple procedure, it is accompanied by a plethora of complications. In addition to the complications of DC, the complications of the subsequent cranioplasty should also be considered [63]. No prospective study assessing the occurrence of complications after DC has been published until now. Most publications have focused on complications in TBI patients. While complications of DC following brain injury are significantly associated with poor outcomes, this has not been demonstrated in stroke patients [64, 65]. Some findings in imaging studies can be considered a consequence of the primary injury or natural sequelae of the DC, rather than a complication of the procedure [65].

From a pathophysiological perspective, DC complications can be divided into hemorrhagic, wound healing-related complications, CSF—related complications, and seizures [63].

Malignant stroke patients are considered a high-risk group for hemorrhagic complications due to antiplatelet medication and IVT. However, it has been shown that only antiplatelet therapy, not IVT or MT, is a risk factor for hemorrhage [66–68]. Hemorrhagic transformation of the ischemic lesion occurs in 30–60% of cases, but a large proportion of them are present even before decompression. It has also not been proven that hemorrhagic transformation has a significant impact on outcomes [67].

The incidence of surgical site infection (SSI) after DC is comparable to that of craniotomies overall. It ranges between 5% and 7% [69]. The risk of SSI increases with the use of artificial dural substitutes [70]. Superficial skin infections may accompany skin necrosis caused by devascularization of the scalp flap. In addition to preserving the superficial temporal artery, proper vascularization of the scalp flap depends on following the base-to-pedicle ratio rule of more than 1 (the with of the flap's base must be wider than its length).

CSF-related complications are mostly delayed and include CSF fistulas, hydrocephalus, hygroma formation (subdural/epidural effusion), the syndrome of the trephined, and paradoxical herniation. There are more data available regarding DC in TBI patients concerning these events. The incidence of hydrocephalus after DC ranges from 0.7% to 86%, depending on the diagnostic criteria and classification [71]. Surprisingly, hydrocephalus occurs most frequently after DC in stroke patients (25.5%) [63, 72]. Alteration of CSF dynamics after hemicraniectomy is the primary cause of both hydrocephalus and hygroma formation. The occurrence of hygromas precedes hydrocephalus and correlates with its subsequent development [73]. After cranioplasty, both hydrocephalus and subdural effusion usually resolve spontaneously. However, 10% of patients with persistent hydrocephalus after cranioplasty require a ventriculoperitoneal shunt [74].

A long-term complication associated with CSF disturbances is trephine syndrome, also known as sinking skin flap syndrome. The pathophysiology of this syndrome is due to the direct effect of atmospheric pressure on the exposed cerebral hemisphere. Alterations in CSF circulation, cortical blood perfusion, and venous drainage occur. The syndrome is characterized by nonspecific symptoms, including headaches, dizziness, irritability, and memory and concentration disorders, accompanied by a sunken hemicraniectomy defect [75]. The so-called paradoxical herniation can be considered the most severe form of sinking skin flap syndrome. Atmospheric pressure on the open intracranial compartment leads to paradoxical downward herniation of the brain. The negative pressure gradient between the intracranial and spinal compartments can be provoked by vertical positioning, lumbar puncture, ventriculo-peritoneal (VP) shunting, administration of mannitol, or hyperventilation [76]. Both trephine syndrome and paradoxical herniation resolve after cranioplasty.

The incidence of seizures after DC in MHI patients ranges between 50–60%, and epilepsy occurs in 45–53% of cases [77, 78]. Seizures are a long-term complication characterized by a clustering of events after cranioplasty.

Mechanical damage to the brain or venous infarcts due to shear injury and impingement of cortical veins against bony edges is a concern in patients with suboptimally sized hemicraniectomy [79]. In such cases, it is referred to as mushroom cup-like herniation [80].

8 Cranioplasty

After decompressive craniectomy, cranial reconstruction is required (Fig. 1c). To date, no prospective data have been published to determine the optimal timing for cranioplasty. This issue remains controversial. Cranioplasty alleviates neurological symptoms, restores brain protection, aesthetics, and also has a positive psychosocial impact [81–85]. Either an autologous bone flap, which has been frozen or subcutaneously preserved, can be replanted, or various alloplastic materials can be used. So far, no consensus has been reported regarding the best material for cranioplasty [86]. Currently, all allogeneic materials allow for the design of personalized skull implants that provide an excellent cosmetic outcome, but their positive influence on clinical outcomes has not yet been proven [86]. Despite being technically straightforward, cranioplasty is associated with a high complication rate of 15–30% [87]. The two most serious and common complications of cranioplasty are SSI and bone flap resorption. When considering decompressive craniectomy, it is essential to account for both the risks of decompression and the high complication rate associated with subsequent cranioplasty. However, no RCTs included the morbidity of cranioplasty in the final clinical outcome.

9 Randomised Controlled Trials

A number of studies investigating the role of decompressive craniectomy versus best medical treatment alone in malignant stroke have been conducted. Until now, eight randomized controlled trials and several subsequent meta-analyses of these RCTs have been published [51, 52, 88–101]. One study continued its follow-up and published long-term outcomes as well after 3 years [103]. One randomized trial was found to have been withdrawn from publication [102]. However, this study was completed, and its results were included in recent meta-analyses [94, 95]. An overview of the RCTs is provided in Table 1.

All studies had a similar design, followed the same surgical decompression technique (hemicraniectomy), and mostly adhered to a standardized medical treatment protocol. However, the studies differed in certain factors, including the definition of malignant infarction, indications and timing of surgery, patient age, and the definition of favorable outcomes.

Malignant infarction was defined using clinical and radiological criteria. The primary clinical criterion assessing stroke severity was either the NIHSS or the Glasgow Coma Scale (GCS). The minimum cut-off NIHSS scores for inclusion varied across the studies. While the lowest minimum NIHSS score was 14 for non-dominant infarctions [89], the highest minimum NIHSS score was 21 for dominant hemisphere involvement [52]. Patients with severe comorbidities and limited life expectancy were excluded. Additional exclusion criteria were prestroke modified Rankin Scale (mRS) >1 or mRS >2 (two trials), as well as the absence of a pupillary reaction.

The radiological inclusion criterion was an infarction affecting the majority of the MCA territory on neuroimaging (at least 50% or 2/3, with or without basal ganglia involvement, or a minimum infarct volume of 145 cm^3 on DWI). In the HeADDFIRST study, a midline shift had to be demonstrated on a repeated CT before randomization [90]. In the study by Slezins et al., an ICP monitor was implanted in patients randomized to DC who did not have a midline shift on CT. DC was indicated only when ICP was elevated [92].

The age criterion varied significantly between the studies. DESTINY and HAMLET included participants aged 60 years or younger, while DECIMAL had a maximum inclusion age of 55, HeMMI 65, and HeADDFIRST

Table 1 Overview of ten randomized controlled trials

Study	Year	No. of patients (n)	Age (y)	Timing of surgery (h)	Primary outcome: Medical Mortality (%)	Medical mRS 0–3 (%)	Surgical Mortality (%)	Surgical mRS 0–3 (%)
DESTINY (Jüttler)	2007	32	18–60	<36	53/53	27/27	18/18	47/48
					at 6/12 months		at 6/12 months	
DECIMAL (Vahedi)	2007	38	18–55	<30	78/78	6/22	25/25	25/50
Vahedi					at 6/12 months		at 6/12 months	
HAMLET (Hofmeijer)	2009	64	18–60	<96	59	25	22	25
					at 12 months		at 12 months	
Zhao	2012	47	18–80	<48	61/70	4/9	13/17	1/25
					at 6/12 months		at 6/12 months	
Slezins	2012	24	>18	<48	92	0	55	45
					at 12 months		at 12 months	
HeADDFIRST (Frank)	2014	24	18–75	<96	40	30	36	29
					at 6 months		at 6 months	
	2014	112	>60	<48	70/76	3/5	33/43	7/6
Jüttler					at 6/12 months		at 6/12 months	
HAMLET (Geurts)	2014	64	18–60	<96	63	25	26	26
					at 36 months		at 36 months	
HeMMI (Chua)	2015	24	18–65	<72	55	38	39	23
					at 6 months		at 6 months	
DEMITUR (Kumral)	–	151	40–80	12–38	79	20	21	64
					at 12 months		at 12 months	

Study characteristics and clinical outcomes of patients undergoing decompressive hemicraniectomy compared to those treated medically
mRS modified Rankin Scale

75 years of age [51, 52, 88, 90, 91]. The Zhao and DEMITUR trials enrolled patients up to 80 years of age [93, 102]. DESTINY II specifically targeted elderly patients aged over 60 years [89].

The timing of randomization also varied between the studies. Most studies randomized patients and indicated DC early, within a maximum of 48 hours from the onset of stroke. HAMLET and HeADDFIRST included participants with stroke symptoms up to 96 hours, while HeMMI included participants up to 72 hours [51, 90, 91].

The most commonly assessed outcome measures were mortality and functional outcomes at 6 or 12 months. Geurts et al. reported the outcomes of the HAMLET study even after 3 years [103]. In all studies, the possibility of dichotomizing the mRS was applied at both 0–3 vs. 4–6 and 0–4 vs. 5–6. A favorable outcome was defined as a mRS score of 0–3 or 0–4, depending on the study.

All studies had small enrollment numbers. The smallest cohort included 24 participants, while the largest cohort, comprising a total of 151 patients, was in the unpublished DEMITUR study [102]. Furthermore, three major European studies (DECIMAL, DESTINY, HAMLET) were terminated early [51, 52, 88]. The reasons for early termination included significantly lower mortality in the surgical group, slow recruitment, and the improbability of achieving a statistically significant difference with the planned sample size. The results of the prematurely terminated studies were pooled into a single analysis [53].

10 Mortality

A consistent finding across RCTs and meta-analyses shows that DC, compared to conservative treatment alone, significantly reduces mortality in MHI [51, 52, 88–101]. Moreover, this effect is quite substantial, with an absolute risk reduction of 41%, and a number needed to treat (NNT) = 2.4 [30]. In all RCTs, differences in the primary outcome were predominantly driven by differences in mortality (Fig. 4).

Diverging from the findings of most RCTs, the HeADDFIRST and HeMMI trials showed no significant difference in mortality between surgical and conservative treatments [90, 91]. This lack of signifikance was attributed to the surprisingly low mortality rate in the conservative treatment group compared to the surgical treatment group, where mortality was consistent with that in other trials [30]. The opti-

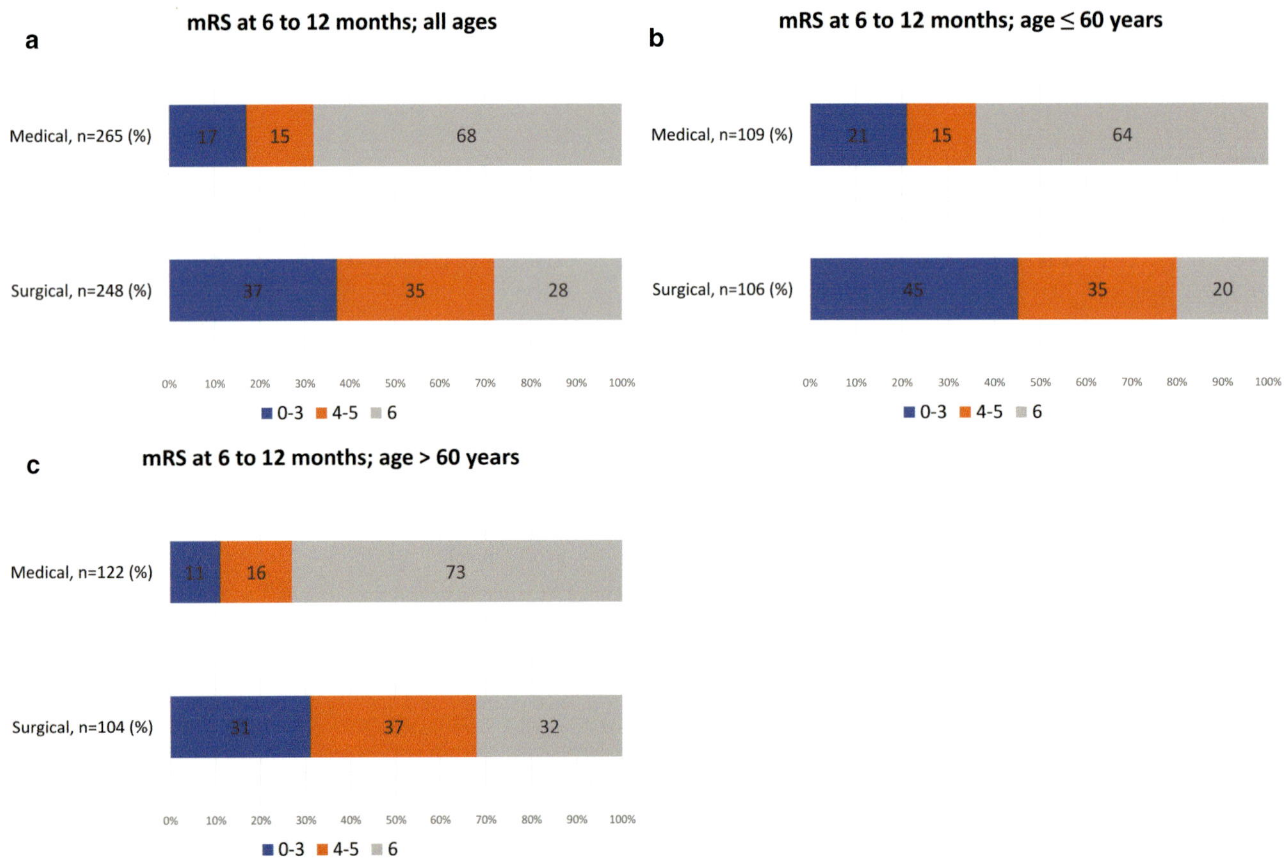

Fig. 4 A pooled analysis of functional outcomes evaluated by the modified Rankin Scale (mRS) at 6–12 months, comparing the medical and hemicraniectomy groups in nine randomized controlled trials: (**a**) All ages; (**b**) ≤60 years; (**c**) >60 years

mized medical treatment used in HeADDFIRST (strictly standardized medical protocol) likely reduced the mortality benefit of DC [90]. This finding pointed to possible gaps and the therapeutic potential of contemporary conservative treatment.

11 Functional Outcome

All studies utilized the mRS to assess functional outcomes. The HeMMI study was the only one that did not present results for the full spectrum of mRS [91]. No patient with an mRS of 0 to 1 was found in any published study, except for one patient with an mRS of 1 in the HeADDFIRST [90]. The pooled analysis of the three European RCTs (DECIMAL, DESTINY, HAMLET) showed a clear absolute risk reduction (ARR) with DC performed within 48 hours in patients younger than 60 years in functional outcomes at 1 year for both mRS score 0–3 (ARR 23%, NNT 4) and mRS 0–4 (ARR 51%, NNT 2) [53]. However, even if we conducted a combined analysis of all RCTs that evaluated functional outcomes at 12 months, we would find convincing superiority of surgical treatment regardless of the timing of surgery and patient age, for both mRS 0–3 (37% vs. 17%) and mRS 0–4 (59% vs. 22%) (Fig. 4).

The data presented convincingly suggests that patients treated with early DC have significantly higher chances of a good functional outcome with survival than medically treated survivors. Early DC effectively reduces mortality and severe disability, with a NNT of 2 and 4, respectively. Better outcomes are likely not only due to preventing lethal brain herniation, but also through the reduction of intracranial pressure and improvement in hemodynamics, which have the potential to salvage the persistent penumbral zone and mitigate secondary cerebral injury [97].

However, through a significant reduction in mortality, early DC paradoxically also increases the risk of survival with an unfavorable outcome (mRS 4–5) (Fig. 4). What constitutes a (un)favorable outcome after DC remains a matter of debate. While mRS 0–2 is clearly considered a good outcome, mRS 5–6 a poor outcome, and mRS 3 a favorable outcome, the perception of mRS 4 (moderate severe disability—unable to meet both own needs and walk without assistance) varies widely. Some studies defined a favorable outcome as mRS 0–3, while others defined it as mRS 0–4. However, this is merely an academic debate. What is crucial is the degree of functional impairment that is still acceptable for the patient and the resulting likelihood of a good quality of life (QOL). The decision-making algorithm should always consider the functional outcome acceptable to the patient and the preferred goal of care.

The pooled functional outcomes from RCTs assessing outcomes after 12 months allow us to determine that, if an mRS of 0–3 was acceptable to the patient, they would have a 37% chance of good QOL, a 35% chance of poor QOL, and a 28% chance of death after DC (Fig. 4). If an mRS of 0–4 was acceptable, they would have a 59% chance of good QOL, a 13% chance of poor QOL, and the chance of death would remain unchanged. Taking age into account (younger vs. older), the mRS distribution shifts either in favor of or against a favorable outcome (Fig. 4). The data suggest that if the patient prefers to maximize functional outcome and survival, DC should be indicated. On the other hand, if the patient's priority is to minimize survival with significant disability, they should be treated medically [97].

Quality of life, however, was not the primary outcome in any RCTs. The mRS primarily focuses on motor impairment but does not adequately assess cognitive function, aphasia, or QOL. Some RCTs evaluated QOL using questionnaires [51, 52, 88, 89]. In an international survey, 79% of 1860 physicians considered a mRS of 3 acceptable, while only 38% considered a mRS of 4 acceptable [104]. In contrast, a systematic review examining patient satisfaction and QOL found that 77% of patients or their caregivers considered an mRS of 4 acceptable and would also retrospectively consent to surgery [105]. The study also revealed that the mean overall reduction in QOL was 45%, and depression affected over half of the respondents [105].

The discrepancy between functional disability and QOL is influenced by the patient's personality, family, social, and cultural background. The challenge lies in determining, prior to surgery, whether the patient is likely to achieve an acceptable level of disability and QOL based on preoperative predictions.

12 Dominant Versus Nondominant Hemispheric Stroke

Another important aspect is the laterality of the stroke. In clinical practice, involvement of the dominant hemisphere is often considered a reason to avoid surgical treatment. This is reflected in the low representation of patients with dominant hemispheric infarcts in meta-analyses [106]. However, no evidence suggests that functional outcomes or QOL are worse in patients undergoing DC for dominant hemispheric infarcts [53, 94, 95, 106].

This perception is likely driven by an overestimation of the impact of aphasia on QOL and an underestimation of the effect of nondominant hemispheric injury, which is often associated with cognitive deficits, neglect syndrome, abulia, and depression [107, 108]. Moreover, patients with aphasia may recover their language function with intensive speech therapy, particularly in younger individuals [109]. Additionally, right hemispheric infarcts are considered a risk factor for cardiovascular complications, as the right insular cortex likely plays a key role in the neural regulation of autonomic functions [110, 111]. However, doubts remain about the ability of patients with aphasia to reliably assess their functional status or QOL.

The mentioned findings are consistent with meta-analyses of studies on both MT and IVT, which report no differences in outcomes between right-hemispheric and left-hemispheric strokes [112, 113]. However, a recent systematic review suggested that aphasia may predict a worse overall clinical outcome, regardless of the treatment for MHI [94]. Overall, we lack sufficient evidence to support withholding DC based on stroke laterality [106].

13 Involvement of an Additional Vascular Territory

Another factor that is often a reason to withhold DC in clinical practice is the involvement of an additional vascular territory (ACA or PCA) [114]. Some studies have shown that larger infarcts are associated with worse functional outcomes [115–117]. Severe disability (mRS 4–5) is significantly more frequent in patients with infarcts exceeding 270 cm^3 [117]. However, the available data have not shown that infarction extending beyond the MCA territory is associated with a lower benefit from DC [95]. On the contrary, patients with more extensive infarcts, which tend to have a more significant space-occupying effect, may benefit more from DC than those with smaller infarcts, where surgery is often prophylactic. In the DECIMAL study, no patient with an infarct volume greater than 210 cm^3 survived without DC [88]. In patients with large infarcts or infarcts involving an additional vascular territory, DC alone may be insufficient. In these cases, adjuvant strokectomy may be performed [54, 118].

14 Decompressive Hemicraniectomy in Elderly Patients

Patients in RCTs were younger than those in the overall malignant stroke population, which means that the results may not be generally applicable [96]. DESTINY, DECIMAL, and HAMLET enrolled patients up to the age of 60, but the mean age in these studies did not even reach 50 years [30, 51, 52, 88]. Other RCTs did include patients over the age of 60, but the average age in these studies was below 65 years [89–93].

Only the DESTINY II study specifically targeted patients over the age of 60. The median age of patients in DESTINY II was 70 years [89]. The study demonstrated that DC is a life-saving procedure even in elderly patients, in whom it increases the chance of survival without complete dependency. However, the significant benefit in the surgical group was mainly due to the large difference in mortality (70% vs. 33% at 6 months). If deceased patients had been excluded, DESTINY II would have been a negative trial. A favorable outcome (mRS 0–3) was achieved by only 6% of hemicraniectomy patients, and no survivor reached a mRS score of 0–2 at 6 months. The majority of survivors in the surgical group, compared to the conservative group, essentially shifted from a mRS of 5 to 4.

Several other prospective observational trials showed comparable results to DESTINY II and concluded that the probability of survival without severe disability in elderly patients is low after DC [119–121]. While the primary benefit of DC in older patients is reducing mortality, the benefit in achieving a favorable functional outcome is small, and the risk of a poor functional outcome is high compared to younger patients.

However, a recent review showed a non-significant effect of age > 60 years compared to age ≤ 60 on death or moderate disability and indicates that elderly patients are likely to have a poorer functional outcome regardless of surgical intervention [94].

All in all, the indication for DC in the elderly is reasonable. However, it must always be considered individually, taking into account the overall prognosis and the expectations of patients and their caregivers.

15 Timing of Decompressive Hemicraniectomy

Patients with MHI generally deteriorate after 48 hours due to the development of malignant edema and usually die within 72–96 hours [122, 123]. The optimal timing for DC after stroke onset, however, remains the subject of ongoing debate. Some authors advocate for prophylactic surgery as soon as the radiographic and clinical parameters of MHI are met, while others recommend waiting for mild drowsiness associated with the progression of edema [122, 124, 125].

The pragmatic cut-off at 48 hours from the onset of infarction for performing DC has been accepted in most RCTs. Only HAMLET, HeMMI, and HeADDFIRST were studies that allowed for randomization after 48 hours [51, 90, 91]. However, data on DC performed later than 48 hours after stroke onset are too limited for reliable conclusions (only 25 participants in the ≥48 hours group versus 440 participants in the <48 hours group) [94, 95]. A recent review showed only a non-significant trend of greater reduction in death in the <48 hours subgroup [94]. The meta-analysis focusing on the timing of DC concluded that the outcome of patients who underwent DC after 48 hours was not worse compared to those operated within 48 hours [122]. Other large retrospective studies also did not find a difference in outcome depending on the timing of surgery [126, 127]. The largest retrospective analysis of 1301 patients found a correlation between later surgery (≥72 hours) and increased mortality, but not for surgery ≥48 hours. Moreover, the correlation found between surgery timing and outcome was only observed when brain herniation was present [105].

These results suggest that the outcome is more influenced by the onset of clinical deterioration than by the timing of surgery. Not every MHI leads to subsequent clinical deterioration; therefore, early surgery may be performed even in patients who could have originally recovered without surgery [128–130]. Rather than blindly following guidelines (early DC <48 hours), it seems more rational to intensively observe patients and perform DC only if clinical deterioration begins. The development of deterioration in patients should correlate with edema progression and midline shift. However, it is crucial to perform surgery in time, before brain herniation develops [105]. Timely, rather than early, DC may be the key factor for a favorable outcome [128]. Given the proven benefit of DC performed within 48 hours, initiating an RCT assessing the timing of surgery (<48 hours versus ≥48 hours) would be considered unethical.

16 Decompressive Craniectomy in Pediatric Population

Ischemic stroke in children is rare (incidence 1.2–3.6 cases per 100,000 per year), and less than 2% are malignant [131]. Due to lower cerebral compliance in children, which reduces the capacity to tolerate edema and mass effect, one could expect the opposite. The low prevalence of malignant infarction is clearly attributed to a lower rate of large vessel occlusion [132]. The causes of cerebral infarction are cardioembolic, hematological, infectious, and vessel wall abnormalities [79, 133]. Even 7% of malignant strokes occur after IVT or MT [133]. Data on the role of DC in the pediatric population are very limited, and evidence-based recommendations are lacking. To date, only 97 well-documented cases have been published [133]. A male predominance (sex ratio 3:1) and a median age of 9.3 years were found.

In the pediatric population, the timely diagnosis of MHI is a significant challenge. A characteristic presentation often includes a combination of age > 2 years, prolonged seizures, high pediatric NIHSS, and anisocoria [134]. Unfortunately, diagnostic delay is common. This is caused both by the number of medical conditions that mimic stroke and by the delayed performance of MRI, which often requires sedation or general anesthesia. The average time interval between the onset of malignant symptoms and imaging is 9.4 hours. Diagnostic delay is also associated with significant treatment delay. A recent case-based review showed that all DCs were performed after the onset of intracranial hypertension signs, and 61–84% of patients even had preoperative mydriasis. Nevertheless, 95.4% of children survived, with the vast majority achieving a good outcome (mRS 0 in 2%, mRS 1–2 in 51%, mRS 3–4 in 40%, and mRS 5–6 in 4%). The median follow-up was 32 months. In contrast, a 67% mortality rate was observed in patients treated medically [133].

Although DC in the pediatric population with malignant infarction is typically performed at the stage of brain herniation, it is associated with significantly better functional outcomes than in adult [133]. This is most likely due to the greater potential for recovery and brain plasticity in childhood. Instead of counterproductive ICP monitoring, which can paradoxically lead to a delayed indication for surgery, early deterioration could be detected through bedside neuromonitoring methods, such as quantitative electroencephalography (EEG), TCD, or pupillometry [135, 136].

In addition to the common complications of DC seen in the adult population, children have an increased risk of significant intraoperative blood loss.

17 Decompressive Craniectomy Combined with Hypothermia

Therapeutic hypothermia has a considerable neuroprotective effect in experimental animal models [137]. In a rat model of permanent MCA occlusion, it was demonstrated that hypothermia in addition to DC has a significantly beneficial effect on both neurological outcomes and the reduction of infarct size [138, 139]. However, translation into the clinical field remains challenging, and hypothermia in patients with MCA infarction is still considered controversial. Some clinical studies have highlighted the positive effects of hypothermia, leading to its usage in combination with DC at selected institutions [140–144]. A trend toward the reduction of short-term mortality is likely associated with the anti-edematous effect of hypothermia, which has the potential to decrease the risk of cerebral herniation [141]. A lower incidence of systemic complications has been described with the use of a local cooling method [140]. In clinical practice, therapeutic hypothermia can be divided into induction, maintenance, and rewarming phases. The rewarming period is risky because rebound edema associated with ICP elevation may occur [145].

However, a pivotal RCT by Neugebauer et al. convincingly showed that moderate hypothermia early after DC did not improve functional outcomes or mortality in MHI patients. Moreover, the study had to be terminated early due to a higher rate of serious adverse events in the hypothermia group [146]. Currently, the application of hypothermia in patients with MHI is not recommended outside of clinical trials [146].

18 Malignant Cerebellar Infarction

It has been estimated that 20% of patients with infratentorial stroke deteriorate clinically due to space-occupying cerebellar edema [147]. Malignant cerebellar infarction (MCI) usually occurs in the territory of the posterior inferior cerebellar artery. Clinical deterioration can be caused by direct compression of the brainstem, tonsillar herniation, upward herniation into the tentorial hiatus, or obstructive hydrocephalus and may develop rapidly in the limited confines of the posterior fossa.

Since the first report of surgical treatment for MCI in 1956, suboccipital decompressive craniectomy (SDC) has been considered a well-accepted life-saving treatment option [13, 14]. The benefit of SDC has been convincingly demonstrated in clinical practice [148]. Although SDC is often performed in severely deteriorated patients, the clinical outcome is usually favorable. Unlike MHI, many patients can survive without neurological deficit (mRS 0). This difference is due to the presence of more eloquent areas in the MCA territory. The mortality rate for patients with MCI and MHI after surgical treatment is comparable [148].

A systematic review showed that SDC is associated with a 20% mortality rate and an unfavorable outcome in 28% of cases [148]. Nevertheless, compared to MHI, there is a lack of high-quality clinical data regarding the role of surgical treatment for cerebellar stroke. Existing data regarding SDC mostly come from retrospective studies, case series, case reports, and only one prospective observational study [147, 149–151]. The methodologies of the clinical studies were heterogeneous, various surgical treatments were performed, and different assessment scales were used. Comparing different surgical techniques is challenging due to significant selection bias [148].

Long-term outcomes in patients after SDC were evaluated in two German retrospective studies. Jüttler et al. studied 56 consecutive patients with MCI treated surgically. SDC was performed in 14% of patients, external ventricular drainage (EVD) in 16%, and a combination of both methods in 70% of patients. Overall mortality was 39%, and a favorable outcome (mRS 0–3) was reported in 52% of the study participants. There were no significant differences in mortality or functional outcomes between the surgical treatment groups [147].

The second trial by Pfefferkorn et al. studied 57 patients with MCI infarction. In all patients, bilateral SDC was performed. Additionally, 82% of patients underwent EVD, and 56% underwent strokectomy. The mortality rate was 40%, and more than half of the survivors had a favorable outcome (40% were independent—mRS 0–2). Poor outcome was associated with brainstem infarction. Neither age over 60 nor the timing of SDC had an impact on the outcome [150].

Tsitsopoulos et al. evaluated the effect of a uniform surgical treatment approach (SDC + strokectomy + EVD) in 32 patients with MCI. Mortality at 6 months was 12.5%. At long-term follow-up, nearly 70% of patients were alive, and among them, 77% had an mRS of 0–2. A good outcome was also observed in the majority of patients over 70 years of age and in one-third of preoperatively comatose patients [151].

The only prospective trial by Jauss et al. included 84 patients with MCI. The patients were assigned to three treatment groups (SDC, EVD, medical treatment) based on the level of consciousness, signs of mass effect on CT, and signs of brainstem involvement. Surprisingly, surgical treatment was found to be superior to medical treatment only in comatose patients. Half of all patients deteriorating to coma and treated with EVD or DC had a meaningful recovery. A total of 76% of operated patients achieved independence (mRS 0–2). The preoperative level of consciousness was the most powerful predictor of clinical outcome [149].

The presented data clearly indicate that the optimal surgical treatment for MCI has not yet been established. Surgical options vary from SDC, strokectomy, and ventriculostomy, either as stand-alone procedures or in combination. Some neurosurgeons consider obstructive hydrocephalus to be the main cause of initial consciousness impairment. Therefore, they primarily perform ventriculostomy and reserve SDC for secondary use in cases of persistent clinical deterioration [152, 153]. Others view this approach as risky due to the potential for ascending herniation and brainstem compression and therefore recommend performing SDC combined with strokectomy as the primary treatment [154, 155]. At some centers, SDC alone is considered a reliable solution for both MCI and hydrocephalus, while at others, SDC is always combined with ventriculostomy [147, 156]. Based on our experience, strokectomy is usually sufficient. SDC is indicated only in cases of insufficient debridement of infarcted tissue or in bilateral MCI. The optimal surgical approach depends on the patient's clinical condition and the extent of the space-occupying effect of the MCI.

The optimal timing for surgical treatment after the onset of MCI is not defined and ranges from 24 to 96 hours [148]. In some institutional practices, SDC is performed as a prophylactic measure, while in others it is used as a salvage procedure for comatose patients after the failure of medical treatment. Differences in timing are also related to the patients clinical status and its dynamics, as well as the heterogeneous nature of cerebellar strokes. Despite the unclear timing, waiting to perform surgery until the patient is comatose is not standard practice. To maximize the chances of neurological recovery and a favorable outcome, SDC should be performed before a significant decrease in consciousness [148].

Poor clinical status is convincingly associated with involvement of the brainstem. However, in clinical practice, it is difficult to distinguish ischemic damage to the brainstem from its reversible compression. MRI is not routinely performed in the acute phase of the infarction. On the other hand, it has not been proven that the type of affected vascular territory influences the outcome [149]. In patients with bilateral MCIs, the rate of favorable outcomes was similar to that observed in unilateral cases. Therefore, bilateral MCIs should not be considered an exclusion criterion for surgical treatment [150, 157].

Although elderly patients with MCI do not have convincingly worse clinical outcome, as seen in MHI, age is considered an independent prognostic factor. It was suggested that age ≤ 60 years, a higher preoperative GCS score (GCS > 9), SDC performed <48 hours after stroke onset, the absence of brainstem compression or infarction, and concomitant EVD or strokectomy are prognostic factors associated with favorable outcome [148].

Although SDC is a well-accepted, life-saving treatment option, the surgical management of MCI is not clearly defined from an evidence-based medicine perspective. No RCT has been published to date, and initiating such a trial would be unethical and result in high crossover rates. The use of prospective registries with central data repositories could help in selecting patients for the optimal surgical treatment modality.

19 Current Guidelines

The American Heart Association and American Stroke Association (AHA/ASA) published the most comprehensive guidelines for the early management of patients with acute ischemic stroke in 2018 and 2019, respectively [158].

The guidelines provided two class I general recommendations:

1. Early transfer of patients at risk for malignant cerebral edema to a center with neurosurgical expertise should be considered.
2. Patient-centered preferences in shared decision-making regarding prognosis, interventions, and limitations of care should be discussed early with patients and their families.

The guidelines provided two class I recommendations for MCI:

1. Ventriculostomy is recommended for patients with obstructive hydrocephalus. Concomitant or subsequent SDC may be necessary depending on the infarction size, the degree of brainstem compression, the neurological condition, and the effectiveness of medical treatment.
2. SDC should be performed in patients who deteriorate due to brainstem compression despite maximal medical therapy.

There are two class IIa recommendations with level A evidence for MHI:

1. It is reasonable to use a decrease in the level of consciousness as a selection criterion for DC. However, the optimal trigger remains unknown.
2. DC is reasonable in patients ≤60 years of age who deteriorate within 48 hours due to cerebral edema associated with MHI despite medical therapy.

There is one class IIb recommendation for MHI:

1. In patients >60 years of age, the same approach may be considered.

20 State of Current Knowledge and Future Directions

MHI has a mortality rate of up to 80% despite maximal medical treatment. DC performed in patients with MHI ≤ 60 years of age has strong evidence for improving survival and functional outcome. Although the beneficial effect of DC has been demonstrated when performed within 48 hours of infarct onset, the optimal trigger for performing DC remains unknown. Timely, rather than early, DC may be the key to achieving optimal surgical timing. Timely surgery in patients with early signs of deterioration associated with progressive malignant edema is more justified than unnecessary surgery in patients without progressive malignant edema, who may benefit from medical therapy alone.

DC in patients >60 years of age should be considered on an individual basis, as the probability of survival without complete dependency is low in this group. However, elderly patients are likely to have poorer functional outcomes regardless of surgical intervention.

The decision-making algorithm, regardless of the patient's age, should always take into account the degree of functional disability and the QOL that is still acceptable to the patient.

The minimum size of DC required to ensure sufficient decompression is 12 cm. When considering surgery, it is essential to account for the high complication rates associated with both DC and subsequent cranioplasty.

Data on the role of DC in the pediatric population are very limited. Although DC is often performed at a late stage, frequently after brain herniation has occurred, the vast majority of children survive, and most achieve a favorable clinical outcome.

SDC is a well-accepted, life-saving treatment option for patients with MCI, despite the absence of high-quality clinical data. Some patients who undergo SDC, unlike those undergoing hemicraniectomy, may survive without neurological deficits.

While RCTs have focused on assessing the benefits of DC itself, current and future research should aim to prevent edema progression and associated secondary brain injury. A deeper understanding of the pathophysiology of malignant infarction is essential for optimizing medical and neurocritical care, as well as for developing better predictive models with the potential to reduce the need for decompressive surgery.

Nationwide trends indicate that, despite the increasing incidence of strokes over time, successful reperfusion of the penumbra through IVT and MT has significantly reduced the need for DC in MHI patients.

Significant improvements are needed in the initial shared decision-making process with patients and their families, aiming to minimize potential differences between the patient's and clinician's preferences.

Ongoing research into new medical treatment options for patients with MHI is focused on glibenclamide, a highly promising candidate currently being evaluated in a phase III clinical trial.

Declarations

Competing Interests The author(s) has no competing interests to declare that are relevant to the content of this manuscript.

Ethics Approval The author(s) declares that this manuscript does not include primary research with human participants.

References

1. Hacke W, Schwab S, Horn M, Spranger M, De Georgia M, von Kummer R. "Malignant" middle cerebral artery territory infarction: clinical course and prognostic signs. Arch Neurol. 1996;53(4):309–15.
2. Malhotra K, Gornbein J, Saver JL. Ischemic strokes due to large-vessel occlusions contribute disproportionately to stroke-related dependence and death: a review. Front Neurol. 2017;8:651.
3. Moulin DE, Lo R, Chiang J, Barnett HJ. Prognosis in middle cerebral artery occlusion. Stroke. 1985;16(2):282–4.
4. Frank JI. Large hemispheric infarction, deterioration, and intracranial pressure. Neurology. 1995;45(7):1286–90.
5. Berrouschot J, Sterker M, Bettin S, Koster J, Schneider D. Mortality of space-occupying ("malignant") middle cerebral artery infarction under conservative intensive care. Intensive Care Med. 1998;24(6):620–3.
6. Cushing HI. Subtemporal decompressive operations for the intracranial complications associated with bursting fractures of the skull. Ann Surg. 1908;47(5):641–644.1.
7. Cushing H. The establishment of cerebral hernia as a decompressive measure for inaccessible brain tumors: with the description of intermuscular methods of making the bone defect in temporal and occipital regions. Surg Gynecol Obstet. 1905;1:297–314.
8. Kocher T. Die Terapie des Hirndruckes. In: Hölder A, editor. Hirnerschütterung, Hirndruck und chirurgische Eingriffe bei Hirnkrankheiten. Vienna: Hölder; 1901. p. 262–6.
9. Babinski J. De la craniectomie décompressive. Rev Neurol. 1910;21:27–8.
10. King AB. Massive cerebral infarction producing ventriculographic changes suggesting a brain tumor. J Neurosurg. 1951;8(5):536–9.
11. Scarcella G. Encephalomalacia simulating the clinical and radiological aspects of brain tumor; a report of 6 cases. J Neurosurg. 1956;13(4):278–92.
12. Ivamoto HS, Numoto M, Donaghy RM. Surgical decompression for cerebral and cerebellar infarcts. Stroke. 1974;5(3):365–70.
13. Fairburn B, Oliver LC. Cerebellar softening; a surgical emergency. Br Med J. 1956;1(4979):1335–6.
14. Lindgren SO. Infarctions simulating brain tumours in the posterior fossa. J Neurosurg. 1956;13(6):575–81.
15. Lehrich JR, Winkler GF, Ojemann RG. Cerebellar infarction with brain stem compression. Diagnosis and surgical treatment. Arch Neurol. 1970;22(6):490–8.
16. Bar M, Mikulik R, Skoloudik D, Czerny D, Lipina R, Klecka L, et al. Nationwide study of decompressive surgery for malignant supratentorial infarction in the Czech Republic: utilization and outcome predictors. Clinical article. J Neurosurg. 2010;113(4):897–900.
17. Rahme R, Curry R, Kleindorfer D, Khoury JC, Ringer AJ, Kissela BM, et al. How often are patients with ischemic stroke eligible for decompressive hemicraniectomy? Stroke. 2012;43(2):550–2.
18. Rumalla K, Ottenhausen M, Kan P, Burkhardt JK. Recent nationwide impact of mechanical thrombectomy on decompressive hemicraniectomy for acute ischemic stroke. Stroke. 2019;50(8):2133–9.
19. Beez T, Steiger HJ. Impact of randomized controlled trials on neurosurgical practice in decompressive craniectomy for ischemic stroke. Neurosurg Rev. 2019;42(1):133–7.
20. Sporns PB, Minnerup J, Warneke N, Dziewas R, Hanning U, Berkemeyer S, et al. Impact of the implementation of thrombectomy with stent retrievers on the frequency of hemicraniectomy in patients with acute ischemic stroke. Clin Neuroradiol. 2017;27(2):193–7.
21. Wu S, Yuan R, Wang Y, Wei C, Zhang S, Yang X, et al. Early prediction of malignant brain edema after ischemic stroke. Stroke. 2018;49(12):2918–27.
22. Mrosk F, Hecht N, Vajkoczy P. Decompressive hemicraniectomy in ischemic stroke. J Neurosurg Sci. 2021;65(3):249–58.
23. Matsukawa H, Kiura Y, Sakai N, Yamagami H, Uchida K, Morimoto T, et al. Effect of endovascular therapy on subsequent decompressive hemicraniectomy in cardioembolic ischemic stroke with proximal intracranial occlusion in the anterior circulation: sub-analysis of the RESCUE-Japan Registry 2. Cerebrovasc Dis. 2019;48(1–2):9–16.
24. Broughton BR, Reutens DC, Sobey CG. Apoptotic mechanisms after cerebral ischemia. Stroke. 2009;40(5):e331–9.
25. Astrup J, Siesjo BK, Symon L. Thresholds in cerebral ischemia – the ischemic penumbra. Stroke. 1981;12(6):723–5.
26. Hossmann KA. Pathophysiology and therapy of experimental stroke. Cell Mol Neurobiol. 2006;26(7–8):1057–83.
27. Sueiras M, Thonon V, Santamarina E, Sanchez-Guerrero A, Poca MA, Quintana M, et al. Cortical spreading depression phenomena are frequent in ischemic and traumatic penumbra: a prospective study in patients with traumatic brain injury and large hemispheric ischemic stroke. J Clin Neurophysiol. 2021;38(1):47–55.
28. Pinczolits A, Zdunczyk A, Dengler NF, Hecht N, Kowoll CM, Dohmen C, et al. Standard-sampling microdialysis and spreading depolarizations in patients with malignant hemispheric stroke. J Cereb Blood Flow Metab. 2017;37(5):1896–905.
29. Jeon SB, Koh Y, Choi HA, Lee K. Critical care for patients with massive ischemic stroke. J Stroke. 2014;16(3):146–60.
30. Lin J, Frontera JA. Decompressive hemicraniectomy for large hemispheric strokes. Stroke. 2021;52(4):1500–10.

31. Suyama K, Horie N, Hayashi K, Nagata I. Nationwide survey of decompressive hemicraniectomy for malignant middle cerebral artery infarction in Japan. World Neurosurg. 2014;82(6):1158–63.
32. Ong CJ, Gluckstein J, Laurido-Soto O, Yan Y, Dhar R, Lee JM. Enhanced detection of edema in malignant anterior circulation stroke (EDEMA) score: a risk prediction tool. Stroke. 2017;48(7):1969–72.
33. Jo K, Bajgur SS, Kim H, Choi HA, Huh PW, Lee K. A simple prediction score system for malignant brain edema progression in large hemispheric infarction. PLoS One. 2017;12(2):e0171425.
34. Krieger DW, Demchuk AM, Kasner SE, Jauss M, Hantson L. Early clinical and radiological predictors of fatal brain swelling in ischemic stroke. Stroke. 1999;30(2):287–92.
35. Park J, Goh DH, Sung JK, Hwang YH, Kang DH, Kim Y. Timely assessment of infarct volume and brain atrophy in acute hemispheric infarction for early surgical decompression: strict cutoff criteria with high specificity. Acta Neurochir. 2012;154(1):79–85.
36. Barber PA, Demchuk AM, Zhang J, Kasner SE, Hill MD, Berrouschot J, et al. Computed tomographic parameters predicting fatal outcome in large middle cerebral artery infarction. Cerebrovasc Dis. 2003;16(3):230–5.
37. MacCallum C, Churilov L, Mitchell P, Dowling R, Yan B. Low Alberta Stroke Program Early CT score (ASPECTS) associated with malignant middle cerebral artery infarction. Cerebrovasc Dis. 2014;38(1):39–45.
38. Ryoo JW, Na DG, Kim SS, Lee KH, Lee SJ, Chung CS, et al. Malignant middle cerebral artery infarction in hyperacute ischemic stroke: evaluation with multiphasic perfusion computed tomography maps. J Comput Assist Tomogr. 2004;28(1):55–62.
39. Oppenheim C, Samson Y, Manai R, Lalam T, Vandamme X, Crozier S, et al. Prediction of malignant middle cerebral artery infarction by diffusion-weighted imaging. Stroke. 2000;31(9):2175–81.
40. Thomalla G, Hartmann F, Juettler E, Singer OC, Lehnhardt FG, Kohrmann M, et al. Prediction of malignant middle cerebral artery infarction by magnetic resonance imaging within 6 hours of symptom onset: a prospective multicenter observational study. Ann Neurol. 2010;68(4):435–45.
41. Gerriets T, Stolz E, Konig S, Babacan S, Fiss I, Jauss M, et al. Sonographic monitoring of midline shift in space-occupying stroke: an early outcome predictor. Stroke. 2001;32(2):442–7.
42. Asil T, Uzunca I, Utku U, Berberoglu U. Monitoring of increased intracranial pressure resulting from cerebral edema with transcranial Doppler sonography in patients with middle cerebral artery infarction. J Ultrasound Med. 2003;22(10):1049–53.
43. Gupta A, Sattur MG, Aoun RJN, Krishna C, Bolton PB, Chong BW, et al. Hemicraniectomy for ischemic and hemorrhagic stroke: facts and controversies. Neurosurg Clin N Am. 2017;28(3):349–60.
44. Sheth KN, Kimberly WT, Elm JJ, Kent TA, Yoo AJ, Thomalla G, et al. Exploratory analysis of glyburide as a novel therapy for preventing brain swelling. Neurocrit Care. 2014;21(1):43–51.
45. Kimberly WT, Bevers MB, von Kummer R, Demchuk AM, Romero JM, Elm JJ, et al. Effect of IV glyburide on adjudicated edema endpoints in the GAMES-RP Trial. Neurology. 2018;91(23):e2163–e9.
46. Sheth KN, Elm JJ, Molyneaux BJ, Hinson H, Beslow LA, Sze GK, et al. Safety and efficacy of intravenous glyburide on brain swelling after large hemispheric infarction (GAMES-RP): a randomised, double-blind, placebo-controlled phase 2 trial. Lancet Neurol. 2016;15(11):1160–9.
47. Munch E, Horn P, Schurer L, Piepgras A, Paul T, Schmiedek P. Management of severe traumatic brain injury by decompressive craniectomy. Neurosurgery. 2000;47(2):315–22; discussion 22–3.
48. Flechsenhar J, Woitzik J, Zweckberger K, Amiri H, Hacke W, Juttler E. Hemicraniectomy in the management of space-occupying ischemic stroke. J Clin Neurosci. 2013;20(1):6–12.
49. Neugebauer H, Fiss I, Pinczolits A, Hecht N, Witsch J, Dengler NF, et al. Large size hemicraniectomy reduces early herniation in malignant middle cerebral artery infarction. Cerebrovasc Dis. 2016;41(5–6):283–90.
50. Lehrieder D, Muller HP, Kassubek J, Hecht N, Thomalla G, Michalski D, et al. Large diameter hemicraniectomy does not improve long-term outcome in malignant infarction. J Neurol. 2023;270(8):4080–9.
51. Hofmeijer J, Kappelle LJ, Algra A, Amelink GJ, van Gijn J, van der Worp HB, et al. Surgical decompression for space-occupying cerebral infarction (the Hemicraniectomy After Middle Cerebral Artery infarction with Life-threatening Edema Trial [HAMLET]): a multicentre, open, randomised trial. Lancet Neurol. 2009;8(4):326–33.
52. Juttler E, Schwab S, Schmiedek P, Unterberg A, Hennerici M, Woitzik J, et al. Decompressive surgery for the treatment of malignant infarction of the middle cerebral artery (DESTINY): a randomized, controlled trial. Stroke. 2007;38(9):2518–25.
53. Vahedi K, Hofmeijer J, Juettler E, Vicaut E, George B, Algra A, et al. Early decompressive surgery in malignant infarction of the middle cerebral artery: a pooled analysis of three randomised controlled trials. Lancet Neurol. 2007;6(3):215–22.
54. Kurten S, Munoz C, Beseoglu K, Fischer I, Perrin J, Steiger HJ. Decompressive hemicraniectomy for malignant middle cerebral artery infarction including patients with additional involvement of the anterior and/or posterior cerebral artery territory-outcome analysis and definition of prognostic factors. Acta Neurochir. 2018;160(1):83–9.
55. Park J, Kim E, Kim GJ, Hur YK, Guthikonda M. External decompressive craniectomy including resection of temporal muscle and fascia in malignant hemispheric infarction. J Neurosurg. 2009;110(1):101–5.
56. Moughal S, Trippier S, Al-Mousa A, Hainsworth AH, Pereira AC, Minhas PS, et al. Strokectomy for malignant middle cerebral artery infarction: experience and meta-analysis of current evidence. J Neurol. 2022;269(1):149–58.
57. Mestre H, Du T, Sweeney AM, Liu G, Samson AJ, Peng W, et al. Cerebrospinal fluid influx drives acute ischemic tissue swelling. Science. 2020;367(6483):eaax7171.
58. Cherian I, Beltran M, Landi A, Alafaci C, Torregrossa F, Grasso G. Introducing the concept of "CSF-shift edema" in traumatic brain injury. J Neurosci Res. 2018;96(4):744–52.
59. Poca MA, Benejam B, Sahuquillo J, Riveiro M, Frascheri L, Merino MA, et al. Monitoring intracranial pressure in patients with malignant middle cerebral artery infarction: is it useful? J Neurosurg. 2010;112(3):648–57.
60. Sauvigny T, Gottsche J, Czorlich P, Vettorazzi E, Westphal M, Regelsberger J. Intracranial pressure in patients undergoing decompressive craniectomy: new perspective on thresholds. J Neurosurg. 2018;128(3):819–27.
61. Jeon SB, Park JC, Kwon SU, Kim YJ, Lee S, Kang DW, et al. Intracranial pressure soon after hemicraniectomy in malignant middle cerebral artery infarction. J Intensive Care Med. 2018;33(5):310–6.
62. Paldor I, Rosenthal G, Cohen JE, Leker R, Harnof S, Shoshan Y, et al. Intracranial pressure monitoring following decompressive hemicraniectomy for malignant cerebral infarction. J Clin Neurosci. 2015;22(1):79–82.
63. Kurland DB, Khaladj-Ghom A, Stokum JA, Carusillo B, Karimy JK, Gerzanich V, et al. Complications associated with decompressive craniectomy: a systematic review. Neurocrit Care. 2015;23(2):292–304.
64. Honeybul S, Ho KM. Decompressive craniectomy for severe traumatic brain injury: the relationship between surgical complications and the prediction of an unfavourable outcome. Injury. 2014;45(9):1332–9.

65. Mracek J, Mork J, Dostal J, Tupy R, Mrackova J, Priban V. Complications following decompressive craniectomy. J Neurol Surg A Cent Eur Neurosurg. 2021;82(5):437–45.
66. Schuss P, Borger V, Vatter H, Singer OC, Seifert V, Guresir E. Antiplatelet therapy, but not intravenous thrombolytic therapy, is associated with postoperative bleeding complications after decompressive craniectomy for stroke. J Neurol. 2013;260(8):2149–55.
67. Al-Jehani H, Petrecca K, Martel P, Sinclair D, Sirhan D. Decompressive craniectomy for ischemic stroke: effect of hemorrhagic transformation on outcome. J Stroke Cerebrovasc Dis. 2016;25(9):2177–83.
68. Fischer U, Taussky P, Gralla J, Arnold M, Brekenfeld C, Reinert M, et al. Decompressive craniectomy after intra-arterial thrombolysis: safety and outcome. J Neurol Neurosurg Psychiatry. 2011;82(8):885–7.
69. Fang C, Zhu T, Zhang P, Xia L, Sun C. Risk factors of neurosurgical site infection after craniotomy: a systematic review and meta-analysis. Am J Infect Control. 2017;45(11):e123–e34.
70. Malliti M, Page P, Gury C, Chomette E, Nataf F, Roux FX. Comparison of deep wound infection rates using a synthetic dural substitute (neuro-patch) or pericranium graft for dural closure: a clinical review of 1 year. Neurosurgery. 2004;54(3):599–603; discussion 603–4.
71. De Bonis P, Sturiale CL, Anile C, Gaudino S, Mangiola A, Martucci M, et al. Decompressive craniectomy, interhemispheric hygroma and hydrocephalus: a timeline of events? Clin Neurol Neurosurg. 2013;115(8):1308–12.
72. Kenning TJ, Gooch MR, Gandhi RH, Shaikh MP, Boulos AS, German JW. Cranial decompression for the treatment of malignant intracranial hypertension after ischemic cerebral infarction: decompressive craniectomy and hinge craniotomy. J Neurosurg. 2012;116(6):1289–98.
73. Kan P, Amini A, Hansen K, White GL Jr, Brockmeyer DL, Walker ML, et al. Outcomes after decompressive craniectomy for severe traumatic brain injury in children. J Neurosurg. 2006;105(5 Suppl):337–42.
74. Finger T, Prinz V, Schreck E, Pinczolits A, Bayerl S, Liman T, et al. Impact of timing of cranioplasty on hydrocephalus after decompressive hemicraniectomy in malignant middle cerebral artery infarction. Clin Neurol Neurosurg. 2017;153:27–34.
75. Ashayeri K, Jackson EM, Huang J, Brem H, Gordon CR. Syndrome of the trephined: a systematic review. Neurosurgery. 2016;79(4):525–34.
76. Akins PT, Guppy KH. Sinking skin flaps, paradoxical herniation, and external brain tamponade: a review of decompressive craniectomy management. Neurocrit Care. 2008;9(2):269–76.
77. Creutzfeldt CJ, Tirschwell DL, Kim LJ, Schubert GB, Longstreth WT Jr, Becker KJ. Seizures after decompressive hemicraniectomy for ischaemic stroke. J Neurol Neurosurg Psychiatry. 2014;85(7):721–5.
78. Brondani R, Garcia de Almeida A, Abrahim Cherubini P, Mandelli Mota S, de Alencastro LC, Antunes ACM, et al. High risk of seizures and epilepsy after decompressive hemicraniectomy for malignant middle cerebral artery stroke. Cerebrovasc Dis Extra. 2017;7(1):51–61.
79. Beez T, Munoz-Bendix C, Steiger HJ, Beseoglu K. Decompressive craniectomy for acute ischemic stroke. Crit Care. 2019;23(1):209.
80. Olivecrona M, Rodling-Wahlstrom M, Naredi S, Koskinen LO. Effective ICP reduction by decompressive craniectomy in patients with severe traumatic brain injury treated by an ICP-targeted therapy. J Neurotrauma. 2007;24(6):927–35.
81. Dujovny M, Fernandez P, Alperin N, Betz W, Misra M, Mafee M. Post-cranioplasty cerebrospinal fluid hydrodynamic changes: magnetic resonance imaging quantitative analysis. Neurol Res. 1997;19(3):311–6.
82. Halani SH, Chu JK, Malcolm JG, Rindler RS, Allen JW, Grossberg JA, et al. Effects of cranioplasty on cerebral blood flow following decompressive craniectomy: a systematic review of the literature. Neurosurgery. 2017;81(2):204–16.
83. Honeybul S, Janzen C, Kruger K, Ho KM. The impact of cranioplasty on neurological function. Br J Neurosurg. 2013;27(5):636–41.
84. Mah JK, Kass RA. The impact of cranioplasty on cerebral blood flow and its correlation with clinical outcome in patients underwent decompressive craniectomy. Asian J Neurosurg. 2016;11(1):15–21.
85. Mee H, Anwar F, Timofeev I, Owens N, Grieve K, Whiting G, et al. Cranioplasty: a multidisciplinary approach. Front Surg. 2022;9:864385.
86. Iaccarino C, Kolias A, Adelson PD, Rubiano AM, Viaroli E, Buki A, et al. Consensus statement from the international consensus meeting on post-traumatic cranioplasty. Acta Neurochir. 2021;163(2):423–40.
87. Yadla S, Campbell PG, Chitale R, Maltenfort MG, Jabbour P, Sharan AD. Effect of early surgery, material, and method of flap preservation on cranioplasty infections: a systematic review. Neurosurgery. 2011;68(4):1124–9; discussion 30.
88. Vahedi K, Vicaut E, Mateo J, Kurtz A, Orabi M, Guichard JP, et al. Sequential-design, multicenter, randomized, controlled trial of early decompressive craniectomy in malignant middle cerebral artery infarction (DECIMAL Trial). Stroke. 2007;38(9):2506–17.
89. Juttler E, Unterberg A, Woitzik J, Bosel J, Amiri H, Sakowitz OW, et al. Hemicraniectomy in older patients with extensive middle-cerebral-artery stroke. N Engl J Med. 2014;370(12):1091–100.
90. Frank JI, Schumm LP, Wroblewski K, Chyatte D, Rosengart AJ, Kordeck C, et al. Hemicraniectomy and durotomy upon deterioration from infarction-related swelling trial: randomized pilot clinical trial. Stroke. 2014;45(3):781–7.
91. Chua AE, Buckley B, Lapitan MCM, Jamora RDG. Hemicraniectomy for malignant middle cerebral artery infarction (HeMMI): a randomized controlled clinical trial of decompressive hemicraniectomy with standardized medical care versus standardized medical care alone. Acta Med Philipp. 2015;49(1):28–33.
92. Slezins J, Keris V, Bricis R, Millers A, Valeinis E, Stukens J, et al. Preliminary results of randomized controlled study on decompressive craniectomy in treatment of malignant middle cerebral artery stroke. Medicina (Kaunas). 2012;48(10):521–4.
93. Zhao J, Su YY, Zhang Y, Zhang YZ, Zhao R, Wang L, et al. Decompressive hemicraniectomy in malignant middle cerebral artery infarct: a randomized controlled trial enrolling patients up to 80 years old. Neurocrit Care. 2012;17(2):161–71.
94. Dower A, Mulcahy M, Maharaj M, Chen H, Lim CED, Li Y, et al. Surgical decompression for malignant cerebral oedema after ischaemic stroke. Cochrane Database Syst Rev. 2022;11(11):CD014989.
95. Reinink H, Juttler E, Hacke W, Hofmeijer J, Vicaut E, Vahedi K, et al. Surgical decompression for space-occupying hemispheric infarction: a systematic review and individual patient meta-analysis of randomized clinical trials. JAMA Neurol. 2021;78(2):208–16.
96. Das S, Mitchell P, Ross N, Whitfield PC. Decompressive hemicraniectomy in the treatment of malignant middle cerebral artery infarction: a meta-analysis. World Neurosurg. 2019;123:8–16.
97. Streib CD, Hartman LM, Molyneaux BJ. Early decompressive craniectomy for malignant cerebral infarction: meta-analysis and clinical decision algorithm. Neurol Clin Pract. 2016;6(5):433–43.
98. Alexander P, Heels-Ansdell D, Siemieniuk R, Bhatnagar N, Chang Y, Fei Y, et al. Hemicraniectomy versus medical treatment with large MCA infarct: a review and meta-analysis. BMJ Open. 2016;6(11):e014390.

99. Wei H, Jia FM, Yin HX, Guo ZL. Decompressive hemicraniectomy versus medical treatment of malignant middle cerebral artery infarction: a systematic review and meta-analysis. Biosci Rep. 2020;40(1):BSR20191448.
100. Gul W, Fuller HR, Wright H, Sen J. A systematic review and meta-analysis of the effectiveness of surgical decompression in treating patients with malignant middle cerebral artery infarction. World Neurosurg. 2018;120:e902–e20.
101. Li YP, Hou MZ, Lu GY, Ciccone N, Wang XD, Dong L, et al. Neurologic functional outcomes of decompressive hemicraniectomy versus conventional treatment for malignant middle cerebral artery infarction: a systematic review and meta-analysis. World Neurosurg. 2017;99:709–25.e3.
102. Kumral E, Sirin H, Sagduyu A, Guler A, Ozdamar N, Kose T. WITHDRAWN: decompressive surgery in patients with malignant middle cerebral artery infarction: a randomized, controlled trial in a Turkish population (Demitur trial). Int J Stroke. 2021:17474930211007671. https://doi.org/10.1177/17474930211007671.
103. Geurts M, van der Worp HB, Kappelle LJ, Amelink GJ, Algra A, Hofmeijer J, et al. Surgical decompression for space-occupying cerebral infarction: outcomes at 3 years in the randomized HAMLET trial. Stroke. 2013;44(9):2506–8.
104. Neugebauer H, Creutzfeldt CJ, Hemphill JC 3rd, Heuschmann PU, Juttler E. DESTINY-S: attitudes of physicians toward disability and treatment in malignant MCA infarction. Neurocrit Care. 2014;21(1):27–34.
105. Rahme R, Zuccarello M, Kleindorfer D, Adeoye OM, Ringer AJ. Decompressive hemicraniectomy for malignant middle cerebral artery territory infarction: is life worth living? J Neurosurg. 2012;117(4):749–54.
106. Raty S, Georgiopoulos G, Aarnio K, Martinez-Majander N, Uhl E, Ntaios G, et al. Hemicraniectomy for dominant vs nondominant middle cerebral artery infarction: a systematic review and meta-analysis. J Stroke Cerebrovasc Dis. 2021;30(11):106102.
107. von Sarnowski B, Kleist-Welch Guerra W, Kohlmann T, Moock J, Khaw AV, Kessler C, et al. Long-term health-related quality of life after decompressive hemicraniectomy in stroke patients with life-threatening space-occupying brain edema. Clin Neurol Neurosurg. 2012;114(6):627–33.
108. Parikh RM, Robinson RG, Lipsey JR, Starkstein SE, Fedoroff JP, Price TR. The impact of poststroke depression on recovery in activities of daily living over a 2-year follow-up. Arch Neurol. 1990;47(7):785–9.
109. Kastrau F, Wolter M, Huber W, Block F. Recovery from aphasia after hemicraniectomy for infarction of the speech-dominant hemisphere. Stroke. 2005;36(4):825–9.
110. Aszalos Z, Barsi P, Vitrai J, Nagy Z. Lateralization as a factor in the prognosis of middle cerebral artery territorial infarct. Eur Neurol. 2002;48(3):141–5.
111. Yoon BW, Morillo CA, Cechetto DF, Hachinski V. Cerebral hemispheric lateralization in cardiac autonomic control. Arch Neurol. 1997;54(6):741–4.
112. Almekhlafi MA, Hill MD, Roos YM, Campbell BCV, Muir KW, Demchuk AM, et al. Stroke laterality did not modify outcomes in the HERMES meta-analysis of individual patient data of 7 trials. Stroke. 2019;50(8):2118–24.
113. Golsari A, Cheng B, Sobesky J, Schellinger PD, Fiehler J, Gerloff C, et al. Stroke lesion volumes and outcome are not different in hemispheric stroke side treated with intravenous thrombolysis based on magnetic resonance imaging criteria. Stroke. 2015;46(4):1004–8.
114. Neugebauer H, Juttler E. Hemicraniectomy for malignant middle cerebral artery infarction: current status and future directions. Int J Stroke. 2014;9(4):460–7.
115. Fatima N, Razzaq S, El Beltagi A, Shuaib A, Saqqur M. Decompressive craniectomy: a preliminary study of comparative radiographic characteristics predicting outcome in malignant ischemic stroke. World Neurosurg. 2020;133:e267–e74.
116. Freyschlag CF, Boehme C, Bauer M, Kerschbaumer J, Pinggera D, Riedmann M, et al. The volume of ischemic brain predicts poor outcome in patients with surgically treated malignant stroke. World Neurosurg. 2019;123:e515–e9.
117. Hecht N, Neugebauer H, Fiss I, Pinczolits A, Vajkoczy P, Juttler E, et al. Infarct volume predicts outcome after decompressive hemicraniectomy for malignant hemispheric stroke. J Cereb Blood Flow Metab. 2018;38(6):1096–103.
118. Marklund N. Decompressive craniectomy, ICP monitoring and secondary necrosectomy as treatment options in patients presenting with malignant ischemic infarctions extending beyond the middle cerebral artery territory. Acta Neurochir. 2018;160(1):91–3.
119. Rahmig J, Wopking S, Juttler E, Uhlmann L, Limprecht R, Barlinn J, et al. Decompressive hemicraniectomy in elderly patients with space-occupying infarction (DECAP): a prospective observational study. Neurocrit Care. 2019;31(1):97–106.
120. Arac A, Blanchard V, Lee M, Steinberg GK. Assessment of outcome following decompressive craniectomy for malignant middle cerebral artery infarction in patients older than 60 years of age. Neurosurg Focus. 2009;26(6):E3.
121. Li J, Zhang P, Tao W, Yi X, Zhang J, Wang C. Age-specific clinical characteristics and outcome in patients over 60 years old with large hemispheric infarction. Brain Behav. 2018;8(12):e01158.
122. Goedemans T, Verbaan D, Coert BA, Kerklaan B, van den Berg R, Coutinho JM, et al. Outcome after decompressive craniectomy for middle cerebral artery infarction: timing of the intervention. Neurosurgery. 2020;86(3):E318–E25.
123. Qureshi AI, Suarez JI, Yahia AM, Mohammad Y, Uzun G, Suri MF, et al. Timing of neurologic deterioration in massive middle cerebral artery infarction: a multicenter review. Crit Care Med. 2003;31(1):272–7.
124. Beucler N. Indications and scientific support for supratentorial unilateral decompressive craniectomy for different subgroups of patients: a scoping review. Acta Neurochir. 2024;166(1):388.
125. Mori K, Nakao Y, Yamamoto T, Maeda M. Early external decompressive craniectomy with duroplasty improves functional recovery in patients with massive hemispheric embolic infarction: timing and indication of decompressive surgery for malignant cerebral infarction. Surg Neurol. 2004;62(5):420–9; discussion 9–30.
126. Gupta R, Connolly ES, Mayer S, Elkind MS. Hemicraniectomy for massive middle cerebral artery territory infarction: a systematic review. Stroke. 2004;35(2):539–43.
127. Hernandez-Duran S, Hautmann X, Rohde V, von der Brelie C, Mielke D. Surgical timing and indications for decompressive craniectomy in malignant stroke: results from a single-center retrospective analysis. Acta Neurochir. 2023;165(12):3815–20.
128. Lin TK, Chen SM, Huang YC, Chen PY, Chen MC, Tsai HC, et al. The outcome predictors of malignant large infarction and the functional outcome of survivors following decompressive craniectomy. World Neurosurg. 2016;93:133–8.
129. Rahmanian A, Seifzadeh B, Razmkon A, Petramfar P, Kivelev J, Alibai EA, et al. Outcome of decompressive craniectomy in comparison to nonsurgical treatment in patients with malignant MCA infarction. Springerplus. 2014;3:115.
130. Schwab S, Steiner T, Aschoff A, Schwarz S, Steiner HH, Jansen O, et al. Early hemicraniectomy in patients with complete middle cerebral artery infarction. Stroke. 1998;29(9):1888–93.
131. Rahme R, Jimenez L, Bashir U, Adeoye OM, Abruzzo TA, Ringer AJ, et al. Malignant MCA territory infarction in the pediatric

population: subgroup analysis of the Greater Cincinnati/Northern Kentucky Stroke Study. Childs Nerv Syst. 2013;29(1):99–103.
132. Bhatia KD, Briest R, Goetti R, Webster R, Troedson C, Dale RC, et al. Incidence and natural history of pediatric large vessel occlusion stroke: a population study. JAMA Neurol. 2022;79(5):488–97.
133. Carlhan-Ledermann A, Bartoli A, Gebistorf F, Beghetti M, Sologashvili T, Rebollo Polo M, et al. Decompressive hemicraniectomy in pediatric malignant arterial ischemic stroke: a case-based review. Childs Nerv Syst. 2023;39(9):2377–89.
134. Andrade A, Bigi S, Laughlin S, Parthasarathy S, Sinclair A, Dirks P, et al. Association between prolonged seizures and malignant middle cerebral artery infarction in children with acute ischemic stroke. Pediatr Neurol. 2016;64:44–51.
135. Harrar DB, Sun LR, Segal JB, Lee S, Sansevere AJ. Neuromonitoring in children with cerebrovascular disorders. Neurocrit Care. 2023;38(2):486–503.
136. Couret D, Boumaza D, Grisotto C, Triglia T, Pellegrini L, Ocquidant P, et al. Reliability of standard pupillometry practice in neurocritical care: an observational, double-blinded study. Crit Care. 2016;20:99.
137. Lanier WL. Cerebral metabolic rate and hypothermia: their relationship with ischemic neurologic injury. J Neurosurg Anesthesiol. 1995;7(3):216–21.
138. Doerfler A, Schwab S, Hoffmann TT, Engelhorn T, Forsting M. Combination of decompressive craniectomy and mild hypothermia ameliorates infarction volume after permanent focal ischemia in rats. Stroke. 2001;32(11):2675–81.
139. Jieyong B, Zhong W, Shiming Z, Dai Z, Kato Y, Kanno T, et al. Decompressive craniectomy and mild hypothermia reduces infarction size and counterregulates Bax and Bcl-2 expression after permanent focal ischemia in rats. Neurosurg Rev. 2006;29(2):168–72.
140. Fan L, Su Y, Zhang Y, Ye H, Chen W, Liu G. Decompressive craniectomy combined with mild hypothermia in patients with large hemispheric infarction: a randomized controlled trial. BMC Neurol. 2021;21(1):114.
141. Chen Z, Zhang X, Liu C. Outcomes of therapeutic hypothermia in patients treated with decompressive craniectomy for malignant Middle cerebral artery infarction: a systematic review and meta-analysis. Clin Neurol Neurosurg. 2020;188:105569.
142. Neugebauer H, Kollmar R, Niesen WD, Bosel J, Schneider H, Hobohm C, et al. DEcompressive surgery Plus hypoTHermia for Space-Occupying Stroke (DEPTH-SOS): a protocol of a multicenter randomized controlled clinical trial and a literature review. Int J Stroke. 2013;8(5):383–7.
143. Els T, Oehm E, Voigt S, Klisch J, Hetzel A, Kassubek J. Safety and therapeutical benefit of hemicraniectomy combined with mild hypothermia in comparison with hemicraniectomy alone in patients with malignant ischemic stroke. Cerebrovasc Dis. 2006;21(1–2):79–85.
144. Park HS, Choi JH. Safety and efficacy of hypothermia (34 degrees C) after hemicraniectomy for malignant MCA infarction. J Korean Neurosurg Soc. 2018;61(2):267–76.
145. Schwab S, Schwarz S, Spranger M, Keller E, Bertram M, Hacke W. Moderate hypothermia in the treatment of patients with severe middle cerebral artery infarction. Stroke. 1998;29(12):2461–6.
146. Neugebauer H, Schneider H, Bosel J, Hobohm C, Poli S, Kollmar R, et al. Outcomes of hypothermia in addition to decompressive hemicraniectomy in treatment of malignant middle cerebral artery stroke: a randomized clinical trial. JAMA Neurol. 2019;76(5):571–9.
147. Juttler E, Schweickert S, Ringleb PA, Huttner HB, Kohrmann M, Aschoff A. Long-term outcome after surgical treatment for space-occupying cerebellar infarction: experience in 56 patients. Stroke. 2009;40(9):3060–6.
148. Ayling OGS, Alotaibi NM, Wang JZ, Fatehi M, Ibrahim GM, Benavente O, et al. Suboccipital decompressive craniectomy for cerebellar infarction: a systematic review and meta-analysis. World Neurosurg. 2018;110:450–9.e5.
149. Jauss M, Krieger D, Hornig C, Schramm J, Busse O. Surgical and medical management of patients with massive cerebellar infarctions: results of the German-Austrian Cerebellar Infarction Study. J Neurol. 1999;246(4):257–64.
150. Pfefferkorn T, Eppinger U, Linn J, Birnbaum T, Herzog J, Straube A, et al. Long-term outcome after suboccipital decompressive craniectomy for malignant cerebellar infarction. Stroke. 2009;40(9):3045–50.
151. Tsitsopoulos PP, Tobieson L, Enblad P, Marklund N. Surgical treatment of patients with unilateral cerebellar infarcts: clinical outcome and prognostic factors. Acta Neurochir. 2011;153(10):2075–83.
152. Raco A, Caroli E, Isidori A, Salvati M. Management of acute cerebellar infarction: one institution's experience. Neurosurgery. 2003;53(5):1061–5; discussion 5–6.
153. Mohsenipour I, Gabl M, Schutzhard E, Twerdy K. Suboccipital decompressive surgery in cerebellar infarction. Zentralbl Neurochir. 1999;60(2):68–73.
154. Chen HJ, Lee TC, Wei CP. Treatment of cerebellar infarction by decompressive suboccipital craniectomy. Stroke. 1992;23(7):957–61.
155. Kase CS, Wolf PA. Cerebellar infarction: upward transtentorial herniation after ventriculostomy. Stroke. 1993;24(7):1096–8.
156. Tohgi H, Takahashi S, Chiba K, Hirata Y. Cerebellar infarction. Clinical and neuroimaging analysis in 293 patients. The Tohoku Cerebellar Infarction Study Group. Stroke. 1993;24(11):1697–701.
157. Tsitsopoulos PP, Tobieson L, Enblad P, Marklund N. Clinical outcome following surgical treatment for bilateral cerebellar infarction. Acta Neurol Scand. 2011;123(5):345–51.
158. Powers WJ, Rabinstein AA, Ackerson T, Adeoye OM, Bambakidis NC, Becker K, et al. Guidelines for the early management of patients with acute ischemic stroke: 2019 update to the 2018 guidelines for the early management of acute ischemic stroke: a guideline for healthcare professionals from the American Heart Association/American Stroke Association. Stroke. 2019;50(12):e344–418.

Cerebral Ischemia in Children

Jaroslava Paulasová Schwabová, Lukáš Paulas,
Pavel Kršek, and Aleš Tomek

1 Introduction and Definitions

Stroke is defined as an acutely occurring neurological symptomatology resulting from haemorrhage or infarction [1, 2].

In paediatrics, stroke is classified into two age categories: perinatal stroke, occurring from the 28th gestational week to the 28th postnatal day, and childhood stroke, occurring from the 28th postnatal day to 18 years of age.

The following text specifically addresses childhood ischemic stroke—encompassing both arterial ischemic stroke (AIS) and venous stroke (cerebral sinovenous thrombosis, CSVT).

2 Incidence

In Western countries, the incidence of arterial ischemic stroke, excluding perinatal stroke cases, is approximately 1–2 per 100,000 children annually [3–7]. Incidence rates vary based on sex, age, and ethnicity, with the highest occurrence observed in children under the age of 5 and a higher incidence in boys compared to girls. Black and Asian children are at a higher risk compared to white children [4–11]. In comparison, haemorrhagic stroke accounts for approximately half of all paediatric stroke cases, with an annual incidence of 1–1.7 per 100,000 children [3, 11]. The highest occurrence of stroke is reported within the first year of life, excluding subarachnoid haemorrhage, which is more commonly associated with adolescence [12]. The risk of stroke recurrence in children receiving antithrombotic therapy is approximately 7% within the first month and 12% within the first year. The most significant predictor of recurrence is the presence of arteriopathy, which has been shown to increase the risk of recurrence by up to fivefold [13].

3 Aetiology and Pathogenesis

The aetiology and pathogenesis of ischemic stroke in children differ significantly from those observed in adults. In adults, stroke is predominantly associated with atherosclerotic risk factors such as arterial hypertension, dyslipidemia, and diabetes mellitus. In contrast, ischemic stroke in children is primarily linked to heart disease, arteriopathies (both extracranial and intracranial), thrombophilia, and systemic diseases (Table 1).

A primary risk factor for ischemic stroke in children is heart disease, whether congenital or acquired, including perioperative complications associated with cardiac surgery. Cardioembolism accounts for approximately 30% of cases of arterial ischemic stroke in the paediatric population [14]. The role of patent foramen ovale (PFO) in paediatric stroke remains controversial. Limited studies have suggested a higher prevalence of PFO in children with cryptogenic stroke [15, 16]. Based on findings from adult studies, paediatric patients with larger PFO and cryptogenic stroke may benefit from PFO closure.

J. P. Schwabová (✉)
Department of Paediatric Neurology, Comprehensive Stroke Center, Second Faculty of Medicine,Charles University and Motol University Hospital, Prague, Czech Republic

Department of Neurology, Comprehensive Stroke Center, Second Faculty of Medicine,Charles University and Motol University Hospital, Prague, Czech Republic
e-mail: jaroslava.schwabova@fnmotol.cz

L. Paulas · P. Kršek
Department of Paediatric Neurology, Comprehensive Stroke Center, Second Faculty of Medicine,Charles University and Motol University Hospital, Prague, Czech Republic
e-mail: lukas.paulas@fnmotol.cz; pavel.krsek@fnmotol.cz

A. Tomek
Department of Neurology, Comprehensive Stroke Center, Second Faculty of Medicine,Charles University and Motol University Hospital, Prague, Czech Republic
e-mail: ales.tomek@fnmotol.cz

V. Beneš, D. Netuka (eds.), *Surgical and Interventional Treatment of Cerebral Ischemia*,
https://doi.org/10.1007/978-3-032-08934-2_31

Table 1 Causes and risk factors of acute ischemic stroke in children

Category	Subgroups	Examples
Cardiac	Congenital cardiac anomaly	Cyanotic congenital heart diseases (CHD), cardiomyopathy, valve replacement, PFO
	Acquired cardiac disease	Endocarditis
	Arrhythmia	
Arteriopathy	Intracranial	FCA-i (VZV)
		FCA-d
		Moyamoya
	Extracranial	CCAD
Thrombophilia	Inherited	FV Leiden
		Prothrombin
		Deficit of protein C, S
	Acquired	Antiphospholipid sy
		Malignancies
		Infections
Systemic disease	Inflammatory	Lupus
		PACNS
		PAN, Wegener disease
	Genetic metabolic	Fabry disease
		MELAS
		POLG1
	Genetic connective tissue	Ehler-Danlos sy
		Loeys-Dietz sy

Note: Some categories may overlap
PFO permanent foramen ovale, *FCA-i* focal cerebral arteriopathy inflammation type, *VZV* varicella zoster virus, *FCA-d* focal cerebral arteriopathy dissection type, *sy* syndrome, *CCAD* craniocervical arterial dissection, *PACNS* primary angiitis of central nervous system, *PAN* polyarteritis nodosa, *MELAS* mitochondrial encephalomyopathy with lactic acidosis and stroke-like episodes, *POLG1* DNA POLymerase subunit Gamma

Arteriopathy is responsible for up to 53% of stroke cases in children [9, 17]. Among these, arteriopathy induced by the varicella-zoster virus accounts for up to 30% of AIS, with an even higher prevalence observed in preschool and younger school-aged children [18]. Another notable form of vasculopathy is craniocervical arterial dissection (CCAD). Identified risk factors for CCAD in paediatric population include male sex, head or neck trauma and connective tissue disorders [17, 19–21]. In patients presenting with multiple lesions in the posterior circulation, digital subtraction angiography (DSA) should be considered for evaluation of the V3 segment of the vertebral artery [22]. Additionally, when dissection is accompanied by sing of hypermobility, connective tissue disease should be considered as a potential underlying aetiology [23].

Arteriopathy is a significant predictor of recurrence, thus crucial for the rational management of secondary prevention—with recurrence risk being up to five times higher in this population [13]. However, it is crucial to differentiate between acute arterial involvement associated with infections (e.g. varicella) or trauma, which typically necessitate short-term treatment, and chronic arterial involvement, often rooted in genetic factors or as a part of chronic systemic conditions (e.g., Takayasu arteritis), which require long-term follow-up and ongoing therapy.

4 Clinical Presentation

The symptoms of ischemic stroke in childhood are similar to those observed in adults but depend on age and the stroke subtype. Seizures occur more frequently in children (particularly before the age of 6), with an incidence of 15–25% [4–6, 8, 24–27].

Cardioembolic stroke is more commonly observed in hospitalised patients between the ages of 6 months and 3 years, and it is distinguished from arteriopathies by its abrupt, non-fluctuating onset [28–32]. Children with Moyamoya syndrome frequently experience recurrent transient ischemic attacks (TIA) and clinically silent infarcts. Ischemic changes can be detected on initial imaging in up to 50% of patients with this diagnosis [33]. Vertebrobasilar stroke typically affects boys aged 7–8 years, often following minor head or neck trauma, and in addition to posterior fossa symptoms mainly presents with headache, vomiting, and altered consciousness [19, 34]. Sinus thrombosis may present with symptoms of intracranial hypertension (headache, nausea and vomiting, lethargy, abducens nerve palsy, and diplopia) or focal neurological deficits depending on the location of venous infarction or hemorrhage.

Neurological deficits in the paediatric population are evaluated using the Pediatric NIH Stroke Scale (PedNIHSS) [35], or in older children, the standard NIH Stroke Scale (NIHSS), which is commonly applied in adults [36].

5 Diagnosis

Diagnosing stroke in children presents significant challenges due to its rarity and the complexity of the differential diagnosis. As previously noted, the advancement of recanalisation techniques has heightened the urgency for rapid stroke diagnosis in the paediatric population. The Thrombolysis in Paediatric Stroke (TIPS) study highlighted that the primary and most critical obstacle in the implementation of recanalisation methods for children is the time delay from symptom onset to stroke diagnosis [37]. Unlike in adults, due to the infrequent occurrence of pediatric stroke, a patient with sudden-onset focal neurological deficits cannot automatically be considered a candidate for recanalisation. Rather, a definite diagnosis must be established, ideally through imaging, with MRI (Magnetic Resonance Imaging) being the preferred modality, although this often necessitates the use of anaesthesia.

The average time from symptom onset to contacting medical assistance is 6 hours. However, the average time for a radiologically confirmed diagnosis is between 15 and 24 hours, with delays being more pronounced during evenings and weekends [38].

Additional challenge in diagnosing paediatric stroke is the differential diagnosis, with initial misdiagnosis occurring in up to 40% of paediatric stroke cases [32, 39]. Clinical diagnostic strategies that are effective in adult populations demonstrate only approximately 60% sensitivity in paediatric patients [39, 40].

As previously noted, the development of recanalisation methods has accentuated the need for prompt stroke diagnosis in children. Therefore, it is advisable to perform acute imaging (including MRI or CT) for children presenting with sudden-onset focal neurological deficits within 24 hours from symptom-onset, particularly if the neurological impairment results in disability.

Routine diagnostic procedures for suspected stroke include non-contrast CT, contrast CT, MRI (Magnetic Resonance Imaging), and MR angiography, with MR venography indicated when CSVT is suspected. While CT is more accessible, faster, and may provide sufficient information to guide therapeutic decisions, MRI is preferred in paediatric cases of sudden-onset focal neurological symptoms due to concerns about radiation exposure and the need for anaesthesia in uncooperative or agitated patients. Additionally, MRI is often required after a negative CT scan. It is also important to note that one-third to half of patients suspected of having a stroke have stroke mimics, i.e. other causes of symptoms than stroke. In these cases, MRI offers superior sensitivity in detecting alternative aetiologies. Brain CT, being a rapidly available modality with a shorter examination time, is always indicated in unstable patients when intracerebral haemorrhage is suspected, or in patients with cochlear implants, pacemakers, or other contraindications to MRI.

Traditional angiography is often regarded as the most precise diagnostic tool; however, it is an invasive procedure. In routine clinical practice, MR or CT angiography are typically sufficient for diagnostic purposes [41]. The risk of vessel damage at the insertion site (femoral artery aneurysm) by dissection or perforation is highest in children during their first year of life. When MR or CT angiography is normal, subsequent angiography is unlikely to reveal any pathology of large calibre vessels. However, digital subtraction angiography (DSA) remains more informative when the small or medium calibre vessels are affected. DSA has clear clinical value, particularly in Moyamoya disease/syndrome cases. While MRA can identify this condition, traditional angiography is more beneficial for the assessment of potential surgical interventions.

6 Differential Diagnosis

Given the low incidence of stroke in children, the initial differential diagnosis of sudden onset focal neurological symptoms includes migraine with aura, peripheral facial nerve paresis, epilepsy (e.g. Todd's paresis), and neuroinfections, particularly herpes encephalitis. Symptoms of secondary ischemia, which may develop due to neuroinfection or traumatic brain injury, could be obscured by the underlying condition. Consequently, acute ischemic stroke (AIS) should be strongly considered if there is a deterioration in the patient's status for unclear reasons during the course of appropriate and ongoing treatment.

7 Acute Therapy

Upon first contact with a patient suspected of having a stroke, all measures aimed at stabilizing the clinical condition of the patient should be implemented. In paediatric patients with arterial hypotension, particularly in those with arteriopathies associated with stenosis, more aggressive treatment may be necessary at borderline pressure levels [12].

The management of intracranial hypertension is tailored as needed, with a primary focus on maintaining adequate cerebral blood flow and managing epileptic seizures, which occur relatively frequently in paediatric stroke cases (over 20% of children post-stroke) [42]. Administration of antiseizure medication is not recommended in the absence of a prior seizure [12]. Depending on the infarct's size and location, monitoring for sings of herniation is essential, particularly in patients with ischemia in the cerebellum, brainstem, or in those with large infarcts in the territory of middle cerebral artery. According to Dasenbrock et al., patients who underwent decompressive craniectomy prior to herniation had a better neurological outcome compared to those for whom craniectomy was performed after herniation occurred. In paediatric patients, early surgical intervention may have an even more significant impact, given the absence of cerebral atrophy [43].

In cases where hyperacute recanalisation therapy is not indicated, initial aspirin or low molecular weight heparin (LMWH) are generally recommended [44]. For patients with CSVT, newer anticoagulants are also available as therapeutic options. Heparin may be considered in exceptional cases for patients with a significantly elevated risk of bleeding.

The treatment approach is based on the aetiology of stroke. In paediatric patients, the most common causes are cardiac conditions, arteriopathies, and coagulopathies—clinical situations in which anticoagulation therapy appears beneficial. However, the efficacy of LMWH administration during the early phase of paediatric stroke has not been conclusively established, and there remains ongoing debate regarding the use of anticoagulants versus antiplatelet agents in this context.

7.1 Hyperacute Recanalization Therapy

Recommendations for the treatment and prevention of stroke in children generally rely more heavily on clinical experience than on evidence from controlled, randomized clinical trials. In some cases, the recommendations are partially informed by findings from studies conducted in adult populations.

Recanalization therapies, including both intravenous and intra-arterial administration of tissue plasminogen activator (tPA) as well as endovascular thrombectomy within a defined therapeutic time window, have demonstrated clear benefits in adult patients [45, 46]. However, the application of these therapeutic modalities in paediatric population remains a subject of ongoing debate [12]. Arguments supporting their consideration include the favourable outcomes observed in adult populations and the thrombus composition [47]. Conversely, certain physiological factors in children, such as greater neuronal plasticity and more efficient leptomeningeal collateral circulation, may mitigate the potential benefits of recanalization therapy [48–50].

7.1.1 Intravenous Thrombolysis

A primary challenge in hyperacute care for paediatric stroke patients lies in an accurate diagnosis of a possible stroke in the time limit (4.5 hours from the onset of symptoms; extended time window is 9 hours) for thrombolysis administration [51, 52]. Due to the rarity of acute ischemic stroke (AIS) in paediatric population, the diagnostic process often takes significantly longer than in adult patients, as evidenced by the prospective Thrombolysis in Paediatric Stroke study [37]. According to the study's findings, only one out of 93 children met all criteria for the rational administration of thrombolysis. In many cases, delayed diagnosis or the inability to confirm AIS precluded timely intervention. Specifically, for over half of the paediatric patients initially suspected of having AIS, the diagnosis could not ultimately be confirmed. Despite these challenges, the study reported no increased risk of bleeding associated with thrombolysis in paediatric patients who met the time window criterion. Furthermore, the safety of revascularization strategies was corroborated by findings from a multicentric retrospective study [53].

7.1.2 Mechanical Recanalization

In paediatric cases, mechanical recanalization may be preferable to thrombolysis due to its extended therapeutic window and the characteristics of the thrombus. The 2015 guidelines of the American Heart Association (AHA)/ American Stroke Association (ASA) suggest that thrombectomy might be considered for patients under the age of 18 who meet adult eligibility criteria, although the risk-benefit profile for paediatric patients remains undefined [54]. Evidence from case studies and larger paediatric cohorts is promising [53, 55–57]. More recently, Sporns et al. reported that thrombectomy in paediatric patients with large- or medium-vessel occlusions was associated with improved functional outcomes when compared to the best medical treatment alone [58].

When assessing eligibility for mechanical recanalization therapy in paediatric patients, careful consideration must be given to the high prevalence of vasculopathies within this population. Particular caution is warranted in very young children, where factors such as the technical specifications of stent retrievers—particularly their size—must be carefully evaluated. Additional constraints include limitations related to the appropriate contrast agent dosage for smaller children and concerns related to radiation exposure.

The indications for mechanical recanalisation in children mirror those in adults and include AIS with sudden onset and clinically significant neurological deficits, provided there is confirmation of symptomatic large-artery occlusion (Fig. 1). The standard therapeutic time window is set at 6 hours. However, based on advanced imaging techniques such as CT perfusion or MRI, this time window may be extended up to 24 hours in selected cases [59]. In paediatric patients, an even longer interval may be considered due to the presence of functional collateral circulation. Recanalisation therapy in paediatric patients should only be performed by an experienced, multidisciplinary team consisting of specialists in paediatric emergency medicine, paediatric neurology, and interventional neuroradiology situated in a centre with advanced cerebrovascular care capabilities such as comprehensive cerebrovascular centre or a certified stroke centre.

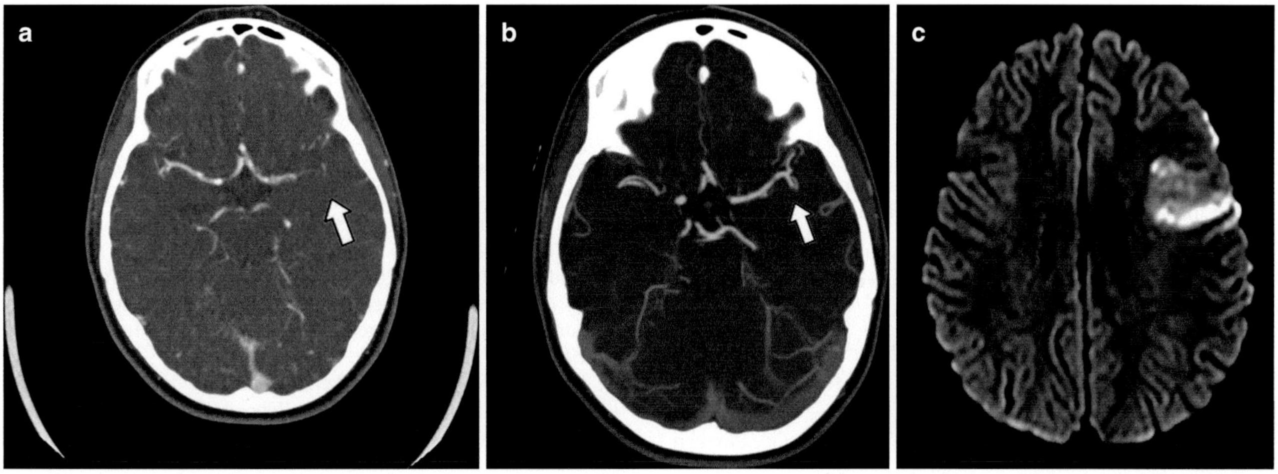

Fig. 1 Successful thrombectomy of the left M1 segment of the middle cerebral artery in a 14-year-old patient. (**a**) CT angiography prior to mechanical thrombectomy. (**b**) CT angiography following mechanical thrombectomy. (**c**) Brain MRI—diffusion-weighted imaging demonstrating the ischemic lesion

8 Prevention of Stroke and Stroke Recurrence

The risk of stroke recurrence (in paediatric patients) is approximately 20% [13]. The highest risk is associated with arteriopathies, particularly Moyamoya disease/syndrome and posterior circulation strokes [60].

Primary prevention of stroke plays a critical role in childhood, as up to 40% of children exhibit known risk factors for ischemia at the time of AIS onset. These risk factors commonly include underlying conditions such as cardiac defects or sickle cell anaemia.

The selection of therapeutic interventions and lifestyle modifications for secondary stroke prevention, as well as the duration of recurrence prevention efforts, are determined by the underlying aetiology of the stroke. Preventive measures include discontinuation of hormonal contraception, implementation of lifestyle modifications for prothrombotic conditions, management and correction of identified prothrombotic factors, and the administration of (preventive) prophylactic antiplatelet or anticoagulant therapy as appropriate.

In the 1990s, in the absence of systematic post-stroke antithrombotic prophylaxis, the risk of recurrence was estimated to range between 30% and 50% [13].

9 Prognosis and Prevention

The mortality rate for childhood ischemic stroke is reported to be approximately 10% [61, 62]. Among surviving paediatric patients, 70% experience persistent neurological deficits, with 36% classified as mild and 10% as severe. Key predictors of poor outcomes include the extent of ischemic damage, the presence of combined cortical and subcortical lesion, involvement of basal ganglia, multiple brain lesions, and hyperglycemia during the acute post-stroke phase.

Hemiparesis is the most common neurological deficit following paediatric stroke, typically presenting as mild in 49% of cases. Dysphasia, although generally mild, is observed in 21% of affected children [63]. Cognitive impairments have also been documented in post-stroke children, particularly in older girls [64]. Difficulties in verbal skills, working memory and processing speed, as well as attention deficits and executive dysfunction, have been noted.

Early initiation of physiotherapy, occupational therapy, and speech therapy, among other interventions, significantly contributes to overall improvement in the patient's condition. In children, improvements may manifest over an extended period, and subsequent deterioration is uncommon.

Acknowledgments We extend our gratitude to the Department of Radiology, Charles University, Second Faculty of Medicine, and Motol University Hospital, Prague, Czech Republic, for providing access to their imaging documentation.

Declarations

Competing Interests The author(s) has no competing interests to declare that are relevant to the content of this manuscript.

Ethics Approval The author(s) declares that this manuscript does not include primary research with human participants.

References

1. Grinnon ST, Miller K, Marler JR, Lu Y, Stout A, Odenkirchen J, et al. National Institute of Neurological Disorders and Stroke Common Data Element Project – approach and methods. Clin Trials. 2012;9(3):322–9.
2. Sacco RL, Kasner SE, Broderick JP, Caplan LR, Connors JJ, Culebras A, et al. An updated definition of stroke for the 21st century: a statement for healthcare professionals from the American Heart Association/American Stroke Association. Stroke. 2013;44(7):2064–89.
3. Lehman LL, Khoury JC, Taylor JM, Yeramaneni S, Sucharew H, Alwell K, et al. Pediatric stroke rates over 17 years: report from a population-based study. J Child Neurol. 2018;33(7):463–7.
4. Steinlin M, Pfister I, Pavlovic J, Everts R, Boltshauser E, Capone Mori A, et al. The first three years of the Swiss Neuropaediatric Stroke Registry (SNPSR): a population-based study of incidence, symptoms and risk factors. Neuropediatrics. 2005;36(2):90–7.
5. Christerson S, Stromberg B. Childhood stroke in Sweden I: incidence, symptoms, risk factors and short-term outcome. Acta Paediatr. 2010;99(11):1641–9.
6. Yock-Corrales A, Mackay MT, Mosley I, Maixner W, Babl FE. Acute childhood arterial ischemic and hemorrhagic stroke in the emergency department. Ann Emerg Med. 2011;58(2):156–63.
7. Simma B, Martin G, Muller T, Huemer M. Risk factors for pediatric stroke: consequences for therapy and quality of life. Pediatr Neurol. 2007;37(2):121–6.
8. Mallick D, Karmakar R, Barui G, Gon S, Chakrabarti S. The prognostic significance of HbF in childhood haematological malignancies. Indian J Hematol Blood Transfus. 2015;31(1):116–20.
9. Wintermark M, Hills NK, deVeber GA, Barkovich AJ, Elkind MS, Sear K, et al. Arteriopathy diagnosis in childhood arterial ischemic stroke: results of the vascular effects of infection in pediatric stroke study. Stroke. 2014;45(12):3597–605.
10. Mallick AA, Ganesan V, Kirkham FJ, Fallon P, Hedderly T, McShane T, et al. Childhood arterial ischaemic stroke incidence, presenting features, and risk factors: a prospective population-based study. Lancet Neurol. 2014;13(1):35–43.
11. Fullerton HJ, Wu YW, Zhao S, Johnston SC. Risk of stroke in children: ethnic and gender disparities. Neurology. 2003;61(2):189–94.
12. Ferriero DM, Fullerton HJ, Bernard TJ, Billinghurst L, Daniels SR, DeBaun MR, et al. Management of stroke in neonates and children: a scientific statement from the American Heart Association/American Stroke Association. Stroke. 2019;50(3):e51–96.
13. Fullerton HJ, Wintermark M, Hills NK, Dowling MM, Tan M, Rafay MF, et al. Risk of recurrent arterial ischemic stroke in childhood: a prospective international study. Stroke. 2016;47(1):53–9.
14. Sinclair AJ, Fox CK, Ichord RN, Almond CS, Bernard TJ, Beslow LA, et al. Stroke in children with cardiac disease: report from the International Pediatric Stroke Study Group Symposium. Pediatr Neurol. 2015;52(1):5–15.
15. Benedik MP, Zaletel M, Meglic NP, Podnar T. Patent foramen ovale and unexplained ischemic cerebrovascular events in children. Catheter Cardiovasc Interv. 2007;70(7):999–1007.
16. Benedik MP, Zaletel M, Meglic NP, Podnar T. A right-to-left shunt in children with arterial ischaemic stroke. Arch Dis Child. 2011;96(5):461–7.
17. Rafay MF, Armstrong D, Deveber G, Domi T, Chan A, MacGregor DL. Craniocervical arterial dissection in children: clinical and radiographic presentation and outcome. J Child Neurol. 2006;21(1):8–16.
18. Gilden D, Cohrs RJ, Mahalingam R, Nagel MA. Varicella zoster virus vasculopathies: diverse clinical manifestations, laboratory features, pathogenesis, and treatment. Lancet Neurol. 2009;8(8):731–40.
19. McCrea N, Saunders D, Bagkeris E, Chitre M, Ganesan V. Diagnosis of vertebral artery dissection in childhood posterior circulation arterial ischaemic stroke. Dev Med Child Neurol. 2016;58(1):63–9.
20. Brandt T, Orberk E, Weber R, Werner I, Busse O, Muller BT, et al. Pathogenesis of cervical artery dissections: association with connective tissue abnormalities. Neurology. 2001;57(1):24–30.
21. Fullerton HJ, Johnston SC, Smith WS. Arterial dissection and stroke in children. Neurology. 2001;57(7):1155–60.
22. Rollins N, Braga B, Hogge A, Beavers S, Dowling M. Dynamic arterial compression in pediatric vertebral arterial dissection. Stroke. 2017;48(4):1070–3.
23. Debette S, Goeggel Simonetti B, Schilling S, Martin JJ, Kloss M, Sarikaya H, et al. Familial occurrence and heritable connective tissue disorders in cervical artery dissection. Neurology. 2014;83(22):2023–31.
24. Wintermark M, Hills NK, DeVeber GA, Barkovich AJ, Bernard TJ, Friedman NR, et al. Clinical and imaging characteristics of arteriopathy subtypes in children with arterial ischemic stroke: results of the VIPS study. AJNR Am J Neuroradiol. 2017;38(11):2172–9.
25. Tuckuviene R, Christensen AL, Helgestad J, Johnsen SP, Kristensen SR. Paediatric arterial ischaemic stroke and cerebral sinovenous thrombosis in Denmark 1994-2006: a nationwide population-based study. Acta Paediatr. 2011;100(4):543–9.
26. Hartman AL, Lunney KM, Serena JE. Pediatric stroke: do clinical factors predict delays in presentation? J Pediatr. 2009;154(5):727–32.
27. McGlennan C, Ganesan V. Delays in investigation and management of acute arterial ischaemic stroke in children. Dev Med Child Neurol. 2008;50(7):537–40.
28. Asakai H, Cardamone M, Hutchinson D, Stojanovski B, Galati JC, Cheung MM, et al. Arterial ischemic stroke in children with cardiac disease. Neurology. 2015;85(23):2053–9.
29. Cheng HH, Rajagopal S, McDavitt E, Wigmore D, Williams K, Thiagarajan R, et al. Stroke in acquired and congenital heart disease patients and its relationship to hospital mortality and lasting neurologic deficits. Pediatr Crit Care Med. 2016;17(10):976–83.
30. Dowling MM, Hynan LS, Lo W, Licht DJ, McClure C, Yager JY, et al. International Paediatric Stroke Study: stroke associated with cardiac disorders. Int J Stroke. 2013;8 Suppl A100:39–44.
31. Ziesmann MT, Nash M, Booth FA, Rafay MF. Cardioembolic stroke in children: a clinical presentation and outcome study. Pediatr Neurol. 2014;51(4):494–502.
32. Braun KP, Rafay MF, Uiterwaal CS, Pontigon AM, DeVeber G. Mode of onset predicts etiological diagnosis of arterial ischemic stroke in children. Stroke. 2007;38(2):298–302.
33. Amlie-Lefond C, Ellenbogen RG. Factors associated with the presentation of moyamoya in childhood. J Stroke Cerebrovasc Dis. 2015;24(6):1204–10.
34. Rollins N, Pride GL, Plumb PA, Dowling MM. Brainstem strokes in children: an 11-year series from a tertiary pediatric center. Pediatr Neurol. 2013;49(6):458–64.

35. Ichord RN, Bastian R, Abraham L, Askalan R, Benedict S, Bernard TJ, et al. Interrater reliability of the Pediatric National Institutes of Health Stroke Scale (PedNIHSS) in a multicenter study. Stroke. 2011;42(3):613–7.
36. Kothari R, Hall K, Brott T, Broderick J. Early stroke recognition: developing an out-of-hospital NIH Stroke Scale. Acad Emerg Med. 1997;4(10):986–90.
37. Rivkin MJ, deVeber G, Ichord RN, Kirton A, Chan AK, Hovinga CA, et al. Thrombolysis in pediatric stroke study. Stroke. 2015;46(3):880–5.
38. Daverio M, Bressan S, Gregori D, Babl FE, Mackay MT. Patient and process factors associated with type of first neuroimaging and delayed diagnosis in childhood arterial ischemic stroke. Acad Emerg Med. 2016;23(9):1040–7.
39. Mackay MT, Monagle P, Babl FE. Improving diagnosis of childhood arterial ischaemic stroke. Expert Rev Neurother. 2017;17(12):1157–65.
40. Mackay MT, Churilov L, Donnan GA, Babl FE, Monagle P. Performance of bedside stroke recognition tools in discriminating childhood stroke from mimics. Neurology. 2016;86(23):2154–61.
41. Stence NV, Fenton LZ, Goldenberg NA, Armstrong-Wells J, Bernard TJ. Craniocervical arterial dissection in children: diagnosis and treatment. Curr Treat Options Neurol. 2011;13(6):636–48.
42. Singh RK, Zecavati N, Singh J, Kaulas H, Nelson KB, Dean NP, et al. Seizures in acute childhood stroke. J Pediatr. 2012;160(2):291–6.
43. Dasenbrock HH, Robertson FC, Vaitkevicius H, Aziz-Sultan MA, Guttieres D, Dunn IF, et al. Timing of decompressive hemicraniectomy for stroke: a nationwide inpatient sample analysis. Stroke. 2017;48(3):704–11.
44. Roach ES, Golomb MR, Adams R, Biller J, Daniels S, Deveber G, et al. Management of stroke in infants and children: a scientific statement from a Special Writing Group of the American Heart Association Stroke Council and the Council on Cardiovascular Disease in the Young. Stroke. 2008;39(9):2644–91.
45. Goyal M, Menon BK, van Zwam WH, Dippel DW, Mitchell PJ, Demchuk AM, et al. Endovascular thrombectomy after large-vessel ischaemic stroke: a meta-analysis of individual patient data from five randomised trials. Lancet. 2016;387(10029):1723–31.
46. Bendszus M, Fiehler J, Subtil F, Bonekamp S, Aamodt AH, Fuentes B, et al. Endovascular thrombectomy for acute ischaemic stroke with established large infarct: multicentre, open-label, randomised trial. Lancet. 2023;402(10414):1753–63.
47. Miller CMF, Price PL, Meyer D. Mass balance analyses of nutrients on California dairies to evaluate data quality for regulatory review. Sci Total Environ. 2017;579:37–46.
48. Sporns PB, Fullerton HJ, Lee S, Kim H, Lo WD, Mackay MT, et al. Childhood stroke. Nat Rev Dis Primers. 2022;8(1):12.
49. Wittenberg GF. Neural plasticity and treatment across the lifespan for motor deficits in cerebral palsy. Dev Med Child Neurol. 2009;51(Suppl 4):130–3.
50. Lee S, Jiang B, Wintermark M, Mlynash M, Christensen S, Strater R, et al. Cerebrovascular collateral integrity in pediatric large vessel occlusion: analysis of the Save ChildS Study. Neurology. 2022;98(4):e352–e63.
51. Harrar DB, Salussolia CL, Kapur K, Danehy A, Kleinman ME, Mannix R, et al. A stroke alert protocol decreases the time to diagnosis of brain attack symptoms in a pediatric emergency department. J Pediatr. 2020;216:136–41.e6.
52. deVeber GA. Delays in the timely diagnosis of stroke in children. Nat Rev Neurol. 2010;6(2):64–6.
53. Kossorotoff M, Kerleroux B, Boulouis G, Husson B, Tran Dong K, Eugene F, et al. Recanalization treatments for pediatric acute ischemic stroke in France. JAMA Netw Open. 2022;5(9):e2231343.
54. Powers WJ, Derdeyn CP, Biller J, Coffey CS, Hoh BL, Jauch EC, et al. 2015 American Heart Association/American Stroke Association focused update of the 2013 guidelines for the early management of patients with acute ischemic stroke regarding endovascular treatment: a guideline for healthcare professionals from the American Heart Association/American Stroke Association. Stroke. 2015;46(10):3020–35.
55. Bhatia K, Kortman H, Blair C, Parker G, Brunacci D, Ang T, et al. Mechanical thrombectomy in pediatric stroke: systematic review, individual patient data meta-analysis, and case series. J Neurosurg Pediatr. 2019;24(5):558–71.
56. Sporns PB, Strater R, Minnerup J, Wiendl H, Hanning U, Chapot R, et al. Feasibility, safety, and outcome of endovascular recanalization in childhood stroke: the Save ChildS Study. JAMA Neurol. 2020;77(1):25–34.
57. Sporns PB, Straeter R, Minnerup J, Wiendl H, Hanning U, Chapot R, et al. Does device selection impact recanalization rate and neurological outcome?: an analysis of the Save ChildS Study. Stroke. 2020;51(4):1182–9.
58. Sporns PB, Bhatia K, Abruzzo T, Pabst L, Fraser S, Chung MG, et al. Endovascular thrombectomy for childhood stroke (Save ChildS Pro): an international, multicentre, prospective registry study. Lancet Child Adolesc Health. 2024;8(12):882–90.
59. Hill MD, Goyal M, Demchuk AM, Fisher M. Ischemic stroke tissue-window in the new era of endovascular treatment. Stroke. 2015;46(8):2332–4.
60. Uohara MY, Beslow LA, Billinghurst L, Jones BM, Kessler SK, Licht DJ, et al. Incidence of recurrence in posterior circulation childhood arterial ischemic stroke. JAMA Neurol. 2017;74(3):316–23.
61. Fullerton HJ, Chetkovich DM, Wu YW, Smith WS, Johnston SC. Deaths from stroke in US children, 1979 to 1998. Neurology. 2002;59(1):34–9.
62. Krishnamurthi RV, deVeber G, Feigin VL, Barker-Collo S, Fullerton H, Mackay MT, et al. Stroke prevalence, mortality and disability-adjusted life years in children and youth aged 0-19 years: data from the global and regional burden of stroke 2013. Neuroepidemiology. 2015;45(3):177–89.
63. Friefeld SJ, Westmacott R, Macgregor D, Deveber GA. Predictors of quality of life in pediatric survivors of arterial ischemic stroke and cerebral sinovenous thrombosis. J Child Neurol. 2011;26(9):1186–92.
64. Westmacott R, Askalan R, MacGregor D, Anderson P, Deveber G. Cognitive outcome following unilateral arterial ischaemic stroke in childhood: effects of age at stroke and lesion location. Dev Med Child Neurol. 2010;52(4):386–93.

Future Directions and Research in Ischemic Stroke

Vladimír Beneš, David Netuka, and Adéla Bubeníková

1 Introduction

Stroke remains a leading cause of death and long-term disability globally, imposing a heavy burden on individuals, families, healthcare systems, and societies [1]. Despite significant advancements in prevention, diagnosis, and treatment, the prevalence of stroke continues to rise, primarily due to an aging population and the growing rates of modifiable risk factors such as hypertension, diabetes, and obesity [2]. These escalating challenges necessitate urgent, innovative, and multidisciplinary approaches to stroke management and research. The future of stroke research is poised to evolve through advancements in technology, precision medicine, and a deeper understanding of the biological, environmental, and social determinants of health. As research moves forward, it will require collaboration between clinicians, researchers, policymakers, and the public to ensure that new therapies, technologies, and treatment protocols translate into better clinical outcomes and enhanced quality of life for stroke survivors.

The landscape of stroke research is rapidly evolving. Emerging trends in the field are expected to drive transformative changes in prevention, acute care, and long-term rehabilitation. At the heart of these changes lies the integration of cutting-edge technologies, including artificial intelligence (AI), big data analytics, and advanced imaging modalities, which have the potential to revolutionize stroke diagnosis, treatment, and rehabilitation. Precision medicine—tailoring therapies to individual genetic and phenotypic profiles—also holds significant promise for optimizing patient care [3]. Additionally, research into the biological mechanisms of neuroprotection and neuroregeneration, alongside new therapeutic agents, could provide novel treatments that extend the window of recovery for stroke patients, improving functional outcomes and long-term survival.

The global nature of the stroke epidemic underscores the need for equitable strategies to ensure that emerging therapies are accessible across diverse populations and healthcare systems. Many regions still face substantial healthcare disparities in stroke care, particularly in low- and middle-income countries, where limited access to advanced diagnostics, treatment, and rehabilitation infrastructure exacerbate the impact of stroke [4]. Therefore, any future innovations must prioritize inclusivity and work towards minimizing these disparities.

This chapter will explore some of the key areas that are expected to shape the future of stroke research, with a particular focus on the potential impact of AI, novel stroke therapies, precision medicine, and advanced rehabilitation strategies. The chapter will also highlight how these innovations can be translated into clinical practice and contribute to improved stroke outcomes.

2 Surgical Precision

The future of stroke management is poised to benefit significantly from advancements in surgical precision, driven by innovations in diagnostic imaging, navigation technologies, and robotic systems. State-of-the-art imaging modalities such as high-resolution MRI, advanced CT angiography, and functional imaging techniques are increasingly enabling earlier and more accurate detection of vascular abnormalities. These diagnostic advancements not only facilitate timely intervention but also provide detailed preoperative roadmaps that inform surgical planning.

Emerging navigation technologies are enhancing the precision and safety of cerebrovascular surgeries. Intraoperative

V. Beneš (✉) · D. Netuka
Department of Neurosurgery and Neurooncology, First Medical Faculty, Charles University, Prague, Czech Republic
e-mail: beneseva@volny.cz

A. Bubeníková
Department of Neurosurgery, Second Faculty of Medicine, Charles University and Motol University Hospital, Prague, Czech Republic

V. Beneš, D. Netuka (eds.), *Surgical and Interventional Treatment of Cerebral Ischemia*,
https://doi.org/10.1007/978-3-032-08934-2_32

navigation systems, integrating real-time imaging with augmented reality (AR), allow surgeons to visualize vascular anatomy in three dimensions with unparalleled accuracy. This technology minimizes the risk of damage to critical neurovascular structures and ensures targeted intervention, particularly in complex cases such as carotid artery aneurysms, dissections, or intracranial stenoses. Additionally, fluorescence-guided imaging and intraoperative Doppler ultrasonography are being employed to assess blood flow dynamics and ensure the efficacy of surgical repairs.

Robotic-assisted platforms represent another frontier in enhancing surgical precision. These systems allow for microscale manipulation of delicate vascular structures with greater stability and control than conventional techniques. Integrated with AI, robotic systems can adapt intraoperatively, responding to unexpected anatomical challenges by recalibrating surgical trajectories. The combination of robotic precision with real-time imaging enables safer, minimally invasive approaches, reducing patient morbidity and recovery times.

3 New Endovascular Techniques

The endovascular approach, already a cornerstone of acute ischemic stroke treatment, continues to benefit from device evolution and procedural refinements. Second-generation stent retrievers, with enhanced flexibility and smaller profiles, are expected to improve the accessibility and success rates of mechanical thrombectomy in distal occlusions and anatomically challenging cases. Additionally, biodegradable scaffolds and drug-eluting devices are being developed to address post-procedural complications, such as restenosis and chronic inflammation. Clot aspiration systems and next-generation thrombolytic agents aim to optimize thrombus removal while minimizing the risk of hemorrhagic transformation. Preclinical studies and early-phase trials are actively investigating these technologies, laying the groundwork for their integration into clinical practice.

4 Optimizing Pre-hospital Care

Time remains a critical factor in stroke management, with significant efforts directed at minimizing delays between symptom onset and definitive treatment. Mobile stroke units (MSUs), equipped with advanced imaging modalities and point-of-care diagnostic tools, enable pre-hospital thrombolysis and rapid triage. Enhanced communication systems linking emergency medical services (EMS) to stroke centers are being designed to streamline patient handoffs and ensure seamless care coordination. AI-driven diagnostic tools capable of analyzing clinical and imaging data in real-time are also being integrated into EMS workflows, potentially improving the accuracy of stroke detection and prioritization. These innovations are pivotal in extending the therapeutic window for interventions such as intravenous thrombolysis and mechanical thrombectomy.

5 Neuroprotection and Regenerative Therapies

Beyond acute interventions, significant research is focused on mitigating ischemic brain injury and promoting recovery through neuroprotective and regenerative strategies. Neuroprotective agents targeting excitotoxicity, oxidative stress, and neuroinflammation are under investigation in preclinical and clinical settings [5]. Stem cell therapies, designed to replace damaged neurons and support neurovascular repair, are emerging as promising adjuncts to conventional stroke treatments. Advances in bioengineering and tissue scaffolding are also contributing to the development of strategies for neuronal regeneration and network reorganization. Such approaches aim to not only reduce infarct size but also enhance functional recovery in stroke survivors [6].

6 Stem Cell Therapy in Stroke Recovery

One of the most exciting areas in stroke research is the potential of stem cell therapy to restore function and repair damaged brain tissue following an ischemic stroke. Stem cell therapy offers a promising alternative to current therapeutic options, especially given the limited effectiveness of existing treatments for neuronal repair [7]. Recent advances in stem cell biology have allowed researchers to harness the regenerative potential of various stem cell types, including induced pluripotent stem cells (iPSCs), neural stem cells (NSCs), and mesenchymal stem cells (MSCs). These stem cells can be directed to promote neurogenesis, angiogenesis, and synaptic repair in the ischemic brain, facilitating the regeneration of neural tissue lost during the stroke [8].

While preclinical studies have demonstrated promising results, translating these findings into clinical therapies remains challenging. The effectiveness of stem cell therapy depends on optimizing multiple factors, including the timing of cell transplantation, the route of administration, the specific cell type used, and the selection of appropriate biomarkers to monitor outcomes [7]. Furthermore, the issue of immune rejection and the potential for tumor formation from transplanted stem cells remain significant concerns that must be addressed through rigorous preclinical studies and clinical trials.

Innovative technologies like 3D bioprinting, organoid models, and non-invasive delivery techniques such as intranasal administration or nanoparticle-based targeting systems are helping to refine stem cell therapy. These technologies aim to improve the safety and efficacy of stem cell transplantation by enhancing the integration of the transplanted cells into the damaged brain tissue. As clinical trials continue to investigate the use of stem cells for stroke recovery, the field is likely to see substantial progress in developing personalized treatment protocols based on individual patient profiles.

7 Neural Repair: A Complement to Neuroprotection

Neural repair is a promising therapeutic approach to stroke rehabilitation, aimed at restoring brain function and connectivity following the acute injury phase. Unlike neuroprotection, which focuses on preventing further neuronal damage, neural repair seeks to rejuvenate and regenerate damaged neural tissue, with a particular emphasis on repairing neuronal circuits, improving synaptic connectivity, and restoring cognitive and motor functions. Neural repair mechanisms are particularly effective when initiated within 24 hours of the stroke, but ongoing research has shown that beneficial effects may continue for weeks or even months after the initial injury [9].

Stem cell therapy plays a central role in neural repair by integrating new cells into damaged areas of the brain, facilitating tissue regeneration. In addition to stem cell-based interventions, neurotrophic factors and pharmacological agents that target growth inhibitors, such as myelin-associated glycoprotein (MAG) and NOGO proteins, are also being explored to enhance neuronal growth and axonal regeneration [10]. Animal studies have demonstrated that these factors can help promote functional recovery, but their clinical application remains limited due to issues with efficacy and safety.

Moreover, pharmacological agents and immunological modulators that target specific receptors involved in neuronal growth and repair are under investigation. These agents could block inhibitory signals that hinder neural regeneration, thereby facilitating the repair of neural circuits and enhancing functional recovery. The growing body of research in neural repair holds great potential for improving long-term outcomes for stroke patients, especially when combined with advances in stem cell therapy and targeted pharmacological treatments [8].

8 The Future of Stroke Rehabilitation

Rehabilitation is a critical component of stroke management, with the goal of restoring independence and improving the quality of life for stroke survivors. The future of stroke rehabilitation will be shaped by advances in two key areas: neuroplasticity-driven therapies and technological innovations. Neuroplasticity refers to the brain's ability to reorganize and form new neural connections, an essential process for recovery following stroke [11].

Neuroplasticity-driven therapies, such as task-specific training, robotic-assisted rehabilitation, and neuromodulation techniques, aim to stimulate neuroplastic changes in the brain [12]. These interventions focus on promoting the reorganization of neural circuits in affected brain regions, encouraging the brain to compensate for lost functions. These therapies have shown promise in clinical trials, particularly for improving motor and cognitive function, and will likely become an integral part of stroke rehabilitation in the future.

In addition to neuroplasticity-based therapies, technological innovations are revolutionizing the delivery and monitoring of stroke rehabilitation. Wearable devices, tele-rehabilitation platforms, and mobile health applications are transforming how rehabilitation services are delivered, enabling continuous, personalized care. These technologies offer real-time feedback to both patients and clinicians, allowing for more tailored interventions that adapt to the evolving needs of stroke survivors. Importantly, these innovations also improve access to rehabilitation services, particularly for patients in remote or underserved areas who may face barriers to in-person therapy.

Furthermore, AI and machine learning hold great potential in stroke rehabilitation. These technologies can analyze large datasets to optimize rehabilitation protocols, providing personalized treatment plans that are tailored to individual patient needs. AI could also help identify early signs of recovery or complications, enabling timely interventions to improve patient outcomes.

9 The Role of Clinical Trials in Advancing Stroke Treatment

Clinical trials are essential for advancing stroke research and refining current treatment strategies. A significant focus of stroke trials is on patients eligible for reperfusion therapies, which are designed to restore blood flow to the brain following an ischemic stroke. However, challenges arise when targeting this patient cohort. Many new therapies are likely to provide only modest improvements compared to existing treatments, requiring larger sample sizes and more advanced study designs [13]. The use of advanced imaging techniques and detailed disability outcome assessments adds complexity to the recruitment and execution of these trials.

Moreover, clinical trials investigating prehospital interventions, including early reperfusion strategies, offer an exciting avenue for exploring how to treat patients before they reach the hospital. These trials face logistical and diagnostic challenges, as accurately distinguishing ischemic strokes from hemorrhagic strokes or stroke mimics remains difficult, even with advanced imaging technologies. Mobile stroke units equipped with imaging capabilities could help address some of these issues, though their availability is still limited by infrastructure constraints.

Another important area of stroke research lies in targeting patients who are ineligible for reperfusion therapies, a large and growing segment of the stroke population. Trials are increasingly focusing on patients with more severe strokes, lower Alberta Stroke Program Early CT Scores (ASPECTS), larger ischemic cores, and preexisting disabilities [14]. Expanding inclusion criteria may increase patient recruitment but may also introduce complexity due to the heterogeneity of stroke presentations.

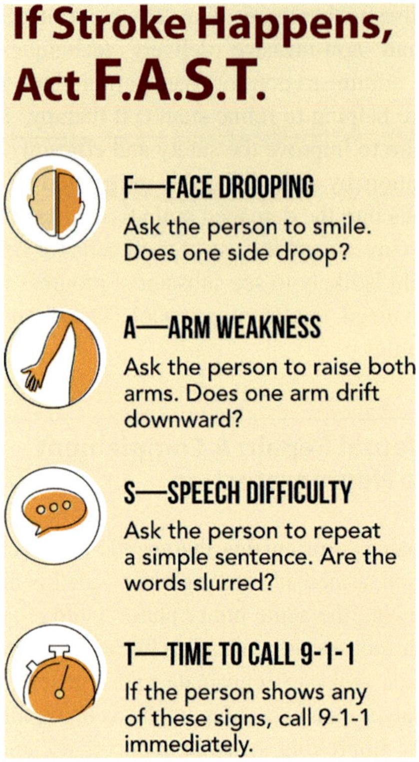

Fig. 1 FAST acronym used in public awareness campaigns. (Reprinted with CC licence)

10 Public Awareness

Public awareness is a cornerstone in reducing the morbidity and mortality associated with stroke. Despite significant advances in stroke care, delays in recognition and treatment remain a major barrier to optimal outcomes. Stroke is a time-critical condition where rapid intervention, particularly for ischemic stroke through reperfusion therapies, significantly improves survival and functional recovery. However, public knowledge of stroke symptoms, risk factors, and the importance of urgent medical attention remains inadequate globally. To address this gap, comprehensive educational initiatives are imperative.

Community-based awareness campaigns should prioritize recognition of stroke symptoms, commonly summarized by acronyms such as FAST (Face drooping, Arm weakness, Speech difficulties, Time to call emergency services, Fig. 1) [15]. These campaigns can leverage diverse platforms, including social media, public service announcements, and collaborations with schools and workplaces, to disseminate information widely. Special emphasis should be placed on high-risk populations, including individuals with hypertension, diabetes, or a history of cardiovascular disease, and underserved communities where access to healthcare and educational resources is limited. Primary prevention remains a cornerstone in reducing the global burden of stroke, and future efforts will likely focus on innovative strategies to enhance public awareness and address modifiable risk factors. Large-scale public health campaigns aimed at promoting healthy lifestyles, increasing awareness of stroke warning signs, and encouraging adherence to preventive measures like smoking cessation and physical activity will be critical. Advances in predictive analytics and artificial intelligence may further enable tailored preventive interventions, identifying high-risk individuals and engaging them in proactive, evidence-based care. These efforts, combined with accessible screening programs, have the potential to transform stroke prevention by shifting the focus toward risk mitigation before disease onset.

Cultural tailoring of messages to align with local beliefs and languages is critical to ensure receptivity and effectiveness. Incorporating stroke education into school curricula and workplace health programs can also embed long-term awareness and promote preventive behaviors. Healthcare systems should support stroke awareness by training first responders and community health workers to reinforce education at the grassroots level. Partnerships with primary care providers to counsel patients on modifiable risk factors, such as smoking cessation, physical activity, and blood pressure control, can further enhance prevention efforts.

Technological innovations, such as mobile health applications, can play a significant role in public education by providing interactive tools to assess stroke risk, recognize symptoms, and offer guidance on emergency responses. Ultimately, sustained and multifaceted public awareness strategies are essential to reduce the global burden of stroke by fostering early recognition, timely treatment, and preventative health behaviors.

11 Conclusion

The future of stroke research is highly promising, driven by advances in stem cell therapy, neural repair strategies, rehabilitation techniques, and clinical trial methodologies. As the field moves toward precision medicine and more personalized treatment approaches, the integration of artificial intelligence and technological innovations will significantly enhance stroke management. Clinical trials will remain central to refining therapies and identifying effective strategies for a broad range of patients, from those eligible for reperfusion therapies to those with milder symptoms or ineligible for these interventions. By addressing challenges in patient recruitment, outcome measurement, and accessibility, the future of stroke care holds the potential for significant improvements in functional recovery and quality of life for stroke survivors worldwide.

Declarations

Competing Interests The author(s) has no competing interests to declare that are relevant to the content of this manuscript.

Ethics Approval The author(s) declares that this manuscript does not include primary research with human participants.

References

1. Donkor ES. Stroke in the 21(st) century: a snapshot of the burden, epidemiology, and quality of life. Stroke Res Treat. 2018;2018:3238165.
2. Wafa HA, et al. Burden of stroke in Europe: thirty-year projections of incidence, prevalence, deaths, and disability-adjusted life years. Stroke. 2020;51(8):2418–27.
3. Chamorro Á, et al. The future of neuroprotection in stroke. J Neurol Neurosurg Psychiatry. 2021;92(2):129–35.
4. Yusuf S, et al. Modifiable risk factors, cardiovascular disease, and mortality in 155 722 individuals from 21 high-income, middle-income, and low-income countries (PURE): a prospective cohort study. Lancet. 2020;395(10226):795–808.
5. Candelario-Jalil E, Dijkhuizen RM, Magnus T. Neuroinflammation, stroke, blood-brain barrier dysfunction, and imaging modalities. Stroke. 2022;53(5):1473–86.
6. Khokale R, et al. Virtual and augmented reality in post-stroke rehabilitation: a narrative review. Cureus. 2023;15(4):e37559.
7. Kawabori M, et al. Clinical trials of stem cell therapy for cerebral ischemic stroke. Int J Mol Sci. 2020;21(19):7380.
8. Rikhtegar R, et al. Stem cell-based cell therapy for neuroprotection in stroke: a review. J Cell Biochem. 2019;120(6):8849–62.
9. Toman NG, Grande AW, Low WC. Neural repair in stroke. Cell Transplant. 2019;28(9–10):1123–6.
10. Uyeda A, Muramatsu R. Molecular mechanisms of central nervous system axonal regeneration and remyelination: a review. Int J Mol Sci. 2020;21(21):8116.
11. Xing Y, Bai Y. A review of exercise-induced neuroplasticity in ischemic stroke: pathology and mechanisms. Mol Neurobiol. 2020;57(10):4218–31.
12. Gnasso R, et al. Robotic-assisted rehabilitation for post-stroke shoulder pain: a systematic review. Sensors (Basel). 2023;23(19):8239.
13. Majersik JJ. Ethics and bias in clinical trial enrollment in stroke. Curr Cardiol Rep. 2019;21(6):49.
14. Nicholson P, et al. Per-region interobserver agreement of Alberta Stroke Program Early CT Scores (ASPECTS). J Neurointerv Surg. 2020;12(11):1069–71.
15. Hughes TAT, Butterworth R. Stroke: think FAST, then SLOW3. Pract Neurol. 2023;23(6):462–3.